Sabine Sarnacki • Luca Pio
Editors

Neuroblastoma

Clinical and Surgical Management

Springer

Editors
Sabine Sarnacki
Department of Pediatric Surgery
Necker - Enfants Malades Hospital
Assistance Publique Hopitaux de Paris
University of Paris
Paris
France

Luca Pio
Department of Pediatric Surgery
Necker - Enfants Malades Hospital
Assistance Publique Hopitaux de Paris
University of Paris
Paris
France

ISBN 978-3-030-18398-1 ISBN 978-3-030-18396-7 (eBook)
https://doi.org/10.1007/978-3-030-18396-7

This Springer imprint is published by the registered company Springer Nature Switzerland AG
The registered company address is: Gewerbestrasse 11, 6330 Cham, Switzerland

Neuroblastoma

Foreword

Sabine Sarnacki and Luca Pio have created a comprehensive text on neuroblastoma. This is a timely submission. The roster of authors are all international experts on the diagnosis and management of neuroblastoma. Drs. Sarnacki and Pio have compiled a text that provides information extending from the epidemiology of this disease to its imaging and, most importantly, the clinical management and surgery. This text will provide the reader a single source of the most current knowledge on all aspects of neuroblastoma. They are to be congratulated for this singular effort providing us a veritable wealth of information on neuroblastoma. I believe it will serve as an invaluable reference text for readers of all levels.

Robert C. Shamberger
Surgery, Boston Children's Hospital
Harvard Medical School
Harvard, MA, USA

Robert E. Gross
Professor of Surgery
Harvard Medical School
Harvard, MA, USA

Chief of Surgery
Boston Children's Hospital
Boston, MA, USA

Contents

Part I

Epidemiology, Biology and Pathology Assessment

1 Epidemiology

Jacqueline Clavel, Brigitte Lacour, and Paula Rios

Neuroblastomas are rare diseases, and as such their surveillance requires specific large-scale reliable population registries. We are more and more able to describe neuroblastomas and other embryonal tumors all over the world, but information is still insufficient and fragile in low-income countries, now prioritized in the international strategies of cancer surveillance. Epidemiological research on risk factors, also, is limited by the rarity of the disease and mostly relies on case–control studies, that is, studies performed at the time of diagnosis, getting information by interview and, in some countries, from databases like birth certificates. Lack of knowledge about risk factors is important, and the international epidemiology consortiums are currently strengthening their efforts on etiological research.

1.1 Descriptive Epidemiology

In the International classification of disease for oncology (ICD-O-3) [1], neuroblastomas are classified into the two morphologic codes 95003 (*neuroblastoma*, the most frequent) and 94903 (*ganglioneuroblastoma*, the best differentiated form of neuroblastoma). Both are grouped in the category IV (*Tumors*), subgroup IV.a (*neuroblastomas*) of the International classification for childhood cancers (ICCC) [2].

J. Clavel (✉) · B. Lacour
CRESS, UMRS1153, INSERM, Université Paris-Descartes, Paris, France

National Registry of Childhood Cancers, APHP Hôpital Paul Brousse, Villejuif, France

CHU de Nancy, Vandoeuvre-lès-Nancy, France
e-mail: jacqueline.clavel@inserm.fr

P. Rios
CRESS, UMRS1153, INSERM, Université Paris-Descartes, Paris, France

S. Sarnacki, L. Pio (eds.), *Neuroblastoma*,
https://doi.org/10.1007/978-3-030-18396-7_1

In this chapter, the epidemiological features of neuroblastomas are described using the 2000–2013 data extracted from the French National Registry of Childhood Cancer (RNCE) (http://rnce.inserm.fr). The RNCE registers 130–150 new cases of neuroblastoma aged under 15 years every year.

1.1.1 Incidence and Epidemiological Features

The annual age-standardized incidence rate is around 14 cases per million of children aged 0–14 years (Table 1.1). Neuroblastomas are mostly diagnosed before the age of 5 years (85%), and 40% occur in infancy. They are very uncommon after the age of 10 years. Annual incidence rates vary from 73 cases per million in infancy to 1 case per million after the age of 10 years. Neuroblastomas are the most frequent tumors diagnosed in neonates (<28 days). One out of ten cases of neuroblastomas is neonate. Most of them (65%) are diagnosed before birth by routine ultrasonography.

According to ICD-O categories, 11% of the French cases are ganglioneuroblastomas and 89% are neuroblastomas. Half of the tumors are located in the adrenal glands, 20% in other abdominal sites, 16% in mediastinum, and the remaining 15% are distributed in pelvis, cervical, or lumbar chains of the sympathetic nervous system.

Almost half of the cases have distant metastases at diagnosis. The proportion is smaller in infants, but most of them (nearly a quarter of the cases under 1 year) are stage 4S, a specific pattern of metastatic disease spread to skin, liver, and bone marrow.

Amplification of *MYCN* oncogene is present in less than 10% of infant neuroblastomas, but in more than 20% of neuroblastomas after the age of 1 year.

In France, incidence has remained stable since 2000, and no spatial heterogeneity has been observed. Increase in incidence has been reported for Europe as a whole over the earlier period of 1978–1997 with an average change of 1.5% per year [3].

Table 1.1 Number of cases of neuroblastomas and annual incidence rates in France from 2000 to 2013, by age groups, according to MYCN status and tumoral extension

	Age groups (years)				
	<1	1–4	5–9	10–14	Total
Incidence rate					
IR (/million year)	73.1	22.2	4.0	1.1	12.5
ASR (/million year)					14.1
Mean annual numbers	55	67	15	4	141
	39.0%	47.5%	10.6%	2.8%	100.0%
MYCN amplification					
Amplified	7.2%	26.4%			16.6%
Nonamplified	78.1%	59.8%			67.8%
Unknown	14.7%	13.8%			15.6%
Tumoral extension					
Nonmetastatic	61.7%	44.8%	49.1%	44.3%	51.8%
Metastatic not 4S	24.4%	54.9%	50.5%	55.7%	42.6%
Metastatic 4S	13.9%	0.2%			5.6%

IR incidence rate, *ASR* age standardized rate

Table 1.2 Five-year overall survival by age groups, according to *MYCN* status and tumoral extension (France, 2000–2013)

	5-year survival [95% CI]		
	<1 year old	≥1 year old	Total
Total	90.3 [88.0–92.2]	66.0 [63.2–68.7]	75.3 [73.3–77.2]
MYCN			
Amplified	40.0 [27.0–52.7]	44.1 [38.0–50.0]	43.3 [37.8–48.7]
Nonamplified	95.1 [93.1–96.6]	71.9 [68.4–75.2]	82.4 [80.2–84.4]
Unknown	89.4 [82.1–93.8]	71.7 [64.6–77.6]	78.1 [72.9–82.4]
Tumor extension			
Nonmetastatic	96.5 [94.3–97.8]	89.7 [86.6–92.2]	93.0 [91.1–94.4]
Metastatic not 4S	71.3 [61.4–79.1]	45.2 [41.2–49.2]	48.7 [44.9–52.4]
Metastatic 4S	84.6 [78.6–89.0]	48.6 [19.2–73.0]	82.5 [76.5–87.1]

The highest incidence rates have been reported in countries with greater medical surveillance such as western Europe, the USA, Canada, Japan, and Australia which may reflect better diagnostic facilities [4]. Incidence rates reported by low- and medium-resource countries are generally lower, which may reflect true risk factors, as well as differences in diagnosis and registration practices [5, 6]. Racial differences have been suggested in previous periods. Nevertheless, annual incidence rate in black children in the USA is now 10.2 per million for 2001–2010, closer to that of white children, while very low rates are reported in the mostly black population of Sub-Saharan Africa [6].

1.1.2 Survival

The overall survival rates in France are 92% at 1 year and 75% at 5 years after diagnosis (Table 1.2). Survival varies strongly with age, with best figures among infants. *MYCN* amplification and metastases are associated with poor prognosis.

Treatment protocols have followed one another over the last 40 years to better account for poor prognostic factors and to intensify the treatment of high-risk groups [4, 7, 8]. However, recent data show a stagnation and even a significant fall in survival for neuroblastoma in Central Europe [9] and the USA [10].

There are still survival disparities between countries, even within Europe [9]. A 5-year overall survival estimate of 59% was recently reported for Southern and Eastern European countries [11]. Disparities could be, at least partly, attributed to differences in detection or registration since more elaborate healthcare systems may capture more low-risk cases, including, for example, spontaneously regressive cases.

1.2 Etiology

Because neuroblastoma is rare, literature on etiology is more limited than for leukemia or brain tumors, and studies often lack power. The characteristics of the cells and the early onset suggest a role of genetic factors and perinatal exposures. In rare cases, neuroblastoma can occur in a context of malformation syndromes (e.g. Hirschsprung's disease) or genetic diseases (e.g. neurofibromatosis type 1) and predisposing constitutional mutations (e.g. *NF1*, *ALK*, or *PHOXB*). These factors are addressed in Sect. 1.1.2. So far, genetic studies are still rare for low-risk low-penetrance susceptibility alleles, and neither gene–environment interactions, nor epigenetic effects of environment are covered yet.

1.2.1 Perinatal Characteristics

1.2.1.1 Gestational Age, Birth Weight, and Size for Gestational Age

Several case–control studies have analyzed the relationship between gestational age, birth weight, and neuroblastoma, some of them based on maternal interview at the time of diagnosis [12–16] and some using information from birth certificates [17–22]. They are summarized in Table 1.3.

Table 1.3 Relative risk estimates for the association between neuroblastoma and birth characteristics

Study	Exposure	Prevalence	Reference group	OR [95% CI]
Interview-based case–control studies				
US-Canada, 1992–1994 504 cases <19 years [12]	<32 weeks	2%	37–42 weeks	1.9 [0.7–4.4]
	33–36 weeks	6%		0.5 [0.3–1.0]
	>42 weeks	1%		0.9 [0.3–3.0]
	<1500 g	1%	2501–4000 g	2.6 [0.7–10.3]
	1500–2500 g	6%		1.1 [0.6–2.0]
	4001–4499 g	11%		1.1 [0.7–1.7]
	≥4500 g	1%		1.4 [0.6–3.2]
Germany, 1988–1994, 183 cases<15 years [13]	<37 weeks	4%	37–42 weeks	2.5 [1.3–4.6]
	<2500 g	3%	2500–4000 g	2.4 [1.2–4.7]
	>4000 g	11%		1.3 [0.8–2.2]
Germany, 1992–1994, 160 cases <14 years [14]	SGA	11%	AGA	1.2 [0.7–2.1]
	LGA	8%		1.6 [0.9–2.7]
Italy, 1998–2001, 207 cases <15 years [15]	≤37 weeks	15%	38–42 weeks	0.8 [0.5–1.3]
	>42 weeks	5%		0.8 [0.3–2.2]
	<2500 g	6%	2500–4000 g	0.6 [0.2–1.6]
	>4000 g	8%		1.1 [0.6–2.0]
France, 2003–2004/2010–2011, 357 cases <6 years [16]	<37 weeks	7%	37–39 weeks	1.2 [0.8–1.9]
	≥42 weeks	2%	2500–400 g	0.4 [0.1–1.3]
	<2500 g	6%	AGA	1.2 [0.9–1.7]
	≥4000 g	9%		1.4 [0.9–2.2]
	SGA	11%		1.4 [1.0–2.0]
	LGA	11%		1.5 [1.1–2.2]

Table 1.3 (continued)

Study	Exposure	Prevalence	Reference group	OR [95% CI]
Record linkage studies				
Norway, 1967–2004, ≤18 months 178 cases <15 years [18]	<37 weeks	N/S	40–41 weeks	0.6 [0.2–2.0]
	>42 weeks	N/S		1.2 [0.7–2.0]
	<2500 g	N/S	3000–3499 g	1.1 [0.3–3.7]
	≥4000 g	N/S		1.8 [1.0–3.1]
>18 months	<37 weeks	N/S	40–41 weeks	0.7 [0.2–2.8]
	>42 weeks	N/S		1.6 [0.8–3.0]
	≥4000 g	N/S	3000–3499 g	0.9 [0.4–1.8]
US New-York state, 1976–1987 155 cases <6 years [17]	<37 weeks	11%	37–42 weeks	0.4 [0.1–0.9]
	>42 weeks	12%		0.3 [0.1–0.7]
	<2500 g	7%	3000–3499	0.9 [0.4–2.2]
	>4000 g	12%		1.2 [0.6–2.2]
US Minnesota state, 1976–2004, 155 cases <14 years [19]	<37 weeks	9%	≥37 weeks	1.0 [0.6–1.8]
	<2500 g	7%	2500–4000 g	1.2 [0.6–2.3]
	>4000 g	15%		1.1 [0.7–1.7]
	SGA	7%	AGA	2.1 [1.1–4.0]
	LGA	24%	AGA	1.0 [0.7–1.5]
US California state, 1988–1997, 508 cases <5 years [21]	<37 weeks	12%	37–41 weeks	0.8 [0.6–1.2]
	>42 weeks	11%		1.1 [0.8–1.5]
	<2500 g	5%	2500–3999 g	1.0 [0.6–1.6]
	≥4000 g	12%		1.2 [0.9–1.7]
	term/<2500 g	2%	term/2500–3999 g	1.4 [0.6–3.0]
	term/≥4000 g	10%		1.2 [0.9–1.8]
US Washington state, 1980–2004, 240 cases <15 years [20]	<37 weeks	8%	37–42 weeks	0.6 [0.3–1.1]
	>42 weeks	4%		1.2 [0.9–1.8]
	<2500 g	5%	2500–3999 g	0.7 [0.4–1.5]
	>4000 g	13%		1.2 [0.9–1.8]
	SGA	9%	AGA	0.9 [0.6–1.5]
	LGA	10%		1.3 [0.8–1.9]
US New-York state, 1983–2001, 529 cases <15 years [22]	<38 weeks	14%	38–40 weeks	0.9 [0.7–1.2]
	<2500 g	7%	2500–4500 g	1.5 [1.0–2.1]
	>4500 g	2%		1.4 [0.7–2.5]
	SGA	6%	AGA	1.0 [0.5–1.9]
	LGA	2%		1.1 [0.8–1.6]

%E proportion of exposed, *SGA* small for gestational age, *LGA* large for gestational age, *AGA* appropriate for gestational age, *N/S* not stated

Regarding gestational age, no pattern of a positive or inverse association has emerged, despite homogeneous definitions. By contrast, a slight positive relationship is observed with high birth weight, with an estimated increase of 20% in a meta-analysis (pooled OR 1.2 [95% CI 1.0–1.4]) [24]. The relation seems less clear in the studies based on interview than in those based on birth certificates, which suggest that a bias in maternal recall or in study sampling is possible. Only six studies [14, 16, 19–22] considered birth weight for gestational age, and they did not show clearer associations.

1.2.2 Maternal Vitamin or Folic Acid Intake Around Pregnancy

Periconceptional folic acid supplementation has been shown to reduce the risk of neural tube defects by almost three-quarters [25]. It was therefore hypothesized that the risk of neuroblastoma could also be reduced by maternal folic acid supplementation before conception and in the first trimester of pregnancy. Five studies [16, 23, 26–28] have investigated the association between vitamin/folic acid supplementation during pregnancy and neuroblastoma, four [16, 23, 26, 27] of which reporting an inverse association with supplementation during preconception or during pregnancy, based on maternal interview.

1.2.3 Breastfeeding

Breastfeeding was reported to reduce risk of neuroblastoma in the COG North-American study (0.6 [0.5–0.9]) [29] and in the French study (0.7 [0.5–1.0]) [16], with no trend with increasing breastfeeding duration. Two other studies [24, 30] based in less than 50 cases did not report significant associations.

1.2.4 Congenital Malformations

Nine studies which investigated the link between congenital malformations and neuroblastoma reported positive associations (Table 1.4). Detailed analyses are limited by small numbers, given the rarity of both congenital malformations and neuroblastomas. The associations with malformations, taken as a whole, are consistently reported by interview-based studies and by studies based on birth certificates. Two studies suggest that the association could be limited to children under 18 months [16, 18].

1.2.5 Parental Smoking and Alcohol Consumption

Overall, literature suggests that maternal tobacco smoking is associated with a slight increase in risk of neuroblastoma (Table 1.5), as suggested by two recent meta-analysis [43, 44]. Fewer studies report data on paternal smoking, and no consistent pattern is observed to date. Findings on maternal alcohol drinking are also heterogeneous.

1.2.6 Pesticides Exposures

Exposures to pesticides have been the most investigated environmental exposures, and published papers are summarized in Table 1.6. Maternal occupational exposures during pregnancy were addressed by five case–control studies, and all but one

Table 1.4 Relative risk estimates for the association between congenital malformations and risk of neuroblastoma

Study	Exposure	%E	RR [95% CI]
Interview-based case–control studies			
US and Canada, 1992–1994, 538 cases <19 years [31]	Any malformation (ICD-10)	5.0%	2.5 [1.6–4.2]
	Major malformation	1.0%	7.5 [2.2–25.5]
Italy, 1998–2001, 207 cases <15 years [15] France, 2003–2004 357 cases <6 years [16] <18 months ≥18 months	N/S Major malformations (ICD-10)	1.3% 2.5%	4.9 [1.8–13.6] 3.6 [1.3–8.9] 0.8 [0.3–2.3]
Record linkage studies			
England, Scotland, and Wales, 1971–1986, 1208 cases <15 years [32]	Spina bifida (ICD-10)	N/S	1.4 (ns)
	Cardiac septal defects (ICD-10)	N/S	1.5 (ns)
	Genitourinary (ICD-10)	N/S	1.5 (ns)
	Spine malformations (ICD-10)	N/S	1.7 (ns)
Canada, 1977–1993 141 cases <15 years [33]	Any malformation (ICD-9)	N/S	$p < 0.001$
Norway, 1978–1997, <18 months	N/S	N/S	3.7 [1.7–8.0]
178 cases<15 years [18] ≥18 months		N/S	0.7 [0.1–4.7]
Australia, 1984–1993, 52 cases <15 years [34]	Any malformation (ICD-9, British Paediatric Association modification)	2.5%	7.9 [3.3–18.8]
US, Washington state, 1980–2004, 240 cases <20 years [20]	Any malformation Major malformations	4.8%	2.1 [1.3–3.4]
		0.6%	6.7 [2.9–16.1]
US, California state, 1988–1997 <5 years	Nonchromosomal malformations	14%	1.0 [0.4–2.7]
508 cases <5 years [21] <1 year		5%	1.6 [0.8–3.3]
US Washington state, 1984–2013 327 cases <20 years [35]			1.9 [1.3–2.8]

%E proportion of exposed, *CI* confidence interval, *N/S* not specified, *RR* relative risk estimate (odds ratio or standardized incidence ratio)

reported increased risk of neuroblastoma with farming or pesticides use. Two cohorts and seven case–control studies investigated paternal exposure with inconsistent results, as summarized by a meta-analysis showing no association with neuroblastoma [53].

Increased risk of neuroblastoma was associated to self-reported use of household pesticides before or after birth [13, 51, 52].

Table 1.5 Relative risk estimates for the association between maternal smoking and alcohol drinking during pregnancy and neuroblastoma

Study	Cases and controls selection				Maternal consumption during pregnancy (ever/never)				
	Cases	Controls			Smoking		Alcohol drinking		Matched factors/Adjustments
Author, country, year of case accrual	Source	*n*	Source	*n*	Crude OR [95% CI][a]	Adjusted OR [95% CI]	Crude OR [95% CI][a]	Adjusted OR [95% CI]	
Data obtained by record linkage									
Johnson et al., 2008 USA (1976–2004) [19]	Cancer Registry Minnesota state	155	Birth Registry	8752	1.4 [0.9–2.2]	1.4 [0.9–2.3]	1.1 [0.4–3.5]	–	Year of birth, sex
Chow et al., 2003 USA (1980–1992) [20]	Cancer Registry Washington state	240	Birth Registry	2400	0.8 [0.6–1.2]	0.8 [0.6–1.2]	–	–	Year of birth, sex/gestational age, birth weight, parental age, ethnicity, maternal residence
McLaughlin et al., 2009 USA (1985–2001) [22]	Cancer Registry New York state	529	Birth Records	12,010	–	1.0 [0.7–1.3]	–	1.2 [0.5–2.6]	Date of birth, sex
Stavrou et al., 2009 Australia (1994–2005) [36]	Cancer Registry New South Wales	122	Midwives data collection	1,045,966	0.8 [0.5–1.3]	1.0 [0.6–1.7]	–	–	Children age and sex, maternal age, birth weight, gestational age, socioeconomics, maternal hypertension, gestational diabetes, preeclampsia
Heck et al., 2016 USA (2007–2013) [37]	Cancer Registry California state	238	Birth certificates	40,356	1.1 [0.5–2.4]	1.2 [0.5–2.5]	–	–	Year of birth/maternal ethnicity, maternal education

Data obtained by Interview									
Kramer et al., 1987 USA (1970–1979) [38]	Cancer Registry Great Delaware valley	93	General population	93	1.3 [0.8–2.1]		1.4 [0.9–2.2]		Date of birth, race, area code,
Buck et al., 2001 USA (1976–1987) [17]	Cancer Registry New York state	155	Birth Registry	310	1.3 [0.8–2.1]	1.4 [0.9–2.1]	1.2 [0.8–1.9]	1.2 [0.8–1.9]	Year of birth, parity, maternal age, smoking and alcohol consumption
Sorahan et al., 1994 UK (1977–1981) [39]	Cancer Registry	93	Birth Registry	93	–	1.0 [0.8–1.3]	–	–	Date of birth, sex
Schwartzbaum et al., 1992 USA (1979–1986) [40]	Hospital Cancer Registry	101	Hospital Cancer Registry	690	–	1.9 [1.1–3.2]	–	0.7 [0.4–1.1]	Age, race, maternal age, social class, exposure to X-ray, miscarriage, others (not specified)
Schuz et al., 2001 Germany (1988–1993) [13]	Cancer Registry	183	Residents database	1785	1.4 [1.0–1.9]	-	0.9 [0.6–1.3]	–	Age, sex, year of birth/SES, degree of urbanization
Pang et al., 2003 UK (1992–1994) [41]	Cancer Registry	188	Family Health Services database	6987	–	0.9 [0.6–1.3]	–	–	Age, sex, parental age, deprivation score
Yang et al., 2000 USA (1992–1994) [42]	Oncology Group	538	General population	538	1.2 [0.9–1.6]	1.1 [0.8–1.4]	1.1 [0.9–1.4]	1.1 [0.8–1.4]	Date of birth/sex, race, maternal education, household income in the birth year
Parodi et al., 2014 Italy (1998–2001) [15]	Oncology Group	153	National health service database	1044	1.4 [0.9–2.2]	1.2 [0.7–2.1]	–	–	Gender, date of birth, area of residence/maternal age, and maternal education
Rios et al., 2019 [43]	Cancer Registry	357	General population	1783	1.3 [1.0–1.7]	1.3 [0.9–1.7]	0.9 [0.7–1.1]	1.0 [0.8–1.4]	Age, sex, maternal age, study of origin

OR [95%CI] odds ratio and its 95% confidence interval

Table 1.6 Relative risk estimates for the association between parental pesticides exposures and neuroblastoma

Study	Exposure	Parent	Period	%E (controls)	RR [95% CI]
Parental occupational exposures—cohorts					
Norway, 1952–1991, 27 cases [45]	Field vegetable farming (agricultural census)	Any parent	Any time Any time	N/S	2.5 [1.0–6.1]
US, 1993–1997, 3 cases [46]	Farming	Any parent		N/S	1.3 [0.4–3.9]
Parental occupational exposures—case–control studies					
US Greater Philadelphia area, 1970–1979, 104 cases [47]	Farming	Any parent	Pregnancy Preconception	N/S N/S	0.7 [0.1–5.8] 3.5 [0.7–35]
US and Canada, 1992–1996, 504 cases [48]	Farming	Maternal	Any time	N/S	2.2 [0.6–8.8]
		Paternal	Any time	N/S	0.9 [0.4–1.8]
US New-York state, 1976–1987, 183 cases [49]	Field vegetable farming	Maternal	Pregnancy	N/S	0.8 [0.2–3.2]
		Paternal	Pregnancy	N/S	1.0 [0.2–3.9]
	Insecticides use	Maternal	Pregnancy	N/S	0.8 [0.2–3.2]
		Paternal	Pregnancy	N/S	2.3 [1.4–3.7]
Germany, 1988–1994, 183 cases [13]	Farming	Maternal	After birth	3%	1.2 [0.4–3.7]
	Any occupational use	Maternal	Any time	1%	5.1 [1.1–23.4]
		Paternal	Any time	4%	1.8 [0.8–3.7]
Great Britain, 1962–1999, 2920 cases [50]	Agriculture	Paternal	Pregnancy	2%	0.9 [0.6–1.3]
	Agrochemical industry	Paternal	Pregnancy	3%	1.0 [0.7–1.4]
Parental nonoccupational exposures—case–control studies					
US and Canada, 1992–1994, 390 cases [51]	Household use	Both parents	Ever	31%	1.6 [1.0–2.3]
			Preconception-pregnancy	18%	1.3 [0.8–3.3]
			After birth	18%	1.4 [0.9–2.2]
	Garden	Both parents	Ever	22%	1.7 [0.9–2.1]
			Preconception-pregnancy	13%	1.3 [0.8–2.0]
			After birth	12%	1.8 [1.0–3.1]
Germany, 1988–1993, 183 cases [13]	Household insecticides use		After birth	6%	1.8 [0.9–3.4]
	Garden pesticides		After birth	10%	0.9 [0.5–1.6]
France, 2003–2004; 2010–2011 357 cases [52]	Household use Insecticides use		Pregnancy Pregnancy	30% 28%	1.5 [1.0–2.1] 1.4 [0.9–2.0]

RR [95%CI] RR estimated (Standardized incidence ratio or odds ratio) and its 95% confidence interval, *N/S* not stated

1.2.7 Other Factors

Associations with maternal medication use, perinatal infections, parental occupational exposures to magnetic fields, hydrocarbons, or other chemicals [46, 48–50], or residential exposure to air pollutants have been investigated reported, and no consistent pattern has emerged yet [54, 55].

References

1. Trott PA. International classification of diseases for oncology. J Clin Pathol. 1977;30:782. http://codes.iarc.fr/. Accessed 14 Feb 2019.
2. Steliarova-Foucher E, Stiller C, Lacour B, Kaatsch P. International classification of childhood cancer, third edition. Cancer. 2005;103:1457–67. https://doi.org/10.1002/cncr.20910.
3. Spix C, Pastore G, Sankila R, et al. Neuroblastoma incidence and survival in European children (1978-1997): report from the Automated Childhood Cancer Information System project. Eur J Cancer. 2006;42:2081–91. https://doi.org/10.1016/j.ejca.2006.05.008.
4. Berthold F, Spix C, Kaatsch P, Lampert F. Incidence, survival, and treatment of localized and metastatic neuroblastoma in Germany 1979–2015. Pediatr Drugs. 2017;19:577–93. https://doi.org/10.1007/s40272-017-0251-3.
5. Kamihara J, Ma C, Fuentes Alabi SL, et al. Socioeconomic status and global variations in the incidence of neuroblastoma: call for support of population-based cancer registries in low-middle–income countries. Pediatr Blood Cancer. 2017;64:321–3. https://doi.org/10.1002/pbc.26244.
6. Steliarova-Foucher E, Colombet M, Ries LAG, et al. International incidence of childhood cancer, 2001–10: a population-based registry study. Lancet Oncol. 2017;18:719–31. https://doi.org/10.1016/S1470-2045(17)30186-9.
7. Haupt R, Garaventa A, Gambini C, et al. Improved survival of children with neuroblastoma between 1979 and 2005: a report of the Italian neuroblastoma registry. J Clin Oncol. 2010;28:2331–8. https://doi.org/10.1200/JCO.2009.24.8351.
8. Moroz V, Machin D, Faldum A, et al. Changes over three decades in outcome and the prognostic influence of age-at-diagnosis in young patients with neuroblastoma: a report from the International Neuroblastoma Risk Group project. Eur J Cancer. 2011;47:561–71. https://doi.org/10.1016/j.ejca.2010.10.022.
9. Gatta G, Botta L, Rossi S, et al. Childhood cancer survival in Europe 1999-2007: results of EUROCARE-5-a population-based study. Lancet Oncol. 2014;15:35–47. https://doi.org/10.1016/S1470-2045(13)70548-5.
10. Coughlan D, Gianferante M, Lynch CF, et al. Treatment and survival of childhood neuroblastoma: evidence from a population-based study in the United States. Pediatr Hematol Oncol. 2017;34:320–30. https://doi.org/10.1080/08880018.2017.1373315.
11. Panagopoulou P, Bouka E, Georgakis MK, et al. Persisting inequalities in survival patterns of childhood neuroblastoma in Southern and Eastern Europe and the effect of socio-economic development compared with those of the US. Eur J Cancer. 2018;96:44–53. https://doi.org/10.1016/j.ejca.2018.03.003.
12. Hamrick SEG, Olshan AF, Neglia JP, Pollock BH. Association of pregnancy history and birth characteristics with neuroblastoma: a report from the Children's Cancer Group and the Pediatric Oncology Group. Paediatr Perinat Epidemiol. 2001;15:328–37. https://doi.org/10.1111/j.1365-3016.2001.0376a.x.
13. Schüz J, Kaletsch U, Meinert R, et al. Risk factors for neuroblastoma at different stages of disease. Results from a population-based case-control study in Germany. J Clin Epidemiol. 2001;54:702–9. https://doi.org/10.1016/S0895-4356(00)00339-5.

14. Schüz J, Forman MR. Birthweight by gestational age and childhood cancer. Cancer Causes Control. 2007;18:655–63. https://doi.org/10.1007/s10552-007-9011-y.
15. Parodi S, Merlo DF, Ranucci A, et al. Risk of neuroblastoma, maternal characteristics and perinatal exposures: the SETIL study. Cancer Epidemiol. 2014;38:686–94. https://doi.org/10.1016/j.canep.2014.09.007.
16. Rios P, Bailey HD, Orsi L, et al. Risk of neuroblastoma, birth-related characteristics, congenital malformations and perinatal exposures: a pooled analysis of the ESCALE and ESTELLE French studies (SFCE). Int J Cancer. 2016;139:1936–48. https://doi.org/10.1002/ijc.30239.
17. Buck GM, et al. Perinatal factors and risk of neuroblastoma. Paediatr Perinat Epidemiol. 2001;15:47–53. https://doi.org/10.1046/j.1365-3016.2001.00307.x.
18. Bjørge T, Engeland A, Tretli S, Heuch I. Birth and parental characteristics and risk of neuroblastoma in a population-based Norwegian cohort study. Br J Cancer. 2008;99:1165–9. https://doi.org/10.1038/sj.bjc.6604646.
19. Johnson KJ, Puumala SE, Soler JT, Spector LG. Perinatal characteristics and risk of neuroblastoma. Int J Cancer. 2008;123:1166–72. https://doi.org/10.1002/ijc.23645.
20. Chow EJ, Friedman DL, Mueller BA. Maternal and perinatal characteristics in relation to neuroblastoma. Cancer. 2007;109:983–92. https://doi.org/10.1002/cncr.22486.
21. Urayama KY, Von Behren J, Reynolds P. Birth characteristics and risk of neuroblastoma in young children. Am J Epidemiol. 2007;165:486–95. https://doi.org/10.1093/aje/kwk041.
22. McLaughlin CC, Baptiste MS, Schymura MJ, et al. Perinatal risk factors for neuroblastoma. Cancer Causes Control. 2009;20:289–301. https://doi.org/10.1007/s10552-008-9243-5.
23. Buck BM, Michalek M, Chen C, Nasca N, Baptiste B. Perinatal factors and risk of neuroblastoma. Paediatr Perinat Epidemiol. 2001;15(1):47–53.
24. Harder T, Plagemann A, Harder A. Birth weight and risk of neuroblastoma: a meta-analysis. Int J Epidemiol. 2010;39:746–56. https://doi.org/10.1093/ije/dyq040.
25. De-Regil LM, Peña-Rosas JP, Fernández-Gaxiola AC, Rayco-Solon P. Effects and safety of periconceptional oral folate supplementation for preventing birth defects. Cochrane Database Syst Rev. 2015;(12):CD007950.
26. French AE, Grant R, Weitzman S, et al. Folic acid food fortification is associated with a decline in neuroblastoma. Clin Pharmacol Ther. 2003;74:288–94. https://doi.org/10.1016/S0009-9236(03)00200-5.
27. Olshan AF, Smith JC, Bondy ML, et al. Maternal vitamin use and reduced risk of neuroblastoma. Epidemiology. 2002;13:575–80. https://doi.org/10.1097/00001648-200209000-00014.
28. Mortensen JHS, Øyen N, Fomina T, et al. Supplemental folic acid in pregnancy and childhood cancer risk. Br J Cancer. 2016;114:71–5. https://doi.org/10.1038/bjc.2015.446.
29. Daniels JL, Olshan AF, Pollock BH, et al. Breast-feeding and neuroblastoma, USA and Canada. Cancer Causes Control. 2002;13:401–5. https://doi.org/10.1023/A:1015746701922.
30. Smulevich VB, Solionova LG, Belyakova SV. Parental occupation and other factors and cancer risk in children: I. Study methodology and non-occupational factors. Int J Cancer. 1999;83:712–7. https://doi.org/10.1002/(SICI)1097-0215(19991210)83:6<712::AID-IJC2>3.0.CO;2-D.
31. Menegaux F, Olshan AF, Reitnauer PJ, et al. Positive association between congenital anomalies and risk of neuroblastoma. Pediatr Blood Cancer. 2005;45:649–55. https://doi.org/10.1002/pbc.20263.
32. Narod SA, Hawkins MM, Robertson CM, Stiller CA. Congenital anomalies and childhood cancer in Great Britain. Am J Hum Genet. 1997;60:474–85.
33. Foulkes WD, Buu PN, Filiatrault D, et al. Excess of congenital abnormalities in French-Canadian children with neuroblastoma: a case series study from montreal. Med Pediatr Oncol. 1997;29:272–9. https://doi.org/10.1002/(SICI)1096-911X(199710)29:4<272::AID-MPO7>3.0.CO;2-J.
34. Altmann AE, Halliday JL, Giles GG. Associations between congenital malformations and childhood cancer. A register-based case-control study. Br J Cancer. 1998;78:1244–9. https://doi.org/10.1038/bjc.1998.662.
35. Norwood MS, Lupo PJ, Chow EJ, et al. Childhood cancer risk in those with chromosomal and non-chromosomal congenital anomalies in Washington State: 1984-2013. PLoS One. 2017;12:e0179006. https://doi.org/10.1371/journal.pone.0179006.

36. Stavrou EP, Baker DF, Bishop JF. Maternal smoking during pregnancy and childhood cancer in New South Wales: a record linkage investigation. Cancer Causes Control. 2009;20:1551–8. https://doi.org/10.1007/s10552-009-9400-5.
37. Heck JE, Contreras ZA, Park AS, et al. Smoking in pregnancy and risk of cancer among young children: a population-based study. Int J Cancer. 2016;139:613–6. https://doi.org/10.1002/ijc.30111.
38. Kramer S, Ward E, Meadows AT, Malone KE. Medical and drug risk factors associated with neuroblastoma: a case-control study. J Natl Cancer Inst. 1987;78:797–804.
39. Sorahan T, Lancashire R, Prior P, et al. Childhood cancer and parental use of alcohol and tobacco. Ann Epidemiol. 2002;5:354–9. https://doi.org/10.1016/1047-2797(95)00032-3.
40. Schwartzbaum JA. Influence of the mother's prenatal drug consumption on risk of neuroblastoma in the child. Am J Epidemiol. 1992;135:1358–67. https://doi.org/10.1093/oxfordjournals.aje.a116247.
41. Pang D, McNally R, Birch JM. Parental smoking and childhood cancer: results from the United Kingdom Childhood Cancer Study. Br J Cancer. 2003;88:373–81. https://doi.org/10.1038/sj.bjc.6600774.
42. Yang Q, Olshan AF, Bondy ML, et al. Parental smoking and alcohol consumption and risk of neuroblastoma. Cancer Epidemiol Biomarkers Prev. 2000;9:967–72.
43. Rios P, Bailey HD, Poulalhon C, et al. Parental smoking, maternal alcohol consumption during pregnancy and the risk of neuroblastoma in children. A pooled analysis of the ESCALE and ESTELLE French studies. Int J Cancer. 2019; https://doi.org/10.1002/ijc.32161.
44. Müller-Schulte E, Kurlemann G, Harder A. Tobacco, alcohol and illicit drugs during pregnancy and risk of neuroblastoma: systematic review. Arch Dis Child Fetal Neonatal Ed. 2018;103:F467–73. https://doi.org/10.1136/archdischild-2017-313615.
45. Kristensen P, Andersen A, Irgens LM, et al. Cancer in offspring of parents engaged in agricultural activities in Norway: incidence and risk factors in the farm environment. Int J Cancer. 1996;65:39–50. https://doi.org/10.1002/(SICI)1097-0215(19960103)65:1<39::AID-IJC8>3.0.CO;2-2.
46. Flower KB, Knott C, Shore DL, et al. Cancer risk and parental pesticide application in children of Agricultural Health Study participants. Environ Health Perspect. 2003;112:631–5. https://doi.org/10.1289/ehp.6586.
47. Bunin GR, Ward E, Kramer S, et al. Neuroblastoma and parental occupation. Am J Epidemiol. 1990;131:776–80.
48. Olshan AF, De Roos AJ, Teschke K, et al. Neuroblastoma and parental occupation. Cancer Causes Control. 1990;10:776–80.
49. Kerr MA, Nasca PC, Mundt KA, et al. Parental occupational exposures and risk of neuroblastoma: a case-control study (United States). Cancer Causes Control. 2000;11:635–43. https://doi.org/10.1023/A:1008951632482.
50. MacCarthy A, Bunch KJ, Fear NT, et al. Paternal occupation and neuroblastoma: a case-control study based on cancer registry data for Great Britain 1962-1999. Br J Cancer. 2010;102:615–9. https://doi.org/10.1038/sj.bjc.6605504.
51. Daniels JL, Olshan AF, Teschke K, et al. Residential pesticide exposure and neuroblastoma. Epidemiology. 2001;12:20–7. https://doi.org/10.1097/00001648-200101000-00005.
52. Rios P, Bailey HD, Lacour B, et al. Maternal use of household pesticides during pregnancy and risk of neuroblastoma in offspring. A pooled analysis of the ESTELLE and ESCALE French studies (SFCE). Cancer Causes Control. 2017;28:1125–32. https://doi.org/10.1007/s10552-017-0944-5.
53. Moore A, Enquobahrie DA. Paternal occupational exposure to pesticides and risk of neuroblastoma among children: a meta-analysis. Cancer Causes Control. 2011;22:1529–36. https://doi.org/10.1007/s10552-011-9829-1.
54. Heck JE, Park AS, Qiu J, et al. An exploratory study of ambient air toxics exposure in pregnancy and the risk of neuroblastoma in offspring. Environ Res. 2013;127:1–6. https://doi.org/10.1016/j.envres.2013.09.002.
55. Kumar SV, Lupo PJ, Pompeii LA, Danysh HE. Maternal residential proximity to major roadways and pediatric embryonal tumors in offspring. Int J Environ Res Public Health. 2018;15:eE505. https://doi.org/10.3390/ijerph15030505.

Biology of Neuroblastoma

2

Gudrun Schleiermacher

2.1 Introduction

To date, the precise etiology of neuroblastoma is unknown, and unlike many adult malignancies, environmental factors are not thought to play a major role, although predisposing effects of prenatal exposures to potentially toxic substances warrant further investigation. However, genetic factors, both at constitutional and somatic levels, are thought to play a major role in neuroblastoma development [1].

2.2 Hereditary Genetic Factors

Several observations corroborate the hypothesis of a role of underlying hereditary genetic factors in the etiology of neuroblastoma.

First, although rare and representing less than 1% of all cases [2], familial neuroblastomas have been described. Mutations of gain of function in the tyrosine kinase domain of the ALK anaplastic lymphoma kinase gene have been detected in the majority of familial cases [3, 4]. This is thought to be associated with an autosomal-dominant pattern of inheritance with incomplete penetrance.

Second, neuroblastoma can appear in association with different clinical syndromes. Neural crest-related developmental disorders associated with an increased risk of developing neuroblastoma have been linked to inactivating mutations in the PHOX2B gene, a major regulator of neural crest development, identified as the first neuroblastoma predisposition mutation [5, 6]. While expansions of the second

G. Schleiermacher (✉)
Recherche Translationnelle en Oncologie Pédiatrique, Institut Curie, Paris Cedex 05, France

SIREDO Département d'Oncologie Pédiatrique, Institut Curie, Paris Cedex 05, France

Inserm U 830, Institut Curie, Paris Cedex 05, France
e-mail: gudrun.schleiermacher@curie.net

S. Sarnacki, L. Pio (eds.), *Neuroblastoma*,
https://doi.org/10.1007/978-3-030-18396-7_2

polyalanine sequence of PHOX2B are mainly observed in patients with a curse of Ondine (also called CCHS, Congenital Central Hypoventilation Syndrome) associated with a low risk of peripheral neuroblastic tumors, non-expansive mutations with Hirschsprung's disease are associated with a higher risk of developing neuroblastoma. Other associations between neuroblastic tumors and cancer susceptibility syndromes include neurofibromatosis type 1 (NF1) [7], characterized by constitutive activation of the RAS–MAPK pathway, as well as Noonan syndrome with PTPN11 gene involvement.

Third, genome-wide association studies have shown that peripheral neuroblastic tumors may occur in the context of underlying genetic factors, as it has been demonstrated that different polymorphic alleles, localized at different genome loci, influence oncogenesis [8–13]. Of a weak individual impact on the initiation of the disease (with a relative risk of 1.5–2.0 compared to the global population), these polymorphic alleles can cooperate in an individual patient to promote malignant transformation during neurological development, and some genes targeted by these polymorphic alleles play a role in the pathogenesis of neuroblastoma, including BARD1, LMO1, DUSP12, DDX4, HACE1, and LIN28B. The polymorphic alleles described show a correlation with high-risk or low-risk disease, indicating that favorable and unfavorable forms of neuroblastoma may represent distinct entities in terms of genetic events that initiate tumorigenesis.

In addition, rare cases with various aberrant constitutional karyotypes have been described in patients with neuroblastoma, including constitutional copy-number abnormalities, balanced and unbalanced translocations, and specific chromosomal deletions, including deletions of chromosome 1p [14]. In total, there are probably as yet undiscovered additional genes that predispose to neuroblastoma when they are altered in the germline. It is important to note that, to date, there are no clinically validated guidelines for determining who should be screened for germline mutations, nor how to monitor patients or families with known susceptibility alleles.

2.2.1 Somatic Genetic Alterations

2.2.1.1 Copy-Number Alterations

With only 1–2% of neuroblastomas occurring in a familial context or predisposition, over 98% of all cases occur sporadically. A large number of recurrent somatic genetic alterations have been found in neuroblastoma, the most common being quantitative genomic alterations with gains or losses in genetic material. These genetic abnormalities are related to distinct biological and clinical subgroups of the disease.

The amplification of the oncogene MYCN, located at chromosome 2p24.1, is observed in about 25% of neuroblastomas and 40% of high-risk tumors [15]. It remains one of the most important genetic alterations associated with advanced stages of disease, with an aggressive phenotype and poor survival [1]. It is the first genetic marker used in clinical practice for risk stratification and treatment adaptation [16]. Closely associated with poor survival in patients with localized disease and in infants, its prognostic impact in metastatic disease of older children with an overall poor outcome is less clear [16, 17]. At a cytogenetic level, amplification of the MYCN oncogene occurs either as double-minute chromosomes (DM) or homogeneously staining regions (HSR), which contain between 10 and over 100 ectopic copies of the *MYCN* oncogene. The oncogenic role of MYCN has been clearly demonstrated as its ectopic expression in the neural crest is sufficient to drive neuroblastoma tumorigenesis in zebrafish and mice models [18]. Its oncogenic role is based on an enhancement of the expression of genes involved in cell proliferation, and on the repression of genes involved in differentiation and apoptosis [19].

Other recurrent amplifications concern the *ALK* gene on chromosome 2p23, as well as amplicons of chromosome 12q13–14 encompassing, among others, the MDM2 and CDK4 genes [20]. Recent data indicate that NB with focal amplifications other than MYCN might present with atypical clinical features and a poorer outcome [21].

Other recurrent structural alterations recurrently observed in neuroblastoma concern segmental chromosome alterations (SCA) corresponding to unbalanced chromosome translocations, including deletions of chromosome arms 1p, 3p, 4p, and 11q, and gains of 1q, 2p, or 17q. Although several recurrently altered chromosome regions have been identified, chromosome breakpoints are not recurrent but lie scattered over wide genomic regions. Deletion of 1p36 is observed in 20–35% of cases and is associated with poor survival in multivariate analyses as well as with aggressive disease markers [22, 23]. Deletions of 11q in a consensus region at 11q23 occur in approximately 40% of cases and are inversely correlated with *MYCN* amplification, identifying a molecularly distinct high-risk patient subset, characterized by advanced stage, older age, as well as a higher genomic instability with a higher number of chromosome breakpoints [24, 25]. Gains of chromosome 17q21-qter represent the most frequent genetic alteration in neuroblastoma, occurring in 70% of tumors. Numerous studies have reported that 17q gain is significantly associated with advanced stage of disease, increased patient age, *MYCN* amplification, as well as other unfavorable genetic parameters [26].

Although intense decade-long research has focused on the identification of hypothetical tumor-suppressor genes or oncogenes in recurrently altered regions of chromosome loss or gain, the smallest regions of overlap remain quite extensive and to date do not point to single-gene candidates as tumor suppressors or oncogenes, suggesting that an overall imbalance of copy-number regions is of importance in neuroblastoma oncogenesis.

Although the individual segmental chromosome alterations have been shown to correlate with outcome, importantly, the overall genomic profile has been shown to be of prognostic impact in neuroblastoma [27–30]. Whereas an overall genomic copy-number profile characterized by numerical chromosome alterations, consisting of gains or losses of whole chromosomes, is associated with a favorable outcome, segmental chromosome alterations of any chromosome region, without or with numerical chromosome alterations, are associated with advanced stage of disease, with an increased age at diagnosis and, importantly, a higher risk of relapse in multivariate analyses [27, 28, 31]. In addition to the determination of MYCN amplifications status, the overall genomic copy-number profile determined by array comparative genomic hybridization (CGH) or single nucleotide polymorphism (SNP) array is now considered part of routine work up in particular in low- and intermediate-risk neuroblastoma and might be used for treatment stratification within prospective clinical protocols [1].

Higher-resolution copy-number analyses have also revealed smaller recurrent interstitial events. Indeed, SNP arrays have identified alterations on chromosome 9p, with homo- or hemizygous deletions encompassing the *CDKN2A* gene [32]. Other sporadic copy-number alterations include focal TERT gains [33] and microdeletions encompassing the *PTPRD* gene [34].

More complex rearrangements resulting from chromothripsis, corresponding to massive genomic rearrangements acquired in a single catastrophic event, have been described in neuroblastoma, but their association with other genomic and clinical subtypes remains to be determined [35, 36].

2.2.1.2 Single-Gene Mutations

Recent next-generation sequencing approaches have indicated that most neuroblastomas harbor only few mutations, with an average of 10–20 predicted nonsynonymous variations in coding regions per genome, indicating an exonic mutation frequency of 0.2–0.4 per Mb. [35, 37–39] The frequency of somatic events strongly correlates with tumor stage, higher-stage tumors harboring a higher number of mutations.

The most frequent recurrent somatic mutation in neuroblastoma concerns the gene *ALK* (anaplastic lymphoma kinase), with mutations activating the tyrosine kinase domain in approximately 10% of all cases at diagnosis. [3, 4] The somatic ALK-1174 mutation appears to contribute to a more aggressive phenotype, but unlike ALK-1275 mutations, these specific mutations are not found in familial neuroblastoma, suggesting that they are not tolerated in the germline [40, 41]. The oncogenic role of activating ALK mutations in neuroblastoma has been demonstrated in vitro and in vivo in both zebrafish and mouse models, with coexpression of ALK-F1174L and MYCN producing a synergistic effect for neuroblastoma tumorigenesis in mice. New-generation small-molecule inhibitors targeting the activated kinase domain of ALK are now available, making this a promising target for molecular therapy, possibly in combination therapies, but still requiring more specific development [40, 42, 43].

Other recurrent mutations in neuroblastoma target distinct cellular pathways and include PTPN11 mutations (in 3% of cases), as well as genes involved in cytoskeleton maintenance, neuritogenesis, and other regulators of the RAC/Rho pathway [35].

Interestingly, genes involved in chromatin remodeling have been found to be targeted in a significant number of cases, either by mutations or by structural variations, including mutations in the ARID1A/ARID1B genes [38]. Somatic alterations of ATRX, consisting either of mutations or small interstitial deletions, are associated with an increase in telomere length and with an absence of the ATRX protein in the nucleus. ATRX alterations appear to be more frequent in older children and occur in mutually exclusive fashion with MYCN amplifications [39]. ATRX mutations are associated with activation of a telomere maintenance mechanism termed alternate lengthening of telomeres (ALT), which may be associated with primary chemotherapy resistance.

Recurrent genomic rearrangements of the promoter region of the telomerase reverse transcriptase (TERT) gene on chromosome 5p15.33 have been described in >10% of neuroblastoma cases, with structural rearrangements of TERT resulting from chromothripsis in some cases [44, 45]. These rearrangements, which are associated with increased TERT expression, target regions immediately up- and downstream of TERT, and position the TERT coding sequence to strong enhancer elements, resulting in massive chromatin remodeling and DNA methylation of the affected region. [44] Occurring in mutually exclusive fashion with *MYCN* amplification and *ATRX* mutations, these rearrangements define a further subgroup of high-risk disease, with TERT rearrangements (23%), ATRX deletions (11%), and MYCN amplifications (37%) identifying three almost non-overlapping groups of high-stage neuroblastoma, each associated with very poor prognosis.

Thus, a large number of high-risk neuroblastomas are affected by genetic alterations of either *MYCN*, *TERT*, or *ATRX*, all of which converge to an activation of telomere-lengthening mechanisms either by direct activation or by ALT, leading to a capacity of near-infinite cell proliferation. [46] Advances in the development of inhibitors of these pathways and their evaluation in clinical trials will lead to new treatment opportunities.

Future studies will determine if the association between these major players in neuroblastoma oncogenesis with distinct genetic profiles and mutational patterns might serve for the definition of different risk groups in particular in high-risk neuroblastoma.

Overall, large-scale sequencing efforts have highlighted distinct mutational signatures which are thought to reflect distinct biochemical cellular processes [47]. In neuroblastoma, in some cases a predominance of C > T transitions, termed mutational signature 1, are observed, with an association with age. Other mutational signatures observed in neuroblastoma, although rarer, concern the canonical double-stranded break signature linked to mutations in *BRCA1* or *BRCA2* or to a "BRCAness" phenotype [48]. Altogether, these studies underline the heterogeneity of somatic genetic alterations in neuroblastoma and highlight the importance to pursue efforts of molecular characterization.

2.2.1.3 Expression Profiles

In addition to genetic changes, neuroblastoma can also be characterized by specific expression profiles. Indeed, to date, a large number of studies have focused on the analysis of differential expression patterns in NB, seeking to identify expression patterns that might be enable to distinguish patients with different clinical courses and thus define different prognostic groups in high-risk disease, and to potentially identify new therapeutic targets.

Thus, different expression signatures, based on 144-gene or 59-gene signatures, reliably distinguished patients with distinct clinical courses, with the strongest difference observed in non-high-risk disease [49, 50]. Using real-time PCR expression data, an expression signature based on only three genes (*CHD5*, *PAFAH1B1*, and

NME1) has been able to discriminate patients with different outcomes [51]. Among high-risk patients, an expression profile based on 55 genes defined patient populations with divergent outcome [52]. Differential expression signature depending on *MYCN* has led to a definition of a 157-gene signature which identified NB patients with poor prognosis independent of the genomic *MYCN* status, those without *MYCN* amplification presenting stabilization of MYCN at the protein level [53].

More recently, based on the hypothesis that tumor-associated inflammatory cells might contribute to the differences in age-dependent outcome of patients with metastatic NB, expression of genes representing tumor-associated macrophages, such as *CD33/CD16/IL6R/IL10/FCGR3*, contributed to a novel 14-gene tumor classification score. Progression-free survival was 47% versus 12% for patients with a low- versus a high-risk score, indicating that interactions between tumor and inflammatory cells may contribute to an aggressive metastatic NB phenotype [54].

In addition to messenger RNA, expression levels of non-coding RNAs are also highly variable. Micro-RNAs function as regulators of gene expression at the post-transcriptional level in diverse cellular processes and constitute the most widely studied non-coding RNA molecules in NB. *MYCN* modulates the expression of several classes of non-coding RNAs, especially some micro-RNAs, and it can also regulate the expression of long non-coding RNAs such as T-UCRs (Transcribed UltraConserved Regions) and non-coding RNA, whereas other long non-coding RNAs remain to be characterized in NB. The landscape of T-UCRs in NB has been studied recently and has revealed a correlation with the *MYCN* status, and preliminary studies have suggested that T-UCR-based expression signatures might distinguish short-from long-term survivors in high risk NB [55].

The miRNA expression pattern can also be used to classify NB patients according to survival [56, 57]. An advantage of the study of miRNA rather than mRNA expression signatures is linked to the greatest stability of miRNAs, and thus to an analytical feasibility even with formalin-fixed, paraffin-embedded (FFPE) samples as opposed to frozen samples [57]. The miRNA expression pattern can also be used to classify NB patients according to survival [56, 57].

The paucity of recurrent genetic mutations as compared to adult tumors indicates that additional mechanisms such as epigenetic alterations may play an important role in the molecular pathogenesis of these developmental tumors. Alterations in DNA methylation represent one of the most common molecular events in neoplasia, and CpG-island hypermethylation of gene promoters is a frequent mechanism for functional inactivation of relevant tumor-associated genes in neuroblastoma. Promoter methylation patterns which are associated with patient subgroups and distinct clinical features have been identified [58]. Further studies are now necessary to determine whether these genome-wide methylation patterns correlate with outcome and other prognostic molecular markers in NB patients.

Taken together, to date, many studies have demonstrated the feasibility of expression profiling of mRNA, miRNA, other non-coding RNAs, or epigenetic modifiers in order to determine different prognostic subgroups among NB patients. However, there is little, if any, overlap between the genes of the different signatures rendering cross-study comparisons unfeasible. Furthermore, although most expression signatures clearly distinguish prognostic groups in the overall population, differences in survival among high-risk patients are frequently not very marked. The routine setup of real-time determination of expression profiles in a prospective clinical trial setting, and their interpretation, remains a clear challenge.

2.2.1.4 Spatial and Temporal Heterogeneity

Neuroblastoma presents important spatial and temporal heterogeneity. Spatial heterogeneity has been recorded for several recurrent somatic genetic alterations in neuroblastoma. Indeed, MYCN alterations might occur only in a subset of neuroblastic cells of a given tumor [59]. Segmental chromosome alterations might also vary between different neuroblastic cell populations [60, 61]. Furthermore, mutations can also be observed at a heterogeneous level. In some tumors, low-level mutated allele fractions for ALK driver mutations have been observed [62].

In neuroblastoma, temporal heterogeneity can also occur. Indeed, genetic alterations may evolve over time and clonal evolution is common, leading to the acquisition of somatic alterations in known oncogenic pathways, some of which may be targeted. ALK-activating mutations, in some instance present in a minor subclone at diagnosis, might emerge at relapse [63]. Furthermore, activation of the MAPK pathway and other signaling pathways for epithelial–mesenchymal transition (EMT) processes may appear during a relapse and represent promising targets for targeted molecular treatment approaches [64, 65]. In total, spatial and temporal genetic heterogeneity plays an important role in neuroblastoma.

However, multi-site tumor biopsies, or sequential biopsies from the same tumor, can only rarely be realized, and recently liquid biopsies have emerged as a very promising tool to explore somatic genetic alterations with regards to both spatial and temporal heterogeneity. Indeed, circulating tumor DNA, a fraction of cell-free DNA, can readily be extracted from plasma of neuroblastoma patients. This can serve for the detection of MYCN amplification [66]. Copy-number alterations or mutations such as ALK can also be detected in ctDNA. [67–69] More recently application of whole-exome sequencing techniques to sequential ctDNA samples from NB patients has provided further evidence of the importance of clonal evolution in the progression of neuroblastoma, enabling the description of resistant clones emerging at the time of relapse [70].

Altogether, as neuroblastoma is in general associated with a low mutational burden and only few recurrently occurring mutations, it might be considered a copy-number disease, with large chromosome segments contributing to oncogenesis by gene dosage effects. Further ongoing efforts will enable to determine whether epigenetic changes also play a role in neuroblastoma oncogenesis.

References

1. Matthay KK, Maris JM, Schleiermacher G, Nakagawara A, Mackall CL, Diller L, Weiss WA. Neuroblastoma. Nat Rev Dis Primers. 2016;2:16078.
2. Shojaei-Brosseau T, Chompret A, Abel A, de Vathaire F, Raquin M-A, Brugières L, Feunteun J, Hartmann O, Bonaïti-Pellié C. Genetic epidemiology of neuroblastoma: a study of 426 cases at the Institut Gustave-Roussy in France. Pediatr Blood Cancer. 2004;42:99–105.

3. Mossé YP, Laudenslager M, Longo L, Cole KA, Wood A, Attiyeh EF, Laquaglia MJ, Sennett R, Lynch JE, Perri P, Laureys G, Speleman F, et al. Identification of ALK as a major familial neuroblastoma predisposition gene. Nature. 2008;455:930–5.
4. Janoueix-Lerosey I, Lequin D, Brugières L, Ribeiro A, de Pontual L, Combaret V, Raynal V, Puisieux A, Schleiermacher G, Pierron G, Valteau-Couanet D, Frebourg T, et al. Somatic and germline activating mutations of the ALK kinase receptor in neuroblastoma. Nature. 2008;455:967–70.
5. Trochet D, Bourdeaut F, Janoueix-Lerosey I, Deville A, de Pontual L, Schleiermacher G, Coze C, Philip N, Frébourg T, Munnich A, Lyonnet S, Delattre O, et al. Germline mutations of the paired-like homeobox 2B (PHOX2B) gene in neuroblastoma. Am J Hum Genet. 2004;74:761–4.
6. Trochet D, O'Brien LM, Gozal D, Trang H, Nordenskjöld A, Laudier B, Svensson P-J, Uhrig S, Cole T, Niemann S, Munnich A, Gaultier C, et al. PHOX2B genotype allows for prediction of tumor risk in congenital central hypoventilation syndrome. Am J Hum Genet. 2005;76:421–6.
7. Brems H, Beert E, de Ravel T, Legius E. Mechanisms in the pathogenesis of malignant tumours in neurofibromatosis type 1. Lancet Oncol. 2009;10:508–15.
8. Bosse KR, Diskin SJ, Cole KA, Wood AC, Schnepp RW, Norris G, Nguyen LB, Jagannathan J, Laquaglia M, Winter C, Diamond M, Hou C, et al. Common variation at BARD1 results in the expression of an oncogenic isoform that influences neuroblastoma susceptibility and oncogenicity. Cancer Res. 2012;72:2068–78.
9. Diskin SJ, Hou C, Glessner JT, Attiyeh EF, Laudenslager M, Bosse K, Cole K, Mossé YP, Wood A, Lynch JE, Pecor K, Diamond M, et al. Copy number variation at 1q21.1 associated with neuroblastoma. Nature. 2009;459:987–91.
10. Maris JM, Mosse YP, Bradfield JP, Hou C, Monni S, Scott RH, Asgharzadeh S, Attiyeh EF, Diskin SJ, Laudenslager M, Winter C, Cole KA, et al. Chromosome 6p22 locus associated with clinically aggressive neuroblastoma. N Engl J Med. 2008;358:2585–93.
11. Capasso M, Devoto M, Hou C, Asgharzadeh S, Glessner JT, Attiyeh EF, Mosse YP, Kim C, Diskin SJ, Cole KA, Bosse K, Diamond M, et al. Common variations in BARD1 influence susceptibility to high-risk neuroblastoma. Nat Genet. 2009;41:718–23.
12. Nguyen LB, Diskin SJ, Capasso M, Wang K, Diamond MA, Glessner J, Kim C, Attiyeh EF, Mosse YP, Cole K, Iolascon A, Devoto M, et al. Phenotype restricted genome-wide association study using a gene-centric approach identifies three low-risk neuroblastoma susceptibility Loci. PLoS Genet. 2011;7:e1002026.
13. Wang K, Diskin SJ, Zhang H, Attiyeh EF, Winter C, Hou C, Schnepp RW, Diamond M, Bosse K, Mayes PA, Glessner J, Kim C, et al. Integrative genomics identifies LMO1 as a neuroblastoma oncogene. Nature. 2011;469:216–20.
14. Vandepoele K, Andries V, Van Roy N, Staes K, Vandesompele J, Laureys G, De Smet E, Berx G, Speleman F, van Roy F. A constitutional translocation t(1;17)(p36.2;q11.2) in a neuroblastoma patient disrupts the human NBPF1 and ACCN1 genes. PLoS One. 2008;3:e2207.
15. Brodeur GM, Seeger RC, Schwab M, Varmus HE, Bishop JM. Amplification of N-myc in untreated human neuroblastomas correlates with advanced disease stage. Science. 1984;224:1121–4.
16. Campbell K, Gastier-Foster JM, Mann M, Naranjo AH, Van Ryn C, Bagatell R, Matthay KK, London WB, Irwin MS, Shimada H, Granger MM, Hogarty MD, et al. Association of MYCN copy number with clinical features, tumor biology, and outcomes in neuroblastoma: a report from the Children's Oncology Group. Cancer. 2017;123:4224–35.
17. Bagatell R, Beck-Popovic M, London WB, Zhang Y, Pearson ADJ, Matthay KK, Monclair T, Ambros PF, Cohn SL, International Neuroblastoma Risk Group. Significance of MYCN amplification in international neuroblastoma staging system stage 1 and 2 neuroblastoma: a report from the International Neuroblastoma Risk Group database. J Clin Oncol Off J Am Soc Clin Oncol. 2009;27:365–70.
18. Weiss WA, Aldape K, Mohapatra G, Feuerstein BG, Bishop JM. Targeted expression of MYCN causes neuroblastoma in transgenic mice. EMBO J. 1997;16:2985–95.

19. Hansford LM, Thomas WD, Keating JM, Burkhart CA, Peaston AE, Norris MD, Haber M, Armati PJ, Weiss WA, Marshall GM. Mechanisms of embryonal tumor initiation: distinct roles for MycN expression and MYCN amplification. Proc Natl Acad Sci U S A. 2004;101:12664–9.
20. Depuydt P, Boeva V, Hocking TD, Cannoodt R, Ambros IM, Ambros PF, Asgharzadeh S, Attiyeh EF, Combaret V, Defferrari R, Fischer M, Hero B, et al. Genomic amplifications and distal 6q loss: novel markers for poor survival in high-risk neuroblastoma patients. J Natl Cancer Inst. 2018;110:1084.
21. Guimier A, Ferrand S, Pierron G, Couturier J, Janoueix-Lerosey I, Combaret V, Mosseri V, Thebaud E, Gambart M, Plantaz D, Marabelle A, Coze C, et al. Clinical characteristics and outcome of patients with neuroblastoma presenting genomic amplification of loci other than MYCN. PLoS One. 2014;9:e101990.
22. Caron H, Spieker N, Godfried M, Veenstra M, van Sluis P, de Kraker J, Voûte P, Versteeg R. Chromosome bands 1p35-36 contain two distinct neuroblastoma tumor suppressor loci, one of which is imprinted. Genes Chromosomes Cancer. 2001;30:168–74.
23. Schleiermacher G, Delattre O, Peter M, Mosseri V, Delonlay P, Vielh P, Thomas G, Zucker J, Magdelénat H, Michon J. Clinical relevance of loss heterozygosity of the short arm of chromosome 1 in neuroblastoma: a single-institution study. Int J Cancer. 1996;69:73–8.
24. Attiyeh EF, London WB, Mossé YP, Wang Q, Winter C, Khazi D, McGrady PW, Seeger RC, Look AT, Shimada H, Brodeur GM, Cohn SL, et al. Chromosome 1p and 11q deletions and outcome in neuroblastoma. N Engl J Med. 2005;353:2243–53.
25. Carén H, Kryh H, Nethander M, Sjöberg R-M, Träger C, Nilsson S, Abrahamsson J, Kogner P, Martinsson T. High-risk neuroblastoma tumors with 11q-deletion display a poor prognostic, chromosome instability phenotype with later onset. Proc Natl Acad Sci U S A. 2010;107:4323–8.
26. Bown N, Cotterill S, Lastowska M, O'Neill S, Pearson AD, Plantaz D, Meddeb M, Danglot G, Brinkschmidt C, Christiansen H, Laureys G, Speleman F, et al. Gain of chromosome arm 17q and adverse outcome in patients with neuroblastoma. N Engl J Med. 1999;340:1954–61.
27. Janoueix-Lerosey I, Schleiermacher G, Michels E, Mosseri V, Ribeiro A, Lequin D, Vermeulen J, Couturier J, Peuchmaur M, Valent A, Plantaz D, Rubie H, et al. Overall genomic pattern is a predictor of outcome in neuroblastoma. J Clin Oncol. 2009;27:1026–33.
28. Schleiermacher G, Michon J, Huon I, d'Enghien C, Klijanienko J, Brisse H, Ribeiro A, Mosseri V, Rubie H, Munzer C, Thomas C, Valteau-Couanet D, et al. Chromosomal CGH identifies patients with a higher risk of relapse in neuroblastoma without MYCN amplification. Br J Cancer. 2007;97:238–46.
29. Vandesompele J, Baudis M, De Preter K, Van Roy N, Ambros P, Bown N, Brinkschmidt C, Christiansen H, Combaret V, Lastowska M, Nicholson J, O'Meara A, et al. Unequivocal delineation of clinicogenetic subgroups and development of a new model for improved outcome prediction in neuroblastoma. J Clin Oncol Off J Am Soc Clin Oncol. 2005;23:2280–99.
30. Tomioka N, Oba S, Ohira M, Misra A, Fridlyand J, Ishii S, Nakamura Y, Isogai E, Hirata T, Yoshida Y, Todo S, Kaneko Y, et al. Novel risk stratification of patients with neuroblastoma by genomic signature, which is independent of molecular signature. Oncogene. 2008;27:441–9.
31. Coco S, Theissen J, Scaruffi P, Stigliani S, Moretti S, Oberthuer A, Valdora F, Fischer M, Gallo F, Hero B, Bonassi S, Berthold F, et al. Age-dependent accumulation of genomic aberrations and deregulation of cell cycle and telomerase genes in metastatic neuroblastoma. Int J Cancer. 2012;131:1591–600.
32. Caren H, Erichsen J, Olsson L, Enerback C, Sjoberg RM, Abrahamsson J, Kogner P, Martinsson T. High-resolution array copy number analyses for detection of deletion, gain, amplification and copy-neutral LOH in primary neuroblastoma tumors: four cases of homozygous deletions of the CDKN2A gene. BMC Genomics. 2008;9:353.
33. Cobrinik D, Ostrovnaya I, Hassimi M, Tickoo SK, Cheung IY, Cheung N-KV. Recurrent pre-existing and acquired DNA copy number alterations, including focal TERT gains, in neuroblastoma central nervous system metastases. Genes Chromosomes Cancer. 2013;52:1150–66.

34. Stallings RL, Nair P, Maris JM, Catchpoole D, McDermott M, O'Meara A, Breatnach F. High-resolution analysis of chromosomal breakpoints and genomic instability identifies PTPRD as a candidate tumor suppressor gene in neuroblastoma. Cancer Res. 2006;66:3673–80.
35. Molenaar JJ, Koster J, Zwijnenburg DA, van Sluis P, Valentijn LJ, van der Ploeg I, Hamdi M, van Nes J, Westerman BA, van Arkel J, Ebus ME, Haneveld F, et al. Sequencing of neuroblastoma identifies chromothripsis and defects in neuritogenesis genes. Nature. 2012;483:589–93.
36. Boeva V, Jouannet S, Daveau R, Combaret V, Pierre-Eugène C, Cazes A, Louis-Brennetot C, Schleiermacher G, Ferrand S, Pierron G, Lermine A, Rio Frio T, et al. Breakpoint features of genomic rearrangements in neuroblastoma with unbalanced translocations and chromothripsis. PLoS One. 2013;8:e72182.
37. Pugh TJ, Morozova O, Attiyeh EF, Asgharzadeh S, Wei JS, Auclair D, Carter SL, Cibulskis K, Hanna M, Kiezun A, Kim J, Lawrence MS, et al. The genetic landscape of high-risk neuroblastoma. Nat Genet. 2013;45:279–84.
38. Sausen M, Leary RJ, Jones S, Wu J, Reynolds CP, Liu X, Blackford A, Parmigiani G, Diaz LA, Papadopoulos N, Vogelstein B, Kinzler KW, et al. Integrated genomic analyses identify ARID1A and ARID1B alterations in the childhood cancer neuroblastoma. Nat Genet. 2013;45:12–7.
39. Cheung N-KV, Zhang J, Lu C, Parker M, Bahrami A, Tickoo SK, Heguy A, Pappo AS, Federico S, Dalton J, Cheung IY, Ding L, et al. Association of age at diagnosis and genetic mutations in patients with neuroblastoma. JAMA. 2012;307:1062–71.
40. Bresler SC, Weiser DA, Huwe PJ, Park JH, Krytska K, Ryles H, Laudenslager M, Rappaport EF, Wood AC, McGrady PW, Hogarty MD, London WB, et al. ALK mutations confer differential oncogenic activation and sensitivity to ALK inhibition therapy in neuroblastoma. Cancer Cell. 2014;26:682–94.
41. De Brouwer S, De Preter K, Kumps C, Zabrocki P, Porcu M, Westerhout EM, Lakeman A, Vandesompele J, Hoebeeck J, Van Maerken T, De Paepe A, Laureys G, et al. Meta-analysis of neuroblastomas reveals a skewed ALK mutation spectrum in tumors with MYCN amplification. Clin Cancer Res. 2010;16:4353–62.
42. Wood AC, Krytska K, Ryles HT, Infarinato NR, Sano R, Hansel TD, Hart LS, King FJ, Smith TR, Ainscow E, Grandinetti KB, Tuntland T, et al. Dual ALK and CDK4/6 Inhibition Demonstrates Synergy against Neuroblastoma. Clin Cancer Res. 2017;23:2856–68.
43. Infarinato NR, Park JH, Krytska K, Ryles HT, Sano R, Szigety KM, Li Y, Zou HY, Lee NV, Smeal T, Lemmon MA, Mossé YP. The ALK/ROS1 inhibitor PF-06463922 overcomes primary resistance to crizotinib in ALK-driven neuroblastoma. Cancer Discov. 2016;6:96–107.
44. Valentijn LJ, Koster J, Zwijnenburg DA, Hasselt NE, van Sluis P, Volckmann R, van Noesel MM, George RE, Tytgat GAM, Molenaar JJ, Versteeg R. TERT rearrangements are frequent in neuroblastoma and identify aggressive tumors. Nat Genet. 2015;47:1411–4.
45. Peifer M, Hertwig F, Roels F, Dreidax D, Gartlgruber M, Menon R, Krämer A, Roncaioli JL, Sand F, Heuckmann JM, Ikram F, Schmidt R, et al. Telomerase activation by genomic rearrangements in high-risk neuroblastoma. Nature. 2015;526:700–4.
46. Hertwig F, Peifer M, Fischer M. Telomere maintenance is pivotal for high-risk neuroblastoma. Cell Cycle. 2016;15:311–2.
47. Alexandrov LB, Nik-Zainal S, Wedge DC, Aparicio SAJR, Behjati S, Biankin AV, Bignell GR, Bolli N, Borg A, Børresen-Dale A-L, Boyault S, Burkhardt B, et al. Signatures of mutational processes in human cancer. Nature. 2013;500:415–21.
48. Gröbner SN, Worst BC, Weischenfeldt J, Buchhalter I, Kleinheinz K, Rudneva VA, Johann PD, Balasubramanian GP, Segura-Wang M, Brabetz S, Bender S, Hutter B, et al. The landscape of genomic alterations across childhood cancers. Nature. 2018;555:321–7.
49. Oberthuer A, Hero B, Berthold F, Juraeva D, Faldum A, Kahlert Y, Asgharzadeh S, Seeger R, Scaruffi P, Tonini GP, Janoueix-Lerosey I, Delattre O, et al. Prognostic impact of gene expression-based classification for neuroblastoma. J Clin Oncol. 2010;28:3506–15.
50. Vermeulen J, De Preter K, Naranjo A, Vercruysse L, Van Roy N, Hellemans J, Swerts K, Bravo S, Scaruffi P, Tonini GP, De Bernardi B, Noguera R, et al. Predicting outcomes for children

with neuroblastoma using a multigene-expression signature: a retrospective SIOPEN/COG/GPOH study. Lancet Oncol. 2009;10:663–71.
51. Garcia I, Mayol G, Ríos J, Domenech G, Cheung N-KV, Oberthuer A, Fischer M, Maris JM, Brodeur GM, Hero B, Rodríguez E, Suñol M, et al. A three-gene expression signature model for risk stratification of patients with neuroblastoma. Clin Cancer Res. 2012;18:2012–23.
52. Asgharzadeh S, Pique-Regi R, Sposto R, Wang H, Yang Y, Shimada H, Matthay K, Buckley J, Ortega A, Seeger RC. Prognostic significance of gene expression profiles of metastatic neuroblastomas lacking MYCN gene amplification. J Natl Cancer Inst. 2006;98:1193–203.
53. Valentijn LJ, Koster J, Haneveld F, Aissa RA, van Sluis P, Broekmans MEC, Molenaar JJ, van Nes J, Versteeg R. Functional MYCN signature predicts outcome of neuroblastoma irrespective of MYCN amplification. Proc Natl Acad Sci U S A. 2012;109:19190–5.
54. Asgharzadeh S, Salo JA, Ji L, Oberthuer A, Fischer M, Berthold F, Hadjidaniel M, Liu CW-Y, Metelitsa LS, Pique-Regi R, Wakamatsu P, Villablanca JG, et al. Clinical significance of tumor-associated inflammatory cells in metastatic neuroblastoma. J Clin Oncol. 2012;30:3525–32.
55. Mestdagh P, Fredlund E, Pattyn F, Rihani A, Van Maerken T, Vermeulen J, Kumps C, Menten B, De Preter K, Schramm A, Schulte J, Noguera R, et al. An integrative genomics screen uncovers ncRNA T-UCR functions in neuroblastoma tumours. Oncogene. 2010;29:3583–92.
56. Schulte JH, Schowe B, Mestdagh P, Kaderali L, Kalaghatgi P, Schlierf S, Vermeulen J, Brockmeyer B, Pajtler K, Thor T, de Preter K, Speleman F, et al. Accurate prediction of neuroblastoma outcome based on miRNA expression profiles. Int J Cancer. 2010;127:2374–85.
57. De Preter K, Mestdagh P, Vermeulen J, Zeka F, Naranjo A, Bray I, Castel V, Chen C, Drozynska E, Eggert A, Hogarty MD, Izycka-Swieszewska E, et al. miRNA expression profiling enables risk stratification in archived and fresh neuroblastoma tumor samples. Clin Cancer Res. 2011;17:7684–92.
58. Decock A, Ongenaert M, Hoebeeck J, De Preter K, Van Peer G, Van Criekinge W, Ladenstein R, Schulte JH, Noguera R, Stallings RL, Van Damme A, Laureys G, et al. Genome-wide promoter methylation analysis in neuroblastoma identifies prognostic methylation biomarkers. Genome Biol. 2012;13:R95.
59. Berbegall AP, Bogen D, Pötschger U, Beiske K, Bown N, Combaret V, Defferrari R, Jeison M, Mazzocco K, Varesio L, Vicha A, Ash S, et al. Heterogeneous MYCN amplification in neuroblastoma: a SIOP Europe Neuroblastoma Study. Br J Cancer. 2018;118:1502.
60. Abbasi MR, Rifatbegovic F, Brunner C, Mann G, Ziegler A, Pötschger U, Crazzolara R, Ussowicz M, Benesch M, Ebetsberger-Dachs G, Chan GCF, Jones N, et al. Impact of disseminated neuroblastoma cells on the identification of the relapse-seeding clone. Clin Cancer Res. 2017;23:4224–32.
61. Karlsson J, Valind A, Holmquist Mengelbier L, Bredin S, Cornmark L, Jansson C, Wali A, Staaf J, Viklund B, Øra I, Börjesson A, Backman T, et al. Four evolutionary trajectories underlie genetic intratumoral variation in childhood cancer. Nat Genet. 2018;50:944–50.
62. Bellini A, Bernard V, Leroy Q, Rio Frio T, Pierron G, Combaret V, Lapouble E, Clement N, Rubie H, Thebaud E, Chastagner P, Defachelles A, et al. Deep sequencing reveals occurrence of subclonal ALK mutations in neuroblastoma at diagnosis. Clin Cancer Res. 2015;21:4913–21.
63. Schleiermacher G, Javanmardi N, Bernard V, Leroy Q, Cappo J, Rio Frio T, Pierron G, Lapouble E, Combaret V, Speleman F, de Wilde B, Djos A, et al. Emergence of new ALK mutations at relapse of neuroblastoma. J Clin Oncol. 2014;32:2727–34.
64. Schramm A, Köster J, Assenov Y, Althoff K, Peifer M, Mahlow E, Odersky A, Beisser D, Ernst C, Henssen AG, Stephan H, Schröder C, et al. Mutational dynamics between primary and relapse neuroblastomas. Nat Genet. 2015;47:872–7.
65. Eleveld TF, Oldridge DA, Bernard V, Koster J, Daage LC, Diskin SJ, Schild L, Bentahar NB, Bellini A, Chicard M, Lapouble E, Combaret V, et al. Relapsed neuroblastomas show frequent RAS-MAPK pathway mutations. Nat Genet. 2015;47:864–71.
66. Combaret V, Audoynaud C, Iacono I, Favrot M-C, Schell M, Bergeron C, Puisieux A. Circulating MYCN DNA as a tumor-specific marker in neuroblastoma patients. Cancer Res. 2002;62:3646–8.

67. Chicard M, Boyault S, Colmet Daage L, Richer W, Gentien D, Pierron G, Lapouble E, Bellini A, Clement N, Iacono I, Bréjon S, Carrere M, et al. Genomic copy number profiling using circulating free tumor DNA highlights heterogeneity in neuroblastoma. Clin Cancer Res. 2016;22:5564–73.
68. Combaret V, Bréjon S, Iacono I, Schleiermacher G, Pierron G, Ribeiro A, Bergeron C, Marabelle A, Puisieux A. Determination of 17q gain in patients with neuroblastoma by analysis of circulating DNA. Pediatr Blood Cancer. 2011;56:757–61.
69. Van Roy N, Van Der Linden M, Menten B, Dheedene A, Vandeputte C, Van Dorpe J, Laureys G, Renard M, Sante T, Lammens T, De Wilde B, Speleman F, et al. Shallow whole genome sequencing on circulating cell-free DNA allows reliable noninvasive copy-number profiling in neuroblastoma patients. Clin Cancer Res. 2017;23:6305–14.
70. Chicard M, Colmet Daage L, Clement N, Danzon A, Bohec M, Bernard V, Baulande S, Bellini A, Deveau P, Pierron G, Lapouble E, Janoueix-Lerosey I, et al. Whole exome sequencing of cell-free DNA reveals temporo-spatial heterogeneity and identifies treatment-resistant clones in neuroblastoma. Clin Cancer Res. 2018;24:939.

Neuroblastoma Pathogenesis

3

Isabelle Janoueix-Lerosey

3.1 Neuroblastoma, a Disease of the Neural Crest

The neural crest is a transient cell type that arises from the neural tube once this tube is closed during development. Through an epithelial-to-mesenchymal transition, neural crest cells (NCCs) are able to delaminate and migrate from their initial location to numerous and distant sites throughout the embryo ([1]; for a review see [2]). NCCs can differentiate into an incredibly diverse range of cell types that contribute to various anatomical structures, including neurons and glia of the peripheral nervous system, pigment cells of the skin, and cartilage and bone cells of the craniofacial skeleton. According to their position along the axial level, four main functional types of NCCs may be distinguished: cranial, cardiac, trunk as well as vagal and sacral [1]. NCCs from the trunk part migrate ventrolaterally toward the dorsal aorta. Cells remaining at this location differentiate into sympathetic progenitor cells in response to extrinsic and intrinsic factors. Adrenal chromaffin progenitors have been described to migrate further ventrally. These progenitor cells will generate the cells of the sympathetic ganglia and the adrenal gland, from where neuroblastoma tumors develop. However, a very recent study revised the current hypothesis regarding the origin of adrenal chromaffin cells describing that they are rather generated from Schwann cell precursors [3]. Therefore, two types of different progenitors may be proposed as the cells of origin of neuroblastoma.

In addition of being a disease of cells derived from the neural crest, neuroblastoma has been shown to be associated with other neural crest derivatives pathologies, named neurocristopathies. In these diseases, an abnormally high frequency of neuroblastic tumors (including ganglioneuroma, ganglioneuroblastoma, and

I. Janoueix-Lerosey (✉)
Institut Curie, SIREDO Oncology Center (Care, Innovation and research for children and AYA with cancer), Inserm U830, PSL Research University, Paris, France
e-mail: janoueix@curie.fr

S. Sarnacki, L. Pio (eds.), *Neuroblastoma*,
https://doi.org/10.1007/978-3-030-18396-7_3

neuroblastoma) is observed compared to the general population. This is the case for the Hirschsprung disease (HSCR, aganglionosis of the colon), the type 1 neurofibromatosis, a well-known condition characterized by a predisposition to a large spectrum of tumors including neuroblastomas and the Congenital Central Hypoventilation Syndrome (CCHS), also called Ondine's curse [4, 5]. Ondine's curse is a disease characterized by respiratory arrest during sleep and impaired or absent response to hypercapnia [6].

Bone morphogenic factors (BMPs) are the major extrinsic factors secreted from the dorsal aorta that are essential for the generation of the sympathoadrenal lineage [7]. Specification of cells toward sympathetic neurons relies on extremely precise transcriptional programs involving a network of cross-regulatory key transcription factors, including ASCL1, PHOX2B, HAND2, and GATA3 among others [8]. The sequential onset of expression starts with Phox2b and Ascl1, followed by Hand2, Phox2a, Gata2/3, and finally the specific enzymes for catecholamine biosynthesis Th (tyrosine hydroxylase) and Dbh (dopamine-β-hydroxylase) and several generic neuronal markers such as SCG10 and NF160. These factors which are crucial for the initial neuron specification and differentiation are also involved in the control of proliferation, survival, and maintenance of differentiated functions of sympathetic neurons [8].

3.2 Key Genes Involved in Neuroblastoma Pathogenesis

3.2.1 PHOX2B, a Transcription Factor Involved in Syndromic and Familial Neuroblastoma Cases

The *PHOX2B* gene has been identified as the causal gene of the Ondine's curse in 2003 [9]. The *PHOX2B* gene encodes a homeobox transcription factor containing a homeodomain domain and two polyalanine repeat domains of 9 and 20 residues, respectively (Fig. 3.1). PHOX2B is a master regulator of the development of the autonomic nervous system composed of the sympathetic and parasympathetic ganglia [14]. Germline mutations observed in patients affected with Ondine's curse are heterozygous and correspond to expansions of 5–13 alanines in the second polyalanine repeat domain [9]. Following the identification of *PHOX2B* mutations in these CCHS syndromic forms, mutations in the same gene were reported in familial forms of neuroblastoma [15–18]. In these patients, germline *PHOX2B* mutations are also heterozygous but are either missense mutations in the homeodomain or missense or frameshift mutations located between the homeodomain and the first polyalanine repeat domain. A large series investigating genotype/phenotype correlations between the occurrence of CCHS with or without Hirschsprung's disease and with or without neuroblastic tumors reported that Ondine's patients with PHOX2B polyalanine expansions rarely developed ganglioneuroma tumors, whereas malignant tumors were observed more frequently in patients with *PHOX2B* missense or frameshift mutations [19].

The functional impact of the various PHOX2B mutations has been investigated in several model systems. A first study showed that the various mutant forms are

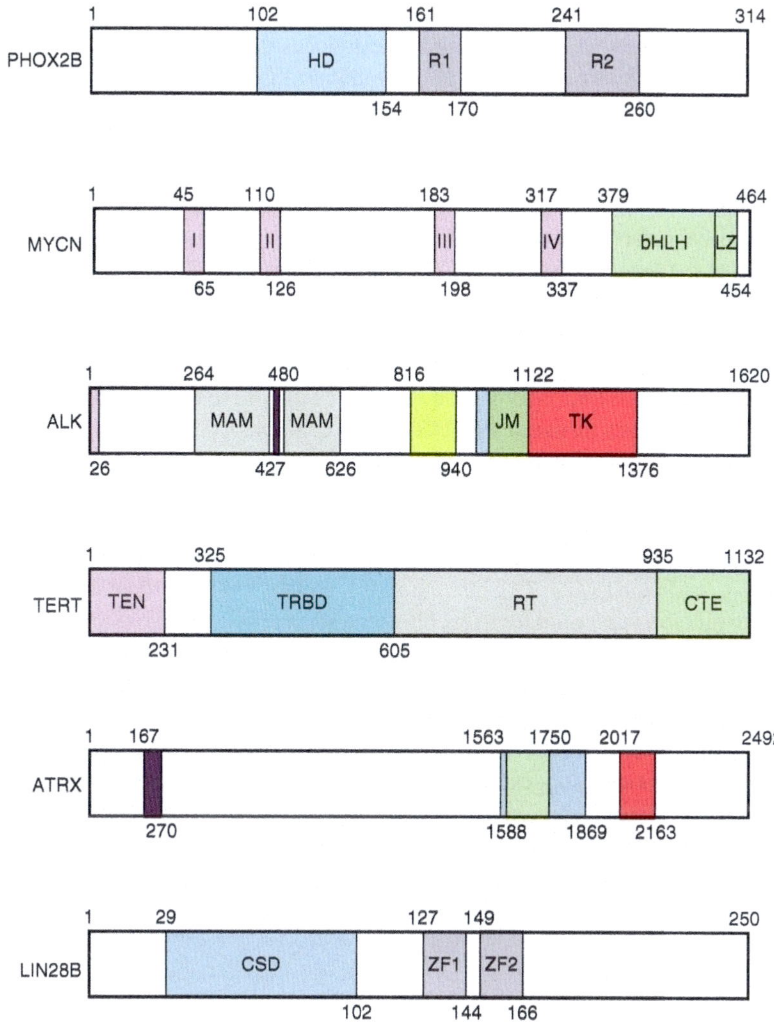

Fig. 3.1 Functional domains of key proteins involved in neuroblastoma pathogenesis. The PHOX2B transcription factor contains a homeodomain (HD) and two repeat domains of 9 and 20 alanines (respectively R1 and R2). In MYCN, the four MYC boxes (I, II, III, IV) [10, 11] are depicted (pink), and the basic helix-loop-helix and leucine zipper domains are indicated. The ALK receptor contains a signal peptide (pink) at its N-terminus. Its extracellular domain includes two MAM (meprin/A5/protein tyrosine phosphatase Mu) domains flanking an LDLa (low-density lipoprotein class A) domain (violet—AA 453–471) and a G-rich region (yellow). The transmembrane domain of the ALK receptor is shown in blue (AA 1030–1058) together with the juxtamembrane (JM, AA 1058–1122) and tyrosine kinase domain (TK) [12]. TERT is composed of a telomerase "essential" N-terminal (TEN) domain, an RNA-binding domain (TRBD), a Reverse Transcriptase (RT) domain, and a C-Terminal extension (CTE). The functional domains of ATRX comprise an ADD (ATRX, DNMT3, DNMT3L) domain (violet) sharing homology with de novo methyltransferases, a SNF2 family N-terminal domain highlighted in blue that includes a DEAD-like helicase superfamily domain shown in green and a helicase C-terminal domain (pink). The LIN28B protein contains several RNA-binding regions, including a cold-shock domain (CSD) and two CCHC Zn finger domains (ZF1 and ZF2) [13]

correctly localized in the nucleus [20]. In vitro, the overexpression of wild-type (WT) PHOX2B decreases proliferation and induces differentiation of sympathetic neuroblasts of the chick cultured at E7, but mutant forms of PHOX2B do not show these properties [21]. However, a concomitant expression of mutated PHOX2B and decreased level of WT PHOX2B results in an increased proliferation, demonstrating that PHOX2B mutations are gain-of-function mutations. Frameshift nonpolyalanine repeat expansion mutations (NPARM) of PHOX2B observed in neuroblastoma cell lines have been further investigated using knock-in (KI) mouse lines bearing the mutation at the heterozygous level [22] (Table 3.1). The two obtained mouse lines showed early postnatal lethality due to breathing disorders and also presented with aganglionosis of the colon, therefore recapitulating the clinical features of CCHS and Hirschsprung disease. The NPARM mutations resulted in reduced sympathetic ganglia, and no overt tumor formation was detected in these mice. Detailed study of the WT and mutated forms of PHOX2B by a combination of various approaches highlighted an impaired regulation of Phox2b on its own transcription as well as a decreased regulation of *Sox10* expression. This imbalance results in an excess and loss of progenitors developing toward the glial and neuron lineages, respectively. These mouse lines therefore do not provide a preclinical model of neuroblastoma linked to germline NPARM *Phox2b* mutations, and the exact mechanism explaining how such mutations account for neuroblastoma susceptibility still remains unknown. Zebrafish has also been used as a model to explore the functional consequences of two neuroblastoma-associated PHOX2B NPARM [30]. Overexpression of the mutant forms impaired terminal differentiation of sympathetic neuron progenitors as revealed by decreased Th and Dbh expression. Altogether, the data obtained in mouse and fish models suggest that Phox2b-mutant forms are responsible for a differentiation blockage that may in turn provide a source of cells vulnerable to additional genetic events.

The role of PHOX2B in neuroblastoma pathogenesis seems mostly linked to its germline mutations since somatic *PHOX2B* mutations occurring in sporadic tumors are extremely rare [15, 17, 31].

3.2.2 MYCN, a Transcription Factor Associated with High-Risk Neuroblastoma

MYCN is the most frequent gene targeted by amplifications in neuroblastoma. First described in 1984, *MYCN* amplification is observed in primary tumors and cell lines, mainly as double minute chromosomes or hsr, and is associated with high level of *MYCN* transcript expression [32, 33]. The *MYCN* gene encodes a transcription factor of the basic-helix-loop-helix-zipper class (Fig. 3.1) that is a master regulator of transcription. *MYCN* exhibits a very restricted expression pattern and is critical in the development of the central and peripheral nervous systems. Disruption of the *MYCN* gene in mouse embryos is lethal between 10.5 and 12.5 days of gestation due to cardiac development abnormalities and reduction of the cranial and spinal ganglia [34]. The conditional disruption of *MYCN* in neural progenitor cells

Table 3.1 Understanding neuroblastoma pathogenesis using GEMMs

a

Model	Reference	Type	Promoter	Gene	Tumor development	Phenotype/features
PHOX2B-NPARM	Nagashimada et al. [22]	Knock-in	Endogenous	Mouse *Phox2b* with NPARM mutations	No	Lethality at birth
						Breathing abnormalities
						Colon aganglionosis
TH-MYCN	Weiss et al. [23]	Transgenic	Rat TH	Human *MYCN*	Neuroblastoma	Long latency, low penetrance,
						Other genetic alterations
						No adrenal tumors
LSL-MYCN;Dbh-iCre	Althoff et al. [24]	Conditional transgenic	CAG	Human *MYCN*	Neuroblastoma	Long latency, low penetrance
						Other genetic alterations
						Adrenal and symp. tumors
TH-ALK^{F1174L}	Berry et al. [25]	Transgenic	Rat TH	Human *ALK*^{F1174L}	No	
ALK^{F1174L}; DBHiCre ALK^{F1174L}; TH-IRES-Cre	Heukamp et al. [26]	Conditional transgenic	Actin	Human *ALK*^{F1174L}	Neuroblastoma	Long latency, Low penetrance
						Other genetic alterations
KI *Alk*^{R1279Q}/KI *Alk*^{F1178L}	Cazes et al. [27]	Knock-in	Endogenous	Mouse *Alk* with R1279Q or F1178L mutation	No	Prolonged neurogenesis in SNS ganglia
						High neonatal lethality of *Alk*^{F1178L} homozygotes
LSL-Lin28b; Dbh-iCre	Molenaar et al. [28]	Conditional transgenic	CAG	Mouse *Lin28b*	Neuroblastoma	Short latency, intermediate penetrance
						Adrenal and symp. tumors

(continued)

Table 3.1 (continued)

b

Breedings of various lines	Reference	Tumor development	Phenotype
TH-ALK^{F1174L} × TH-MYCN	Berry et al. [25]	Neuroblastoma	Short latency, full penetrance
			No other alterations
ALK^{F1174L}; DBHiCre × TH-MYCN	Heukamp et al. [26]	Neuroblastoma	Short latency, full penetrance
			Few other alterations
KI *Alk*^{R1279Q}/KI *Alk*^{F1178L} × TH-MYCN	Cazes et al. [27]	Neuroblastoma	Short latency, full penetrance
			No other alterations
			F1178L>R1279Q
TH-MYCN × casp8 KO	Teitz et al. [29]	Neuroblastoma	Short latency, full penetrance
			Increased bone marrow metastasis

(**A**) Several genetically engineered mouse models (GEMMs) have been generated with the aim to explore the role of important genes in neuroblastoma oncogenesis and to obtain relevant preclinical models of the disease. *CAG* chicken β-actin gene, *Dbh* dopamine β-hydroxylase, *KI* knock-in, *KO* knockout, *NPARM* nonpolyalanine repeat expansion mutations, *TH* tyrosine hydroxylase

(**B**) Some of these mouse lines have been bred to further decipher the role of alterations occurring concomitantly in patient tumors such as *MYCN* amplification or *ALK* mutations or to obtain neuroblastoma with metastasis demonstrates its crucial role during neurogenesis with proliferation and differentiation defects of progenitor cells [35].

Several in vitro and in vivo models have sought to model *MYCN* amplification through overexpression in mammalian cells.

Overexpression of MYCN has been studied in one model of murine neural crest progenitor cells called JoMa-1 cells, generated by immortalization of neural crest cells by a tamoxifen-inducible Myc-ER^T [36, 37]. Expression of MYCN allowed cells to grow independently of Myc-ER^T in vitro, and injection of these cells in mice resulted in formation of neuroblastoma-like tumors [38]. More recently, MYCN overexpression was investigated in neural crest cells isolated from mouse embryonic day 9.5 trunk neural tube explants [39], derived from wild-type or p53$^{+/-}$ mice. Cells were injected subcutaneously into nude or C57Bl/6 mice, and tumor development was assessed in the mice. Overexpression of *MYCN* in WT neural crest led to the development of tumors exhibiting features of neuroblastoma in around one third of the mice. The obtained tumors presented with copy-number aberrations syntenic to those observed in human tumors with *MYCN* amplification, including 17q gain and 1p loss. Yet, when using p53$^{+/-}$ neural crest cells, primitive neuroectodermal tumors with various differentiations were observed, among which osteosarcoma. Macroscopic metastases were observed in a subset of these mice in lymph nodes, lung, and liver and frequently showed a mixed morphology similarly to the primary tumors.

The first mouse line characterized by MYCN overexpression (referred to as TH-MYCN) was engineered by Weiss and colleagues who generated transgenic mice exhibiting the human *MYCN* gene under the control of the rat Tyrosine Hydroxylase promoter in order to drive *MYCN* expression in neural crest cells [23] (Table 3.1). Tumors resembling human neuroblastoma in terms of histology, location, and acquisition of genetic abnormalities in regions syntenic to those seen in patients with *MYCN*-amplified tumors indeed developed in this mouse line. Although an incomplete penetrance of tumor development was observed in this model, this first study demonstrated that *MYCN* is an oncogenic driver in neuroblastoma. However, the occurrence of other chromosomal aberrations in the obtained tumors suggested that MYCN alone is not sufficient to drive transformation. This model has been and is still largely used by the scientific community to explore many aspects of neuroblastoma biology and investigate novel therapies. However, two main limitations of these models may be highlighted, with respect to the characteristics of the human disease: first, the absence of metastasis in the mice in which only locally aggressive tumors are observed and also the absence of tumors occurring in the adrenal medulla, a very frequent localization in neuroblastoma patients (47%) [40, 41]. Of note, the initial study reported the crucial role of the genetic background in tumor development, suggesting that intrinsic factors in various mouse strains may act as modifiers of MYCN-induced oncogenesis [23]. More recently, a different model has been set up by the team of J. Schulte [24] (Table 3.1). This model allows expression of a MYCN-IRES-Luciferase cassette downstream of the chicken β-actin gene (CAG) promoter in Dbh-expressing cells (LSL-MYCN;Dbh-iCre). This resulted in the development of tumors from the adrenals as well as from the superior cervical or celiac ganglia that may be detected by bioluminescent imaging. Chromosomal aberrations in this model were syntenic to those observed in human neuroblastomas, as it has been shown for the TH-MYCN model.

Zebrafish has also been used to model neuroblastoma. Indeed, the peripheral sympathetic nervous system of this fish includes a superior cervical ganglia and an interrenal gland, analogous to the superior cervical ganglia and adrenal medulla of mammals, respectively [42]. *MYCN* overexpression in the sympathetic nervous system of this animal model was obtained using a Dbh promoter fragment [43]. Tumors exhibiting neuroblastoma features developed in the interrenal gland of the transgenic Dbh-MYCN line but with a low penetrance below 20%. One interesting property of the Zebrafish model is linked to the possibility of high-throughput screenings of chemical compounds.

There is no doubt on the oncogenic properties of MYCN in neuroblastoma, which could therefore serve as an interesting therapeutic target. As a proof of principle, Burkhart and colleagues demonstrated that MYCN antisense oligonucleotides impaired tumorigenesis in the murine TH-MYCN model [44]. Unfortunately, there are currently no drugs that could target MYC or MYCN proteins directly. Indeed, these proteins can adopt many conformations and therefore do not present with druggable pockets. One interesting alternative may be to act indirectly on the stability of these proteins. In the case of MYCN, this can be achieved by using different types of molecules involved in the control of MYCN stability. It has been shown indeed that the stability of MYC proteins (comprising MYC, MYCN, and MYCL) is regulated by phosphorylation within conserved sequence motifs called MYC boxes (Fig. 3.1) and further ubiquitinylation and proteolysis. MYCN has been shown to be first phosphorylated by the CDK1/Cyclin B complex on Ser62 and then phosphorylated on Thr58 by GSK3β [45]. Dephosphorylation of the Ser62 by the PP2A phosphatase then allows MYCN ubiquitination by the E3 ubiquitin ligase SCF^{FBxW7} [46, 47] resulting in its degradation. Consistently with these observations, PI3K inhibition, that results in GSK3β activation, has been shown to destabilize MYCN protein and block tumor progression in the TH-MYCN model [48].

MYCN stability is also controlled by the cell-cycle-regulated serine/threonine kinase Aurora-A. Aurora kinases (A, B, and C) are key regulators of chromosomal segregation and cytokinesis during mammalian cell division [49]. Several small-molecule inhibitors of Aurora kinases have been discovered as anticancer drugs and may be of interest to treat neuroblastoma with *MYCN* amplification. Indeed, in 2009, *AURKA* was identified as a gene that is required for the growth of *MYCN*-amplified neuroblastoma cells but largely dispensable for cells lacking *MYCN* amplification [50]. The mechanism underlying this effect relies on Aurora-A forming a complex with MYCN, resulting in MYCN being protected from proteasomal degradation during mitosis. This effect of Aurora-A on MYCN stability does not depend on the catalytic serine/threonine kinase activity of Aurora-A.

The pan Aurora inhibitor CCT137690 is able to inhibit cell proliferation of *MYCN*-amplified neuroblastoma cell lines in vitro and decreases MYCN protein levels [51]. The efficacy of this compound was also demonstrated in the TH-MYCN model. MLN8237 (Alisertib) is a small-molecule inhibitor specific of Aurora-A, that has been tested in the Pediatric Preclinical Testing Program (PPTP) in vivo panel [52]. Antitumor effects of this inhibitor were reported in three of seven neuroblastoma xenograft models. A phase I trial in children with refractory/recurrent solid tumors was performed to define the maximum-tolerated dose, toxicities, and pharmacokinetic properties of MLN8237 [53]. In this study, two patients with neuroblastoma had prolonged stable disease. MLN8054 is another selective small-molecule Aurora-A kinase inhibitor [54]. Both MLN8054 and MLN8237 inhibitors have been shown to disrupt the Aurora-A/MYCN complex and promote degradation of MYCN mediated by the SCF^{FbxW7} ubiquitin ligase [55]. This study demonstrated that disruption of the Aurora-A/MYCN complex inhibits MYCN-dependent transcription and induces tumor regression and prolonged survival in the TH-MYCN mouse neuroblastoma model. Another compound, CD532 is an ATP-mimetic ligand that binds Aurora-A and maintains the protein in its inactive conformation. It blocks both its kinase-dependent and -independent functions [56]. CD532 is efficient at low nanomolar concentrations to induce the proteolytic degradation of MYCN. However, this compound has not been evaluated in in vivo models of neuroblastoma. Recently, a direct interaction has been identified between the catalytic domain of Aurora-A and a site flanking Myc Box I (residues 61–89) that also binds SCF^{FbxW7} [57]. Both MLN8237 (Alisertib) and CD132 compounds induce a conformation of Aurora-A that is not compatible with MYCN binding, allowing binding of MYCN with SCF^{FbxW7} that triggers MYCN Lys48-linked polyubiquitination, leading to proteasomal degradation.

Additional in vitro and in vivo studies have shown that Aurora-A kinase inhibitors result in enhanced cytotoxicity when used in combination with chemotherapy [58]. A phase I study of alisertib with irinotecan and temozolomide in patients with advanced neuroblastoma has recently reported promising response and progression-free survival rates [59]. A phase II trial of this combination (ClinicalTrials.gov Identifier: NCT01601535) is ongoing. The data obtained with Aurora-A inhibitors in neuroblastoma preclinical models as well as those from early clinical trials suggest that these compounds may be of benefit for neuroblastoma patients. It remains however to determine whether these compounds do not induce significant damages to normal tissues through their general function in the control of the mitotic spindle.

In addition to the compounds acting on MYCN stability through the control of its posttranslational modifications, the BET (Bromodomain and extraterminal) inhibitor JQ1 has been identified as a promising candidate for clinical development for neuroblastoma patients with *MYCN* amplification [60]. Open chromatin and transcriptional activation are associated with acetylation of lysine residues on histone tails [61]. Acetylated lysines are mostly recognized by bromodomains that are present in many proteins including the BET family composed of BRD2, BRD3, BRD4, and BRDT. JQ1 is a thienotriazolo-1,4-diazepine that is able to displace BET bromodomains from chromatin by competitive binding to the acetyl lysine recognition pocket. BET inhibition has been identified as a therapeutic strategy in several types of adult cancers including numerous hematologic malignancies. A high-throughput screening of more than 650 cancer cell lines revealed neuroblastoma as among the most JQ1-sensitive cell lines and *MYCN* amplification as the most predictive marker of sensitivity [60]. Further analysis demonstrated that JQ1 induced cell-cycle arrest and apoptosis in *MYCN*-amplified neuroblastoma cell lines. BET inhibition was associated with downregulation of the MYCN transcriptional program accompanied by suppression of *MYCN* transcription. JQ1 treatment impaired tumor growth in several types of neuroblastoma preclinical models. Treatment of a cell line established from a murine neuroblastoma tumor derived from the LSL-MYCN;Dbh-iCre mouse neuroblastoma model with JQ1 demonstrated oncogene addiction to MYCN [24]. It should be noted, however, that JQ1 acts not only at the *MYCN* enhancer and not only on cells with *MYCN* amplification [62, 63].

The *MYCN* locus also encodes an antisense transcript called *MYCNOS* (MYCN Opposite strand) and encoding the N-CYM protein [64]. *MYCNOS* is always coexpressed with *MYCN*. The N-CYM protein is able to inhibit GSK3β involved in the posttranslational control of MYCN stability, resulting in stabilization of the MYCN protein [65]. In addition, it has been showed that treatment with BET inhibitors reduced *NCYM* expression, suggesting that such inhibitors are relevant for therapy of neuroblastoma exhibiting amplification of both *MYCN* and *NCYM* [66].

3.2.3 Implication of the ALK Tyrosine Kinase Receptor in Sporadic, Familial, and Syndromic Cases of Neuroblastoma

The *ALK* (Anaplastic Lymphoma Kinase) gene was identified as a major neuroblastoma gene in 2008, following the discovery of germline and somatic activating mutations in a subset of familial and sporadic cases, respectively [67–70]. This gene encodes a tyrosine kinase receptor (Fig. 3.1) belonging to the insulin receptor subfamily, the *LTK* and *ROS* genes being its closest homologs [12]. Importantly, mutated ALK rapidly appeared as a tractable therapeutic target for precision medicine in neuroblastoma patients with ALK-mutated tumors since inhibition of the mutant receptors led to growth inhibition. Importantly, further analysis by next-generation sequencing technologies revealed the presence of subclonal ALK mutations in a number of cases at diagnosis and relapse [71, 72].

The *ALK* gene is extremely conserved throughout evolution. ALK homologs are present in Drosophila, zebrafish, and chick among other species. In mammals, ALK expression is mostly restricted to the developing central and peripheral nervous system, including thalamic nuclei, several motor nuclei of the brainstem, and sympathetic and enteric ganglia (for a review, [73]). *Alk* knockout mice are viable and do not display any strong phenotype [74–77]. Yet few abnormalities have been reported, including reduced hippocampal neurogenesis, subtle behavioral defects, and defects in the testis function in males. However, no precise evaluation of the sympathetic ganglia and adrenal medulla has been performed in these loss-of-function models. The absence of a strong phenotype in *Alk* and *Alk*/*Ltk* knockout mice may be explained by compensatory mechanisms involving the third member of the Alk subfamily, that is, Ros or other members of the insulin receptor subfamily.

In mammals, the ALK receptor has been considered as an orphan receptor for quite a long time, and the identification of its ligand(s) has been for long a matter of debate. Midkine (MK) and pleiotrophin (PTN), two heparin-binding growth factors, have been described as activating ligands for the ALK receptor [78, 79]. However, other groups did not confirm ALK activation upon PTN treatment in neuroblastoma cells or ALK-transfected cells [80–82]. More recently, heparin (but not MK and PTN) was described as an ALK ligand able to induce its dimerization, autophosphorylation, and subsequent downstream signaling [83]. Also, FAM150A and FAM150B, two highly basic proteins, have been described as ALK and LTK ligands [84, 85]. Interestingly, FAM150B is able to transform ALK-expressing NIH3T3 cells and allows the growth of Ba/F3 cells expressing ALK in the absence of IL-3 [85].

Evidences demonstrating a physiological function of the normal Alk receptor in sympathetic neurogenesis have been obtained using the chick embryo as a model. Indeed, in vitro and in vivo knockdown of Alk in chick sympathetic neuroblasts led to a decreased proliferation [86]. The same study also documented high expression of Mk in chick sympathetic ganglia and functional effect of Mk knockdown.

The *ALK* gene has been initially identified through the characterization of a t(2;5) translocation in anaplastic large-cell non-Hodgkin's lymphoma leading to a NPM–ALK fusion protein [87]. Many translocations involving the *ALK* gene and various partners have been extensively characterized in a variety of children and adult cancers, leading to fusion proteins bearing a constitutive activation of the ALK tyrosine kinase domain [12]. In neuroblastoma, ALK activation results from point mutations in the full-length ALK receptor. Figure 3.1 shows the structure of the ALK receptor: in sporadic cases, the great majority of the mutations are observed in the kinase domain with three main hotspots of mutations at positions 1174, 1245, and 1275 [88]. Several ALK inhibitors, including NVP-TAE684 [89] and crizotinib [90], characterized through their effect on ALK fusion proteins were already described when ALK mutations were reported in neuroblastoma in 2008. These small molecules are competitive inhibitors of the ATP binding within the kinase domain. The availability of these molecules allowed the setup of a first phase I/II clinical trial of crizotinib in neuroblastoma patients at the relapse stage [91]. Although the ALK status was not systematically known in this first trial, the results showed that a number of neuroblastoma patients may benefit from ALK-targeted therapies but also informed that inhibition of full-length ALK was more difficult to achieve compared to ALK fusion proteins.

Of note, the spectrum of germline *ALK* mutations in familial cases is different from that of the somatic mutations in sporadic cases. Indeed, only mutations at position R1275, one of the three hotspots of somatic mutations, have been recurrently observed in familial cases [69, 70]. No germline mutations have been reported in familial forms of the disease at positions 1245 and 1174, the two other somatic hotspots. This suggested that germline mutations at these two positions may be embryonic lethal and potentially more aggressive than mutations at position R1275. This hypothesis revealed to be at least partially true with the discovery of ALK germline and de novo mutations at positions 1174 and 1245 in two unrelated patients affected by severe neurological disorders and congenital neuroblastoma [92].

Several lines of evidences also further documented the lower kinase activity and oncogenic potential of ALK R1275 mutants compared to ALK F1174 mutants, both in vitro [88] and in vivo (see below). Interestingly, the characterization of the genomes of more than 1000 children affected with cancer by next-generation sequencing redemonstrated the involvement of *ALK* germline mutations in neuroblastoma [93].

Several in vitro and in vivo models have been developed to investigate the role of ALK-activating mutations in neuroblastoma oncogenesis. Overexpression of WT or mutated ALK was studied in two different lines of murine neural crest progenitor cells, the MONC-1 cells, generated by immortalization of neural crest cells by v-Myc [36, 37] or the JoMa-1 cells. In vitro, ALK overexpression induced proliferation and survival even in the absence of Myc signaling [38, 94]. Whereas the parental MONC-1 cells were able to generate various tumor types including neuroblastoma after orthotopic injections, only highly malignant undifferentiated tumors developed from MONC-1 cells expressing ALK F1174L, suggesting that activated ALK altered their differentiation capacity [94]. In this study, undifferentiated tumors were also obtained upon injection of JoMa-1 cells expressing WT ALK, ALK F1174L, and ALK R1275Q, providing the first and still only demonstration that WT ALK can drive malignant transformation when expressed in neural crest cell progenitors. Using the same JoMa-1 model, Schulte and colleagues described a weak tumorigenic potential of ALK F1174L but obtained neuroblastoma-like tumors in vivo [38]. The differences observed between both studies may be linked to passage numbers of JoMa-1 cells or different ALK expression levels.

In the chick model, sympathetic neuron proliferation is increased upon overexpression of WT or activated Alk [62, 86]. In this model, Mk is expressed in early sympathetic ganglia, and its expression decreases during chick embryonic development. In vitro, sympathetic neuron proliferation depends on Mk levels, and the effect on proliferation of Mk knockdown may be rescued by ALK^{F1174L} but not by ALK^{WT}. A subsequent study investigating long-term effect of MYC, MYCN, and ALK^{F1174L} overexpression demonstrated that MYC and MYCN overexpression elicits increased proliferation but does not sustain neuroblast survival [62]. In contrast, activated ALK^{F1174L} leads to a transient proliferation increase followed by cell-cycle arrest and neuronal differentiation, resulting in increased survival. The combined expression of ALK^{F1174L} and MYC proteins results in both neuroblast proliferation and survival. Proliferating $MYCN/ALK^{F1174L}$ neuroblasts show a differentiated phenotype similar to ALK^{F1174L} neuroblasts but differ from them by the upregulation of *SKP2*, *CCNA2*, *E2F8*, and *DKC1* among other genes. Furthermore inhibition of *SKP2*, which targets the CDK inhibitor p27 for degradation, reduced proliferation of $MYCN/ALK^{F1174L}$ cells [62, 86]. Together, these in vitro data provide evidences of MYCN/ALK cooperation leading to neuroblast proliferation and survival, that may be critical steps in neuroblastoma development.

Different genetically engineered mouse models (GEMMs) have been set up by various teams to study the function of mutated ALK in vivo. The role of ALK mutations in development and oncogenesis has been addressed using KI mice bearing the two most frequent mutations observed in neuroblastoma patients (ALK R1275Q and ALK F1174L, corresponding to Alk R1279Q and Alk F1178L in the mouse Alk receptor), expressed in a physiological context under the control of its endogenous promoter [27] (Table 3.1a). The analysis of the sympathetic ganglia of the KI Alk^{F1178L} animals, at several stages of development, at birth and at adult stages, documented an enhanced proliferation from E14.5 to birth in sympathetic ganglia and an extended neurogenesis period. However, these KI mice did not develop any tumor. These observations may explain how constitutional ALK mutations may predispose to neuroblastoma and are consistent with the incomplete penetrance of germline *ALK* mutations observed in neuroblastoma families. Two transgenic mouse lines have been generated to induce the expression of the ALK^{F1174L}-mutant receptor in sympathetic neuroblasts. A strong expression of ALK^{F1174L} under the control of the β-actin promoter in Th- or Dbh-expressing cells elicited neuroblastoma formation with a low penetrance and long latency, and many other genetic alterations occurred in the obtained tumors, showing that activated ALK alone is not sufficient for the oncogenic transformation [26] (Table 3.1a). The expression of the same mutant driven by the rat tyrosine hydroxylase promoter was not able to induce mouse tumors [25]. Both the KI and transgenic models were used to demonstrate a strong oncogenic cooperation between ALK mutations and *MYCN* overexpression. Indeed, breedings of ALK-mutated GEMMs with TH-MYCN mice resulted in full tumor penetrance and short latency associated with an absence of additional genetic alterations in the obtained tumors [25–27] (Table 3.1b). The comparison of the KI Alk^{F1178L} and Alk^{R1279Q} mouse lines provided the first in vivo evidence that the Alk^{F1178L} mutant exhibits a higher oncogenic potential compared to the Alk^{R1279Q} mutant, in a *MYCN* overexpression context [27]. A detailed characterization of murine MYCN and MYCN/Alk-mutated tumors highlighted a number of specific features of the latter, including a more differentiated histology and an increased expression of the Ret tyrosine kinase receptor, associated with a sensitivity to the RET inhibitor vandetanib [27]. A further dissection of the underpinning mechanism revealed that an ALK/ERK/ETV5 pathway is involved in the control of *RET* expression [95].

It is also worth mentioning that whereas the Alk^{R1279Q} KI mouse line was viable and did not show any major phenotype at the heterozygous and homozygous state, homozygous KI Alk^{F1178L} mice showed a high neonatal lethality associated with a strongly reduced milk intake, reminiscent of the severe feeding difficulties observed in the patients with the most aggressive *ALK* germline mutations [96].

3.2.4 Telomere Dysfunction Linked to *TERT* and *ATRX* Genomic Aberrations

Whole-genome sequencing of neuroblastoma cell lines and tumors has identified recurrent rearrangements and/or mutations leading to somatic loss of function of *ATRX*, located on the X chromosome [97, 98] and overexpression of *TERT* located on chromosome 5p15.33 [99, 100]. TERT and ATRX abnormalities are mutually exclusive to *MYCN* amplification in most cases. The *ATRX* and *TERT* genes encode a SWI/SNF chromatin-remodeling ATP-dependent RNA helicase and the telomerase reverse transcriptase, respectively (Fig. 3.1), both being involved in the control of telomere length. Germline mutations of the *ATRX* gene are observed in the developmental disorder called α-thalassemia, mental retardation, X-linked syndrome [101, 102]. A number of neuroblastoma cell lines and tumors exhibit *TERT* rearrangements that juxtapose *TERT* to strong enhancer elements, defined as super-enhancer, which results in elevated *TERT* mRNA expression and increased enzymatic telomerase activity compared with cell lines without such alterations [99, 100]. This excess of telomerase activity likely provides cancer cells the ability of maintaining long telomeres and sustained proliferation capacity. Strong upregulation of *TERT* expression is also observed in neuroblastoma with *MYCN* amplification. In high-risk tumors without *MYCN* amplification or *TERT* rearrangements, activation of the alternative lengthening of telomeres (ALT) pathway has been reported. In a subset of these cases, *ATRX* mutations have been characterized. These mutations are preferentially observed in tumors from adolescent and young adult patients [97]; they are associated with an absence of the ATRX protein in the nucleus and with long telomeres. *ATRX* mutations observed in neuroblastoma have not yet been modeled in the mouse, but loss of *ATRX* in a mouse model is embryonic lethal, and postnatal conditional loss of *ATRX* in the forebrain impairs cortex development but does not induce brain tumors [103, 104]. Whereas no molecular therapies have yet been proposed to target the ALT pathway, the development of telomerase inhibitors represents a novel opportunity to target tumors exhibiting increased telomerase activity that are associated to a particularly bad prognosis.

3.2.5 LIN28B

Lin28A/B proteins are RNA-binding proteins (Fig. 3.1) highly expressed in early development. They are involved in the maintenance of progenitor cells by blocking the biogenesis and subsequent differentiation function of Let-7 microRNAs [105, 106]. *LIN28B* amplifications have been observed in only a few percent of high-risk neuroblastoma tumors; however, high expression of this gene is frequent in these tumors [28]. The role of LIN28 in neuroblastoma pathogenesis has been demonstrated using transgenic mouse models exhibiting *Lin28b* overexpression in cells of the sympathoadrenal lineage that express Dbh [28]. Indeed, neuroblastoma tumors developed in sympathetic ganglia and adrenal medulla of the transgenic mice. In these tumors, *Lin28b* upregulation led to Let-7 suppression and *MYCN* overexpression [28]. However, no modification of neuroblast proliferation, sympathetic ganglion and adrenal medulla size, and Let-7 expression was observed during early postnatal development in these transgenic mice [107]. These observations therefore suggest that Lin28b functions in a Let-7-independent manner in early development of neuroblastoma in this mouse model. In vitro, it has been now demonstrated that Lin28A/B and Let-7 are essential for sympathetic neuroblast proliferation during normal development in the chick [107]. Indeed, *Lin28* knockdown decreases proliferation, whereas Let-7 inhibition increases the proportion of proliferating neuroblasts. *Lin28B* overexpression enhances proliferation in E8 sympathetic neuroblasts, but such an effect was not observed in E7 or E9 neuroblasts.

Interestingly, common variants in *LIN28B* have been shown to influence neuroblastoma susceptibility [108]. Expression of *LIN28B* and let-7 miRNA correlated with rs17065417 genotype in neuroblastoma cell lines, and a significant growth inhibition has been reported upon depletion of LIN28B, specifically in neuroblastoma cells that were homozygous for the risk allele.

The signaling networks directed by LIN28B have been further explored and highlighted the role of the RAN protein [109]. RAN (RAS-related nuclear protein) is a member of the RAS family of small GTPases involved in nuclear trafficking and also able to promote Aurora-A phosphorylation [110, 111]. LIN28B directly induces RAN expression by two distinct mechanisms. One the one hand, LIN28B binds directly to RAN transcript and, on the other hand, LIN28B represses Let-7 resulting in a RANBP2 increase that stabilizes RAN. LIN28B also induces high levels of phosphorylated Aurora-A leading to kinase activation. Moreover, Aurora-A is also regulated by Let-7. A complex network connecting LIN28B, RAN, Aurora-A, and MYCN therefore emerges from this analysis [112]. Additional studies will allow deciphering whether modulating this pathway by single agents or more likely combinatorial approaches could provide benefit for neuroblastoma patients.

Of note, another study has explored the role of let-7 disruption in neuroblastoma pathogenesis [113]. This study documented a frequent genetic loss of let-7 in neuroblastoma, inversely associated with *MYCN* amplification and independently associated with poor outcome. More precisely, chromosome 3p and chromosome 11q losses are frequently observed in tumors without *MYCN* amplification. These regions contain the *let-7g* and *let-7a2* loci, respectively. In addition, high levels of *MYCN* transcripts were shown to be able to sponge let-7 microRNA levels. These data therefore suggest that that let-7 disruption is a common aberration involved in neuroblastoma pathogenesis that may occur through different mechanisms including high LIN28B activity, genetic loss, or MYCN sponging.

3.3 Noncoding RNAs in Neuroblastoma Pathogenesis

Noncoding RNAs (microRNAs, lncRNAs, and piRNAs) have now emerged as important players in the regulation of the transcriptome in a variety of biological processes including stem cell biology, development, and cancer. A number of microRNAs and lncRNAs likely play important functions in neuroblastoma pathogenesis.

The importance of miRNAs in neuroblastoma was first highlighted by the demonstration that different miRNA expression profiles are associated with different prognostic subgroups of neuroblastoma [114]. Then, evidence was obtained showing that miR-17-5p-92 family members exhibit oncogenic properties while miR-34a has tumor-suppressor functions in neuroblastoma. The *miR-17-92* cluster is a direct target of MYCN that induces tumorigenesis of *MYCN*-nonamplified neuroblastoma cells by downregulating p21, a negative regulator of the cell cycle and BIM, a proapoptotic gene [115, 116]. Treatment of mice presenting with xenografts of *MYCN*-amplified cells with a specific antagomir-17-5p impaired tumor growth [115]. A following study documented that each individual miRNA of the cluster is upregulated in *MYCN*-amplified samples and that increased activity of miR-17-92 is proportionally correlated to both poor overall and event-free survival [117]. Functional analysis uncovered that miR-17-92 activation represses the TGF-β pathway by acting on multiple key effectors along the signaling cascade and by direct inhibition of TGF-β-responsive genes. The cytostatic signals of active TGF-β signaling are therefore inhibited by miR-17-92 activation, which results in a proliferation phenotype. Whereas *miR-17-92* is activated by MYCN, *miR-34a* directly targets *MYCN* resulting in a decreased expression of the MYCN protein and subsequent growth inhibition through increased apoptosis and decreased DNA synthesis [118]. The global MYCN-miRNA interactome has been further deciphered in order to establish miRNAs controlling *MYCN* expression levels [119]. Interestingly, some of the MYCN-targeting miRNAs showed a decreased expression during murine MYCN-driven neuroblastoma tumor development in the TH-MYCN and LSL-MYCN;Dbh-iCre models, suggesting that these miRNAs are preferentially downregulated in MYCN-driven neuroblastoma to maintain MYCN expression.

Several microRNAs are correlated or inversely correlated with unfavorable outcome in neuroblastoma patients. As an example, the miR181 family has been shown to be associated with neuroblastoma aggressiveness as miR181-a and -b are both upregulated in high-risk neuroblastomas [120]. This family of microRNA regulates the expression of the dependence receptor CDON (cell-adhesion molecule-related/downregulated by oncogenes) that acts as a receptor for SHH (Sonic Hedgehog). High miR181 expression results in low expression of CDON. Reexpression of CDON in neuroblastoma cell lines induces apoptosis in vitro and impairs tumor growth in vivo after engraftment of cells to the chorioallantoic membrane of chick embryos, indicating that CDON acts as a tumor suppressor in neuroblastoma. In contrast, miR-542-3p is downregulated in tumors from patients with adverse outcome [121]. An inverse correlation between its expression and the expression of survivin has been reported, and a direct regulation of survivin by miR-542-3p has been further demonstrated. Ectopic expression of miR-542-3p in neuroblastoma cell lines in vitro results in decreased proliferation and induces tumor apoptosis in xenograft models in vivo. Some microRNAs have been also identified as regulators of ALK expression [122]. Comparison of neuroblastoma cell lines and tumors expressing *ALK* high or low levels revealed higher expression of miR-424-5p and miR-503-5p in the ALK low-level groups. Furthermore, direct binding of miR-424-5p on *ALK* 3′-UTR was demonstrated.

LncRNAs participate in diverse cellular processes with distinct regulatory roles, and some have been implicated in tumorigenesis. A differential expression analysis of lncRNAs between low- and high-risk (or *MYCN*-amplified) neuroblastomas revealed several nonannotated lncRNAs, including LOC729177 (GENCODE annotation, also referred to as CASC14) lncRNA as one of the top-ranked candidates [123]. Interestingly, previous genome-wide association studies revealed that neuroblastoma patients with homozygous risk G allele at the SNP rs6939340 located in intronic region of this lncRNA at 6p22 are likely to have metastatic disease and poor event-free survival [124]. Due to its association with neuroblastoma prognosis, LOC729177 lncRNA was subsequently named neuroblastoma-associated transcript 1 (NBAT-1). Low expression of *NBAT-1* significantly correlated with poor overall and event-free survival probability in neuroblastoma patients [123]. Functional analysis documented that loss of NBAT-1 increases cellular proliferation and invasion and also impairs differentiation of neuronal precursors.

The *lncUSMycN* gene is coamplified with *MYCN* in around 25% of human neuroblastoma tumors [125]. This lncRNA upregulates *MYCN* mRNA through a post-transcriptional mechanism by binding to the RNA-binding protein NonO and increases neuroblastoma cell proliferation. Treatment with antisense oligonucleotides targeting lncUSMycN in *MYCN*-amplified neuroblastoma xenografts impaired tumor progression, providing the first evidence that amplification of lncRNA genes can contribute to tumorigenesis. *LncUSMycN* is also involved in the control of *NCYM* expression by activating its gene transcription, and *NCYM* RNA upregulates MYCN expression by binding to NonO [66].

3.4 Metastasis Study in Neuroblastoma Models

Treatment of patients with stage 4 metastatic disease remains a challenge. Several teams have sought to generate animal models presenting with metastasis that could represent relevant models of the metastatic disease frequently observed in patients. As mentioned above, the TH-MYCN mouse model unfortunately did not recapitulate this form of the disease since only locally invasive tumors develop in the mice. Breeding of this mouse line with a caspase-8-deficient mouse line did not modify tumor penetrance, but bone marrow metastasis was much more frequently observed [29] (Table 3.1b). However, this model has so far not been used in preclinical studies. Xenografts of human neuroblastoma cell lines or fresh tumor material from patients into the mouse represent an alternative to GEMMs in the development of metastatic models of the disease. More recently, the zebrafish and chick models have been shown to be of special interest in the context of the analysis of the neuroblastoma metastatic process, revealing the critical role of *LMO1* and *SEMA3C* genes.

3.4.1 Orthotopic Xenografts in the Mouse

Orthotopic xenografts of human neuroblastoma cell lines in the adrenal medulla of immunodeficient mice have provided a few models in which metastases have been described [126–129]. Metastatic spread after orthotopic graft of *MYCN*-amplified neuroblastoma was observed mainly to the lung, liver, spleen, and adrenals [126]. Such models using cancer cell lines previously established in vitro have been largely used in preclinical studies aiming at testing various anticancer drugs. However, in many cases, the efficacy observed in preclinical studies could not be confirmed in clinical trials. Patient-derived xenografts (PDXs) are generated by direct subcutaneous or orthotopic engraftment of intact patient tumor fragments or biopsies directly into immunodeficient mice. PDXs of various cancer types recapitulate the histopathological features and mutational patterns of the corresponding patient tumors [130]. Importantly, these models have been shown to be predictive of clinical outcomes highlighting their relevance for preclinical drug evaluation and personalized medicine strategies. Recently, a series of pediatric solid tumors have been used to generate orthotopic PDXs [131]. Para-adrenal injections were performed for neuroblastoma, and several models could be established. At that stage, metastasis has not been yet investigated in these models. One limitation of these approaches is related to the immunodeficient background of the mice and potential mouse-specific tumor evolution during passages [132].

3.4.2 LMO1

In 2011, the *LMO1* (LIM domain only 1) gene has been identified as a high-risk neuroblastoma susceptibility gene through a genome-wide association study [133]. This gene encodes a cysteine-rich transcriptional regulator with two LIM zinc-binding domains that is mainly expressed in the nervous system. In sporadic tumors, LMO1 gains are observed in 12% of cases, and this abnormality is significantly more common in tumors from patients with metastatic disease or advanced age [133]. Whereas LMO1 inhibition in neuroblastoma cells expressing high levels of LMO1 results in growth inhibition, overexpression of LMO1 in cells with low levels of LMO1 induces increased growth, suggesting that LMO1 may function as an oncogene in a subset of human neuroblastoma [133]. Further analysis demonstrated that the LMO1 SNPs associated with high-risk neuroblastoma drive high expression of *LMO1* by a direct modulation *in cis* through the formation of a super-enhancer in the first intron of the *LMO1* gene [134].

Recently, the characterization of transgenic zebrafish lines expressing human *LMO1* under the control of the zebrafish Dbh promoter revealed that *LMO1* alone was not able to induce tumors in the fish [135]. However, the overexpression of *LMO1* not only synergizes with *MYCN* to induce neuroblastoma tumors by increasing the proliferation of sympathoadrenal neuroblast cells, but *LMO1* overexpression was also associated with metastasis [135]. Indeed, LMO1 promoted hematogenous dissemination and distant metastasis in multiple organs including orbit and spleen, which are common sites in neuroblastoma metastatic patients. In vitro invasion and migration assays with *MYCN*-amplified neuroblastoma cell lines documented increased invasive properties and greater migratory capacity of cells expressing high *LMO1* levels. The concomitant expression of *MYCN* and *LMO1* leads to increased levels of extracellular matrix regulator genes, including *LOXL3*, *ITGA2b*, *ITGA3*, and *ITGA5*, which should result in remodeling of the extracellular matrix and subsequent enhanced invasion and motility, explaining the synergy between *MYCN* and *LMO1* in neuroblastoma metastasis. *LMO1* therefore appears as an important oncogene involved in neuroblastoma initiation, progression, and widespread metastatic dissemination.

3.4.3 SEMA3C

Recently, C. Delloye-Bourgeois and colleagues developed an elegant avian embryonic model fully replicating human neuroblastoma tumorigenesis and dissemination [136]. This model relies on the engraftment of neuroblastoma cell lines into HH14 chick embryos at the sympathoadrenal crest level (between somite 18 and somite 24). Two days after cell graft, almost all cells have migrated away from the initial site and accumulated mostly in the sympathetic ganglia and the adrenal gland, which are the natural sites that are specifically targeted by endogenous sympathoadrenal neural crest cells [137]. The grafted neuroblastoma cells therefore recapitulated a collective migratory behavior that is typical of neural crest cells. Seven days after the graft of HH14 chick embryos, not only massive tumors were observed in sympathoadrenal derivatives, but loco-regional invasion was observed as well as invasion to more distant sites. These observations indicate that this model recapitulates features of neuroblastoma metastasis. The comparison of the transcriptomic profiles of tumor masses obtained in sympathetic ganglia 2 days after engraftment with that of neuroblastoma cells that had not been engrafted uncovered a decreased expression of *SEMA3C*, *SEMA3D*, and *SEMA3F* genes. These genes belong to the Semaphorin gene family known to regulate axon and cell migration [138]. Further experiments documented that the collective migration of neuroblastoma cells and targeting of embryonic structures were impaired upon SEMA3C downregulation, showing that SEMA3C provides a procohesion autocrine signal that constrains the tumor mass. The downregulation of SEMA3C results in detachment, allowing neuroblastoma cells to collectively evade the tumor. Engraftment experiments with fresh tumor biopsies from localized neuroblastoma tumors or bone marrow aspirates from metastatic patients showed distant disseminations exclusively for samples derived from metastatic cases, although primary tumor masses were detected for all cases in the sympathoadrenal derivatives. Furthermore, the analysis of this model showed that embryonic aorta and nerves are the primary dissemination routes of neuroblastoma cells. This avian embryonic model appears as a promising model to further explore the metastatic process in neuroblastoma and perform preclinical studies.

3.5 Cell Identity and Plasticity in Neuroblastoma

Besides the alterations of the cancer genomes that have been extensively characterized for decades, more recently several studies highlighted that specific epigenetic states, associated with particular histone modifications and/or DNA methylation, may contribute to cancer phenotype. Whereas silencing of tumor-suppressor genes may indeed result from chromatin repression and/or promoter hypermethylation [139, 140], coordinated long-range epigenetic activation of regions harboring oncogenes and/or microRNAs is associated with gain of active chromatin marks and loss of repressive marks [141].

A recent study reported an integrative analysis of methylomes, transcriptomes, and copy-number variations of 105 neuroblastoma cases complemented by the analysis of several histone marks for a subset of primary tumors and cell lines [142]. Distinct genome-wide DNA methylation patterns were observed in various patient subgroups with respect to survival and clinical and biological features, including *MYCN* amplification. The obtained data further identified intragenic enhancer methylation as a mechanism for high-risk-associated transcriptional deregulation and described a catalog of candidate genes for being transcriptionally deregulated by aberrant methylation in high-risk neuroblastomas.

It has also been demonstrated that information on cell lineage identity can be obtained through the characterization of the super-enhancer landscape of the cells of interest. Super-enhancers are clustered enhancers that can be defined by ChIP (chromatin immunoprecipitation)-seq of the H3K27ac histone acetylation mark [143]. Core regulatory circuitries (CRCs) containing the key transcription factors that govern the gene expression program of a specific cell type may be defined from the super-enhancer landscape [144]. The analysis of the super-enhancer landscape of a panel of neuroblastoma cell lines and PDXs has recently highlighted two different types of cell identity and two distinct transcription factor networks: a sympathetic noradrenergic identity, defined by a CRC module including the PHOX2B, HAND2, and GATA3 transcription factors, and a more undifferentiated identity, close to human neural crest cells driven by a CRC module containing AP-1 transcription factors [145, 146]. Importantly, this analysis identified cell lines with an intermediate pattern of super-enhancers, including in particular the SK-N-SH cell line. This cell line has been described as phenotypically heterogeneous, and two different cell lines SH-EP and SH-SY5Y have been subcloned from it [147]. The analysis of the super-enhancer landscape revealed that the SH-EP and SH-SY5Y displayed a NCC-like and a sympathetic noradrenergic identity, respectively. These two distinct identities are consistent with SH-SY5Y cells displaying neurite-like processes and expressing the noradrenergic biosynthetic enzymes Th and Dbh, corresponding to a so-called N phenotype, whereas SH-EP cells exhibit a substrate-adherent S phenotype without expression of Th and Dbh. Other pairs of cell lines have been obtained by the group of R. Versteeg presenting with the same characteristics as the SH-EP/SH-SY5Y pair. Indeed, this group derived cell lines sharing the same genomic alterations and exhibiting divergent phenotypes, expression profiles, and super-enhancer landscapes, corresponding to the two aforementioned identities [146, 148]. Both studies documented that cells of NCC-like/mesenchymal identity were more resistant to chemotherapy than cells of noradrenergic identity in vitro. Additional data documented that sorted cells of each identity were able to reconstitute both types of identity when injected in the mouse [146]. These observations motivated the analysis of pairs of diagnosis and relapse samples from neuroblastoma patients. Whereas one study obtained evidences suggesting that mesenchymal cells are enriched in posttherapy patient samples [146], the other one did not document a systematic enrichment of NCC-like/mesenchymal at the relapse stage [145]. These observations suggest that neuroblastoma cells may be able to shift from a noradrenergic to NCC-like cells under chemotherapy, and from a NCC-like to noradrenergic identity after treatment. Further analysis on larger series of patients at different time points during disease's course will probably provide additional information on neuroblastoma intratumor heterogeneity and plasticity. The mechanisms underlying the plasticity of cell identity still remain to be characterized. Interestingly, it has been suggested that the overexpression of the mesenchymal transcription factor PRRX1 in noradrenergic cells was able to reprogram such cells toward a mesenchymal identity, with an increase in expression of specific proteins and concomitant decrease of the proteins specific of the noradrenergic identity [146]. Finally, functional analysis demonstrated a growth dependency of noradrenergic neuroblastoma cell lines on PHOX2B, HAND2, and GATA3 transcription factors, evocative of lineage addiction [145]. Altogether, these recent data illuminate how epigenetic deregulation may contribute to neuroblastoma pathogenesis, with novel implications for diagnosis and disease treatment.

Previous studies based on the analysis of tumor alterations at diagnosis and relapse using microarrays or more recently next-generation sequencing technologies have documented the accumulation of segmental alterations in neuroblastoma and increase of the mutational burden in relapsing tumors [71, 72, 149–151]. Clonal mutation selection during disease progression was also reported. Understanding the interplay between epigenetic rewiring and genetic alterations during tumor evolution will be crucial to improve neuroblastoma response to therapy and patients outcome.

Acknowledgments I am grateful to my colleagues Caroline Louis-Brennetot, Hermann Rohrer, and Olivier Delattre for their helpful comments on this chapter.

References

1. Le Douarin N. The neural crest. Cambridge: Cambridge University Press; 1982.
2. Bronner ME, Simões-Costa M. The neural crest migrating into the twenty-first century. Curr Top Dev Biol. 2016;116:115–34.
3. Furlan A, Dyachuk V, Kastriti ME, et al. Multipotent peripheral glial cells generate neuroendocrine cells of the adrenal medulla. Science. 2017;357:eaal3753. https://doi.org/10.1126/science.aal3753.
4. Qualman SJ, Green WR, Brovall C, Leventhal BG. Neurofibromatosis and associated neuroectodermal tumors: a congenital neurocristopathy. Pediatr Pathol. 1986;5:65–78.
5. Roshkow JE, Haller JO, Berdon WE, Sane SM. Hirschsprung's disease, Ondine's curse, and neuroblastoma--manifestations of neurocristopathy. Pediatr Radiol. 1988;19:45–9.
6. Spengler CM, Gozal D, Shea SA. Chemoreceptive mechanisms elucidated by studies of congenital central hypoventilation syndrome. Respir Physiol. 2001;129:247–55.
7. Schneider C, Wicht H, Enderich J, Wegner M, Rohrer H. Bone morphogenetic proteins are required in vivo for the generation of sympathetic neurons. Neuron. 1999;24:861–70.
8. Rohrer H. Transcriptional control of differentiation and neurogenesis in autonomic ganglia. Eur J Neurosci. 2011;34:1563–73.
9. Amiel J, Laudier B, Attie-Bitach T, et al. Polyalanine expansion and frameshift mutations of the paired-like homeobox gene PHOX2B in congenital central hypoventilation syndrome. Nat Genet. 2003;33:459–61.
10. Cowling VH, Chandriani S, Whitfield ML, Cole MD. A conserved Myc protein domain, MBIV, regulates DNA binding, apoptosis, transformation, and G2 arrest. Mol Cell Biol. 2006;26:4226–39.

11. Sarid J, Halazonetis TD, Murphy W, Leder P. Evolutionarily conserved regions of the human c-myc protein can be uncoupled from transforming activity. Proc Natl Acad Sci. 1987;84:170–3.
12. Hallberg B, Palmer RH. The role of the ALK receptor in cancer biology. Ann Oncol. 2016;27(Suppl 3):iii4–iii15.
13. Balzeau J, Menezes MR, Cao S, Hagan JP. The LIN28/let-7 pathway in cancer. Front Genet. 2017;8:31. https://doi.org/10.3389/fgene.2017.00031.
14. Pattyn A, Morin X, Cremer H, Goridis C, Brunet JF. The homeobox gene Phox2b is essential for the development of autonomic neural crest derivatives. Nature. 1999;399:366–70.
15. McConville C, Reid S, Baskcomb L, Douglas J, Rahman N. PHOX2B analysis in non-syndromic neuroblastoma cases shows novel mutations and genotype-phenotype associations. Am J Med Genet A. 2006;140:1297–301.
16. Mosse YP, Laudenslager M, Khazi D, Carlisle AJ, Winter CL, Rappaport E, Maris JM. Germline PHOX2B mutation in hereditary neuroblastoma. Am J Hum Genet. 2004;75:727–30.
17. Raabe EH, Laudenslager M, Winter C, Wasserman N, Cole K, LaQuaglia M, Maris DJ, Mosse YP, Maris JM. Prevalence and functional consequence of PHOX2B mutations in neuroblastoma. Oncogene. 2008;27:469–76.
18. Trochet D, Bourdeaut F, Janoueix-Lerosey I, et al. Germline mutations of the paired-like homeobox 2B (PHOX2B) gene in neuroblastoma. Am J Hum Genet. 2004;74:761–4.
19. Trochet D, O'Brien LM, Gozal D, et al. PHOX2B genotype allows for prediction of tumor risk in congenital central hypoventilation syndrome. Am J Hum Genet. 2005;76:421–6.
20. Trochet D, Hong SJ, Lim JK, Brunet J-F, Munnich A, Kim K-S, Lyonnet S, Goridis C, Amiel J. Molecular consequences of PHOX2B missense, frameshift and alanine expansion mutations leading to autonomic dysfunction. Hum Mol Genet. 2005;14:3697–708.
21. Reiff T, Tsarovina K, Majdazari A, Schmidt M, del Pino I, Rohrer H. Neuroblastoma phox2b variants stimulate proliferation and dedifferentiation of immature sympathetic neurons. J Neurosci. 2010;30:905–15.
22. Nagashimada M, Ohta H, Li C, Nakao K, Uesaka T, Brunet J-F, Amiel J, Trochet D, Wakayama T, Enomoto H. Autonomic neurocristopathy-associated mutations in PHOX2B dysregulate Sox10 expression. J Clin Invest. 2012;122:3145–58.
23. Weiss WA, Aldape K, Mohapatra G, Feuerstein BG, Bishop JM. Targeted expression of MYCN causes neuroblastoma in transgenic mice. EMBO J. 1997;16:2985–95.
24. Althoff K, Beckers A, Bell E, et al. A Cre-conditional MYCN-driven neuroblastoma mouse model as an improved tool for preclinical studies. Oncogene. 2015;34:3357–68.
25. Berry T, Luther W, Bhatnagar N, et al. The ALK(F1174L) mutation potentiates the oncogenic activity of MYCN in neuroblastoma. Cancer Cell. 2012;22:117–30.
26. Heukamp LC, Thor T, Schramm A, et al. Targeted expression of mutated ALK induces neuroblastoma in transgenic mice. Sci Transl Med. 2012;4:141ra91.
27. Cazes A, Lopez-Delisle L, Tsarovina K, et al. Activated Alk triggers prolonged neurogenesis and Ret upregulation providing a therapeutic target in ALK-mutated neuroblastoma. Oncotarget. 2014;5:2688–702.
28. Molenaar JJ, Domingo-Fernández R, Ebus ME, et al. LIN28B induces neuroblastoma and enhances MYCN levels via let-7 suppression. Nat Genet. 2012;44:1199–206.
29. Teitz T, Inoue M, Valentine MB, et al. Th-MYCN mice with caspase-8 deficiency develop advanced neuroblastoma with bone marrow metastasis. Cancer Res. 2013;73:4086–97.
30. Pei D, Luther W, Wang W, Paw BH, Stewart RA, George RE. Distinct neuroblastoma-associated alterations of PHOX2B impair sympathetic neuronal differentiation in zebrafish models. PLoS Genet. 2013;9:e1003533.
31. van Limpt V, Schramm A, van Lakeman A, Sluis P, Chan A, van Noesel M, Baas F, Caron H, Eggert A, Versteeg R. The Phox2B homeobox gene is mutated in sporadic neuroblastomas. Oncogene. 2004;23:9280–8.
32. Brodeur GM, Seeger RC, Schwab M, Varmus HE, Bishop JM. Amplification of N-myc in untreated human neuroblastomas correlates with advanced disease stage. Science. 1984;224:1121–4.

33. Seeger RC, Brodeur GM, Sather H, Dalton A, Siegel SE, Wong KY, Hammond D. Association of multiple copies of the N-myc oncogene with rapid progression of neuroblastomas. N Engl J Med. 1985;313:1111–6.
34. Charron J, Malynn BA, Fisher P, Stewart V, Jeannotte L, Goff SP, Robertson EJ, Alt FW. Embryonic lethality in mice homozygous for a targeted disruption of the N-myc gene. Genes Dev. 1992;6:2248–57.
35. Knoepfler PS, Cheng PF, Eisenman RN. N-myc is essential during neurogenesis for the rapid expansion of progenitor cell populations and the inhibition of neuronal differentiation. Genes Dev. 2002;16:2699–712.
36. Maurer J, Fuchs S, Jäger R, Kurz B, Sommer L, Schorle H. Establishment and controlled differentiation of neural crest stem cell lines using conditional transgenesis. Differ Res Biol Divers. 2007;75:580–91.
37. Rao MS, Anderson DJ. Immortalization and controlled in vitro differentiation of murine multipotent neural crest stem cells. J Neurobiol. 1997;32:722–46.
38. Schulte JH, Lindner S, Bohrer A, et al. MYCN and ALKF1174L are sufficient to drive neuroblastoma development from neural crest progenitor cells. Oncogene. 2013;32:1059–65.
39. Olsen RR, Otero JH, García-López J, Wallace K, Finkelstein D, Rehg JE, Yin Z, Wang Y-D, Freeman KW. MYCN induces neuroblastoma in primary neural crest cells. Oncogene. 2017;36:5075. https://doi.org/10.1038/onc.2017.128.
40. Brisse HJ, Blanc T, Schleiermacher G, et al. Radiogenomics of neuroblastomas: relationships between imaging phenotypes, tumor genomic profile and survival. PLoS One. 2017;12:e0185190.
41. Vo KT, Matthay KK, Neuhaus J, et al. Clinical, biologic, and prognostic differences on the basis of primary tumor site in neuroblastoma: a report from the international neuroblastoma risk group project. J Clin Oncol Off J Am Soc Clin Oncol. 2014;32:3169–76.
42. Casey MJ, Stewart RA. Zebrafish as a model to study neuroblastoma development. Cell Tissue Res. 2017;372:223. https://doi.org/10.1007/s00441-017-2702-0.
43. Zhu S, Lee JS, Guo F, et al. Activated ALK collaborates with MYCN in neuroblastoma pathogenesis. Cancer Cell. 2012;21:362–73.
44. Burkhart CA, Cheng AJ, Madafiglio J, Kavallaris M, Mili M, Marshall GM, Weiss WA, Khachigian LM, Norris MD, Haber M. Effects of MYCN antisense oligonucleotide administration on tumorigenesis in a murine model of neuroblastoma. J Natl Cancer Inst. 2003;95:1394–403.
45. Sjostrom SK, Finn G, Hahn WC, Rowitch DH, Kenney AM. The Cdk1 complex plays a prime role in regulating N-myc phosphorylation and turnover in neural precursors. Dev Cell. 2005;9:327–38.
46. Adhikary S, Eilers M. Transcriptional regulation and transformation by Myc proteins. Nat Rev Mol Cell Biol. 2005;6:635–45.
47. Welcker M, Orian A, Jin J, Grim JE, Grim JA, Harper JW, Eisenman RN, Clurman BE. The Fbw7 tumor suppressor regulates glycogen synthase kinase 3 phosphorylation-dependent c-Myc protein degradation. Proc Natl Acad Sci U S A. 2004;101:9085–90.
48. Chesler L, Schlieve C, Goldenberg DD, Kenney A, Kim G, McMillan A, Matthay KK, Rowitch D, Weiss WA. Inhibition of phosphatidylinositol 3-kinase destabilizes mycn protein and blocks malignant progression in neuroblastoma. Cancer Res. 2006;66:8139–46.
49. Giet R, Prigent C. Aurora/Ipl1p-related kinases, a new oncogenic family of mitotic serine-threonine kinases. J Cell Sci. 1999;112(Pt 21):3591–601.
50. Otto T, Horn S, Brockmann M, et al. Stabilization of N-Myc is a critical function of Aurora A in human neuroblastoma. Cancer Cell. 2009;15:67–78.
51. Faisal A, Vaughan L, Bavetsias V, et al. The aurora kinase inhibitor CCT137690 downregulates MYCN and sensitizes MYCN-amplified neuroblastoma in vivo. Mol Cancer Ther. 2011;10:2115–23.
52. Maris JM, Morton CL, Gorlick R, et al. Initial testing of the aurora kinase A inhibitor MLN8237 by the Pediatric Preclinical Testing Program (PPTP). Pediatr Blood Cancer. 2010;55:26–34.

53. MosséYP, Lipsitz E, Fox E, Teachey DT, Maris JM, Weigel B, Adamson PC, Ingle MA, Ahern CH, Blaney SM. Pediatric phase I trial and pharmacokinetic study of MLN8237, an investigational oral selective small-molecule inhibitor of Aurora kinase A: a Children's Oncology Group Phase I Consortium study. Clin Cancer Res. 2012;18:6058–64.
54. Manfredi MG, Ecsedy JA, Meetze KA, et al. Antitumor activity of MLN8054, an orally active small-molecule inhibitor of Aurora A kinase. Proc Natl Acad Sci U S A. 2007;104:4106–11.
55. Brockmann M, Poon E, Berry T, et al. Small molecule inhibitors of aurora-a induce proteasomal degradation of N-myc in childhood neuroblastoma. Cancer Cell. 2013;24:75–89.
56. Gustafson WC, Meyerowitz JG, Nekritz EA, et al. Drugging MYCN through an allosteric transition in Aurora kinase A. Cancer Cell. 2014;26:414–27.
57. Richards MW, Burgess SG, Poon E, Carstensen A, Eilers M, Chesler L, Bayliss R. Structural basis of N-Myc binding by Aurora-A and its destabilization by kinase inhibitors. Proc Natl Acad Sci U S A. 2016;113:13726–31.
58. Lipsitz EG, Nguyen V, Zhao H, Ecsedy J, Maris JM, Adamson PC, Mosse YP. Modeling MLN8237, an aurora kinase a inhibitor, with irinotecan (IRN) and temozolomide (TMZ) in neuroblastoma (NB). J Clin Oncol. 2010;28:10593.
59. DuBois SG, Marachelian A, Fox E, et al. Phase I study of the aurora a kinase inhibitor alisertib in combination with irinotecan and temozolomide for patients with relapsed or refractory neuroblastoma: a NANT (New Approaches to Neuroblastoma Therapy) trial. J Clin Oncol Off J Am Soc Clin Oncol. 2016;34:1368–75.
60. Puissant A, Frumm SM, Alexe G, et al. Targeting MYCN in neuroblastoma by BET bromodomain inhibition. Cancer Discov. 2013;3:308–23.
61. Chen T, Dent SYR. Chromatin modifiers and remodellers: regulators of cellular differentiation. Nat Rev Genet. 2014;15:93–106.
62. Kramer M, Ribeiro D, Arsenian-Henriksson M, Deller T, Rohrer H. Proliferation and survival of embryonic sympathetic neuroblasts by MYCN and activated ALK signaling. J Neurosci. 2016;36:10425–39.
63. Tang Y, Gholamin S, Schubert S, et al. Epigenetic targeting of Hedgehog pathway transcriptional output through BET bromodomain inhibition. Nat Med. 2014;20:732–40.
64. Armstrong BC, Krystal GW. Isolation and characterization of complementary DNA for N-cym, a gene encoded by the DNA strand opposite to N-myc. Cell Growth Differ. 1992;3:385–90.
65. Suenaga Y, Islam SMR, Alagu J, et al. NCYM, a Cis-antisense gene of MYCN, encodes a de novo evolved protein that inhibits GSK3β resulting in the stabilization of MYCN in human neuroblastomas. PLoS Genet. 2014;10:e1003996.
66. Liu PY, Atmadibrata B, Mondal S, Tee AE, Liu T. NCYM is upregulated by lncUSMycN and modulates N-Myc expression. Int J Oncol. 2016;49:2464–70.
67. Chen Y, Takita J, Choi YL, et al. Oncogenic mutations of ALK kinase in neuroblastoma. Nature. 2008;455:971–4.
68. George RE, Sanda T, Hanna M, et al. Activating mutations in ALK provide a therapeutic target in neuroblastoma. Nature. 2008;455:975–8.
69. Janoueix-Lerosey I, Lequin D, Brugieres L, et al. Somatic and germline activating mutations of the ALK kinase receptor in neuroblastoma. Nature. 2008;455:967–70.
70. Mosse YP, Laudenslager M, Longo L, et al. Identification of ALK as a major familial neuroblastoma predisposition gene. Nature. 2008;455:930–5.
71. Bellini A, Bernard V, Leroy Q, et al. Deep sequencing reveals occurrence of subclonal ALK mutations in neuroblastoma at diagnosis. Clin Cancer Res. 2015;21:4913–21.
72. Eleveld TF, Oldridge DA, Bernard V, et al. Relapsed neuroblastomas show frequent RAS-MAPK pathway mutations. Nat Genet. 2015;47:864–71.
73. Janoueix-Lerosey I, Lopez-Delisle L, Delattre O, Rohrer H. The ALK receptor in sympathetic neuron development and neuroblastoma. Cell Tissue Res. 2018;372:325. https://doi.org/10.1007/s00441-017-2784-8.
74. Bilsland JG, Wheeldon A, Mead A, et al. Behavioral and neurochemical alterations in mice deficient in anaplastic lymphoma kinase suggest therapeutic potential for psychiatric indications. Neuropsychopharmacology. 2008;33:685–700.

75. Lasek AW, Lim J, Kliethermes CL, et al. An evolutionary conserved role for anaplastic lymphoma kinase in behavioral responses to ethanol. PLoS One. 2011;6:e22636.
76. Weiss JB, Xue C, Benice T, Xue L, Morris SW, Raber J. Anaplastic lymphoma kinase and leukocyte tyrosine kinase: functions and genetic interactions in learning, memory and adult neurogenesis. Pharmacol Biochem Behav. 2012;100:566–74.
77. Witek B, El Wakil A, Nord C, Ahlgren U, Eriksson M, Vernersson-Lindahl E, Helland Å, Alexeyev OA, Hallberg B, Palmer RH. Targeted disruption of ALK reveals a potential role in hypogonadotropic hypogonadism. PLoS One. 2015;10:e0123542.
78. Stoica GE, Kuo A, Aigner A, et al. Identification of anaplastic lymphoma kinase as a receptor for the growth factor pleiotrophin. J Biol Chem. 2001;276:16772–9.
79. Stoica GE, Kuo A, Powers C, Bowden ET, Sale EB, Riegel AT, Wellstein A. Midkine binds to anaplastic lymphoma kinase (ALK) and acts as a growth factor for different cell types. J Biol Chem. 2002;277:35990–8.
80. Mathivet T, Mazot P, Vigny M. In contrast to agonist monoclonal antibodies, both C-terminal truncated form and full length form of Pleiotrophin failed to activate vertebrate ALK (anaplastic lymphoma kinase)? Cell Signal. 2007;19:2434–43.
81. Miyake I, Hakomori Y, Shinohara A, Gamou T, Saito M, Iwamatsu A, Sakai R. Activation of anaplastic lymphoma kinase is responsible for hyperphosphorylation of ShcC in neuroblastoma cell lines. Oncogene. 2002;21:5823–34.
82. Moog-Lutz C, Degoutin J, Gouzi JY, Frobert Y, Brunet-de Carvalho N, Bureau J, Creminon C, Vigny M. Activation and inhibition of anaplastic lymphoma kinase receptor tyrosine kinase by monoclonal antibodies and absence of agonist activity of pleiotrophin. J Biol Chem. 2005;280:26039–48.
83. Murray PB, Lax I, Reshetnyak A, et al. Heparin is an activating ligand of the orphan receptor tyrosine kinase ALK. Sci Signal. 2015;8:ra6.
84. Guan J, Umapathy G, Yamazaki Y, et al. FAM150A and FAM150B are activating ligands for anaplastic lymphoma kinase. Elife. 2015;4:e09811.
85. Reshetnyak AV, Murray PB, Shi X, Mo ES, Mohanty J, Tome F, Bai H, Gunel M, Lax I, Schlessinger J. Augmentor α and β (FAM150) are ligands of the receptor tyrosine kinases ALK and LTK: hierarchy and specificity of ligand-receptor interactions. Proc Natl Acad Sci U S A. 2015;112:15862–7.
86. Reiff T, Huber L, Kramer M, Delattre O, Janoueix-Lerosey I, Rohrer H. Midkine and Alk signaling in sympathetic neuron proliferation and neuroblastoma predisposition. Development. 2011;138:4699–708.
87. Morris SW, Naeve C, Mathew P, James PL, Kirstein MN, Cui X, Witte DP. ALK, the chromosome 2 gene locus altered by the t(2;5) in non-Hodgkin's lymphoma, encodes a novel neural receptor tyrosine kinase that is highly related to leukocyte tyrosine kinase (LTK). Oncogene. 1997;14:2175–88.
88. Bresler SC, Weiser DA, Huwe PJ, et al. ALK mutations confer differential oncogenic activation and sensitivity to ALK inhibition therapy in neuroblastoma. Cancer Cell. 2014;26:682–94.
89. Galkin AV, Melnick JS, Kim S, et al. Identification of NVP-TAE684, a potent, selective, and efficacious inhibitor of NPM-ALK. Proc Natl Acad Sci U S A. 2007;104:270–5.
90. Zou HY, Li Q, Lee JH, et al. An orally available small-molecule inhibitor of c-Met, PF-2341066, exhibits cytoreductive antitumor efficacy through antiproliferative and antiangiogenic mechanisms. Cancer Res. 2007;67:4408–17.
91. Mossé YP, Lim MS, Voss SD, et al. Safety and activity of crizotinib for paediatric patients with refractory solid tumours or anaplastic large-cell lymphoma: a Children's Oncology Group phase 1 consortium study. Lancet Oncol. 2013;14:472–80.
92. de Pontual L, Kettaneh D, Gordon CT, et al. Germline gain-of-function mutations of ALK disrupt central nervous system development. Hum Mutat. 2011;32:272–6.
93. Zhang J, Walsh MF, Wu G, et al. Germline mutations in predisposition genes in pediatric cancer. N Engl J Med. 2015;373:2336–46.
94. Montavon G, Jauquier N, Coulon A, et al. Wild-type ALK and activating ALK-R1275Q and ALK-F1174L mutations upregulate Myc and initiate tumor formation in murine neural crest progenitor cells. Oncotarget. 2014;5:4452–66.

95. Lopez-Delisle L, Pierre-Eugène C, Louis-Brennetot C, et al. Activated ALK signals through the ERK-ETV5-RET pathway to drive neuroblastoma oncogenesis. Oncogene. 2018;37:1417. https://doi.org/10.1038/s41388-017-0039-5.
96. Lopez-Delisle L, Pierre-Eugène C, Bloch-Gallego E, et al. Hyperactivation of Alk induces neonatal lethality in knock-in AlkF1178L mice. Oncotarget. 2014;5:2703–13.
97. Cheung N-KV, Zhang J, Lu C, et al. Association of age at diagnosis and genetic mutations in patients with neuroblastoma. JAMA. 2012;307:1062–71.
98. Pugh TJ, Morozova O, Attiyeh EF, et al. The genetic landscape of high-risk neuroblastoma. Nat Genet. 2013;45:279–84.
99. Peifer M, Hertwig F, Roels F, et al. Telomerase activation by genomic rearrangements in high-risk neuroblastoma. Nature. 2015;526:700–4.
100. Valentijn LJ, Koster J, Zwijnenburg DA, et al. TERT rearrangements are frequent in neuroblastoma and identify aggressive tumors. Nat Genet. 2015;47:1411–4.
101. Dyer MA, Qadeer ZA, Valle-Garcia D, Bernstein E. ATRX and DAXX: mechanisms and mutations. Cold Spring Harb Perspect Med. 2017;7:a026567. https://doi.org/10.1101/cshperspect.a026567.
102. Gibbons RJ, Picketts DJ, Villard L, Higgs DR. Mutations in a putative global transcriptional regulator cause X-linked mental retardation with alpha-thalassemia (ATR-X syndrome). Cell. 1995;80:837–45.
103. Bérubé NG, Mangelsdorf M, Jagla M, Vanderluit J, Garrick D, Gibbons RJ, Higgs DR, Slack RS, Picketts DJ. The chromatin-remodeling protein ATRX is critical for neuronal survival during corticogenesis. J Clin Invest. 2005;115:258–67.
104. Garrick D, Sharpe JA, Arkell R, Dobbie L, Smith AJH, Wood WG, Higgs DR, Gibbons RJ. Loss of Atrx affects trophoblast development and the pattern of X-inactivation in extraembryonic tissues. PLoS Genet. 2006;2:e58.
105. Heo I, Joo C, Cho J, Ha M, Han J, Kim VN. Lin28 mediates the terminal uridylation of let-7 precursor MicroRNA. Mol Cell. 2008;32:276–84.
106. Viswanathan SR, Daley GQ, Gregory RI. Selective blockade of microRNA processing by Lin28. Science. 2008;320:97–100.
107. Hennchen M, Stubbusch J, Abarchan-El Makhfi I, et al. Lin28B and Let-7 in the control of sympathetic neurogenesis and neuroblastoma development. J Neurosci. 2015;35:16531–44.
108. Diskin SJ, Capasso M, Schnepp RW, et al. Common variation at 6q16 within HACE1 and LIN28B influences susceptibility to neuroblastoma. Nat Genet. 2012;44:1126–30.
109. Schnepp RW, Khurana P, Attiyeh EF, et al. A LIN28B-RAN-AURKA signaling network promotes neuroblastoma tumorigenesis. Cancer Cell. 2015;28:599–609.
110. Trieselmann N, Armstrong S, Rauw J, Wilde A. Ran modulates spindle assembly by regulating a subset of TPX2 and Kid activities including Aurora A activation. J Cell Sci. 2003;116:4791–8.
111. Tsai M-Y, Wiese C, Cao K, Martin O, Donovan P, Ruderman J, Prigent C, Zheng Y. A Ran signalling pathway mediated by the mitotic kinase Aurora A in spindle assembly. Nat Cell Biol. 2003;5:242–8.
112. Schnepp RW, Diskin SJ. LIN28B: an orchestrator of oncogenic signaling in neuroblastoma. Cell Cycle. 2016;15:772–4.
113. Powers JT, Tsanov KM, Pearson DS, et al. Multiple mechanisms disrupt the let-7 microRNA family in neuroblastoma. Nature. 2016;535:246–51.
114. Chen Y, Stallings RL. Differential patterns of microRNA expression in neuroblastoma are correlated with prognosis, differentiation, and apoptosis. Cancer Res. 2007;67:976–83.
115. Fontana L, Fiori ME, Albini S, et al. Antagomir-17-5p abolishes the growth of therapy-resistant neuroblastoma through p21 and BIM. PLoS One. 2008;3:e2236.
116. Mestdagh P, Fredlund E, Pattyn F, et al. MYCN/c-MYC-induced microRNAs repress coding gene networks associated with poor outcome in MYCN/c-MYC-activated tumors. Oncogene. 2010;29:1394–404.
117. Mestdagh P, Boström A-K, Impens F, et al. The miR-17-92 microRNA cluster regulates multiple components of the TGF-β pathway in neuroblastoma. Mol Cell. 2010;40:762–73.

118. Wei JS, Song YK, Durinck S, et al. The MYCN oncogene is a direct target of miR-34a. Oncogene. 2008;27:5204–13.
119. Beckers A, Van Peer G, Carter DR, et al. MYCN-targeting miRNAs are predominantly downregulated during MYCN-driven neuroblastoma tumor formation. Oncotarget. 2015;6:5204–16.
120. Gibert B, Delloye-Bourgeois C, Gattolliat C-H, et al. Regulation by miR181 family of the dependence receptor CDON tumor suppressive activity in neuroblastoma. J Natl Cancer Inst. 2014;106:dju318. https://doi.org/10.1093/jnci/dju318.
121. Althoff K, Lindner S, Odersky A, et al. miR-542-3p exerts tumor suppressive functions in neuroblastoma by downregulating Survivin. Int J Cancer. 2015;136:1308–20.
122. De Mariano M, Stigliani S, Moretti S, Parodi F, Croce M, Bernardi C, Pagano A, Tonini GP, Ferrini S, Longo L. A genome-wide microRNA profiling indicates miR-424-5p and miR-503-5p as regulators of ALK expression in neuroblastoma. Oncotarget. 2017;8:56518–32.
123. Pandey GK, Mitra S, Subhash S, et al. The risk-associated long noncoding RNA NBAT-1 controls neuroblastoma progression by regulating cell proliferation and neuronal differentiation. Cancer Cell. 2014;26:722–37.
124. Maris JM, Mosse YP, Bradfield JP, et al. Chromosome 6p22 locus associated with clinically aggressive neuroblastoma. N Engl J Med. 2008;358:2585–93.
125. Liu PY, Erriquez D, Marshall GM, et al. Effects of a novel long noncoding RNA, lncUSMycN, on N-Myc expression and neuroblastoma progression. J Natl Cancer Inst. 2014;106:dju113. https://doi.org/10.1093/jnci/dju113.
126. Daudigeos-Dubus E, LE Dret L, Rouffiac V, Bawa O, Leguerney I, Opolon P, Vassal G, Geoerger B. Establishment and characterization of new orthotopic and metastatic neuroblastoma models. In Vivo. 2014;28:425–34.
127. Dickson PV, Hamner B, Ng CYC, Hall MM, Zhou J, Hargrove PW, McCarville MB, Davidoff AM. In vivo bioluminescence imaging for early detection and monitoring of disease progression in a murine model of neuroblastoma. J Pediatr Surg. 2007;42:1172–9.
128. Joseph J-M, Gross N, Lassau N, Rouffiac V, Opolon P, Laudani L, Auderset K, Geay J-F, Mühlethaler-Mottet A, Vassal G. In vivo echographic evidence of tumoral vascularization and microenvironment interactions in metastatic orthotopic human neuroblastoma xenografts. Int J Cancer. 2005;113:881–90.
129. Sartelet H, Durrieu L, Fontaine F, Nyalendo C, Haddad E. Description of a new xenograft model of metastatic neuroblastoma using NOD/SCID/Il2rg null (NSG) mice. Vivo Athens Greece. 2012;26:19–29.
130. Hidalgo M, Amant F, Biankin AV, et al. Patient-derived xenograft models: an emerging platform for translational cancer research. Cancer Discov. 2014;4:998–1013.
131. Stewart E, Federico SM, Chen X, et al. Orthotopic patient-derived xenografts of paediatric solid tumours. Nature. 2017;549:96–100.
132. Ben-David U, Ha G, Tseng Y-Y, et al. Patient-derived xenografts undergo mouse-specific tumor evolution. Nat Genet. 2017;49:1567–75.
133. Wang K, Diskin SJ, Zhang H, et al. Integrative genomics identifies LMO1 as a neuroblastoma oncogene. Nature. 2011;469:216–20.
134. Oldridge DA, Wood AC, Weichert-Leahey N, et al. Genetic predisposition to neuroblastoma mediated by a LMO1 super-enhancer polymorphism. Nature. 2015;528:418–21.
135. Zhu S, Zhang X, Weichert-Leahey N, et al. LMO1 Synergizes with MYCN to Promote Neuroblastoma Initiation and Metastasis. Cancer Cell. 2017;32:310–323.e5.
136. Delloye-Bourgeois C, Bertin L, Thoinet K, et al. Microenvironment-driven shift of cohesion/detachment balance within tumors induces a switch toward metastasis in neuroblastoma. Cancer Cell. 2017;32:427–443.e8.
137. Le Douarin N, Kalcheim C. The neural crest. Cambridge: Cambridge University Press; 1999.
138. Jongbloets BC, Pasterkamp RJ. Semaphorin signalling during development. Development. 2014;141:3292–7.

139. Coolen MW, Stirzaker C, Song JZ, et al. Consolidation of the cancer genome into domains of repressive chromatin by long-range epigenetic silencing (LRES) reduces transcriptional plasticity. Nat Cell Biol. 2010;12:235–46.
140. Esteller M. Epigenetic gene silencing in cancer: the DNA hypermethylome. Hum Mol Genet. 2007;16(Spec 1):R50–9.
141. Bert SA, Robinson MD, Strbenac D, Statham AL, Song JZ, Hulf T, Sutherland RL, Coolen MW, Stirzaker C, Clark SJ. Regional activation of the cancer genome by long-range epigenetic remodeling. Cancer Cell. 2013;23:9–22.
142. Henrich K-O, Bender S, Saadati M, et al. Integrative genome-scale analysis identifies epigenetic mechanisms of transcriptional deregulation in unfavorable neuroblastomas. Cancer Res. 2016;76:5523–37.
143. Hnisz D, Abraham BJ, Lee TI, Lau A, Saint-André V, Sigova AA, Hoke HA, Young RA. Super-enhancers in the control of cell identity and disease. Cell. 2013;155:934–47.
144. Saint-André V, Federation AJ, Lin CY, Abraham BJ, Reddy J, Lee TI, Bradner JE, Young RA. Models of human core transcriptional regulatory circuitries. Genome Res. 2016;26:385–96.
145. Boeva V, Louis-Brennetot C, Peltier A, et al. Heterogeneity of neuroblastoma cell identity defined by transcriptional circuitries. Nat Genet. 2017;49:1408–13.
146. van Groningen T, Koster J, Valentijn LJ, et al. Neuroblastoma is composed of two super-enhancer-associated differentiation states. Nat Genet. 2017;49:1261–6.
147. Ross RA, Spengler BA, Biedler JL. Coordinate morphological and biochemical interconversion of human neuroblastoma cells. J Natl Cancer Inst. 1983;71:741–7.
148. Bate-Eya LT, Ebus ME, Koster J, et al. Newly-derived neuroblastoma cell lines propagated in serum-free media recapitulate the genotype and phenotype of primary neuroblastoma tumours. Eur J Cancer. 2014;50:628–37.
149. Schleiermacher G, Janoueix-Lerosey I, Ribeiro A, et al. Accumulation of segmental alterations determines progression in neuroblastoma. J Clin Oncol. 2010;28:3122–30.
150. Schleiermacher G, Javanmardi N, Bernard V, et al. Emergence of new ALK mutations at relapse of neuroblastoma. J Clin Oncol. 2014;32:2727–34.
151. Schramm A, Köster J, Assenov Y, et al. Mutational dynamics between primary and relapse neuroblastomas. Nat Genet. 2015;47:872–7.

Neuroblastoma Pathology

4

Hiroyuki Shimada, Angela R. Sementa, Bruce R. Pawel, and Naohiko Ikegaki

4.1 Introduction

Peripheral neuroblastic tumors, or tumors of the neuroblastoma group, include neuroblastoma, ganglioneuroblastoma, and ganglioneuroma. As well defined by Willis [1], these are embryonal tumors of neural crest origin. Tumors in this group are composed of biologically different subsets. While biologically favorable tumors often show spontaneous regression or maturation, biologically unfavorable tumors are frequently refractory to chemotherapy/irradiation therapy and show aggressive progression. Recent advances in research indicate that molecular/genomic properties of the individual tumors are closely associated with their unique clinical behaviors [2–4]. It is important to note that tumors in this group offer one of the best models for investigating the biologically significant relationship between their genetic/molecular properties and morphological manifestations [5]. According to

H. Shimada (✉)
Department of Pathology and Pediatrics, Stanford University Medical Center, Stanford, CA, USA
e-mail: hshimada@chla.usc.edu

A. R. Sementa
U.O.C. Anatomia Patologica, Dipartimento Ricerca Traslazionale, Medicina di Laboratorio, Diagnostica e Servizi, IRCCS Istituto Giannina Gaslini, Genova, Italy
e-mail: angelaritasementa@gaslini.org; angelasementa@gaslini.org

B. R. Pawel
Department of Pathology & Laboratory Medicine, Children's Hospital of Philadelphia, University of Pennsylvania Perelman School of Medicine, Philadelphia, PA, USA
e-mail: pawelb@email.chop.edu

N. Ikegaki
Department of Anatomy & Cell Biology, College of Medicine, University of Illinois at Chicago, Chicago, IL, USA
e-mail: ikegaki@uic.edu

S. Sarnacki, L. Pio (eds.), *Neuroblastoma*,
https://doi.org/10.1007/978-3-030-18396-7_4

our experience of COG (Children's Oncology Group) Neuroblastoma studies, biologically favorable tumors tend to remain biologically favorable, and biologically unfavorable tumors tend to remain biologically unfavorable during the clinical course of individual patients. Accordingly, determining the histological/biological characteristics of the tumors at the time of diagnosis is critical for patient stratification and appropriate protocol assignment. With regard to biologically unfavorable tumors, however, molecular characteristics detected at the time of diagnosis may not necessarily be the same as those seen at the time of recurrence.

4.2 Historical Considerations

The first pathology description of a tumor we now recognize as neuroblastoma was, perhaps not surprisingly, provided by the groundbreaking German pathologist, Rudolph Virchow. In his 1864 treatise "Hyperplasie der Zirbel und der Nebennieren," he described a childhood abdominal tumor, suggested that the tumor was of neural origin, and diagnosed it as a "glioma" [6]. Dalton, in 1885, was the first to publish a case with such microscopic detail that we can confidently diagnose it as a neuroblastoma, despite his diagnosis of "lymphosarcoma" [7]. Interestingly, it was Dalton, and not James Homer Wright (see below), who first gave attention to neurites and the neuroblastic rosette, writing that "cells are mingled with a peculiar finely-granular and, in places, perhaps slightly fibrillated substance. In some places the round cells are scattered uniformly through this material; in others they are arranged around the borders of a small mass of it, something like the nuclei of a giant cell" [7, 8].

Six years after Dalton, the German pathologist Felix Marchand contributed to our understanding of neuroblastoma by observing that neuroblastoma cells were histologically similar to developing cells of the fetal sympathetic ganglia and moreover suggesting that mature ganglion cells develop from the more undifferentiated tumor cells [9]. However, the theory that neuroblastomas arose from sympathetic neural precursors (neuroblasts) was not universally accepted, with many still believing the tumors to be sarcomas or holding to Virchow's original idea of glial origin. It was James Homer Wright, director of pathology at Massachusetts General Hospital, who effectively disposed of both the sarcoma and glial origin theories. In his 1910 landmark paper "Neurocytoma or neuroblastoma, a kind of tumor not generally recognized," he described and illustrated histologic features of twelve cases he personally observed or studied from the literature. Wright championed the neuroblastic lineage theory of origin by emphasizing that (1) the fibrillar material did not stain like neuroglia or collagen, (2) tumor cells associated with neuropil had similar morphology to sympathetic nervous system/adrenal medulla precursors, and (3) tumor architecture often mimicked the architecture of the sympathetic nervous system at various stages of development [10]. He provided a detailed description of the neuroblastic rosettes, which had been previously described by Dalton and others [7, 11], and due to the greater impact of his paper, these henceforth became known as Homer Wright "pseudo" rosettes. Wright was also the first to use the term "neuroblastoma" to describe these tumors [8].

Following Wright's influential paper, a flurry of manuscripts provided support for the embryonic sympathetic neuroblast origin of neuroblastoma, tracing transitional forms between neuroblasts and mature ganglion cells [12–14]. In 1913, Herxheimer, using silver impregnation techniques, demonstrated that neuropil in neuroblastoma was composed of primitive nerve fibers arising from tumor cells [15]. Building upon observations of others that these tumors often had mixed histology, with both malignant neuroblastic and benign ganglioneuromatous components, Robertson in 1915 suggested the term ganglioneuroblastoma to include mixed types with large amounts of embryonic tissue [16].

The relationship between neuroblastoma and ganglioneuroma was further elucidated by Cushing and Wolbach in 1927, with their description of an extradural neuroblastoma that, over a period of 10 years, matured into a benign ganglioneuroma [17]. That tumor, extensively sampled, showed no evidence of any residual malignant neuroblastic component. Wolbach described it as solely composed of ganglion cells, Schwann cells, and "capsular" or fibroblastic cells. Although the initial tumor was treated with Coley's (bacterial) toxins, a standard treatment at the time, the authors could not ascribe the tumor's maturation to treatment effect. By 1940, the relationship between the forms of peripheral neuroblastic tumors was firmly established, and, as described by Willis, "every ganglioneuroma must have begun as a neuroblastoma, and every nerve cell tumour which is still growing, however mature most of its cells, must still contain immature neuroblasts, i.e. must be a ganglioneuroblastoma" [1].

Concurrent with increased knowledge of the histologic and embryologic underpinnings of neuroblastomas and ganglioneuromas came better understanding of clinical behavior. As early as 1910 and 1917, the propensity of neuroblastoma to cause massive liver involvement in infants (Pepper syndrome) [18] and to metastasize to the orbits and skull (Hutchinson syndrome) [19] was described. The first half of the twentieth century also saw vast improvements in surgical techniques, as well as the introduction of ancillary diagnostic testing techniques for neuroblastoma, such as urine catecholamine metabolite analysis, first described in 1957 [20]. This period also saw the introduction of modern chemotherapy and radiation therapy techniques. Despite these advances, it was not until the second half of the century that histologic grading began to be applied for prognostic purposes. In 1968, Beckwith and Martin proposed a four-tier grading system, ranging from Grade I (predominantly differentiated) to Grade IV (undifferentiated). Despite a limited dataset gleaned from one institutional tumor registry, they were able to recognize that differentiation played an important part in prognosis, but were still unable to fully account for the more favorable outcome in infancy [21].

The next 15 years witnessed advances in the understanding of neuroblastoma biology, including the establishment of the first staging system and elucidation of Stage 4S neuroblastoma, as well as the first observations of neuroblastoma cytogenetics, with descriptions of gene amplification, chromosome 1p deletions, and discovery of the *MYCN* oncogene. However, it was not until 1984 that a histopathology classification schema that correlated well with clinical behavior was introduced by Shimada and colleagues [22]. In 1999, the International Neuroblastoma Pathology

Classification (INPC), based upon Shimada system, was established, and it is this system which is still in use for neuroblastoma grading. As described in greater detail later in the chapter, the INPC subdivides tumors into either favorable or unfavorable categories, based upon patient age on diagnosis, degree of neuroblastic differentiation, content of Schwannian stroma, and mitosis-karyorrhexis index [5, 23].

With the advent of the age of "personalized" medicine in the last few decades, pathologic evaluation of neuroblastomas, as with many other tumor types, has broadened to include molecular analysis. Careful histopathologic characterization remains critically important, but can no longer be considered sufficient. Interrogation of *MYCN* amplification status and ploidy has been a standard since the 1980s, and more recently molecular diagnostics has opened avenues to novel therapies, an example being the discovery of *ALK* as the main familial neuroblastoma gene [24, 25]. So, while the modern pathologist dealing with a neuroblastoma still uses many of the same nineteenth-century tools of Virchow, he or she must also be prepared to carefully triage and preserve valuable tumor tissue for twenty-first-century molecular studies.

4.3 Pathology Diagnosis

4.3.1 Tumor Sampling/Handling

At the time of biopsy/surgery, it is critical to secure enough material for histological examination, so that pathologists are able not only to make the correct diagnosis but also to classify the individual cases into Favorable Histology Group or Unfavorable Histology Group (please see Sect. 4.4). To determine the molecular characteristics of a given tumor, it is important to save snap-frozen material. Making touch preparations is also recommended for *MYCN* and other analyses, such as segmental chromosomal losses/gains, by means of the FISH (fluorescence-based in situ hybridization) method.

4.3.2 Differential Diagnosis

It is beyond the scope of this chapter to describe the molecular tests used for the differential diagnosis of soft tissue tumors in general in the pediatric age group. For practical purposes in routine surgical pathology, immunohistochemical stains can be utilized to support/confirm the diagnosis of neuroblastoma. Historically, many laboratories used neuronal markers (NSE, PGP9.5, synaptophysin, chromogranin, CD56, etc.) and so-called neuroblastoma marker (NB84). However, these markers are not specific/reliable for neuroblastoma diagnosis. For example, these neuronal markers are positive for tumors of neuronal phenotype, such as Ewing/PNET. On the other hand, markers for neural crest tumors with neuronal and neuroendocrine differentiation, which include TH (tyrosine hydroxylase; cytoplasmic stain) and Phox2b (nuclear stain), are more specific for neuroblastoma diagnosis

[26–28]. Of these two neural crest markers, Phox2b is more stable and can be used for the staining of bone and bone marrow samples after decalcification [29]. Furthermore, Phox2b is more sensitive than TH, and is positive for all neuroblastomas, including the undifferentiated subtype [29, 30]. In contrast, in some tumors of the undifferentiated subtype, TH is positive only in sporadic cells, or may even be negative. It should be noted that both Phox2b and TH are positive for neural crest tumors of neuroendocrine differentiation, i.e., pheochromocytomas and paragangliomas [30]. It is also important to note that neuroblastomas are usually negative for muscle markers, lymphoma markers, keratins, and CD99. However, rare neuroblastomas can be positive for vimentin, and even for desmin.

4.4 International Neuroblastoma Pathology Classification (INPC)

The International Neuroblastoma Pathology Classification (INPC), which classifies individual cases into Favorable Histology Group or Unfavorable Histology Group, is applied only to tumor specimens obtained before chemotherapy/irradiation therapy is started [5, 23]. After chemotherapy, tumor samples, especially of biologically unfavorable cases, show acute chemotherapy effects, such as large areas of necrosis and extensive hemosiderin deposition. Cytological/morphological changes of the tumors after chemotherapy, which could mainly represent epigenetic phenomena, are often unreliable in predicting the clinical behaviors of individual tumors. However, we should conduct further study on recurrent tumors, since they could demonstrate different genetic/molecular characteristics from those detected at the time of diagnosis due possibly to clonal selection/evolution or long-term therapy effects during the individual clinical courses.

4.4.1 Histological Categories and Subtypes

The International Neuroblastoma Pathology Classification distinguishes four categories in this group of tumors. The first three categories, i.e., Neuroblastoma (Schwannian stroma-poor), Ganglioneuroblastoma, Intermixed (Schwannian stroma-rich), and Ganglioneuroma (Schwannian stroma-dominant), represent the morphologically defined maturational sequences according to the grade of neuroblastic differentiation and the degree of Schwannian stromal development [5, 23, 31]. We believe that all ganglioneuromas were once neuroblastomas in their early stage of tumor development. Tumor maturation from Neuroblastoma to Ganglioneuroma is prompted by the "cross-talk" supported by various signaling pathways, including TrkA/NGF signaling and Nrg1/ErbB signaling [32–34], between neuroblasts and Schwannian stromal cells. The fourth category is Ganglioneuroblastoma, Nodular (composite, Schwannian stroma-rich/stroma-dominant and stroma-poor), which is defined as multi-clonal tumor.

1. Neuroblastoma (Schwannian stroma-poor)—NB: Tumors in this category include three subtypes: undifferentiated, poorly differentiated, and differentiating. NBs are characterized by the typical growth pattern of neuroblastic cells, which form groups or nests demarcated by thin fibrovascular stromal tissue septa. In these tumors, no or limited (<50% of tumor tissue) Schwannian cell proliferation/development is observed.
   (a) Neuroblastoma, undifferentiated (NB-UD) subtype is rare and supplementary procedures, such as immunohistochemistry and/or molecular tests, are required in order to establish the diagnosis. As mentioned above, positive Phox2b immunostaining can be useful to support the diagnosis. The proliferating cells are uniformly primitive, without clearly recognizable neurite formation (Fig. 4.1a). NB-UD is often associated with biologically unfavorable indicators, such as *MYCN* oncogene amplification, diploid pattern, and/or 1pLOH.
   (b) Neuroblastoma, poorly differentiated (NB-PD) subtype is the most common histological form among the peripheral neuroblastic tumors, and is composed of neuroblasts which display varying amounts of neurite production, with or without Homer Wright rosette formation. It is important to note that neurites are not "stroma," but are cytoplasmic extensions from the tumor cell bodies. By definition, less than 5% of tumor cells have cytomorphological features of differentiating neuroblasts [see (c) NB-D]. Neuroblasts in this subtype are often described as having "salt-and-pepper" (sprinkles of heterochromatin and a few inconspicuous nucleoli) nuclei (Fig. 4.1b). It should be noted, however, that some tumors in this subtype, and more in the undifferentiated subtype, show the presence of one to few prominent nucleoli (nucleolar hypertrophy), especially when the *MYCN* oncogene is amplified (Fig. 4.1c).
   (c) Neuroblastoma, differentiating (NB-D) subtype is often characterized by the presence of abundant neurites. By definition, more than 5% of tumor cells in this subtype have an appearance of differentiating neuroblasts (Fig. 4.1d). These differentiating neuroblasts are defined by synchronous differentiation of both the nucleus (enlarged, eccentrically located with a vesicular chromatin pattern and usually a single prominent nucleolus) and the cytoplasm (eosinophilic/amphophilic with a diameter of twice that of the nucleus, or more). Nissl substance can be seen in the periphery of the cytoplasm.
2. Ganglioneuroblastoma, Intermixed (Schwannian stroma-rich)—GNB-I: This is a transitional form between Neuroblastoma and Ganglioneuroma. Tumors in this category have a ganglioneuromatous appearance, but contain well-defined microscopic nests of neuroblastic cells whose neuritic processes around their cell bodies are still naked and not covered with Schwannian stromal cells. These nests are composed of a mixture of neuroblastic cells in various stages of differentiation, often dominated by differentiating neuroblasts (Fig. 4.1e). Some apoptotic cells may also be seen in the nests. The nests are intermixed or randomly distributed in the ganglioneuromatous tissue, i.e., Schwannian stroma containing individually embedded ganglion cells. By definition, more than 50%

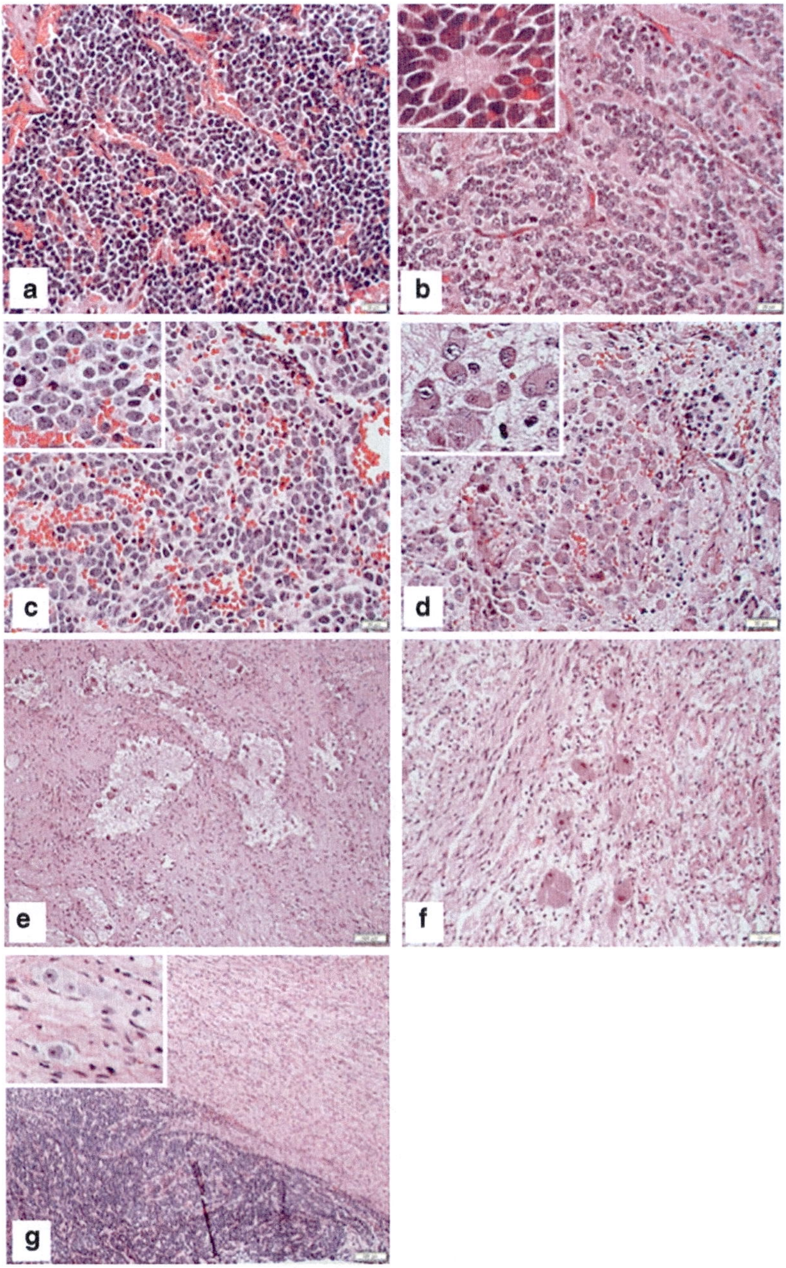

Fig. 4.1 Histological features of peripheral neuroblastic tumors: Neuroblastoma, undifferentiated subtype (**a**); Neuroblastoma, poorly differentiated subtype (**b**, inset—Homer Wright rosette); *MYCN*-amplified neuroblastoma showing an appearance of poorly differentiated subtype with a high mitosis-karyorrhexis index (**c**, inset—neuroblasts with nucleolar hypertrophy); Neuroblastoma, differentiating subtype (**d**, inset—high-power view of differentiating neuroblasts); Ganglioneuroblastoma, Intermixed (**e**); Ganglioneuroma (**f**); and Ganglioneuroblastoma, Nodular (**g**, inset—ganglion cells in ganglioneuromatous component)

of tumor tissue should have a ganglioneuromatous appearance with Schwannian proliferation/development (Schwannian stroma-rich) in this category. Otherwise, the tumor should be called Neuroblastoma (Schwannian stroma-poor). GNB-I is regarded as one step behind of the final tumor maturation (Ganglioneuroma—GN; see below), and both GNB-I and GN invariably display a biologically and clinically benign behavior [35, 36].

3. Ganglioneuroma (Schwannian stroma-dominant)—GN: Tumors in this category are characterized by the presence of individually distributed ganglion cells in Schwannian stroma (Fig. 4.1f). Since the neuritic processes produced by these ganglion cells are immediately incorporated into the cytoplasm of Schwannian stromal cells, there are no recognizable naked neurites without Schwannian coverage. Two subtypes, maturing and mature, are included in this category. The maturing subtype contains both maturing and mature ganglion cells, whereas the mature subtype contains only mature ganglion cells covered with satellite cells. The stromal portion is usually well organized and shows a fascicular profile of Schwann cells bundled with perineurial cells.
4. Ganglioneuroblastoma, Nodular (composite, Schwannian stroma-rich/stroma-dominant and stroma-poor)—GNB-N: The term "composite" implies that the tumor in this category is made up of biologically different histological components (clones). Tumors are characterized by the presence of grossly visible, often hemorrhagic and/or necrotic, NB nodule(s) (stroma-poor component), co-existing with GNB-I (stroma-rich component) or with GN (stroma-dominant component) (Fig. 4.1g).

4.4.2 Prognostic Grouping (Favorable Histology vs. Unfavorable Histology)

The INPC classifies two prognostic groups, Favorable Histology Group and Unfavorable Histology Group (Fig. 4.2) [5, 23, 31, 37]. In order to distinguish these two groups, each tumor is evaluated and placed either within or outside an age-appropriate framework defined by morphological indicators. Morphological indicators used in this classification are tumor differentiation/maturation and mitotic and karyorrhectic activities. With regard to tumor differentiation/maturation, the categories and subtypes described above are utilized. Another morphological indicator, mitotic and karyorrhectic activities of neuroblastic cells, is applied only to tumors in the NB category [38]. On the basis of these activities, each NB tumor is assigned to one of three MKI (mitosis-karyorrhexis index) classes: Low (<100/5000 cells), Intermediate (100–200/5000 cells), and High (>200/5000 cells). Determination of MKI class is based on averaging the activities by counting mitotic and karyorrhectic cells in multiple representative microscopic fields. In other words, MKI class is not determined by counting the activities from the hottest, i.e., most condensed, fields. Cells with nuclear fragmentation (i.e., karyorrhectic) are included in the counting, while simply hyperchromatic (darkly stained) nuclei are not included.

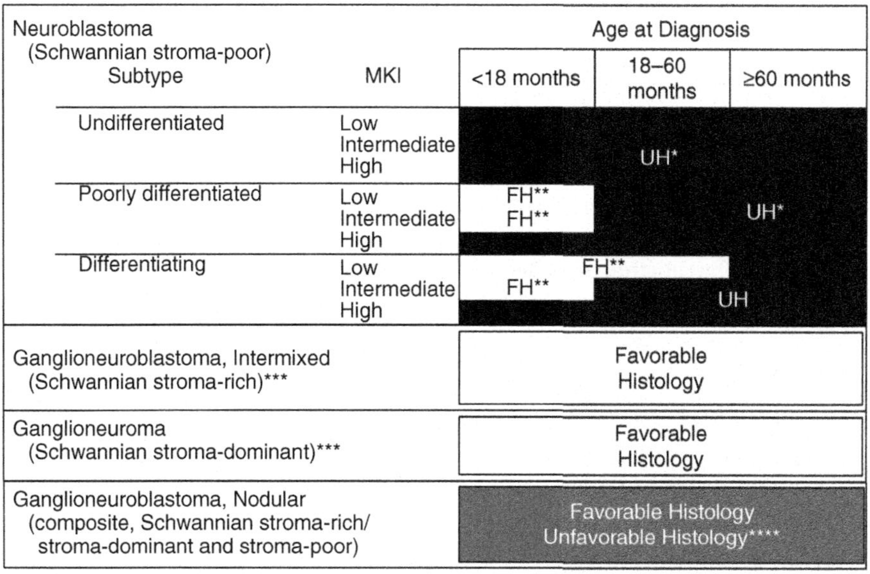

Fig. 4.2 International Neuroblastoma Pathology Classification: ∗UH (black areas in Neuroblastoma category) = Unfavorable Histology; ∗∗FH (white areas in Neuroblastoma category) = Favorable Histology; ∗∗∗Ganglioneuroblastoma, Intermixed and Ganglioneuroma are usually diagnosed in older children and young adults and associated with an excellent prognosis; ∗∗∗∗Prognosis of Ganglioneuroblastoma, Nodular depends on the characteristics of neuroblastoma nodule (please see the text)

1. Favorable Histology Group: Tumors in the Favorable Histology Group can fit into an age-appropriate framework and display differentiation/maturation from NB-PD to NB-D, then to GNB-I, and finally to GN, as a result of the "cross-talk" between tumor cells and Schwannian stromal cells. In order to observe tumor differentiation/maturation, however, a certain period of time, i.e., in vivo latent period, seems to be required in each phase. The INPC defines two critical time points: "up to 18 months" from NB-PD subtype to NB-D subtype and "up to 60 months" to GNB-I or GN. In other words, even though the tumors in the Favorable Histology Group have a potential of differentiation/maturation, they follow the age-appropriate framework. Accordingly, (1) patients <18 months of age on diagnosis with NB-PD, (2) patients <60 months on diagnosis with NB-D, and (3) all GNB-I and GN (usually diagnosed in older children and young adults) fall into the Favorable Histology Group with an excellent prognosis [35, 36]. The prognostic implications of MKI are also age-dependent: (1) Low MKI tumors in patients <60 months of age on diagnosis, and (2) Intermediate MKI tumors in patients <18 months of age on diagnosis come within the framework of the Favorable Histology Group.

   GNB-I and GN tumors are generally well circumscribed. However, microscopic examination may disclose the presence of Schwannian stromal component in an "infiltrative" interface with the peri-tumoral tissues or in the inked surgical margins. Furthermore, clear and complete resection of those tumors in the para-vertebral location is not feasible due to direct adhesion to the vertebral bodies. As long as more than 95% of tumor mass is resected and no grossly visible NB nodule formation is observed, the case is evaluated GNB-I or GN in the Favorable Histology Group and has an excellent prognosis [36].

2. Unfavorable Histology Group: Tumors of the NB-UD subtype in any age group, tumors of the NB-PD subtype in patients over 18 months of age, and tumors of the NB-D subtype in those over 60 months of age are considered to have no or limited differentiating potential: they are outside the age-appropriate framework. Moreover, High MKI NB tumors in any age group, Intermediate MKI tumors ≥18 months of age at diagnosis, and Low MKI tumors ≥60 months of age at diagnosis are also outside the framework. A significant correlation between *MYCN* amplification and High MKI has been reported in NB tumors [39, 40]. Those tumors with morphology indicators outside the frame are assigned to the Unfavorable Histology Group.

   While tumors in the GNB-I and GN category are always assigned to the Favorable Histology Group [23, 35, 36], tumors in the GNB-N category are classified as belonging to either the Favorable Histology Group or the Unfavorable Histology Group, according to the characteristics of the NB nodule(s) [31]. For this purpose, the same criteria of age-linked evaluation of the grade of neuroblastic differentiation and the MKI class that are utilized for the prognostic distinction of NB tumors are applied to the NB nodule(s) in GNB-N. It should be noted here that reaching the correct diagnosis of GNB-N is often difficult on biopsy or partial tumor resection, since the NB nodule could be hidden and not sampled for pathology examination. In such situations, it is advisable to add the disclaimer "Based on Review of Limited Material" in the diagnosis line after "GN or GNB-I, Favorable Histology" in the surgical pathology report and to initiate discussion with the oncology team in order to look for possible hidden NB nodules. A hidden NB nodule may be hemorrhagic/necrotic and MIBG-avid, hence potentially identifiable by imaging study. The nodule can constitute a source of highly elevated serum/urinary VMA/HVA levels and even metastasize to the bone marrow or other sites. We have experienced multiple occasions of diagnosis change from GNB-I/GN to GNB-N after additional biopsy/surgery or even needle biopsy targeting the nodular lesion with help from radiologist colleagues.

4.4.3 Age Factor in Neuroblastoma

In neuroblastoma, the patient's age at diagnosis is one of the prognostic indicators. In the past, 1 year of age was used as the cut-off for distinguishing between groups with better (<356 days) and worse (≥365 days) prognosis. London et al. reported that (1) the prognostic contribution of age to the clinical outcome is continuous in nature: whichever age cut-off is adopted, survival rate of younger patients is always better than that of older patients, and (2) there is statistical evidence of an age cut-off greater than 1 year for risk stratification [41]. The COG is now in the process of raising the cut-off for prognostic distinction from 1 year (365 days) to 18 months (548 days). The age factor should be regarded as a surrogate for other genetic/biologic risk markers. The INPC already has a built-in age cut-off of 18 months, and Sano et al. demonstrated that the INPC was able to add independent prognostic information beyond the prognostic contribution of age [42]. In other words, the INPC clearly distinguishes two prognostic groups (Favorable Histology Group and Unfavorable Histology Group, the former identifying significantly better prognosis than the latter) in different age groups, such as < vs. ≥12 months (365 days), < vs. ≥18 months (548 days), and < vs. ≥24 months (730 days) of age at diagnosis.

4.5 Bone Marrow Involvement in Neuroblastoma

At the time of diagnosis, about 50% of peripheral neuroblastic tumors present with metastatic disease, and bone marrow (BM) is the most common site (70.5%) of tumor spread [43]. Moreover, it is a frequent site of disease recurrence. The BM tissue includes many different cell types: they are both stromal cells and hematopoietic cells. Factors that are released by these cells may play an important role in the "homing" of NB cells to the BM by creating a microenvironment favorable to the metastatic process [44]. These factors may include clusterin [45], the proto-oncoprotein c-myb, the PRAF2 oncogene [46, 47], vascular endothelial growth factor-B, and the X-linked inhibitor of apoptosis [48]. Mesenchymal stem cells (MSCs) are reported to show transcriptional upregulation of IL-6 production, following collaborative interaction with a galectin protein (Gal-3) secreted by NB cells in the BM microenvironment [49]. Recent studies have also shown that BM-infiltrating NB cells display up- or downregulation of various proteins, causing difficulty in patient management. Upregulated proteins include B7H3, CD56, c-Kit, HLA-G, and calprotectin [50, 51], and downregulated proteins include CXCL12 and other immune-regulating proteins [52].

BM involvement by NB cells at disease onset is well known to have an adverse prognostic effect. The persistence of NB cell infiltration in the BM throughout the course of the disease and after treatment is also predictive of poor outcome [53, 54]. The presence of NB cells in the BM is usually detected by means of imaging techniques, including ^{123}I-metaiodobenzylguanidine (MIBG) scintigraphy, and by morphological examination. For many years, the cytology of BM aspirates and the histology of trephine biopsies have constituted the gold standard for the assessment of neuroblastoma disease [43, 55, 56]. However, these methods have limited sensitivity, especially when the NB cell population is <10% of background cells, and could seriously underestimate the prevalence of BM infiltration [57]. Alternative and more sensitive methods of analyzing BM infiltration by NB cells have been developed in the last decade, and their potential prognostic value has been the subject of various investigations. These techniques are the flow cytometry evaluation of whole BM aspirates, the immunocytochemistry of BM mononuclear cells (MNCs), and the molecular analysis of whole BM aspirates [58] by qualitative or quantitative reverse transcriptase polymerase chain reaction (RT-PCR) [60].

With regard to flow cytometry, this method has been used to quantify NB cell content in BM aspirates. However, since the need to analyze large numbers of cells reduces its sensitivity, this approach is not currently recommended in the clinical setting [58]. The most significant improvement in the sensitivity and specificity of NB cell detection in BM aspirates is offered by immunocytology (IC) and quantitative Reverse Transcription Polymerase Chain Reaction (qRT-PCR), which have proved able to detect a single neuroblastoma cell among one million (10^6) normal cells. Most importantly, the quantitative approach provided by these two methods has shown that the percentage of NB cells detected either by IC or qRT-PCR in BM is predictive of outcome.

In 2017, an article entitled "Recommendations for the Standardization of Bone Marrow Disease Assessment and Reporting in Children with Neuroblastoma on Behalf of the International Neuroblastoma Response Criteria Bone Marrow Working Group" [57] presented detailed guidelines for collecting and analyzing BM samples in neuroblastoma. It should be noted that these are designed mainly for the evaluation of the response of BM disease during the clinical course of NB patients. These recommendations are briefly summarized below:

4.5.1 Sample Collection for Testing

Representative bilateral core needle biopsies for histology/immunohistochemistry (IHC) and bilateral bone marrow aspirates for cytology, IC, and qRT-PCR are taken from all children at the time of diagnosis and, in high-risk children, at the time of response assessment at the end of induction therapy. In very young or small infants, core needle biopsies are not recommended, as the size and quality of the biopsy is unlikely to be adequate for analysis. When there is insufficient aspirate to complete all analyses, the priority for investigations is cytology, followed by qRT-PCR, and, finally, IC.

4.5.2 Trephine Biopsies

The recommendation is to report the estimated percentage areas occupied by tumor cells in marrow spaces, in order to minimize the errors that arise when the number of hematopoietic cells (background or denominator of non-NB nucleated cells) is reduced (hypoplastic marrow) after chemotherapy. Tumor histology should be classified as undifferentiated, poorly differentiated, or differentiating subtype (Fig. 4.3a, b). In rare cases, metastatic tumors may display ganglioneuromatous maturation. MKI class is not evaluated in the BM sample, since the amount of tumor tissue is usually insufficient for determination, and mitotic and karyorrhectic activities are not always the same as those seen in extra-BM tumor tissue in the same patient.

Although it is generally accepted that NB cells can be identified more accurately in BM biopsies than in aspirates, it is recommended that analysis of both should be performed in order to achieve the most accurate interpretation of BM disease. Besides H&E staining, IHC with at least two antibodies should be performed in order to detect NB cells in the biopsy specimen. With regard to the IHC test, it is

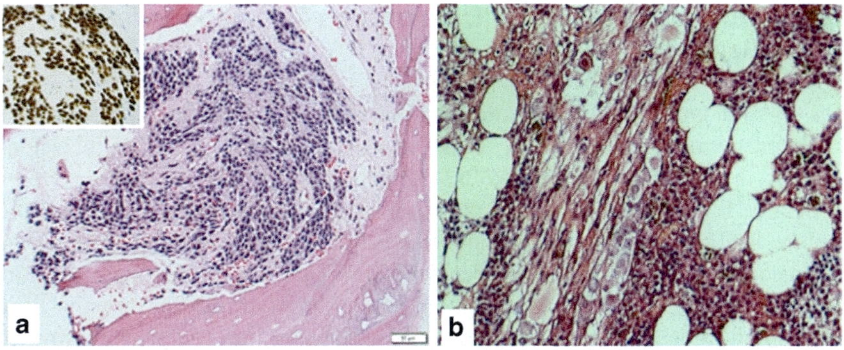

Fig. 4.3 Histology of bone marrow trephine. Metastatic tumor with poorly differentiated subtype (**a** H&E stain, inset—positive nuclear stain for Phox2b, immunostain). Infiltration by differentiating neuroblasts in a post-chemotherapy sample (**b** H&E stain)

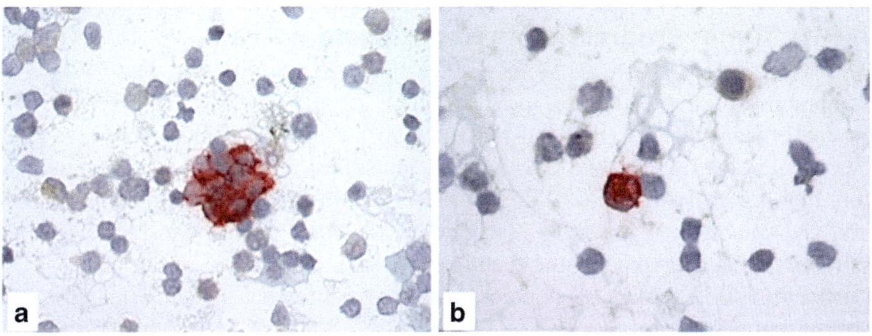

Fig. 4.4 Immunocytology (IC) on bone marrow aspirate stained for anti-GD2. A clump of criteria-positive cells (**a** immunostain) and a single positive cell (**b** immunostain)

strongly recommended that anti-Phox2b antibody be used for NB cell detection (*please see* Fig. 4.3a, *inset*). A BM biopsy is regarded as negative for tumor in the absence of NB cells after reviewing both H&E and IHC slides.

In reporting the results of BM trephine biopsy analysis, a threshold of 5% BM infiltration is considered to be the attainable level of reliable tumor detection. A new category of minimal disease is defined by the presence of BM infiltration ≤5%. Cases falling into this category may hopefully benefit from the timely introduction of emerging therapies that may prove effective in the long term.

4.5.3 Immunocytology (IC)

It should be stressed that, in order to reach a sensitivity of one neuroblastoma cell in 1×10^6 MNCs, IC should be reported on 3×10^6 MNCs per aspirate, using a monoclonal anti-GD2 disialoganglioside antibody, namely, the clone 14G2a. We refer the reader to the published criteria for the reliable light-microscopy identification of NB cells on immunocytochemically stained slides (Fig. 4.4) [59, 60].

4.5.4 Quantitative Reverse Transcription Polymerase Chain Reaction (qRT-PCR)

It is recommended that RNA extracted from BM aspirates taken on diagnosis be amplified by means of qRT-PCR for the expression of at least the neuroblastoma mRNAs, including tyrosine hydroxylase and Phox2b [61, 62].

Finally, BM infiltrated by NB cells is an excellent source of material for tumor genome analysis. For example, results of genomic profiling by SNP array for disseminated NB cells in BM have been reported [63]. High-throughput mutation analysis using next-generation sequencing technology is suitable for formalin-fixed, paraffin-embedded material of various solid tumors [64, 65] and bone marrow trephines [66] in NB cases. The availability of archival material from BM trephine biopsies from patients with metastatic NB may enormously expand the potential for such analyses.

4.6 Tumor Progression in Neuroblastoma

Importantly, the survival rate of the FH group is estimated to be around or over 90%, whereas that of the UH group has remained 50–40% or less [23, 37, 42]. This indicates that at least one in two UH group patients dies from the disease, despite current high-intensity multimodal therapy. Detailed information of clinical behaviors and genomic/molecular factors associated with tumor progression is provided in other sections, and some of the factors are briefly listed here. First of all, *MYCN* oncogene amplification has been reported to be the strongest indicator of aggressive neuroblastoma progression [67]. *MYCN* amplification also causes genetic instability in NB cells, leading to secondary genetic aberrations at the chromosomal level. Some of these aberrations may further support tumor progression and metastasis [68]. Apart from *MYCN* amplification, other chromosomal alterations in NB cells, such as loss of chromosome 1p, 3p, or 11q and the unbalanced gain of chromosome 17q, appear to promote tumor progression and increase the metastatic potential of NB cells [69–72]. Overexpression of TrkB, whose preferred ligand is the brain-derived neurotrophic factor, is reported to upregulate several matrix metalloproteinases (MMPs) and serine proteases, such as urokinase and tissue plasminogen activators. These proteases contribute to the invasiveness of NB cells by degrading the extracellular matrix [73].

4.7 New Directions of Neuroblastoma Pathology Research

New innovative therapeutic approaches are needed for those in the UH group. To address this problem, we have been attempting to identify the expression of potentially drug-targetable proteins that appear to lay the foundation for the aggressive behavior of certain neuroblastomas existing in the UH group. We are aiming to refine the current INPC by incorporating immunohistochemical detection/evaluation of these target proteins and to develop a more precise system of pathology classification for future patient stratification and protocol assignment.

4.7.1 Potential "Actionable/Druggable" Targets in Neuroblastoma

1. ALK (anaplastic lymphoma kinase) overexpression: ALK is a receptor tyrosine kinase and expressed in the developing sympathoadrenal lineage of the neural crest. In neuroblastoma, mutations in the *ALK* gene account for the majority of familial neuroblastoma cases [25]. *ALK* mutations/overexpression and amplification are also found in around 10% of sporadic neuroblastoma cases [74, 75]. *ALK* abnormalities (mutations and amplification) resulting in its protein overexpression seem to cause dysregulation of multiple pathways, including the PI3K, AKT, MEKK3, and MEK5 signaling transduction pathways, allowing uncontrolled proliferation of neuroblasts [76]. In addition, *ALK* gene amplification and F1174 mutations, which are among the most active forms of the mutations in in vitro assay, are associated with MYCN amplification [77]. However, the prognostic significance of *ALK* mutations/overexpression has been controversial, and although ALK protein overexpression can be associated with neuroblastoma aggressiveness, it may not be an independent prognostic factor. Passoni et al. first reported immunohistochemical detection of ALK protein in neuroblastoma, and higher levels of the expression were associated with adverse outcome of the disease in 2009 [78]. However, Regairaz M et al. later showed that the expression of ALK and its active form pALK were observed immunohistochemically in many neuroblastomas independently from *ALK* mutation/amplification [79].
2. MYC family protein overexpression: *MYCN* oncogene is considered a major oncogenic driver of neuroblastoma. *MYCN* amplification is seen in approximately 20% of all neuroblastomas, and the vast majority of *MYCN*-amplified tumors overexpress MYCN protein. Notably, MYC (aka C-Myc) protein overexpression is not associated with *MYCN* amplification and is observed in ~10% of all neuroblastomas. Since *MYC* oncogene amplification seems extremely rare in neuroblastoma [80], further studies are indicated to determine the mechanism(s) of MYC protein overexpression in this disease [81]. Apparently, MYCN/MYC-MAX protein heterodimers both activate downstream molecular targets through binding to E-box sequences, which consequently leads to aggressive tumor growth. Indeed, patients with neuroblastomas expressing immunohistochemically detectable and higher level of MYC family protein (MYCN and MYC) expression exhibit dismal outcome, and therefore we have defined these neuroblastomas as "MYC family-driven neuroblastomas." Histologically, these neuroblastoma cells often show prominent nucleolar formation (nucleolar hypertrophy) [82], which is indicative of hyperactive rRNA synthesis and protein translation (Fig. 4.5a, b). The extreme form of the "MYC family-driven neuroblastoma" displays large cell appearance with bull's-eye-like vesicular nuclei containing

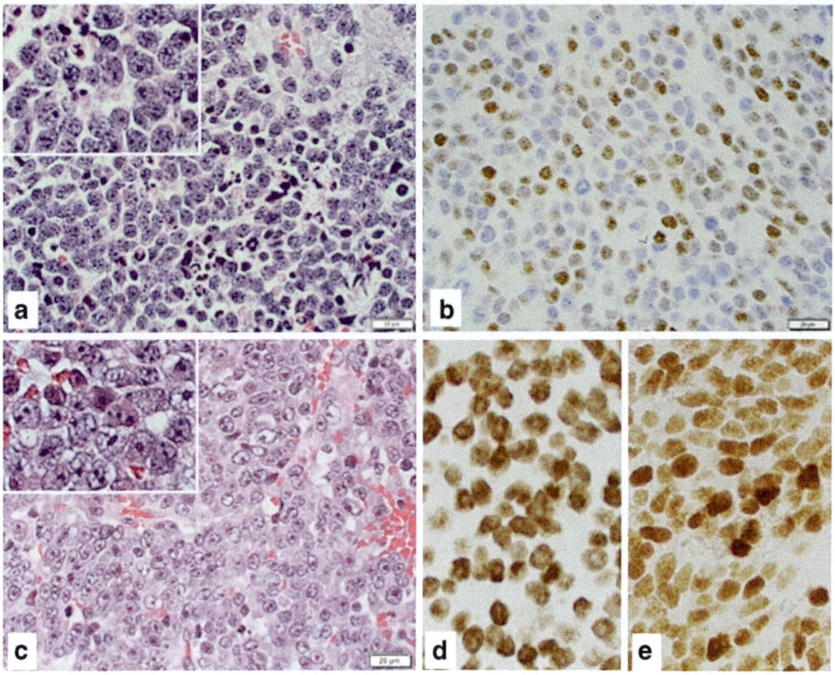

Fig. 4.5 MYC family-driven neuroblastomas: MYC protein overexpressing neuroblastoma (**a** H&E stain, inset—neuroblasts with nucleolar hypertrophy. **b** immunostain for MYC protein); large cell neuroblastoma (**c** H&E stain, inset—neuroblasts with vesicular nuclei and prominent nucleoli. **d** immunostain for Phox2b. **e** immunostain for MYCN protein)

one to few very prominent nucleoli [83] (Fig. 4.5c–e). Large cell neuroblastoma is also reported to express augmented stem cell markers [84].

3. Telomere maintenance aberrations: In addition to the fact that MYC family protein overexpression is the driver of unfavorable and therapy-resistant neuroblastomas, recent studies have shown that telomere maintenance aberrations may account for additional mechanisms that drive therapy-resistant neuroblastomas [85–87]. Telomere maintenance and elongation could prevent neuroblasts from replication senescence and cellular death due to telomere erosion. Accordingly, neuroblasts could acquire infinite proliferating capability.
   (a) Telomere elongation by increased TERT (telomere reverse transcriptase) activity:

      Using immunohistochemical assays, we can identify tumors overexpressing TERT (Fig. 4.6a, b) in both MYC family protein-driven and non-MYC family protein-driven neuroblastomas in any age groups [88]. These observations suggest that there are multiple mechanisms for upregulation of TERT expression; it can be associated with MYCN/MYC protein overexpression, *TERT* rearrangements, or rare promoter hypermethylation [85, 86, 89].

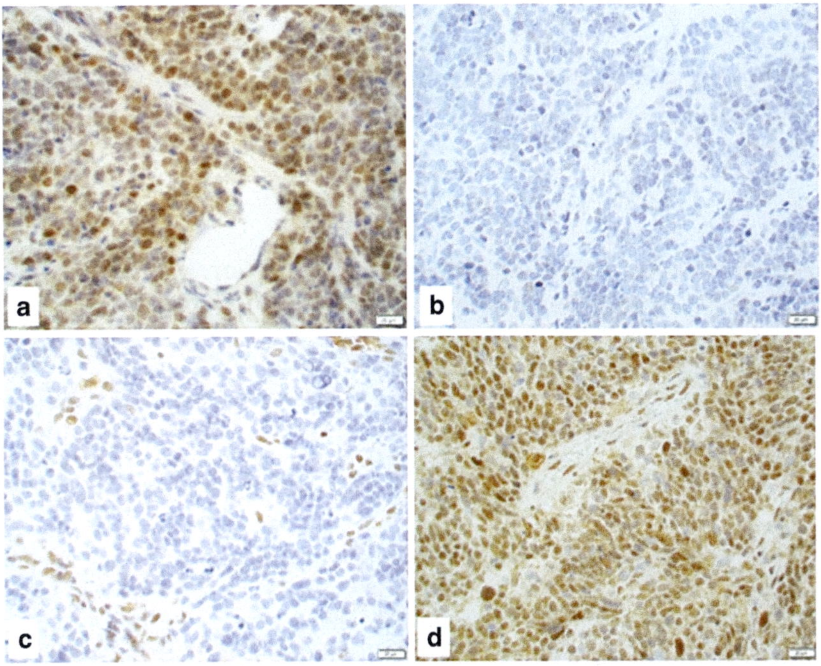

Fig. 4.6 Neuroblastomas with telomere maintenance aberration: Neuroblastoma with (**a** immunostain) or without (**b** immunostain) TERT (telomerase reverse transcriptase) overexpression. Neuroblastoma with ATRX (alpha-thalassemia/mental retardation syndrome X-linked) loss (**c** immunostain) or ATRX retained (**d** immunostain)—note ATRX is retained in the endothelial cells

(b) Alternative lengthening of telomere (ALT) by ATRX (alpha-thalassemia/mental retardation syndrome X-linked) loss: *ATRX* mutations are reported in older children with neuroblastoma (>5 years of age at diagnosis) who have a very poor prognosis [88]. These tumors are almost exclusively found in non-MYC family protein-driven neuroblastomas with Unfavorable Histology. Most of the tumors with *ATRX* mutations show the ALT phenotype [90]. *ATRX* mutations causing loss of ATRX expression can easily be detected by immunohistochemistry (Fig. 4.6c, d). It has also been reported that there are very rare neuroblastomas with *DAXX* mutations, which can also cause ALT as well [91].

4. Proposed subgroups of Unfavorable Histology neuroblastoma for "precision medicine": As we are gaining additional knowledge about the potential molecular targets that underlie the therapy-resistant phenotypes in Unfavorable Histology neuroblastoma, incorporating such information into the INPC may support "precision prognosis and therapy stratification." By using three (or four) immunohistochemical stains with anti-pan-MYC antibody (or anti-MYCN and anti-MYC), anti-TERT antibody, and anti-ATRX antibody, we are planning to classify Unfavorable Histology neuroblastomas into four subgroups. On the

basis of the proposed sub-grouping (Table 4.1), it is expected that non-responders (MYC, TERT, and ALT subgroups) to the current high-intensity multimodal therapy could be identified and separated from the responders (Null subgroup) with a high probability, prior to the initiation of therapy. Accordingly, the next question would be: "What therapeutic options could be available for the non-responder subgroups?" In the following, we will address some of these issues.

4.7.2 Molecular Targeting Therapies for Unfavorable Histology Neuroblastoma Resistant to the Current Therapy

Mutually exclusive relationships likely exist among MYC family protein overexpression, ATRX loss leading to ALT, and TERT overexpression due to *TERT* gene rearrangements, which constitute the vast majority of therapy-resistant and Unfavorable Histology tumors. Thus, targeted therapies against MYC family proteins, TERT, and ALT should improve the outcome of therapy-resistant tumors.

1. Targeting of MYC family-driven neuroblastoma. In order to develop treatment strategies for the "MYC family-driven neuroblastomas," new targets and potential therapeutic agents should be clearly defined. However, direct targeting of MYC family proteins with small molecules has turned out to be a highly formidable task [92]. Hence, many have sought indirect approaches to downregulate MYC family protein expression in cancer cells. The strategies currently under consideration include, but are not limited to, transcriptional repression of MYCN/MYC genes by BET bromodomain inhibitors [93, 94] and CDK (cyclin-dependent kinase) inhibitors [95, 96] or destabilization of MYCN by Aurora kinase A inhibitors [97].

   We have recognized that Unfavorable Histology tumors with high levels of MYC family protein expression tend to exhibit hypertrophic nucleoli [82], indicating that the tumor cells are highly active in rRNA synthesis and protein translation. Small molecule inhibitors, including CX-5461 (a potent RNA Pol I inhibitor) and halofuginone (a potent protein translation inhibitor) could therefore effectively target these pathophysiological features. As we have shown, these inhibitors in fact downregulate MYC family protein expression in neuroblastoma cells [98].
2. Targeting of TERT-overexpressing neuroblastoma: TERT is the protein component of telomerase, which also includes TERC (telomerase RNA component). For those patients with TERT-overexpressing neuroblastoma, telomerase inhibitors can be considered. Imetelstat (GRN163L) [99] potently and specifically inhibits telomerase by binding with high affinity to TERC. Interestingly, sorafenib has been shown to synergize with imetelstat to inhibit the growth of mouse xenografts of human cancer [100]. Sorafenib is a FDA-approved kinase inhibitor [101], but its synergistic effect with imetelstat appears to be due to the p21 attenuating activity [100]. Based on these observations, a combination of imetelstat and sorafenib may prove more efficacious than imetelstat alone in those neuroblastomas with elevated telomerase activity.

Table 4.1 Proposed subgroups of Unfavorable Histology neuroblastoma

		Immunohistochemistry (IHC) markers				Predicted survival based on current therapy
	Subgroups	Pan-MYC or (MYCN/MYC)	TERT	ATRX	Morphological characteristics	
MYC family protein-driven neuroblastoma	MYC (MYCN/MYC)	Overexpression	Overexpression or no overexpression	Retention	Nucleolar hypertrophy (including large cell neuroblastoma)	Dismal
Non-MYC family protein-driven neuroblastoma	TERT	No overexpression	Overexpression	Retention	Salt-and-pepper nuclei Conventional neuroblastoma	Dismal
	ALT	No overexpression	No overexpression	Loss	Salt-and-pepper nuclei Conventional neuroblastoma	Dismal
	Null	No overexpression	No overexpression	Retention	Salt-and-pepper nuclei Conventional neuroblastoma	Better response

MYC subgroup is characterized by augmented MYC family protein expression and exhibits prominent nucleolar formation and hypertrophic cell morphology. It is also expected that a considerable number of MYC family-driven neuroblastomas are associated with TERT overexpression, because *TERT* is a direct gene target of MYC family proteins, and others have little or no TERT overexpression. *TERT subgroup*: Higher levels of TERT expression are observed in this group, with low-level expression of MYC or MYCN proteins. The activation of TERT expression in this case is likely due to genomic rearrangements. *TERT* promoter hypermethylation might also be its activating mechanism. *ALT subgroup* is characterized by ATRX loss, which results in the ALT phenotype. ATRX is rarely mutated in the MYC subgroup and TERT subgroup. Because one of the normal ATRX functions is to insert the variant histone H3, namely, H3.3, into chromatin to maintain transcriptionally active euchromatin, the absence of ATRX may result in a more heterochromatic state globally. Thus, the histological appearance of the ALT subgroup could be the salt and pepper type. *Null subgroup*: There are still UH neuroblastomas without MYCN/MYC overexpression, TERT overexpression, or ATRX loss. Unless any other aggravating factors are found, patients in the Null subgroup should respond to the current high-risk treatment regimens

3. Targeting of ALT (alternative lengthening of telomere)-phenotype neuroblastoma. ALT inhibition could also be considered for those patients with neuroblastoma that have ATRX loss. However, because ATRX loss is due to structural alterations in *ATRX* gene [102], it would be difficult to regain the expression of ATRX expression in neuroblastoma. If so, is there any other way through which the ALT phenotype can be suppressed? To address this question, we need to understand the mechanism of how ATRX loss leads to ALT. It has become evident that the acquisition of the ALT phenotype utilizes the DNA replication stress response [103], which involves a cascade of events, including the obligatory activation of ATR (Ataxia Telangiectasia and Rad3 related) kinase. AZD6738 is a novel potent and selective inhibitor of ATR kinase with IC_{50} values of less than 1 μM in cell-based assays [104] and would effectively target ALT tumor cells.

4.8 Conclusions

Tumors of the neuroblastoma group are the most common extra-cranial solid tumors in the pediatric age group. Although many patients with neuroblastoma do well, those with biologically unfavorable characteristics continue to have a guarded prognosis. Currently, pathologists play a crucial role in the diagnosis and treatment of these patients by applying the International Neuroblastoma Pathology Classification (INPC) and identifying bone marrow involvement, as these are critical steps in assigning these patients to appropriate treatment regimens. In response to the challenge of treating high-risk neuroblastoma, we are prompted to explore a new direction of pathology research toward precise pathway-targeting medicine for personalized treatment options. In other words, we are shifting our focus from "Looking for Prognostic Factors" to "Searching for Actionable/Druggable Targets." In this chapter, based on our recent efforts, we propose to modify the INPC by incorporating the immunohistochemical status of potentially druggable targets, such as MYCN/MYC protein overexpression, TERT (telomerase reverse transcriptase) overexpression, and ALT (alternative lengthening of telomere) phenotype.

References

1. Willis RA. The borderland of embryology and pathology. 2nd ed. London: Butterworths; 1962.
2. Brodeur GM, Hogarty MD, Moose YP, Maris JM. Neuroblastoma. In: Pizzo PA, Poplack DG, editors. Principles and practice of pediatric oncology. Philadelphia, PA: Lippincott Williams & Wilkins; 2011. p. 886–922.
3. Bosse KR, Maris JM. Advances in the translational genomics of neuroblastoma: from improving risk stratification and revealing novel biology to identifying actionable genomic alterations. Cancer. 2016;122(1):20–33.
4. Matthay KK, Maris JM, Schleiermacher G, Nakagawara A, Mackall CL, Diller L, Weiss WA. Neuroblastoma. Nat Rev Dis Primers. 2016;2:16078.

5. Shimada H, Ambros I, Dehner PL, Hata J, Joshi VV, Roald B. Terminology and morphologic criteria of neuroblastic tumors: recommendation by the International Neuroblastoma Pathology Committee. Cancer. 1999;86(2):349–63.
6. Virchow R. Hyperplasie der Zirbel und der Nebennieren. Die Krankhaften Geschwulste, vol. 2. Berlin: Verlag von August Hirschwald; 1964–65. p. 149–50.
7. Dalton N. Infiltrating growth in liver and suprarenal capsule. Trans Path Soc Lond. 1885;XXXVI:247.
8. Lehman EP. Neuroblastoma. With report of a case. J Med Res. 1917;XXXVI:309–26.
9. Marchand F. Beitrage zur Kenntnis der normalen und pathologischen Anatomie der Glandula carotica und der Nebennieren. Internat Beitr z Wissensch Med Festschr R Virchow. 1891;6:535–81.
10. Wright JH. Neurocytoma or neuroblastoma: a kind of tumor not generally recognized. J Exp Med. 1910;12:556–61.
11. Weisel J. Bemerkungen zu der arbeit H. Kusters Virchow's Arch. 1905;clxxx:117.
12. Pick L. Das ganglioma embryonale sympatheticum. Berlin Klin Wochenschr. 1912;xlix:16.
13. Landau M. Die malignen Neuroblastome des Sympathetikus. Frank Zeitschr F Path. 1912;xi:26.
14. Wahl HR. Neuroblastomata, with a study of a case illustrating the three types. J Med Res. 1914;xxx(n.s., xxv):205.
15. Herxheimer G. Uber Tumoren des Nebennierenmarkes insbesondere das Neuroblastoma Sympathetikum. Beitr Z Path Anat U z allg Path. 1913;lvii:112.
16. Robertson HE. Das ganglioneuroblastome, ein besonderer Typus im system der Neurome. Virchows Arch. 1915;ccxx(2):147.
17. Cushing H, Wolbach SB. The transformation of a malignant paravertebral sympathicoblastoma into a benign ganglioneuroma. Am J Pathol. 1927;3:203–16.
18. Pepper W. A study of congenital sarcoma of the liver and suprarenal with the report of a case. Am J Med Sci. 1901;121:287–99.
19. Hutchinson R. Suprarenal sarcoma in children with metastases to skull. Quart J Med. 1907;1:33–8.
20. Mason GA, Hart-Mercer J, Millar EJ, Strang LB, Wynne NA. Adrenaline-secreting neuroblastoma in an infant. Lancet. 1957;273(6990):322–5.
21. Beckwith JB, Martin RF. Observations on the histopathology of neuroblastomas. J Pediatr Surg. 1968;3:106–10.
22. Shimada H, Chatten J, Newton WA Jr, Sachs N, Hamoudi AB, Chiba T, Marsden HB, Misugi K. Histopathologic prognostic factors in neuroblastic tumors: definitions of subtypes of ganglioneuroblastoma and an age-linked classification of neuroblastoma. J Nat Cancer Inst. 1984;73:405–16.
23. Shimada H, Ambros IA, Dehner LP, Hata J, Joshi VV, Roald B, Stram DO, Gerbing RB, Lukens JN, Matthay KK, Castleberry RP. The International Neuroblastoma Pathology Classification (the Shimada System). Cancer. 1999;86:364–72.
24. Brodeur GM, Seeger RC, Schwab M, Varmus HE, Bishop JM. Amplification of N-myc in untreated human neuroblastomas correlates with advanced disease stage. Science. 1984;224:1121–4.
25. Mosse YP, Laudenslager M, Longo L, Cole KA, Wood A, Attiyeh EF, Laquaglia MJ, Sennett R, Lynch JE, Perri P, Laureys G, Speleman F, Kim C, Hou C, Hakonarson H, Torkamani A, Schork NJ, Brodeur GM, Tonini GP, Pappaport E, Devoto M, Maris JM. Identification of ALK as the major familial neuroblastoma predisposition gene. Nature. 2008;455:930–5.
26. Parsons LN, Gheorghe G, Yan K, Simpson P, Jarzembowski JA. Improving detection of metastatic neuroblastoma in bone marrow core biopsies: a proposed immunohistochemical approach. Pediatr Dev Pathol. 2016;19:230–6.
27. Bielle F, Freneaux P, Jeanne-Pasquier C, Maran-Gonzalez A, Rousseau A, Lamant L, Paris R, Nicolas AV, Sastre-Garau X, Delattre O, Bourdeaut F, Peuchmaur M. PHOX2B immunolabeling: a novel tool for the diagnosis of undifferentiated neuroblastomas among childhood small round blue-cell tumors. Am J Surg Pathol. 2012;36:1141–9.

28. Hata JL, Correa H, Krishnan C, Esbenshade AJ, Black JO, Chung DH, Mobley BC. Diagnostic utility of PHOX2B in primary and treated neuroblastoma and in neuroblastoma metastatic to the bone marrow. Arch Pathol Lab Med. 2015;139:543–6.
29. Warren M, Shimada H. Importance of Phox2B immunohistochemical stain for detecting metastatic neuroblastoma cells in bone marrow specimens. Pediatr Dev Pathol. 2016;19:254–5.
30. Warren M, Tran H, Matsuno R, Shimada H. Utility of PHOX2B immunohistochemical stain in neural crest tumours and non-neural crest tumors in paedriaric pateints. Histopathology. 2018;72:685–96.
31. Peuchmaur M, d'Amore ES, Joshi VV, Hata J, Roald B, Dehner LP, Gerbing RB, Stram DO, Lukens JN, Matthay KK, Shimada H. Revision of the international neuroblastoma pathology classification: confirmation of favorable and unfavorable prognostic subsets in ganglioneuroblastoma, nodular. Cancer. 2003;98:2274–81.
32. Liu S, Tian Y, Chlenski A, Yang Q, Zage P, Salwen HR, Cohn SL. Cross-talk between Schwann cells and neuroblasts influences the biology of neuroblastoma xenografts. Am J Pathol. 2005;166:891–900.
33. Brodeur GM, Minturn JE, Ho R, Simpson AM, Iyer R, Varela CR, Light JE, Kolla V, Evans AE. Trk receptor expression and inhibition in neuroblastomas. Clin Cancer Res. 2009;15:3244–50.
34. Pajtler KW, Mahlow E, Odersky A, Lindner S, Stephan H, Bendix I, Eggert A, Schramm A, Schulte JH. Neuroblastoma in dialog with its stroma: NTRK1 is a regulator of cellular cross-talk with Schwann cells. Oncotarget. 2014;5:11180–92.
35. DeBernardi B, Gambini C, Haupt R, Granata C, Rizzo A, Conte M, Tonini GP, Bianchi M, Giuliano M, Luksch R, Prete A, Viscardi E, Garaventa A, Sementa AR, Bruzzi P, Angelini P. Retrospective study of childhood ganglioneuroma. J Clin Oncol. 2008;26:1710–6.
36. Okamatsu C, London WB, Naranjo A, Hogarty MD, Gastier-Foster JM, Look AT, LaQuaglia M, Maris JM, Cohn SL, Matthay KK, Seeger RC, Saji T, Shimada H. Clinicopathological characteristics of ganglioneuroma and ganglioneuroblastoma: a report from the CCG and COG. Pediatr Blood Cancer. 2009;53:563–9.
37. Shimada H, Umehara S, Monobe Y, Hachitanda Y, Nakagawa A, Goto S, Gerbing RB, Stram DO, Lukens JN, Matthay KK. International neuroblastoma pathology classification for prognostic evaluation of peripheral neuroblastic tumors: a report from the Children's Cancer Group. Cancer. 2001;92:2451–61.
38. Teshiba R, Kawano S, Wang LL, He L, Naranjo A, London WB, Seeger RC, Gastier-Foster JM, Look AT, Hogarty MD, Cohn SL, Maris JM, Park JR, Shimada H. Age-dependent prognostic effect by mitosis-karyorrhexis index (MKI) in neuroblastoma: a report from the Children's Oncology Group. Pediatr Dev Pathol. 2014;17:441–9.
39. Shimada H, Stram D, Chatten J, Joshi VV, Hachitanda Y, Brodeur GM, Lukens JN, Matthay KK, Seeger RC. Identification of subsets of neuroblastomas combined histopathologic and N-myc analysis. J Natl Cancer Inst. 1995;87:1470–6.
40. Goto S, Umehara S, Gerbing RB, Stram DO, Brodeur GM, Seeger RC, Lukens JN, Matthay KK, Shimada H. Histopathology and MYCN status in peripheral neuroblastic tumors: a report from the Children's Cancer Group. Cancer. 2001;92:2699–708.
41. London WB, Castleberry RP, Matthay KK, Look AT, Seeger RC, Shimada H, Thorner P, Brodeur G, Maris JM, Reynolds CP, Cohn SL. Evidence for age cutoff greater than 365 days for neuroblastoma risk group stratification in the Children's Oncology Group. J Clin Oncol. 2005;23:6459–65.
42. Sano H, Bonadio J, Gerbing RB, London WB, Matthay KK, Lukens JN, Shimada H. International neuroblastoma pathology classification adds independent prognostic information beyond the prognostic contribution of age. Eur J Cancer. 2006;42:1113–9.
43. Cohn SL, Pearson AD, London WB, Monclair T, Ambros PF, Brodeur GM, Faldum A, Hero B, Iehara T, Machin D, Mosseri V, Simon T, Garaventa A, Castel V, Matthay KK, INRG Task Force. The International Neuroblastoma Risk Group (INRG) classification system: an INRG Task Force report. J Clin Oncol. 2009;27:289–97.

44. Ara T, Song L, Shimada H, Keshelava N, Russell HV, Metelista LS, Groshen SG, Seeger RC, DeClerck YA. Interleukin-6 in the bone marrow microenvironment promotes the growth and survival of neuroblastoma cells. Cancer Res. 2009;69:329–37.
45. Morandi F, Corrias MV, Levreri I, Scaruffi P, Raffaghello L, Carlini B, Bocca P, Prigione I, Stigliani S, Amoroso L, Ferrone S, Pistoia V. Serum levels of cytoplasmic melanoma-associated antigen at diagnosis may predict clinical relapse in neuroblastoma patients. Cancer Immunol Immunother. 2011;60:1485–95.
46. Tanno B, Sesti F, Cesi V, et al. Expression of slug is regulated by c-Myb and is required for invasion and bone marrow homing of cancer cells of different origin. J Biol Chem. 2010;285:29434–45.
47. Yco LP, Geerts D, Koster J, Bachmann AS. PRAF2 stimulates cell proliferation and migration and predicts poor prognosis in neuroblastoma. Int J Oncol. 2013;42:1408–16.
48. Osman J, Galli S, Hanafy M, Tang X, Ahmed A. Identification of novel biomarkers in neuroblastoma associated with the risk for bone marrow metastasis: a pilot study. Clin Transl Oncol. 2013;15:953–8.
49. Silverman AM, Nakata R, Shimada H, Sposto R, DeClerck YA. A galectin-3-dependent pathway upregulates interleukin-6 in the microenvironment of human neuroblastoma. Cancer Res. 2012;72:2228–38.
50. Amiot L, Ferrone S, Grosse-Wilde H, Seliger B. Biology of HLA-G in cancer: a candidate molecule for therapeutic intervention? Cell Mol Life Sci. 2011;68:417–31.
51. Morandi F, Scaruffi P, Gallo F, et al. Bone Marrow infiltrating human neuroblastoma cells express high levels of calprotectin and HLA-G proteins. PLoS One. 2012;7:e299922.
52. Scaruffi P, Morandi F, Gallo F, Stigliani S, Parodi S, Moretti S, Bonassi S, Fardin P, Garaventa A, Zanazzo G, Pistoia V, Tonini GP, Corrias MV. Bone marrow of neuroblastoma patients shows down-regulation of CXCL12 expression and presence of IFN signature. Pediatr Blood Cancer. 2012;59:44–51.
53. Seeger RC, Reynolds CP, Gallego R, Stram DO, Gerbing RB, Matthay KK. Quantitative tumor cell content of bone marrow and blood as a predictor of outcome in stage IV neuroblastoma: a Children's Cancer Group study. J Clin Oncol. 2000;18:4067–76.
54. Choi YB, Bae GE, Lee NH, Kim JS, Lee SH, Yoo KH, Sung KW, Koo HH. Clinical significance of persistent tumor in bone marrow during treatment of high-risk neuroblastoma. J Korean Med Sci. 2015;30:1062–7.
55. Brodeur GM, Pritchard J, Berthold F, Carlsen NL, Castel V, Castleberry RP, De Bernardi B, Evans AE, Favrot M. Hedborg F Revisions of the international criteria for neuroblastoma diagnosis, staging, and response to treatment. J Clin Oncol. 1993;11:1466–77.
56. Monclair T, Brodeur GM, Ambros PF, Brisse PF, Cechetto G, Holmes K, Kaneko M, London WB, Matthay KK, Nuchtern JG, von Schweinitz D, Simon T, Cohn SL, Pearson AD, INRG Task Force. The International Neuroblastoma Risk Group (INRG) staging system: an INRG Task Force report. J Clin Oncol. 2009;27:298–303.
57. Burchill SA, Beiske K, Shimada H, Ambros PF, Seeger R, Tytgat GA, Brock PR, Haber M, Park JR, Berthold F. Recommendations for the standardization of bone marrow disease assessment and reporting in children with neuroblastoma on behalf of the International Neuroblastoma Response Criteria Bone Marrow Working Group. Cancer. 2017;123:1095–105.
58. Ifversen MR, Kagedal B, Christensen LD, Rechnitzer C, Petersen BL, Heilmann C. Comparison of immunocytochemistry, real-time quantitative RT-PCR and flow cytometry for detection of minimal residual disease in neuroblastoma. Int J Oncol. 2005;27:121–9.
59. Swerts K, Ambros PF, Brouzes C, Navarro JM, Gross N, Rampling D, Schumacher-Kuckelkorn R, Sementa AR, Ladenstein R, Beiske K. Standardization of the immunocytochemical detection of neuroblastoma cells in bone marrow. J Histochem Cytochem. 2005;53:1433–40.
60. Beiske K, Burchill SA, Cheung IY, Hiyama E, Seeger RC, Cohn SL, Pearson AD, Matthay KK, International Neuroblastoma Risk Group Task Force. Consensus criteria for sensitive detection of minimal neuroblastoma cells in bone marrow, blood and stem cell preparations

by immunocytology and QRT-PCR: recommendations by the International Neuroblastoma Risk Group Task Force. Br J Cancer. 2009;100:1627–37.
61. Stutterheim J, Gerritsen A, Zappeij-Kannegieter L, Kleijn I, Dee R, Hooft L, van Noesel MM, Bierings M, Berthold F, Versteeg R, Caron HN, van der Schoot CE, Tytgat GA. PHOX2B is a novel and specific marker for minimal residual disease testing in neuroblastoma. J Clin Oncol. 2008;26:5443–9.
62. Viprey VF, Corrias MV, Kagedal B, Oltra S, Swerts K, Vicha A, Ladenstein R, Burchill SA. Standardisation of operating procedures for the detection of minimal disease by QRT-PCR in children with neuroblastoma: quality assurance on behalf of SIOPEN-R-NET. Eur J Cancer. 2007;43:341–50.
63. Abbasi MR, Rifatbegovic F, Brunner C, Ladenstein R, Ambros IM, Ambros PF. Bone marrow from neuroblastoma patients: an excellent source for tumor genome analyses. Mol Oncol. 2015;9:545–54.
64. Hadd AG, Houghton J, Choudhary A, Sah S, Chen L, Marko AC, Sanford T, Buddavarapu K, Krosting J, Garmire L, Wylie D, Shinde R, Beaudenon S, Alexander EK, Mambo E, Adai AT, Latham GJ. Targeted, high-depth next-generation sequencing of cancer genes in formalin-fixed, paraffin-embedded and fine-needle aspiration tumor specimens. J Mol Diagn. 2013;15:234–47.
65. Kerick M, Isau M, Timmermann B, Sueltmann H, Herwig R, Krobitsch S, Schaefer G, Verdorfer I, Bartsch G, Klocker H, Lehrach H, Schweiger MR. Targeted high-throughput sequencing in clinical cancer settings: formaldehyde-fixed, paraffin-embedded (FFPE) tumor tissues, input amount and tumour heterogeneity. BMC Med Genomics. 2011;4:68.
66. Hasemeier B, Geffers R, Bartels S, Schlegelberger B, Kreipe H, Lehmann U. Archival bone marrow trephines are suitable for high-throughput mutation analysis using next generation sequencing technology. Haematologica. 2013;98:e115–6.
67. Schwab M. Amplification of N-myc as a prognostic marker for patients with neuroblastoma. Semin Cancer Biol. 1993;4:13–8.
68. Wan TS, Ma ES, Chan GC, Chan LC. Investigation of MYCN status in neuroblastoma by fluorescence in situ hybridization. Int J Mol Med. 2004;14:981–7.
69. Caron H, van Sluis P, de Kraker J, Boekkerink J, Egeler M, Laureys G, Slater R, Westerveld A, Voute PA, Versteer R. Allelic loss of chromosome 1p as a predictor of unfavorable outcome in patients with neuroblastoma. N Engl J Med. 1996;334:225–30.
70. Ejeskaer K, Aburatani H, Abrahamsson J, Kogner P, Martinsson T. Loss of heterozygosity of 3p markers in neuroblastoma tumours implicate a tumour-suppressor locus distal to the FHIT gene. Br J Cancer. 1998;77:1787–91.
71. Luttikhuis ME, Powell JE, Rees SA, Genus T, Chughtai S, Ramani P, Mann JR, McConville CM. Neuroblastomas with chromosome 11q loss and single copy MYCN comprise a biologically distinct group of tumours with adverse prognosis. Br J Cancer. 2001;85:531–7.
72. Bown N, Cotterill S, Lastowska M, et al. Gain of chromosome arm 17q and adverse outcome in patients with neuroblastoma. N Engl J Med. 1999;340:1954–61.
73. Hecht M, Schulte JH, Eggert A, Wilting J, Schweigerer L. The neurotrophin receptor TrkB cooperates with c-Met in enhancing neuroblastoma invasiveness. Carcinogenesis. 2005;26:2105–15.
74. Chmielecki J, Bailey M, He J, Elvin J, Vergilio JA, Ramkissoon S, Suh J, Frampton GM, Sun JX, Morley S, Spritz D, Ali S, Gay L, Erlich RL, Ross JS, Buxhaku J, Davies H, Faso V, Germain A, Glanville B, Miller VA, Stephens PJ, Janeway KA, Maris JM, Meshinchi S, Pugh TJ, Shern JF, Lipson D. Genomic profiling of a large set of diverse pediatric cancers identifies known and novel mutations across tumor spectra. Cancer Res. 2017;77:509–19.
75. Bellini A, Bernard V, Leroy Q, Rio Frio T, Pierron G, Combaret V, Lapouble E, Clement N, Rubie H, Thebaud E, Chastagner P, Defachelles AS, Bergeron C, Buchbinder N, Taque S, Auvrignon A, Valteau-Couanet D, Michon J, Janoueix-Lerosey I, Delattre O, Schleiermacher G. Deep sequencing reveals occurrence of subclonal ALK mutations in neuroblastoma at diagnosis. Clin Cancer Res. 2015;21:4913–21.

76. Umapathy G, El Wakil A, Witek B, Chesler L, Danielson L, Deng X, Gray NS, Johansson M, Kvarnbrink S, Ruuth K, Schonherr C, Palmer RH, Hallberg B. The kinase ALK stimulates the kinase ERK5 to promote the expression of the oncogene MYCN in neuroblastoma. Sci Signal. 2014;7:ra102.
77. De Brouwer S, De Preter K, Kumps C, Zabrocki P, Porcu M, Westerhout EM, Lakeman A, Vandesompele J, Hoebeeck J, Van Maerken T, De Paepe A, Laureys G, Schulte JH, Schramm A, Van Den Broecke C, Vermeulen J, Van Roy N, Beiske K, Renard M, Noguera R, Delattre O, Janoueix-Lerosey I, Kogner P, Martinsson T, Nakagawara A, Ohira M, Caron H, Eggert A, Cools J, Versteeg R, Speleman F. Meta-analysis of neuroblastomas reveals a skewed ALK mutation spectrum in tumors with MYCN amplification. Clin Cancer Res. 2010;16:4353–62.
78. Passoni L, Longo L, Collini P, Coluccia AM, Bozzi F, Podda M, Gregorio A, Gambini C, Garaventa A, Pistoia V, Del Grosso F, Tonini GP, Cheng M, Gambacorti-Passerini C, Anichini A, Fossati-Bellani F, Di Nicola M, Luksch R. Mutation-independent anaplastic lymphoma kinase overexpression in poor prognosis neuroblastoma patients. Cancer Res. 2009;69:7338–46.
79. Regairaz M, Munier F, Sartelet H, Castaing M, Marty V, Renauleaud C, Doux C, Delbe J, Courty J, Fabre M, Ohta S, Vielh P, Michiels S, Valteau-Couanet D, Vassal G. Mutation-independent activation of the anaplastic lymphoma kinase in neuroblastoma. Am J Pathol. 2016;186:435–45.
80. Matsuno R, Gifford AJ, Fang J, Warren M, Lukeis R, Trahair T, Sugimoto T, Marachelian A, Asgharzadeh S, Maris JM, Ikegaki N, Shimada H. Rare *MYC*-amplified neuroblastoma with large cell histology. Pediatr Dev Pathol. 2018;21:461. https://doi.org/10.1177/1093526617749670.
81. Zimmerman MW, Liu Y, He S, Durbin AD, Abraham BJ, Easton J, Shao Y, Xu B, Zhu S, Zhang X, Li Z, Weichert-Leahey N, Young RA, Zhang J, Look AT. c-MYC drives a subset of high-risk pediatric neuroblastomas and is activated through mechanisms including enhancer hijacking and focal enhancer amplification. Cancer Discov. 2018;8:320. https://doi.org/10.1158/2159-8290.CD-17-0993. pii: CD-17-0993.
82. Wang LL, Teshiba R, Ikegaki N, Tang XX, Naranjo A, London WB, Hogarty MD, Gastier-Foster JM, Look AT, Park JR, Maris JM, Cohn SL, Seeger RC, Asgharzadeh S, Shimada H. Augmented expression of MYC and/or MYCN protein defines highly aggressive MYC-driven neuroblastoma: a Children's Oncology Group study. Br J Cancer. 2015;113:57–63.
83. Tornoczky T, Kalman E, Kajtar PG, Nyari T, Pearson ADJ, Board J, Shimada H. Large cell neuroblastoma: a distinct phenotype with aggressive clinical behavior. New entity? Cancer. 2004;100:390–7.
84. Ikegaki N, Shimada H, Fox AM, Regan PL, Jacobs J, Kicks SL, Rappaport EF, Tang XX. Transient treatment with epigenetic modifiers yields stable neuroblastoma stem cells resembling aggressive large-cell neuroblastomas. Proc Natl Acad Sci U S A. 2013;110:6097–102.
85. Peifer M, Hertwig F, Roels F, Dreidax D, Gartlgruber M, Menon R, Kramer A, Roncaioli JL, Sand F, Heuckmann JM, Ikram F, Schmidt R, Ackermann S, Engesser A, Kahlert Y, Vogel W, Altmuller J, Nurnberg P, Thierry-Mieg J, Thierry-Mieg D, Mariappan A, Heynck S, Mariotti E, Henrich KO, Gloeckner C, Bosco G, Leuschner I, Schweiger MR, Savelyeva L, Watkins SC, Shao C, Bell E, Hofer T, Achter V, Lang U, Theissen J, Volland R, Saadati M, Eggert A, de Wilde B, Berthold F, Peng Z, Zhao C, Shi L, Ortmann M, Buttner R, Perner S, Hero B, Schramm A, Schulte JH, Herrmann C, O'Sullivan RJ, Westermann F, Thomas RK, Fischer M. Telomerase activation by genomic rearrangements in high-risk neuroblastoma. Nature. 2015;526:700–4.
86. Valentijn LJ, Koster J, Zwijnenburg DA, Hasselt NE, van Sluis P, Volckmann R, van Noesel MM, George RE, Tytgat GA, Molenaar JJ, Versteeg R. TERT rearrangements are frequent in neuroblastoma and identify aggressive tumors. Nat Genet. 2015;47:1411–4.
87. Kawashima M, Kojima M, Ueda Y, Kurihara S, Hiyama E. Telomere biology including TERT rearrangements in neuroblastoma: a useful indicator for surgical treatments. J Pediatr Surg. 2016;51:2080–5.

88. Nael A, Matsuno R, Shows J, Warren M, Gastier-Foster J, Ikegaki N, Shimada H. TERT overexpression in neuroblastoma. In: Proceedings Society for Pediatric Pathology Spring meeting, Fall meeting, Denver, CO; 2017.
89. Lindsey JC, Schwalbe EC, Potluri S, Bailey S, Williamson D, Clifford SC. TERT promoter mutation and aberrant hypermethylation are associated with elevated expression in medulloblastoma and characterise the majority of non-infant SHH subgroup tumours. Acta Neuropathol. 2014;127:307–9.
90. Cheung NK, Zhang J, Lu C, Parker M, Bahrami A, Tickoo SK, Heguy A, Pappo AS, Federico S, Dalton J, Cheung IY, Ding L, Fulton R, Wang J, Chen X, Becksfort J, Wu J, Billups CA, Ellison D, Mardis ER, Wilson RK, Downing JR, Dyer MA, St Jude Children's Research Hospital-Washington University Pediatric Cancer Genome P. Association of age at diagnosis and genetic mutations in patients with neuroblastoma. JAMA. 2012;307:1062–71.
91. Kurihara S, Hiyama E, Onitake Y, Yamaoka E, Hiyama K. Clinical features of ATRX or DAXX mutated neuroblastoma. J Pediatr Surg. 2014;49:1835–8.
92. Darnell JE Jr. Transcription factors as targets for cancer therapy. Nat Rev Cancer. 2002;2:740–9.
93. Delmore JE, Issa GC, Lemieux ME, Rahl PB, Shi J, Jacobs HM, Kastritis E, Gilpatrick T, Paranal RM, Qi J, Chesi M, Schinzel AC, McKeown MR, Heffernan TP, Vakoc CR, Bergsagel PL, Ghobrial IM, Richardson PG, Young RA, Hahn WC, Anderson KC, Kung AL, Bradner JE, Mitsiades CS. BET bromodomain inhibition as a therapeutic strategy to target c-Myc. Cell. 2011;146:904–17.
94. Puissant A, Frumm SM, Alexe G, Bassil CF, Qi J, Chanthery YH, Nekritz EA, Zeid R, Gustafson WC, Greninger P, Garnett MJ, McDermott U, Benes CH, Kung AL, Weiss WA, Bradner JE, Stegmaier K. Targeting MYCN in neuroblastoma by BET bromodomain inhibition. Cancer Discov. 2013;3:308–23.
95. Christensen CL, Kwiatkowski N, Abraham BJ, Carretero J, Al-Shahrour F, Zhang T, Chipumuro E, Herter-Sprie GS, Akbay EA, Altabef A, Zhang J, Shimamura T, Capelletti M, Reibel JB, Cavanaugh JD, Gao P, Liu Y, Michaelsen SR, Poulsen HS, Aref AR, Barbie DA, Bradner JE, George RE, Gray NS, Young RA, Wong KK. Targeting transcriptional addictions in small cell lung cancer with a covalent CDK7 inhibitor. Cancer Cell. 2014;26:909–22.
96. Chipumuro E, Marco E, Christensen CL, Kwiatkowski N, Zhang T, Hatheway CM, Abraham BJ, Sharma B, Yeung C, Altabef A, Perez-Atayde A, Wong KK, Yuan GC, Gray NS, Young RA, George RE. CDK7 inhibition suppresses super-enhancer-linked oncogenic transcription in MYCN-driven cancer. Cell. 2014;159:1126–39.
97. Gustafson WC, Meyerowitz JG, Nekritz EA, Chen J, Benes C, Charron E, Simonds EF, Seeger R, Matthay KK, Hertz NT, Eilers M, Shokat KM, Weiss WA. Drugging MYCN through an allosteric transition in Aurora kinase A. Cancer Cell. 2014;26:414–27.
98. Niemas-Teshiba R, Matsuno R, Wang LL, Tang XX, Chiu B, Zeki J, Coburn J, Ornell K, Naranjo A, Van Ryn C, London WB, Hogarty MD, Gastier-Foster JM, Look AT, Park JR, Maris JM, Cohn SL, Seeger RC, Asgharzadeh S, Ikegaki N, Shimada H. MYC-family protein overexpression and prominent nucleolar formation represent prognostic indicators and potential therapeutic targets for aggressive high-MKI neuroblastomas: a report from the Children's Oncology Group. Oncotarget. 2018;9:6416–32.
99. Dikmen ZG, Gellert GC, Jackson S, Gryaznov S, Tressler R, Dogan P, Wright WE, Shay JW. In vivo inhibition of lung cancer by GRN163L: a novel human telomerase inhibitor. Cancer Res. 2005;65:7866–73.
100. Gupta R, Dong Y, Solomon PD, Wettersten HI, Cheng CJ, Min JN, Henson J, Dogra SK, Hwang SH, Hammock BD, Zhu LJ, Reddel RR, Saltzman WM, Weiss RH, Chang S, Green MR, Wajapeyee N. Synergistic tumor suppression by combined inhibition of telomerase and CDKN1A. Proc Natl Acad Sci U S A. 2014;111:E3062–71.
101. Wilhelm S, Carter C, Lynch M, Lowinger T, Dumas J, Smith RA, Schwartz B, Simantov R, Kelley S. Discovery and development of sorafenib: a multikinase inhibitor for treating cancer. Nat Rev Drug Discov. 2006;5:835–44.

102. Cheung NK, Dyer MA. Neuroblastoma: developmental biology, cancer genomics and immunotherapy. Nat Rev Cancer. 2013;13:397–411.
103. Flynn RL, Cox KE, Jeitany M, Wakimoto H, Bryll AR, Ganem NJ, Bersani F, Pineda JR, Suva ML, Benes CH, Haber DA, Boussin FD, Zou L. Alternative lengthening of telomeres renders cancer cells hypersensitive to ATR inhibitors. Science. 2015;347:273–7.
104. Vendetti FP, Lau A, Schamus S, Conrads TP, O'Connor MJ, Bakkenist CJ. The orally active and bioavailable ATR kinase inhibitor AZD6738 potentiates the anti-tumor effects of cisplatin to resolve ATM-deficient non-small cell lung cancer in vivo. Oncotarget. 2015;6:44289–305.

Part II

Imaging

Radiology

5

Hervé J. Brisse, Martijn Verhagen, Kieran McHugh, and Claudio Granata

5.1 Introduction

Medical imaging plays an essential role in the management of neuroblastic tumours. Imaging is usually the first step for initial diagnosis and disease staging, including identification of image-defined risk factors (see Sect. 5.4). Imaging is used during percutaneous needle biopsy procedures to guide the needle tract and select the optimal target areas (see Sect. 5.4). Response assessment during chemotherapy is based on both anatomical (tumour volume) and functional imaging (nuclear medicine). Imaging is used for postoperative assessment to identify potential residual disease and surgical complications. The treatment planning for radiation therapy that is recommended for high-risk neuroblastoma (NB) is based on imaging data. Finally, long-term post treatment follow-up includes recurrent imaging which should be adjusted to the risk of local or distant relapse.

Different imaging modalities can be employed to evaluate disease and have clinical usefulness in different ways. This chapter will give insights into the workings of the varying imaging modalities to help the reader understand when to employ which modality. The goal is to improve understanding, communication and cooperation between paediatric surgeons, paediatric oncologists, radiation oncologists and radiologists.

H. J. Brisse
Institut Curie, Paris, France
e-mail: herve.brisse@curie.fr

M. Verhagen · K. McHugh
Great Ormond Street Hospital, London, UK
e-mail: Kieran.McHugh@gosh.nhs.uk

C. Granata (✉)
IRCCS Istituto Giannina Gaslini, Genova, Italy
e-mail: cgranata@sirm.org

S. Sarnacki, L. Pio (eds.), *Neuroblastoma*,
https://doi.org/10.1007/978-3-030-18396-7_5

5.2 Imaging Modalities: Technical Aspects and Rational for Use

5.2.1 Plain Films

The role of conventional radiology in NB patients is limited. However, some typical radiological patterns should be recognized as they can reveal the disease.

In the **chest**, NB can manifest as an opacity or mass in the posterior mediastinum (Fig. 5.1a, b) and plain radiography is usually relatively sensitive for the detection [1]. A posterior mediastinal mass is suspected in case of disturbance of

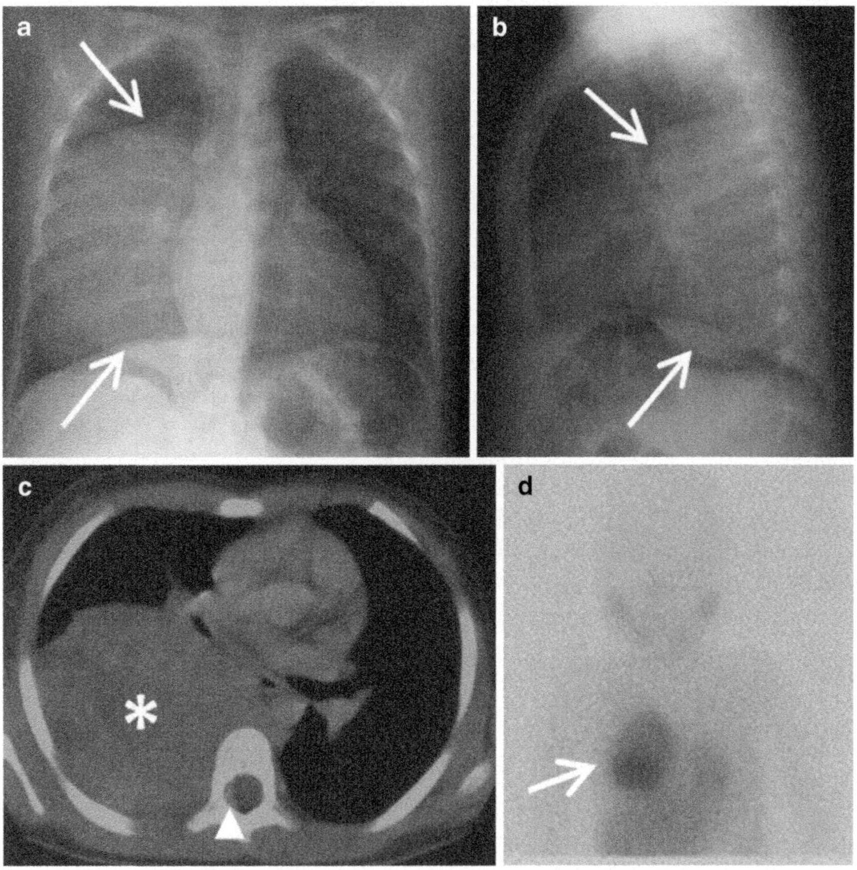

Fig. 5.1 A 3-year-old girl with localized chest nodular ganglioneuroblastoma (INSS stage 1, INRGSS L2). Chest X-ray (**a**, **b**) showing a typical right posterior mediastinal mass (arrows). Contrast-enhanced CT-scan (**c**) transverse view. The tumour (asterisks) arises from the right paravertebral sympathetic chain and contains stippled calcifications. It displaces anteriorly the right bronchus. Intraspinal epidural invasion is visible as a thin enhanced crescent (arrowhead). MIBG scan (**d**) shows tumour uptake (arrow) without distant metastasis

the paraspinal lines or an abnormal contour behind the normal cardio-mediastinal opacity. Other manifestations are widened or subtle erosion of the posterior ribs or vertebral pedicles, the latter indicating extension into the vertebral canal [1]. Thoracic NB can demonstrate calcification on plain film (coarse or finely stippled) in 30% of cases, and such finding in young children leads to a high likelihood of NB [2].

In the **abdomen**, plain radiographs have very limited usefulness and should be avoided as a general rule, ultrasound examination being a far more useful test in the setting of a palpable mass. NB in the abdomen usually manifests as a nonspecific mass. Calcification may be seen in up to 10% at diagnosis.

Bone metastases may be picked up on skeletal plain films. Bone metastases occur in about one half of NB patients; therefore, they are a frequent manifestation of the disease. Initial presentation may be with bone pain or a pathological fracture. Bone metastases are generally lytic and ill-defined, with or without a periosteal reaction. Sclerotic metastases are uncommon. Bone metastases occur in the most vascularized growing areas of bones. Therefore, in long bones they occur in the metaphysis and may mimic osteomyelitis. Less frequently, they present as lucent zones instead of more focal round lesions, mimicking leukemic infiltration [1]. The axial skeleton is also frequently involved, especially the pelvic bones, the spine, the skull and skull base, typically along cranial sutures. The orbital wall includes many sutures and is frequently involved, leading to the classic "raccoon eyes" (periorbital eyelid ecchymoses) [3] or exophtalmia with periorbital and cranial bumps (Hutchinson syndrome). Intracranial epidural infiltration is common, leading to sutural widening [1].

5.2.2 Ultrasonography

Ready availability, real-time imaging and lack of ionizing radiation make ultrasonography (US) an effective tool for the study of NB in children. Traditionally, US is the first choice imaging modality for the initial evaluation of a possible abdominal or cervical NB. US is also the method of choice for image-guided needle biopsy.

The limitations of the technique are (1) a relatively low interobserver reproducibility, (2) the acoustic shadowing caused by intestinal gas and large calcifications and (3) a marked limitation in retrospective review of the data which is mandatory for data collection and follow-up in clinical trials. Consequently, NB patients require in most cases additional imaging with MRI and/or CT for staging and treatment planning.

Abdominal NB commonly appears as an inhomogeneous or homogeneous, slightly hyperechoic retroperitoneal mass. It may have well-defined margins and be limited in size (Fig. 5.2a), or it can be very large, crossing the midline. Calcifications are frequently observed (Fig. 5.3a). On colour Doppler, the mass usually appears vascularized (Fig. 5.2b). The tumour may include necrotic areas. A cystic pattern is frequently observed in adrenal NB in newborns and infants (Fig. 5.4).

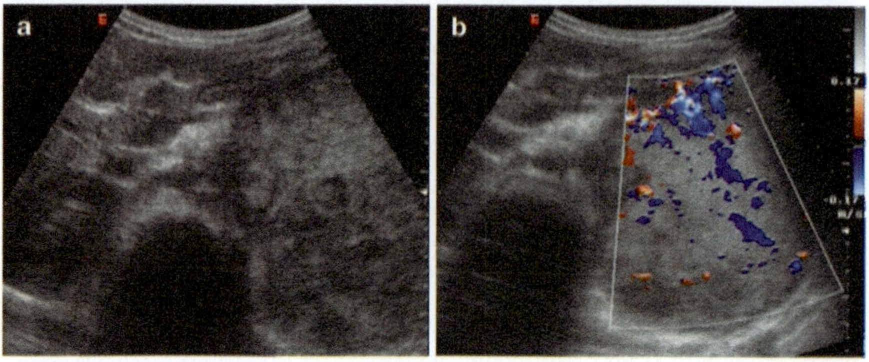

Fig. 5.2 A 10-month-old boy with left adrenal neuroblastoma. Ultrasonography showed a left oval, slightly hyperechoic suprarenal mass with sharp margins (**a**), richly vascularized on colour Doppler (**b**)

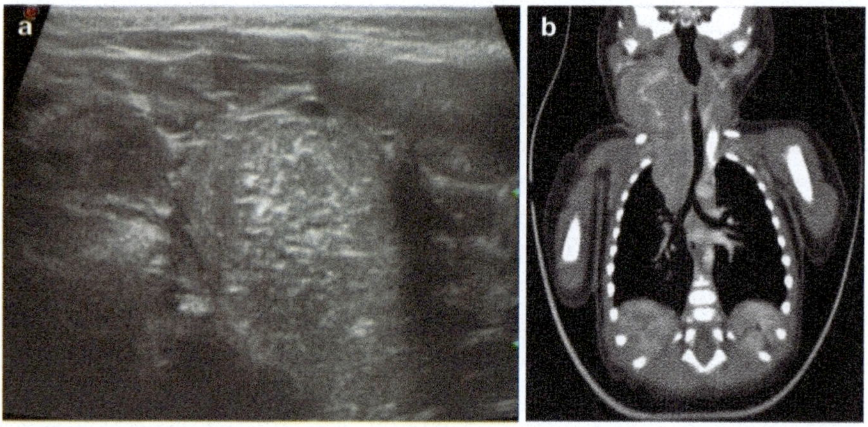

Fig. 5.3 An 18-month-old boy with cervicothoracic neuroblastoma. Ultrasonography showed a solid cervical mass with sharp margins and scattered calcifications. The common carotid artery and internal jugular vein were not seen (**a**). On contrast-enhanced CT, coronal image (**b**) showed a large right-sited thoracic mass extending from the postero-superior mediastinum to the neck

In addition to mass size, site, echostructure and vascularization, the involvement of adjacent vessels and organs (mainly liver and kidneys) can be preliminarily assessed.

The liver should be carefully assessed for possible secondary involvement, usually represented by multiple hypoechoic nodules of varying size.

The kidney can be displaced by a large NB, sometimes causing hydronephrosis, but also directly invaded through the hilum or the cortex.

Primary cervical NB is rare and usually observed in infants. Very rarely, a cervical NB may be part of a thoracic tumour extending to the neck. On US, it is generally echogenic but, if necrosis occurs, scattered hypoechoic foci may be seen.

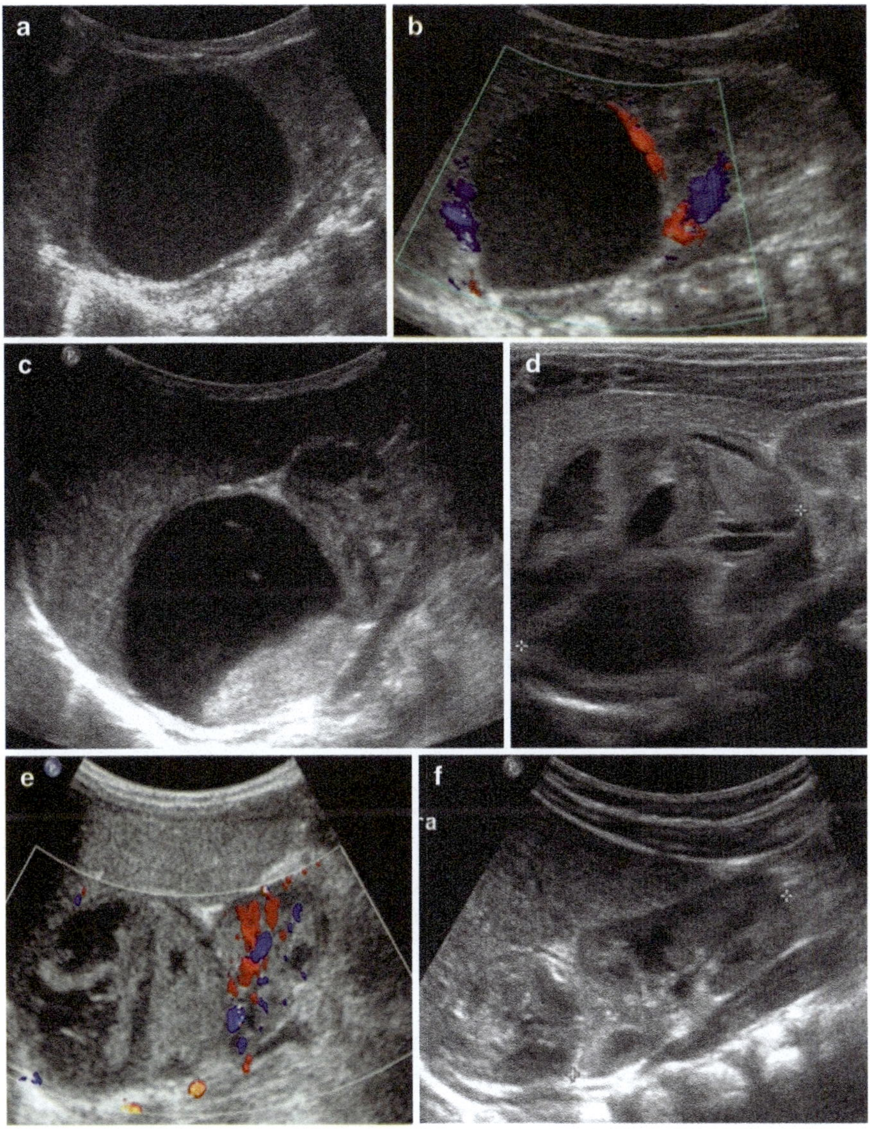

Fig. 5.4 A 6-day-old newborn with detection on ultrasonography of a right cystic suprarenal mass (**a**), associated with slightly increased excretion of urinary catecholamines. Vascularization was only peripheral on colour Doppler (**b**). After 2 weeks, the size of the mass appeared unchanged, whereas a large amount of debris was present (**c**). After 6 weeks, the mass appeared partially solid (**d**), with no evidence of vascularization on colour Doppler (**e**). At 23 weeks of age, the mass appeared mostly solid and slightly reduced in size (**f**). At 31 weeks of age, the mass was smaller and hyperechoic with tiny calcifications (**g**). Finally, at 45 weeks of age, CT contrast-enhanced coronal image showed an almost complete regression of the mass (**h**). These findings and their evolution show the spontaneous regression of a neonatal adrenal neuroblastoma

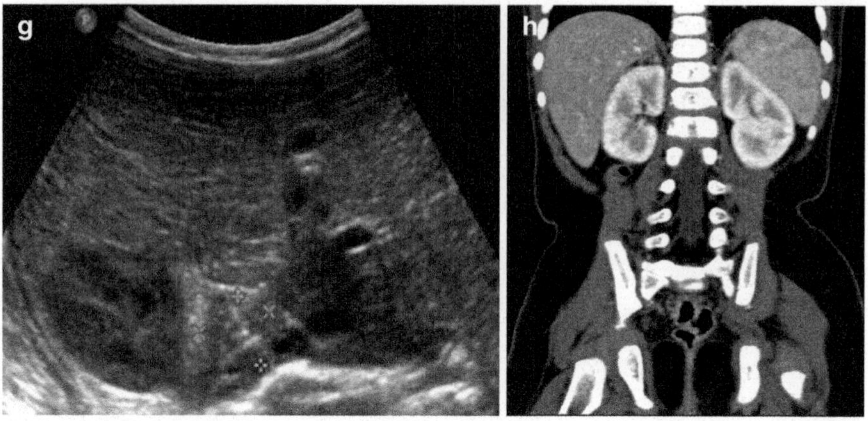

Fig. 5.4 (continued)

The relationship of the mass with the carotid artery and internal jugular vein should also be assessed during the examination (Fig. 5.3).

In newborns and infants, the spinal canal content can be assessed by US. Although MRI is the optimal method, assessment of the spinal canal may be immediately performed for young children with neurological signs and suspected chest or lumbar NB.

5.2.3 Computed Tomography

Computed tomography (CT) is widely available and can usually be rapidly obtained in emergency situations. Multi-detector row CT machines allow extremely fast acquisitions (about 5–10 s) allowing performing the examination of the whole trunk without any sedation and providing excellent image quality without motion artefacts. Post-processing softwares allow multiplanar reconstructions (MPR) providing accurate coronal and sagittal views (Fig. 5.5) and maximum intensity projection (MIP) reconstructions for vascular analysis (Fig. 5.6d). The spatial resolution of CT is high allowing the analysis of small structures, especially small vessels. For patients requiring radiation therapy, most treatment planning systems still use CT data. Finally, compared to MRI, the quality of CT scan is still much more reproducible among centres. As a result, CT is frequently the preferred technique among non-radiologist physicians involved in cancer management.

The use of intravenous iodine contrast agent is mandatory in order to enhance the soft tissue contrast and for assessing relationships between the tumour and adjacent vessels. Except in case of renal failure, contrast agents are well tolerated by children and adverse allergic reactions remain exceptional.

However, a major limitation of CT is the associated radiation exposure. Repeated examinations may lead to substantial cumulative doses, and children are known to have a higher inherent sensitivity to ionizing radiations [4]. Although the risk

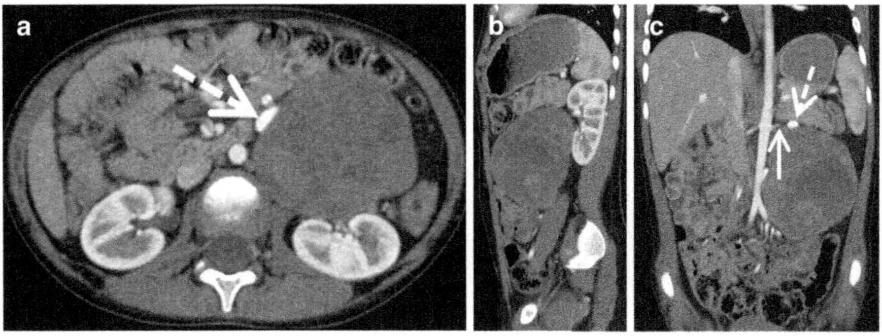

Fig. 5.5 A 4-year-old girl with localized prerenal neuroblastoma (MYCN non-amplified, segmental chromosome alterations, INSS stage 3, INRGSS L2). Contrast-enhanced transverse CT scan (**a**), sagittal (**b**) and coronal (**c**) views. The tumour demonstrates moderate and heterogeneous enhancement. The tumour arises from the periarterial sympathetic fibres. It displaces upwards and forward the left renal pedicles (artery, arrow; vein, dotted arrow)

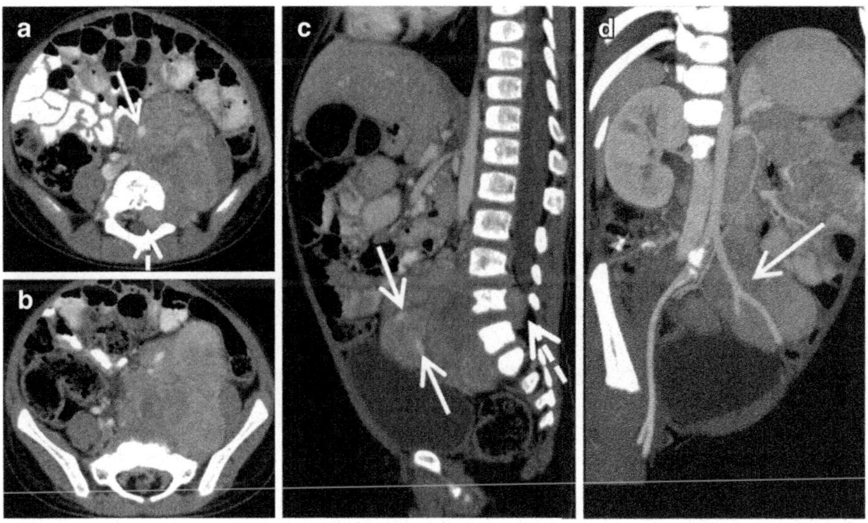

Fig. 5.6 A 4-year-old boy with localized lumbar ganglioneuroblastoma (numeric chromosome alterations, INSS stage 3, INRGSS L2). Contrast-enhanced transverse CT scan (**a**, **b**), sagittal (**c**) and MIP coronal (**d**) views. The tumour demonstrates intense and heterogeneous enhancement. The tumour arises from the left paravertebral lumbar sympathetic chain. It encases left primitive, internal and external iliac arteries (arrows), infiltrates the L5-S1 left foramina and adjacent epidural space (dotted arrows)

associated with low-dose exposures is still a matter of debate [5], CT scanning should be used as sparingly as possible especially in children exposed in parallel to drugs which can cause genetic mutations. If done, the CT dose must be optimized for each examination; repeated examinations should be avoided by using alternative methods such as US and MRI.

In daily practice, sedation is no more used, provided there is adequate immobilization of young children. The use of oral contrast agent (or water) to delineate the digestive tract is no more required. Unenhanced series better depict subtle intratumoural calcifications but are not mandatory and should only be used in doubtful cases and focused on the tumour only. One contrast-enhanced series is usually sufficient to assess the tumour extent. Well-tolerated contrast agents (low osmolarity, nonionic with 300–350 mg/L iodine concentration) should be used with a total volume of 1.5–2 mL/kg. The perfusion rate should be adapted to patients' age and to the IV line diameter, usually between 0.8 and 2 mL/s to ensure appropriate enhancement and preferably performed with an automatic injection device. The scan delay should be adjusted in order to get both arterial and venous enhancement and depends on the patient's age, the anatomic region assessed and the acquisition time. The beam collimation depends on the CT machine, but the nominal slice thickness should be 0.5–1.5 mm and the reconstruction thickness between 2 and 4 mm. Recommended pitch values are between 1 and 1.5 providing a reasonable compromise between a short acquisition time and sufficient z-resolution. Tube voltage and current should be adapted to the patient's age and weight and to the anatomic region studied. The tube voltage is usually set between 70 and 100 kVp. The mAs must be adjusted to obtain a final mean absorbed dose (CTDIvolume) in agreement with the current paediatric recommendations or dose reference levels [6, 7] without jeopardizing image quality. Iterative reconstruction is very useful to increase the signal-to-noise ratio and the low-contrast detectability and optimize the radiation dose [8].

The CT pattern of NB is very variable according to the patients' age, histologic subtype and tumour size. Slow-growing and well-differentiated tumours appear as well-delineated homogeneous soft tissue masses (Fig. 5.7), with or without calcifications and usually with limited and low enhancement. Rapidly growing large NBs are more frequently heterogeneous, commonly contain necrosis and calcifications (Fig. 5.8.). As

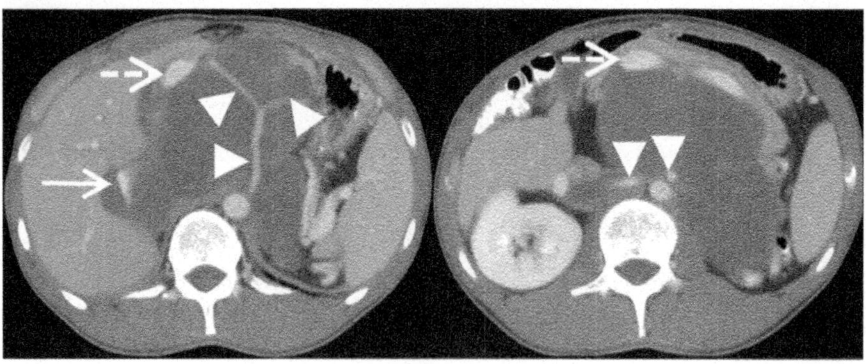

Fig. 5.7 A 16-year-old boy with retroperitoneal ganglioneuroma (INSS stage 3, INRGSS L2). Contrast-enhanced transverse CT scan views. The tumour arises from the periaortic sympathetic chains and typically demonstrates low density with little enhancement. The mass encases (arrowheads) the major aortic branches (celiac, hepatic, splenic, superior mesenteric and the right renal arteries), as well as the inferior vena cava (arrow). The duodenopancreatic bloc and the portal vein (dotted arrow) are anteriorly displaced

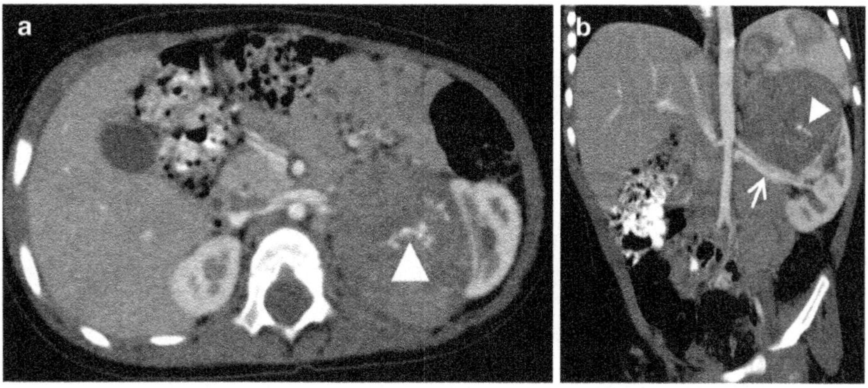

Fig. 5.8. A 14-month-old boy with localized left adrenal neuroblastoma (MYCN non-amplified, segmental chromosome alterations, INSS stage 3, INRG L2). Contrast-enhanced transverse CT scan (**a**) and MPR coronal (**b**) views. The tumour demonstrates low central calcifications (arrowheads) and moderate and heterogeneous enhancement. The mass displaces the upper pole of the left kidney and the renal pedicle (arrows)

previously described for US, a cystic pattern is common in newborns and infants with adrenal primaries. The enhancement after contrast injection of the solid part of the tumour is variable and usually moderate. These findings are nonspecific. The radiological diagnosis of NB is not based on specific measurable densities or enhancement but rather on the anatomic location of the mass and typical pattern of locoregional or distant extensions, interpreted with the background clinical information.

5.2.4 Magnetic Resonance Imaging

MRI has been long recognized as an effective imaging method for assessing neuroblastoma (NB) [2, 9–13]. Compared to CT, MRI provides a higher contrast resolution in soft tissues and offers the main advantage of not using ionizing radiation. In patients with intraspinal extension, MRI is the recommended imaging modality because of the excellent visualization of the spinal cord, nerve roots and subarachnoid spaces [13].

However, MRI is also associated with some limitations: (1) a lower availability in many countries, compared to CT, and (2) the need for sedation or general anaesthesia in young children because of a long acquisition time (several minutes) and a high sensitivity to motion artefacts. A downside of anaesthesia is the complex logistics such as providing MRI-safe equipment, an anaesthesiologic team and arranging for pre-MRI sedation and post-MRI recovery. Another possible disadvantage is a potential neurotoxic effect of anaesthesia on the developing central nervous system, although this is still controversial [14–16]. Therefore, the risk associated with sedation or general anaesthesia must be balanced with the risk of radiation exposure from CT. This safety issue is currently a matter of debate in the paediatric radiology literature [17]. As such, anaesthesia should be employed whenever necessary, but alternative measures such as a child-friendly environment allowing the child to try out the MRI before the examination itself can in some cases avoid anaesthesia. Babies up to 6 months usually do not need anaesthesia because they tend to do well by using the "feed and wrap" technique. This is done by feeding the baby just before the MRI and wrapping them comfortably, causing them to sleep through the examination with little to no movement artefacts.

The need for intravenous gadolinium contrast injection to assess NB extension is still a matter of debate [13]. Gadolinium actually improves the assessment of infiltration into adjacent tissues and tumour vascularity. However, T1- and T2-weighted sequences provide excellent contrast resolution, and sufficient display of vessels can be achieved without the use of contrast media [9]. In one study, the accuracy of T2-weighted and post-gadolinium T1-weighted sequences in defining local regional extent were compared, and no difference was found [18]. The increasing use of diffusion-weighted imaging (DWI) may also reduce the need for injected contrast agents in a near future. In one recent study [19], lesion conspicuity, as measured by signal intensity ratio, was found to be superior on DWI compared to contrast-enhanced T1 sequences. Moreover, recent safety concerns raised since the repeated use of gadolinium-based contrast agents can lead to free gadolinium deposits in normal tissues, especially in the brain [20, 21]. Since reported cases were associated with "linear" agents, the so-called "macrocyclic" gadolinium contrast agents are now preferred [22–24]. Lastly, gadolinium should be avoided in children with renal function impairment because of the risk of secondary nephrogenic systemic fibrosis [25].

In routine practice, safety rules include systematic auditory protection (to reduce the noise from gradient commutators) and monitoring of the specific absorption rate (SAR), especially in infants and newborns. Although no radiation is involved, the radiofrequency pulses contain energy and will give off part of that energy as heat. This is measured using the SAR (expressed in W kg^{-1}, 1 W kg^{-1} applied for 1 h would increase the body temperature by 1 °C). All MRIs are built in such a way that the amount of energy given in the form of radiofrequency pulses is monitored and limited according to the patients' weight. In addition, the imaging protocols and sequences will take this limitation into account, and the radiographer controlling the machine monitors the SAR reading.

There are a variety of MR sequences that can be utilized. Sequences and settings vary between manufacturers, specific machines, technical specifications and the preferences of the local radiologist. However, T1- and T2-weighted sequences still are the basis of any protocol. Table 5.1 is an example of a routine protocol used in a paediatric MR unit. Most sequences are—unlike CT—not 3D datasets but instead acquired as slabs of data with small gaps of missing data in between slices. Three dimensional datasets can be acquired with MRI and then, like CT, allow for multiplanar reconstruction, but 3D sequences are more time consuming and therefore more susceptible to movement artefacts. For each sequence, a compromise must be obtained between spatial resolution, signal-to-noise ratio and acquisition time. When performed, gadolinium-enhanced sequences are always T1-weighted, and a fat-suppression technique (based on spectral saturation or selective water excitation,

Table 5.1 Example of MRI protocol

Sequence	Plane	Gadolinium	Fat suppression	Voxel dimensions (mm)
STIR	Coronal	No	Yes	0.6 × 0.6 × 6
	Transverse	No	Yes	0.5 × 0.5 × 9
3D-T2	Isotropic	No	No	0.9 × 0.9 × 0.9
DWI	Transverse	No	No	2 × 2 × 5
T1	Transverse	No	No	0.5 × 0.5 × 5
T1 TSE	Transverse	No	Yes	1.2 × 1.2 × 5
	Transverse	Yes[a]	Yes	1.2 × 1.2 × 5

[a]Optional

inversion-recovery or Dixon technique) is ideally applied to allow for better detection of enhancement, especially against fatty tissues. T2-weighted sequences can also benefit from fat suppression.

Artefacts are related to diaphragmatic or cardiac movement and vessel pulsation. Cardiac and diaphragmatic movement artefacts can be reduced or resolved by gating the heart rate and diaphragmatic movement (heart gating, respiratory triggering or echo-navigator).

Acquisition planes should always include the axial plane and at least one longitudinal (mostly coronal) plane [13]. A three-plane study is recommended for paraspinal NBs to assess foraminal and intraspinal invasion with coronal views showing all foraminal and intraspinal tumour extent on the same image [13] and a sagittal view to precisely define the vertebral levels involved.

Signal intensity of NB is usually high on T2 and intermediate on T1 at diagnosis [2]. After treatment, the tumour may be fibrotic and variably calcific, which results in a decrease of signal intensity on both T1 and T2 sequences [26]. The mass lesions may contain calcifications or necrosis and so may have a heterogeneous appearance on all sequences. The lesions demonstrate homogeneous or heterogeneous enhancement after gadolinium administration.

Diffusion-weighted imaging (DWI) is a functional MRI technique increasingly used, especially in oncology. Since the acquisition time is short, those sequences can be easily added to routine protocols. DWI assesses the random movement (so-called Brownian motion) of water protons located in the extracellular space of living tissues [27]. In a relative unrestricted container of water (e.g. the urinary bladder), a high degree of free movement will be shown. However, in a tightly packed piece of tissue with a high concentration of small cells such as a malignant tumour, diffusion in the extracellular spaces will be restricted and thus a high signal will be seen [28]. Information is provided by both native sequences obtained with variable motion-probing gradients ("*b*-values", expressed in sec mm^{-2}) and reconstructed parametric maps based on the calculated ADC values (apparent diffusion coefficient, expressed in mm^2 sec^{-1}). In oncology, DWI is considered as an in vivo marker strongly related to cellular density (Fig. 5.9b). However, interpretation of DWI should always be performed by comparison with conventional T1 and T2 sequences. Possible pitfalls include tumour necrosis which, both at presentation and in response to treatment, can have restricted diffusion because of cell degradation products limiting water

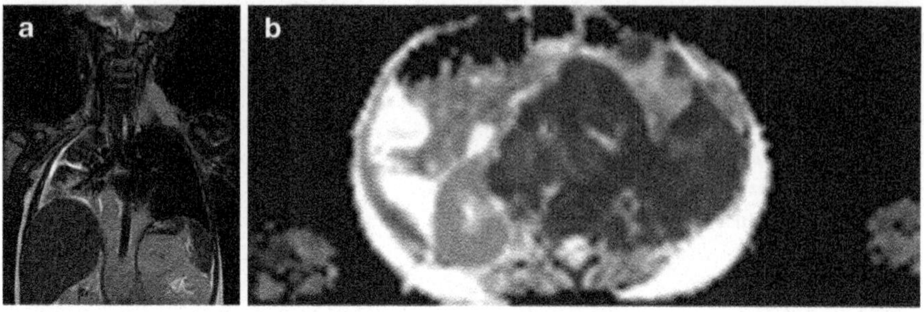

Fig. 5.9 (**a**) Coronal T2W image shows a central lower and upper abdominal mass lesion, which is encasing the descending thoracic aorta. There is a right pleural effusion, oedema in the right chest and lymphadenopathy in the left supraclavicular area, a further area of neuroblastoma. (**b**) Axial ADC map of the same patient at the left of the right kidney shows widespread dark signal indicating restricted diffusion and high cellularity in the neuroblastoma masses

diffusion, fibrosis which also lead to apparent restriction because of low water content or haemorrhage which can mimic restrictive diffusion because of blood degradation products.

Several studies specifically focused on DWI in neuroblastic tumours. One preliminary study [29] reported ADC values and confirmed the link between ADC and cellular density. Another study [30] demonstrated a significant difference of the ADC of NB compared to the ADC of ganglioneuroma/ganglioneuroblastoma. Recent studies [19, 31] suggested that DWI can distinguish between NB and ganglioneuroblastoma versus ganglioneuromas with high certainty and could provide plausible quantitative data (ADC) on tumour response to therapy. The rationale for use of this technique for NB is still a matter of research but could further help for both diagnostic and response assessment.

5.2.5 Nuclear Medicine

^{123}I-metaiodobenzylguanidine (mIBG) scintigraphy is a major imaging technique for the study of NB, especially to assess the metastatic disease. Guidelines have been published for mIBG scanning in children [32–34]. Since there is no physiological uptake of mIBG in the bone and bone marrow, mIBG is an accurate method for detecting osteomedullary metastases, its sensitivity and specificity being estimated at 90% and 100%, respectively [35, 36].

The role of nuclear medicine in NB is described in Part III.

5.2.6 DICOM Data Storage

Since almost all NB patients are included in national or international trials including retrospective reviews of imaging, it is of major importance that all imaging data are stored in a picture archiving and communication system (PACS). The recommended format is the internationally accepted DICOM format (Digital Imaging and Communications in Medicine, http://medical.nema.org/).

5.3 Diagnostic Imaging at Diagnosis

5.3.1 Classical Imaging Patterns

Imaging patterns of neuroblastic tumours have been thoroughly described [1–3, 9–11, 37–40]. Ganglioneuroma is a slow-growing localized and usually relatively homogeneous tumour and without significant enhancement or MIBG uptake. Apart from this specific benign histologic subtype, the anatomical imaging characteristics of other neuroblastic tumours are relatively similar [1]. The histological subtypes cannot be discriminated by imaging and still rely on pathologic analysis.

However, the diagnosis of neuroblastic tumour is usually suspected with a high degree of confidence on the basis of both the patient's age and the anatomic location:

- The median age at diagnosis is about 16 months, and 95% occur by 7 years of age [41, 42].
- The most common sites of origin are the adrenal region (48%), extraadrenal retroperitoneum (25%) and chest (16%). Less common sites are the neck (3%) and the pelvis (3%) [41].

Recent studies [43] suggested using an anatomic classification based on the sympathetic origin of the tumour rather than the anatomic compartment only. Actually, imaging efficiently depicted the sympathetic origin of the tumour and is significantly related to the tumour genomic profile and patients' outcome [43]:

- Cervical NBs typically arise from the superior cervical sympathetic chain (Fig. 5.10) located in the vascular (retrostylian) space behind the internal carotid artery. These tumours extend anteriorly and laterally, displacing the carotid artery and internal jugular vein, or medially, compressing the airway and upwards to the skull base.
- Cervicothoracic NBs arising from the stellate ganglion (located above the subclavian artery at the level of the origin of the vertebral artery) are rare but associated with particular imaging patterns [44]. Foraminal and intraspinal extensions may be associated.
- Chest NBs chiefly arise from the paraspinal sympathetic chains in the posterior mediastinum (Fig. 5.1). The descending aorta may be displaced or even encased. Foraminal and intraspinal extensions ("dumbbell" tumours) are often present and may lead to spinal cord compression. Infiltrating mediastinal tumours arising from the periaortic sympathetic plexuses occur less commonly.
- Abdominal NBs arise either from the adrenal gland (Figs. 5.8., 5.11, 5.12, and 5.13), from sympathetic ganglia (celiac, superior and inferior mesenteric ganglia) or from sympathetic fibres and plexuses located along the aorta and its main

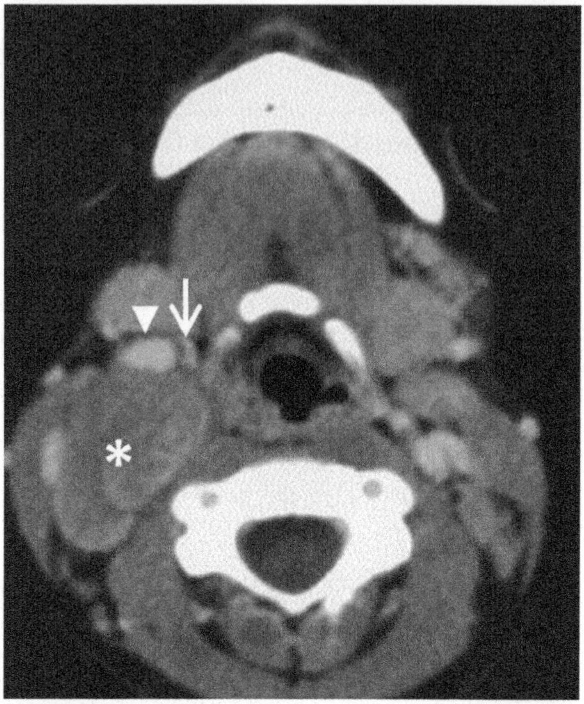

Fig. 5.10 A 3-year-old girl with localized cervical intermixed ganglioneuroblastoma (INSS stage 1, INRG L1). Contrast-enhanced transverse CT scan view. The tumour (asterisk) arises from the right cervical sympathetic chain and displaces anteriorly the carotid artery (arrow) and the internal jugular vein (arrowhead). The tumour is not calcified and partially enhanced by iodine contrast

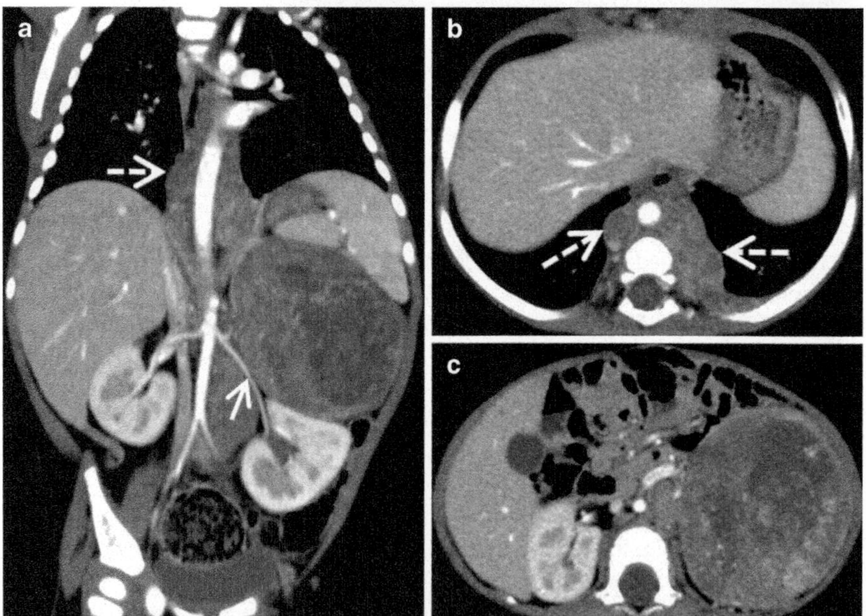

Fig. 5.11 An 11-month-old boy with metastatic left adrenal neuroblastoma (MYCN amplified, INSS stage 4, INRGSS M). Contrast-enhanced CT-scan coronal (**a**) and transverse views (**b**, **c**). The tumour demonstrates moderate and heterogeneous enhancement. The mass displaces the upper pole of the left kidney and encases the renal pedicle (arrows). Regional lymph node involvement in the lower mediastinum is visible (dotted arrows)

branches (Figs. 5.5, 5.7, and 5.14). Therefore, detailed analysis of all arteries and veins is critical (aorta, celiac axis, superior and inferior mesenteric arteries, renal arteries and veins, inferior vena cava, iliac arteries and veins, portal vein). The tumour may invade the adjacent organs and structures (liver parenchyma or hilum, diaphragm, kidneys, duodeno-pancreatic block). The mesentery may be infiltrated, especially by tumours arising from the Zuckerkandl organ (at the origin of the inferior mesentery artery) (Fig. 5.15).

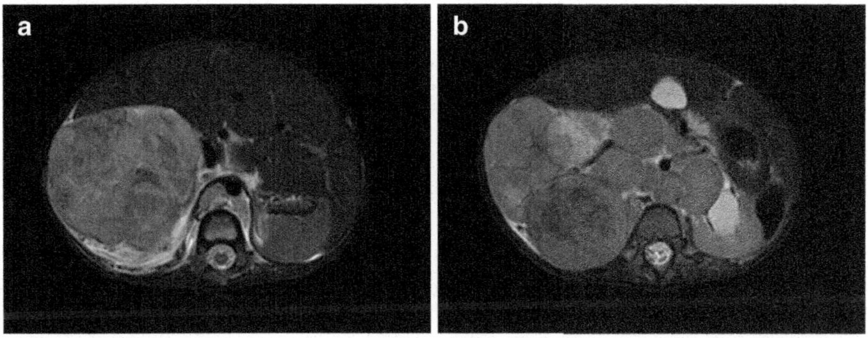

Fig. 5.12 (**a**) Axial T2W image in a 19-month-old child shows a right suprarenal mass and retrocrural tumour also. (**b**) More inferiorly the mass is seen to be displacing the aorta anteriorly with encasement of the aorta and IVC also. Tumour extends to the left renal hilum with left-sided hydronephrosis

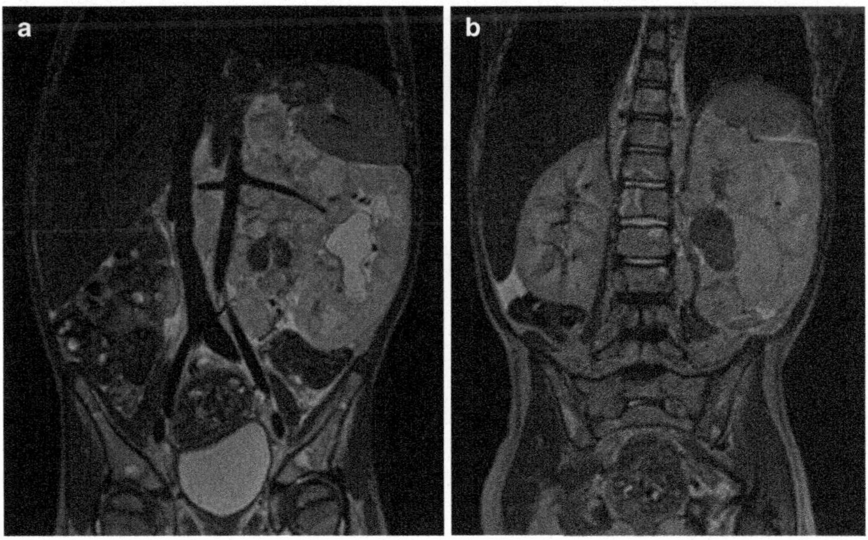

Fig. 5.13 (**a**) Coronal T2W image showing a mainly left-sided mass encasing the abdominal aorta and both renal arteries. The mass is causing left-sided hydronephrosis. (**b**) More posteriorly the heterogeneous appearances to the vertebral marrow are due to vertebral bone marrow metastases

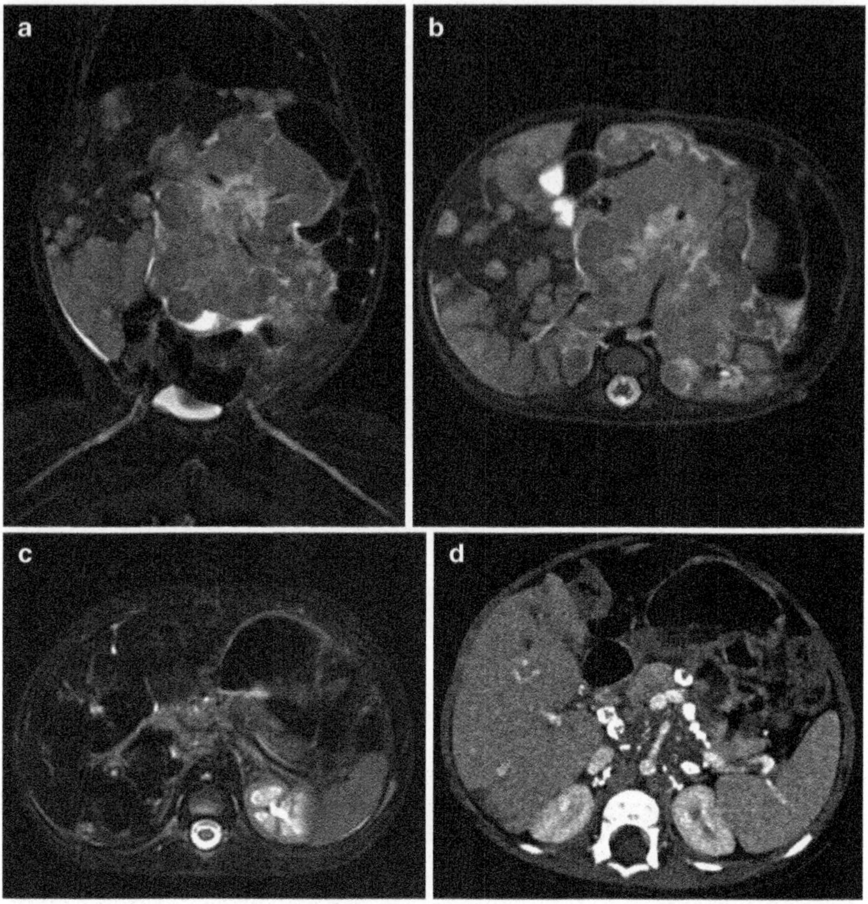

Fig. 5.14 (**a**) Coronal T2W image showing numerous liver metastases (the darker liver signal is normal liver) with a central abdominal mass in a 2-year-old. (**b**) Axial T2W image in the same patient better depicting the central abdominal mass which is encasing the aorta and superior mesenteric artery. (**c**) Follow-up MRI at day 70. There has been considerable tumour shrinkage and the mass is less conspicuous than at diagnosis. (**d**) Contrast-enhanced CT done at the same time, for surgical planning purposes, reveals widespread calcification in the residual tumour, which was not apparent on the MRI

- Lumbar paraspinal NBs are less common. Frequently classified as "abdominal" locations because of their anterior extension (Fig. 5.6), these tumours are associated with foraminal and intraspinal extension (dumbbell tumours) sharing the same pattern as mediastinal primaries.
- Pelvic NBs mainly arise from either the upper hypogastric sympathetic plexus or presacral sympathetic ganglia. Pelvic organs are usually anteriorly displaced. Extensions occur along the iliac vessels and into lumbosacral foramina and, less frequently, laterally into the gluteal region through the greater sciatic foramen.
- Multifocal primary NBs are rare and may be familial [45, 46]. They can manifest as synchronous or metachronous non-contiguous tumours.

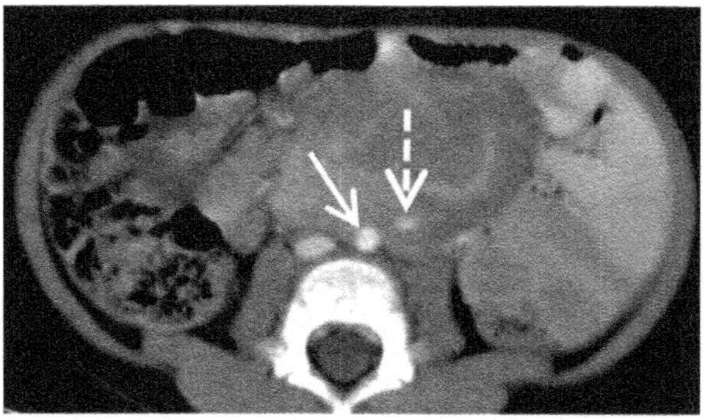

Fig. 5.15 A 4-year-old boy with localized abdominal intermixed ganglioneuroblastoma (INSS stage 1, INRGSS L1). Contrast-enhanced transverse CT scan view. The tumour demonstrates moderate and heterogeneous enhancement. It probably arises from the Zuckerkandl organ and encases partially the aorta (arrow) and totally the inferior mesenteric artery (dotted arrow)

5.3.2 Specific Diagnostic Issues

5.3.2.1 Differential Diagnosis of Retroperitoneal Solid Tumours During Childhood

A common challenge for radiologists is the differential diagnosis between renal and extrarenal retroperitoneal tumours, i.e. between NB and nephroblastoma, since both occur within the same age group [47]. Actually, nephroblastoma may be exophytic and associated with enlarged lymph nodes, whereas NB may directly invade the renal parenchyma leading to relatively similar radiological patterns (Fig. 5.16). In nephroblastoma, the mass rarely crosses the midline, the vessels are much more frequently displaced than encased, and calcifications are rarely seen. Although those criteria are helpful, none is 100% specific. Therefore, in difficult cases the final diagnosis relies on specific tests (urinary catecholamines, MIBG scan) or on histology after percutaneous needle biopsy.

5.3.2.2 Suprarenal Masses of the Foetus and Newborns

Imaging has gained a pivotal role in the antenatal evaluation of suprarenal masses. The routine use of foetal US has made the observation of prenatally detected suprarenal masses a relatively common situation. In most cases, they are observed in the third trimester of pregnancy [48]. Not all suprarenal foetal masses are NBs, but most NBs observed in the foetus or newborn appear as suprarenal masses [49]. The differential diagnosis of these masses mostly includes benign conditions such as adrenal haemorrhage, congenital adrenal hyperplasia, subdiaphragmatic extralobar pulmonary sequestration and bronchogenic cysts.

Prenatally detected or neonatal NB represents a relatively benign condition, the survival rate being more than 90%, with INSS stage 1 at presentation in most cases, with generally favourable biological and histological features in most cases [50].

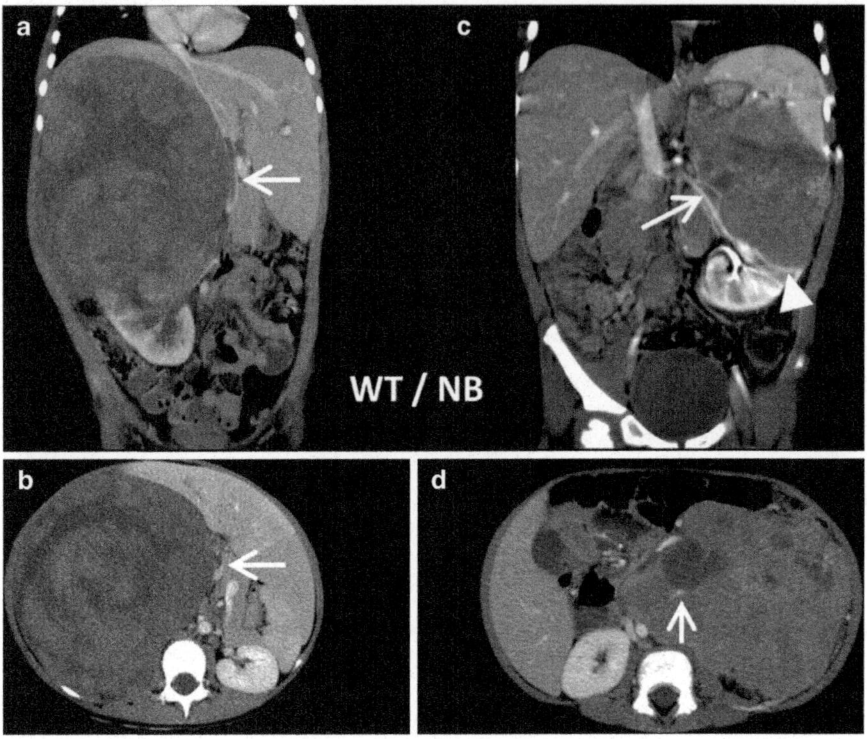

Fig. 5.16 The differential diagnosis between neuroblastoma and Wilms tumour may be difficult. Contrast-enhanced transverse CT scan (**b**, **d**) and coronal (**a**, **c**) MPR views. (**a**, **b**) A 6-year-old girl with exophytic upper pole Wilms tumour of the right kidney (intermediate-risk histology, local stage 3, lung metastases). Inferior vena cava thrombosis (arrows) is seen in about 10% of Wilms tumour and remains exceptional in neuroblastoma. (**c**, **d**) A 3.5-year-old boy with left adrenal neuroblastoma (MYCN non-amplified, segmental chromosome alterations, INSS stage 3, INRGSS L2). The renal pedicle is encased within the tumour (arrows) which is uncommon in Wilms tumour. The cortex of the left kidney (arrowhead) is still visible in relation to extrarenal origin of the tumour

On US, the appearance of prenatal or neonatal adrenal NB can be cystic (55%), solid (17.5%) or heterogeneous (27.5%) [51]. However, these findings may not differ from those observed in other suprarenal neonatal masses, especially adrenal haemorrhage (Fig. 5.17). Furthermore, the role of urinary assay in pinpointing NB is very limited, having a sensitivity of 52% and a negative predictive power 46% in newborns and 36% and 72%, respectively, in prenatally detected NB [48]. Similarly, the sensitivity and negative predictive power of MIBG may be limited, being 70% and 55%, respectively [48].

Therefore, the differential diagnosis of a neonatal suprarenal mass can be difficult at the first observation. In order to facilitate the diagnosis, a series of features should be thoroughly assessed with US including mass size and echostructure and their evolution during follow-up, and mass vascularization [52]. A palpable or large (diameter >5 cm) mass is probably a NB [48]. During follow-up, a mass remaining

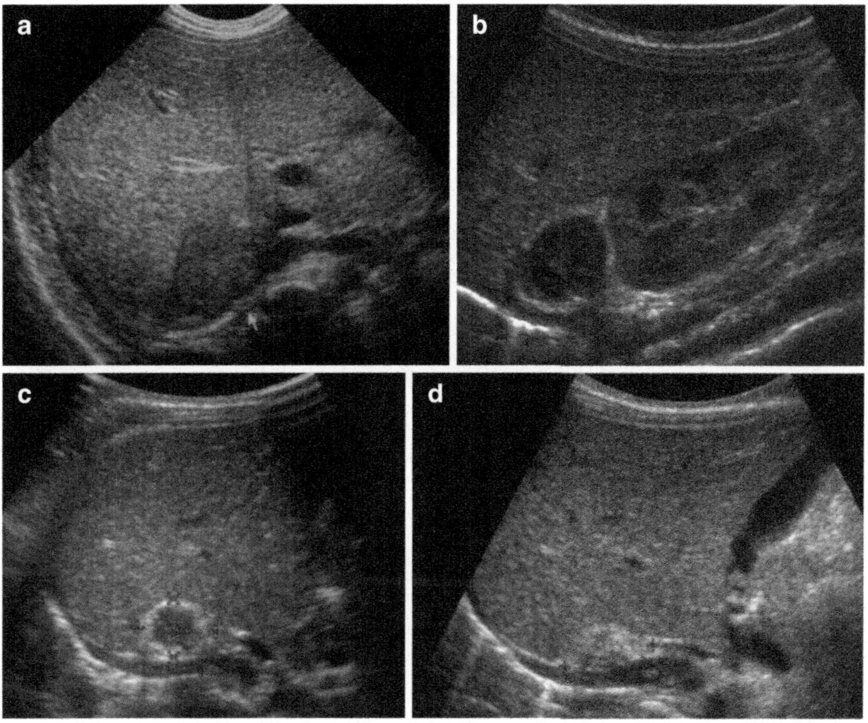

Fig. 5.17 A 5-day-old newborn with adrenal haemorrhage. At 5 days of age, ultrasonography showed a solid mass in the right suprarenal region (**a**). After 40 days, the same mass appeared more hypoechoic and surrounded by a hyperechoic shell; vascularization of the mass was not seen with colour Doppler (**b**). After further 2 months, the suprarenal mass was smaller, whereas the echostructure appeared unchanged (**c**). At 6 months of age, ultrasonography showed a very small, calcific mass (**d**)

stable or increasing in size is probably a NB, while a mass becoming heterogeneous with internal echoes and late appearance of calcifications and/or progressively decreasing in size on serial US is very probably an adrenal haemorrhage [53] (Fig. 5.17). Even a non-metastatic neonatal adrenal NB can regress in a few months, especially when it is initially cystic [54] (Fig. 5.4).

US Doppler may also play a role in differential diagnosis, showing vascularization within a solid NB, peripheral vascularization in a cystic NB, a systemic vessel originating from the aorta in an extralobar pulmonary sequestration [54] (Fig. 5.18) or the absence of vascularization within an adrenal haemorrhage. However, none of these findings are pathognomonic or consistently observed.

The awareness that foetal or neonatal asymptomatic suprarenal masses—non-metastatic NB included—have a benign course in most cases and may often regress led to a recent trial based on the European Low and Intermediate Risk NB protocol (https://clinicaltrials.gov/ct2/show/NCT01728155). According to this protocol, an observational approach is recommended in case of suprarenal masses

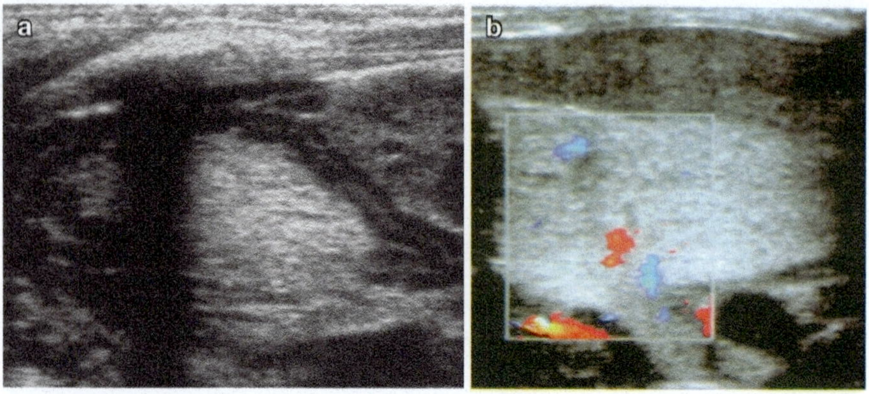

Fig. 5.18 A 5-day-old newborn with left pulmonary subdiaphragmatic sequestration. Ultrasonography showed a hyperechoic mass in close relationship with the adrenal gland (**a**); the hyperechogenicity of the lesion results from the many interfaces produced by multiple microscopically dilated structures such as bronchioles, ducts and alveoli. A systemic arterial vessel feeds the mass (**b**)

smaller than 5 cm and observed during pregnancy or within 90 days from birth. This approach is based on a wait-and-see attitude until 48 weeks of age, a period in which there could be a spontaneous regression of the mass, making it possible to avoid surgical resection and its possible complications. US plays a pivotal role during this observation period in detecting mass shrinkage, or persistence, or increase in size. The mass will be resected in case of persistence after 48 weeks of age or increase in size.

5.3.2.3 Occult Neuroblastoma: Imaging Strategy

Imaging has a major role in the depiction of the primary tumour especially in case of disease revealed by metastases, or in patients presenting with paraneoplastic opsoclonus-myoclonus syndrome (OMS) [39]. Although chest X-ray and abdominal US are traditionally performed upfront, CT/MR imaging of the chest and abdomen are considered the most accurate tests to detect occult neuroblastoma [55]. MIBG is also usually performed in OMS [56], but poorer sensitivities have been noted for MIBG and urine catecholamines, reflecting the low metabolic activity of these tumours [55].

5.4 Imaging for Initial Staging

The rationale for use of the various imaging techniques is currently based on the international consensus published in 2011 [13] although these recommendations will certainly be further updated according to technical improvement. Imaging guidelines of the numerous trials should rely on such consensus reports to ensure appropriate recommendations.

The mandatory examinations for initial staging are:

- MRI or contrast-enhanced CT of the primary tumour compartment
- Chest X-ray
- MIBG scan

Optional examinations are:

- FDG-PET if the primary tumour is not MIBG avid or has been previously removed [57]
- Localized bone plain film if single equivocal skeletal uptake on MIBG
- Liver imaging (US, CT or MRI) if not assessed with the primary (outside the abdomen)
- Contrast-enhanced chest CT if pleuro-pulmonary clinical or radiological abnormalities
- Brain MRI or contrast-enhanced CT if abnormal neurologic symptom (other than spinal cord compression) or abnormal skull base or orbit uptake on MIBG

Disease staging is based on two different classifications (see tables Part II) which are currently used in parallel: (1) the International Neuroblastoma Staging System (INSS) developed in 1988 [58] and modified in 1993 [59] and based on surgico-pathological findings and (2) the International Neuroblastoma Risk Group Staging System (INRGSS) published in 2009, designed for staging before any treatment [60] and allowing better comparison between international trials. Both classifications are relatively similar for metastatic stages, whereas, for localized tumours, the INRGSS is totally based on imaging and considered more robust and reproducible than the INSS [13].

5.4.1 Primary Tumour Assessment

MRI and CT are routinely used depending on local availability, physicians' preference, patient's age and tumour location.

Radiologists have to assess:

- The primary anatomic location of the tumour (anatomic compartment and, as far as possible, the most probable origin of the tumour, i.e. the adrenal gland or the paravertebral, periarterial or cervical sympathetic chains [43])
- The initial tumour volume (three dimensions or at least the longest tumour diameter in accordance with the INRC and RECIST guidance [57])
- The potential invasion of adjacent compartments (Figs. 5.3 and 5.11)
- The potential invasion of the spinal canal for paravertebral primaries
- The relationships between the tumour and adjacent vessels (Fig. 5.19), organs (Fig. 5.20) and structures with a specific attention to IDRFs (see Part II)
- The occurrence of regional or distant lymph nodes (occurring in about 30%)

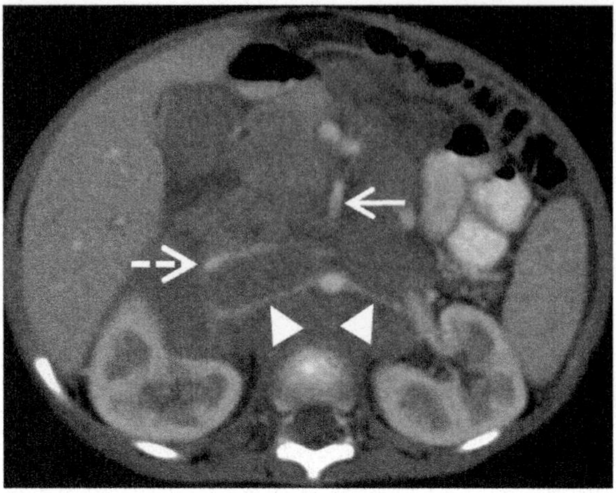

Fig. 5.19 A 2-year-old boy with metastatic abdominal neuroblastoma (MYCN amplified, INSS stage 4, INRGSS M). Contrast-enhanced transverse CT scan view. The tumour demonstrates moderate and homogeneous enhancement. It arises from the periaortic sympathetic fibres and encases both renal pedicles (arrowhead), the superior mesenteric artery (arrow) and the inferior vena cava (dotted arrow)

- The potential metastases included in the field of view (mainly in the bone and liver)

5.4.2 Metastatic Disease

Metastatic disease is observed in 48% of patients at diagnosis [41]. Distant metastases are mainly located in the bone marrow (56%) or bone (47%); metastatic disease involving soft tissue sites includes lymph nodes (24%), liver (21%) and, less commonly, skin (4%), lung (3%) and CNS (1%) [57].

Bone and bone marrow involvement is currently assessed by bilateral bone marrow aspirate and biopsy and by ^{123}I-metaiodobenzylguanidine (mIBG) scintigraphy [32–34] (see Part III). Whole-body MRI (WB-MRI) is not recommended although one small series [61] provided encouraging results, although because of its low specificity it has only limited value in assessing therapeutic response compared to MIBG.

Skeletal surveys are no more recommended in infants; however, painful bone location should be assessed by plain films to depict pathologic fractures.

Skull metastases depicted by MIBG do not require specific imaging unless there are neurologic symptoms. However, brain MRI or CT should be obtained when skull base or orbit involvement is clinically suspected or depicted on MIBG in order to detect optic nerve compression [62] which may require emergency treatment (Figs. 5.21 and 5.22).

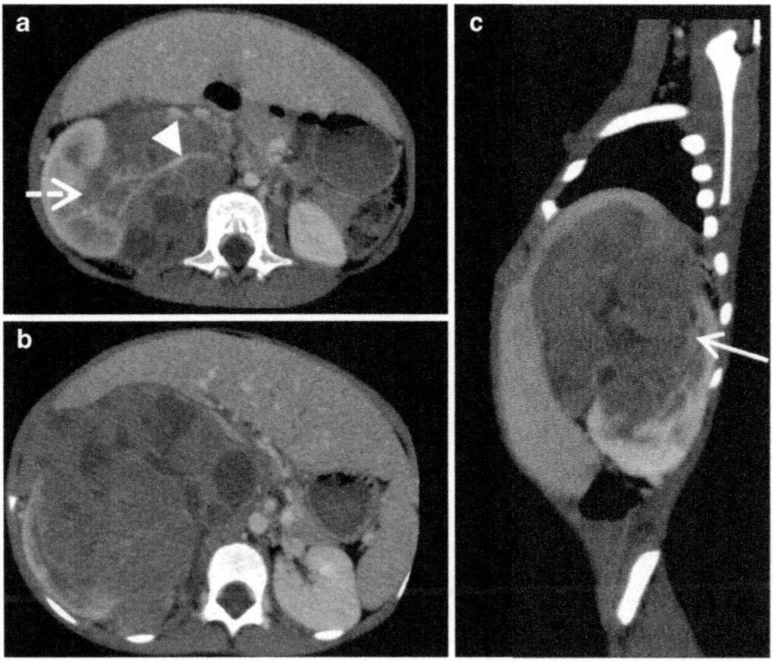

Fig. 5.20 A 4-year-old girl with localized right adrenal neuroblastoma (MYCN amplified, INSS stage 3, INRGSS L2). Contrast-enhanced transverse CT scan (**a**, **b**) and MPR sagittal views (**c**). The tumour demonstrates moderate and heterogeneous enhancement with necrotic low densities. The mass infiltrates the upper pole (arrow) and the hilum (dotted arrow) of the right kidney and encases the renal pedicle (arrowhead)

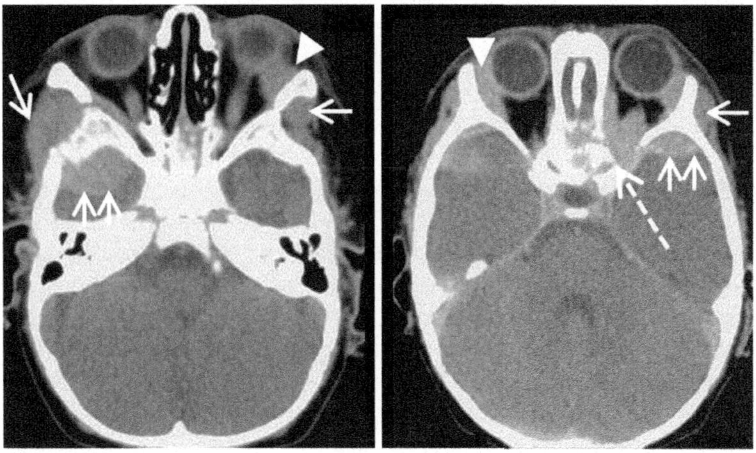

Fig. 5.21 A 10-month-old boy with metastatic adrenal neuroblastoma (MYCN amplified, INSS stage 4, INRGSS M). Contrast-enhanced transverse CT scan views of the brain and orbits. Typical bone metastases occurring along bone fissures of the skull and facial bones. Soft tissue invasion is visible in the external temporal fossa (arrow), in the epidural space along the great sphenoid wings (double arrows) and in the orbit (arrowheads). Invasion of the left optic canal (dotted arrow) represents an emergency situation because of possible optic nerve compression

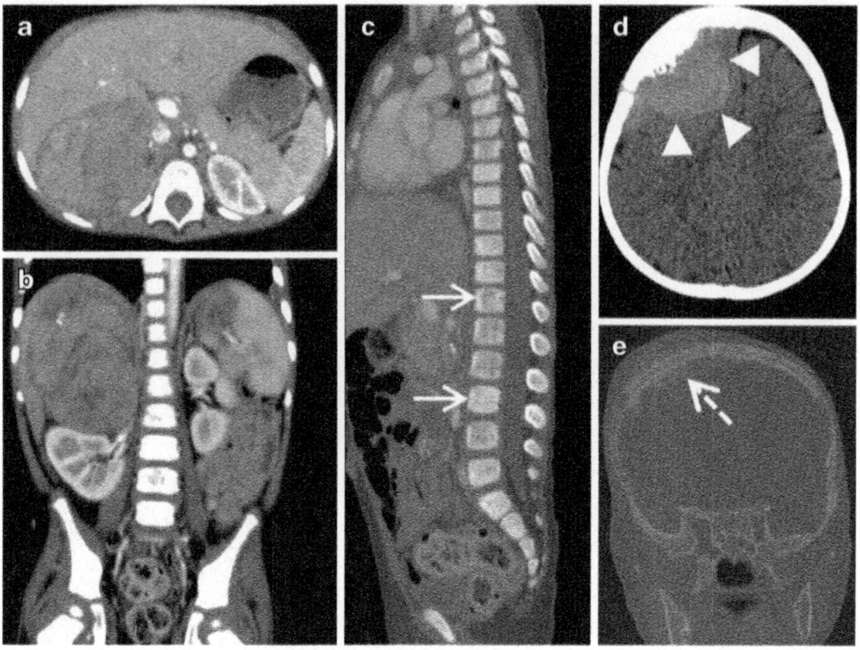

Fig. 5.22 A 27-month-old boy with metastatic abdominal neuroblastoma (MYCN non-amplified, segmental chromosome alteration, INSS stage 4, INRGSS M). Contrast-enhanced transverse CT scan (**a**) and coronal (**b**) views of the abdomen, sagittal (**c**) view of the spine and transverse (**d**) and coronal (**e**) views of the brain and skull. The primary tumour arises from the right adrenal gland (**a**, **b**). Spinal bone and bone marrow metastases (**c**) are depicted by CT which demonstrates both decreased and increased density areas (arrows). Skull metastases (**d**, **e**) typically occur around the coronal fissure: the right frontal and parietal bones appear heterogeneous with cortical destruction and spiculated periosteal reaction (dotted arrows). In this patient, intracranial soft tissue invasion crosses the dura and directly invades the frontal lobe (arrowheads)

Liver and **subcutaneous** metastases are mainly observed in infants (Pepper syndrome, stage 4S/MS) [63]. Liver metastases are assessed by either US, CT or MRI. Liver metastases may present as focal masses or diffuse infiltration (Figs. 5.14 and 5.23).

Distant (non-regional) **lymph nodes** depicted by CT, MRI or MIBG scan (e.g. supraclavicular lymph node associated with a retroperitoneal primary) are considered metastatic disease (Fig. 5.9a).

Lung and pleural metastases are uncommon and usually observed among patients with MNA tumours [64] and therefore are not routinely screened for by CT unless there is an abnormal chest X-ray.

Pleural disease is associated with reduced survival rates in patients with metastatic disease [65]. However, an isolated pleural effusion is not considered metastatic disease.

CNS parenchymal or meningeal metastatic spread is exceptional and usually observed in metastatic patients with recurrences [66, 67]. Therefore, it is usually not

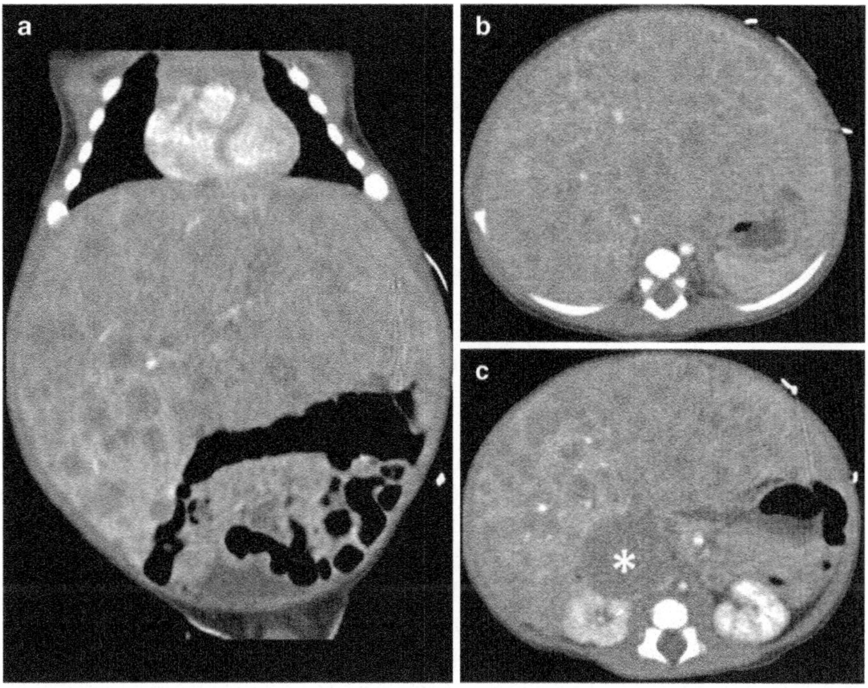

Fig. 5.23 A 2-month-old boy with metastatic abdominal neuroblastoma (INSS stage 4S, INRGSS MS). Contrast-enhanced CT-scan coronal (**a**) and transverse (**b**, **c**) views. The primary tumour arises from the right adrenal gland and demonstrates low density and limited enhancement (asterisk). The liver is dramatically enlarged and diffusely invaded by multiple metastases appearing as low-density nodules compared to normal parenchyma on portal phase

systematically screened for at diagnosis unless specific symptoms are present. The radiologic features of CNS metastases vary from single, large, parenchymal lesions with possible cystic or haemorrhagic features or calcifications, to diffuse meningeal involvement [66, 68–70].

5.5 Prognostic Value of Imaging

Apart from stage, imaging data can provide additional information related to prognosis. The primary tumour location is a prognostic criterion. Abdominal locations are associated with poorer prognosis. Adrenal tumours are more likely than non-adrenal tumours to have MYCN amplification, and thoracic tumours are less likely than non-thoracic tumours to have MYCN amplification [71].

Chest location is associated with better outcome among the extra-abdominal sites [72, 73]; however, multivariate analysis did not identify the chest location as an independent prognostic factor [74].

Cervical and pelvic NBs are also associated with better prognosis although this information is based on limited data [75–80].

Links between initial tumour volume, tumour shape, volume decrease and genomic profile and outcome have been recently described: a small tumour volume, a single mass (as opposed to multiple confluent masses), and a limited number of IDRFs are associated with better prognosis [43]. Tumour volume reduction during the early phase of induction chemotherapy in high-risk NBs was reported as associated with a better outcome [81], but this critera was not confirmed by another study including any risk-group tumours [43].

5.6 Disease Assessment During Treatment

The International Neuroblastoma Response Criteria (INRC) have been defined and recently updated by an international working group [57].

For metastatic disease, the follow-up during treatment is based on both bone marrow aspirate/biopsies and on MIBG with specific scoring systems [57, 82, 83] (see Part III).

For the primary tumour, 1D, 2D or 3D measurements can be obtained. Unidimensional measurements according to RECIST (Response Evaluation Criteria in Solid Tumours) have been proposed for tumour response assessment [57, 84, 85]. However, this is still a matter of debate since a 3D assessment provides a more realistic tumour volume, especially for infiltrative tumours. In a recent study [86], 3D measurements (versus volumetric change) were found to most accurately quantify NB size response in patients with stage 3 and 4 NB, whereas 1D and 2D measurements underrepresented tumour response.

5.7 Imaging for Long-Term Follow-Up

Since patients' follow-up potentially results in high cumulative exposure to ionizing radiation, mostly because of repeated CT, the role of surveillance imaging in the detection of relapse is a major issue.

Surveillance of the primary tumour site in localized disease should be performed, as far as possible, by techniques not using ionizing radiation, i.e. US or MRI. There is currently no consensus about the periodicity of examinations, usually provided by protocol guidelines. This periodicity should be driven by the occurrence or not of a local residue, and the risk of local relapse, which should be based on the major prognostic criteria such as the age at diagnosis, initial stage, histology and genomic abnormalities.

US should be preferred for children less than 5 years who require sedation for MRI, provided that the initial tumour area can be assessed by this technique (i.e. abdomen or lower cervical area). When the primary tumour occurred in the upper cervical chains, in the chest or in the presacral pelvic area, or is associated with intraspinal residue, MRI is the preferred technique.

In infants with liver metastases, usually associated with adrenal primary, US is the method of choice.

Among non-thoracic high-risk NB, progression or recurrence in the chest is rare and often presents with symptoms or is identified using standard non-CT imaging modalities [87]. Therefore, chest CT can be omitted without compromising disease detection.

Among children with high-risk NB, a recent series [88] assessed a cohort of 183 patients in which 50 experienced a recurrence. Most patients (92%) had metastatic relapse. The mean cumulative effective dose prior to relapse was 125.2 mSv (range, 24.5–259.7), 64% of which was from computed tomography (CT) scans. Among relapse patients, 74% had clinically evident or measurable disease detected by X-ray, US or urinary catecholamines. The addition of MIBG identified eight additional recurrences. Thus, cross-sectional imaging (CT/MRI) was only required to identify 10% of relapses. These results support the rationale of a reduced use of CT imaging in post-therapy surveillance and refinement of surveillance imaging, which may be further guided by risk stratification, disease sites and potentially biomolecular markers.

References

1. Lonergan GJ, Schwab CM, Suarez ES, Carlson CL. Neuroblastoma, ganglioneuroblastoma, and ganglioneuroma: radiologic-pathologic correlation. Radiographics. 2002;22:911–34.
2. Hiorns MP, Owens CM. Radiology of neuroblastoma in children. Eur Radiol. 2001;11:2071–81.
3. Swift CC, Eklund MJ, Kraveka JM, Alazraki AL. Updates in diagnosis, management, and treatment of neuroblastoma. Radiographics. 2018;38:566–80.
4. Brody AS, Frush DP, Huda W, et al. Radiation risk to children from computed tomography. Pediatrics. 2007;120:677–82.
5. Journy N, Roue T, Cardis E, et al. Childhood CT scans and cancer risk: impact of predisposing factors for cancer on the risk estimates. J Radiol Prot. 2016;36:N1–7.
6. Brisse HJ, Aubert B. Niveaux d'exposition en tomodensitométrie multicoupes pédiatrique: résultats de l'enquête dosimétrique SFIPP/IRSN 2007-2008 [CT exposure from pediatric MDCT: results from the 2007-2008 SFIPP/ISRN survey]. J Radiol. 2009;90:207–15.
7. Goske MJ, Applegate KE, Boylan J, et al. The image gently campaign: working together to change practice. Am J Roentgenol. 2008;190:273–4.
8. Gay F, Pavia Y, Pierrat N, et al. Dose reduction with adaptive statistical iterative reconstruction for paediatric CT: phantom study and clinical experience on chest and abdomen CT. Eur Radiol. 2014;24:102–11.
9. Sofka CM, Semelka RC, Kelekis NL, et al. Magnetic resonance imaging of neuroblastoma using current techniques. Magn Reson Imaging. 1999;17:193–8.
10. Siegel MJ, Jaju A. MR imaging of neuroblastic masses. Magn Reson Imaging Clin N Am. 2008;16:499–513. vi.
11. Berdon WE, Ruzal-Shapiro C, Abramson SJ, Garvin J. The diagnosis of abdominal neuroblastoma: relative roles of ultrasonography, CT, and MRI. Urol Radiol. 1992;14:252–62.
12. Siegel MJ, Ishwaran H, Fletcher BD, et al. Staging of neuroblastoma at imaging: report of the Radiology Diagnostic Oncology Group. Radiology. 2002;223:168–75.
13. Brisse HJ, McCarville MB, Granata C, et al. Guidelines for imaging and staging of neuroblastic tumors: consensus report from the International Neuroblastoma Risk Group Project. Radiology. 2011;261:243–57.

14. Brown RE Jr. Safety considerations of anesthetic drugs in children. Expert Opin Drug Saf. 2017;16:445–54.
15. Sinner B, Becke K, Engelhard K. General anaesthetics and the developing brain: an overview. Anaesthesia. 2014;69:1009–22.
16. Vutskits L, Xie Z. Lasting impact of general anaesthesia on the brain: mechanisms and relevance. Nat Rev Neurosci. 2016;17:705–17.
17. Callahan MJ, MacDougall RD, Bixby SD, et al. Ionizing radiation from computed tomography versus anesthesia for magnetic resonance imaging in infants and children: patient safety considerations. Pediatr Radiol. 2018;48:21–30.
18. Kornreich L, Horev G, Kaplinsky C, et al. Neuroblastoma: evaluation with contrast enhanced MR imaging. Pediatr Radiol. 1991;21:566–9.
19. Neubauer H, Li M, Muller VR, et al. Diagnostic value of diffusion-weighted MRI for tumor characterization, differentiation and monitoring in pediatric patients with neuroblastic tumors. Rofo. 2017;189:640–50.
20. Olchowy C, Cebulski K, Lasecki M, et al. The presence of the gadolinium-based contrast agent depositions in the brain and symptoms of gadolinium neurotoxicity - a systematic review. PLoS One. 2017;12:e0171704.
21. Flood TF, Stence NV, Maloney JA, Mirsky DM. Pediatric brain: repeated exposure to linear gadolinium-based contrast material is associated with increased signal intensity at unenhanced T1-weighted MR imaging. Radiology. 2017;282:222–8.
22. McDonald RJ, McDonald JS, Dai D, et al. Comparison of gadolinium concentrations within multiple rat organs after intravenous administration of linear versus macrocyclic gadolinium chelates. Radiology. 2017;0:161594.
23. Runge VM. Critical questions regarding gadolinium deposition in the brain and body after injections of the gadolinium-based contrast agents, safety, and clinical recommendations in consideration of the EMA's pharmacovigilance and risk assessment committee recommendation for suspension of the marketing authorizations for 4 linear agents. Invest Radiol. 2017;52:317–23.
24. Tibussek D, Rademacher C, Caspers J, et al. Gadolinium brain deposition after macrocyclic gadolinium administration: a pediatric case-control study. Radiology. 2017;0:161151.
25. Mendichovszky IA, Marks SD, Simcock CM, Olsen OE. Gadolinium and nephrogenic systemic fibrosis: time to tighten practice. Pediatr Radiol. 2008;38:489.
26. Dumba M, Jawad N, McHugh K. Neuroblastoma and nephroblastoma: a radiological review. Cancer Imaging. 2015;15:5.
27. Le Bihan D, Breton E, Lallemand D, et al. MR imaging of intravoxel incoherent motions: application to diffusion and perfusion in neurologic disorders. Radiology. 1986;161:401–7.
28. Humphries PD, Sebire NJ, Siegel MJ, Olsen OE. Tumors in pediatric patients at diffusion-weighted MR imaging: apparent diffusion coefficient and tumor cellularity. Radiology. 2007;245:848–54.
29. Uhl M, Altehoefer C, Kontny U, et al. MRI-diffusion imaging of neuroblastomas: first results and correlation to histology. Eur Radiol. 2002;12:2335–8.
30. Gahr N, Darge K, Hahn G, et al. Diffusion-weighted MRI for differentiation of neuroblastoma and ganglioneuroblastoma/ganglioneuroma. Eur J Radiol. 2011;79:443.
31. Demir S, Altinkaya N, Kocer NE, et al. Variations in apparent diffusion coefficient values following chemotherapy in pediatric neuroblastoma. Diagn Interv Radiol. 2015;21:184–8.
32. Olivier P, Colarinha P, Fettich J, et al. Guidelines for radioiodinated MIBG scintigraphy in children. Eur J Nucl Med Mol Imaging. 2003;30:B45–50.
33. Franzius C, Schmidt M, Hero B, et al. Procedure guidelines for MIBG-scintigraphy in children. Nuklearmedizin. 2008;47:132–8.
34. Matthay KK, Shulkin B, Ladenstein R, et al. Criteria for evaluation of disease extent by (123)I-metaiodobenzylguanidine scans in neuroblastoma: a report for the International Neuroblastoma Risk Group (INRG) Task Force. Br J Cancer. 2010;102:1319–26.

35. Lumbroso J, Guermazi F, Hartmann O, et al. Sensitivity and specificity of meta-iodobenzylguanidine (mIBG) scintigraphy in the evaluation of neuroblastoma: analysis of 115 cases. Bull Cancer. 1988;75:97–106.
36. Jacobs A, Delree M, Desprechins B, et al. Consolidating the role of *I-MIBG-scintigraphy in childhood neuroblastoma: five years of clinical experience. Pediatr Radiol. 1990;20:157–9.
37. McHugh K. Renal and adrenal tumours in children. Cancer Imaging. 2007;7:41–51.
38. Mehta K, Haller JO, Legasto AC. Imaging neuroblastoma in children. Crit Rev Comput Tomogr. 2003;44:47–61.
39. Brisse H, Edeline V, Michon J, et al. Current strategy for the imaging of neuroblastoma. J Radiol. 2001;82:447–54.
40. Papaioannou G, McHugh K. Neuroblastoma in childhood: review and radiological findings. Cancer Imaging. 2005;5:116–27.
41. Cohn SL, Pearson AD, London WB, et al. The International Neuroblastoma Risk Group (INRG) classification system: an INRG Task Force report. J Clin Oncol. 2009;27:289–97.
42. Moroz V, Machin D, Faldum A, et al. Changes over three decades in outcome and the prognostic influence of age-at-diagnosis in young patients with neuroblastoma: a report from the International Neuroblastoma Risk Group Project. Eur J Cancer. 2011;47:561–71.
43. Brisse HJ, Blanc T, Schleiermacher G, et al. Radiogenomics of neuroblastomas: relationships between imaging phenotypes, tumor genomic profile and survival. PLoS One. 2017;12:e0185190.
44. Sauvat F, Brisse H, Magdeleinat P, et al. The transmanubrial approach: a new operative approach to cervicothoracic neuroblastoma in children. Surgery. 2006;139:109–14.
45. Maris JM, Kyemba SM, Rebbeck TR, et al. Molecular genetic analysis of familial neuroblastoma. Eur J Cancer. 1997;33:1923–8.
46. Hiyama E, Yokoyama T, Hiyama K, et al. Multifocal neuroblastoma: biologic behavior and surgical aspects. Cancer. 2000;88:1955–63.
47. Wu YH, Song B, Xu J, et al. Retroperitoneal neoplasms within the perirenal space in infants and children: differentiation of renal and non-renal origin in enhanced CT images. Eur J Radiol. 2010;75:279–86.
48. Sauvat F, Sarnacki S, Brisse H, et al. Outcome of suprarenal localized masses diagnosed during the perinatal period: a retrospective multicenter study. Cancer. 2002;94:2474–80.
49. Granata C, Fagnani AM, Gambini C, et al. Features and outcome of neuroblastoma detected before birth. J Pediatr Surg. 2000;35:88–91.
50. Nadler EP, Barksdale EM. Adrenal masses in the newborn. Semin Pediatr Surg. 2000;9:156–64.
51. Curtis MR, Mooney DP, Vaccaro TJ, et al. Prenatal ultrasound characterization of the suprarenal mass: distinction between neuroblastoma and subdiaphragmatic extralobar pulmonary sequestration. J Ultrasound Med. 1997;16:75–83.
52. Deeg KH, Bettendorf U, Hofmann V. Differential diagnosis of neonatal adrenal haemorrhage and congenital neuroblastoma by colour coded Doppler sonography and power Doppler sonography. Eur J Pediatr. 1998;157:294–7.
53. Lin JN, Lin GJ, Hung IJ, Hsueh C. Prenatally detected tumor mass in the adrenal gland. J Pediatr Surg. 1999;34:1620–3.
54. Daneman A, Baunin C, Lobo E, et al. Disappearing suprarenal masses in fetuses and infants. Pediatr Radiol. 1997;27:675–81.
55. Brunklaus A, Pohl K, Zuberi SM, de Sousa C. Investigating neuroblastoma in childhood opsoclonus-myoclonus syndrome. Arch Dis Child. 2012;97:461–3.
56. Swart JF, de Kraker J, van der Lely N. Metaiodobenzylguanidine total-body scintigraphy required for revealing occult neuroblastoma in opsoclonus-myoclonus syndrome. Eur J Pediatr. 2002;161:255–8.
57. Park JR, Bagatell R, Cohn SL, et al. Revisions to the international neuroblastoma response criteria: a consensus statement from the National Cancer Institute Clinical Trials Planning Meeting. J Clin Oncol. 2017;35:2580–7.

58. Brodeur GM, Seeger RC, Barrett A, et al. International criteria for diagnosis, staging, and response to treatment in patients with neuroblastoma. J Clin Oncol. 1988;6:1874–81.
59. Brodeur GM, Pritchard J, Berthold F, et al. Revisions of the international criteria for neuroblastoma diagnosis, staging, and response to treatment. J Clin Oncol. 1993;11:1466–77.
60. Monclair T, Brodeur GM, Ambros PF, et al. The International Neuroblastoma Risk Group (INRG) staging system: an INRG Task Force report. J Clin Oncol. 2009;27:298–303.
61. Goo HW, Choi SH, Ghim T, et al. Whole-body MRI of paediatric malignant tumours: comparison with conventional oncological imaging methods. Pediatr Radiol. 2005;35:766–73.
62. Lau JJ, Trobe JD, Ruiz RE, et al. Metastatic neuroblastoma presenting with binocular blindness from intracranial compression of the optic nerves. J Neuroophthalmol. 2004;24:119–24.
63. DuBois SG, Kalika Y, Lukens JN, et al. Metastatic sites in stage IV and IVS neuroblastoma correlate with age, tumor biology, and survival. J Pediatr Hematol Oncol. 1999;21:181–9.
64. Dubois SG, London WB, Zhang Y, et al. Lung metastases in neuroblastoma at initial diagnosis: a report from the International Neuroblastoma Risk Group (INRG) project. Pediatr Blood Cancer. 2008;51:589–92.
65. Kammen BF, Matthay KK, Pacharn P, et al. Pulmonary metastases at diagnosis of neuroblastoma in pediatric patients: CT findings and prognosis. AJR Am J Roentgenol. 2001;176:755–9.
66. Matthay KK, Brisse H, Couanet D, et al. Central nervous system metastases in neuroblastoma: radiologic, clinical, and biologic features in 23 patients. Cancer. 2003;98:155–65.
67. D'Ambrosio N, Lyo JK, Young RJ, et al. Imaging of Metastatic CNS Neuroblastoma. Am J Roentgenol. 2010;194:1223–9.
68. Aronson MR, Smoker WR, Oetting GM. Hemorrhagic intracranial parenchymal metastases from primary retroperitoneal neuroblastoma. Pediatr Radiol. 1995;25:284–5.
69. Kellie SJ, Hayes FA, Bowman L, et al. Primary extracranial neuroblastoma with central nervous system metastases characterization by clinicopathologic findings and neuroimaging. Cancer. 1991;68:1999–2006.
70. Quackenbush KE, Luna-Fineman S, Magee JF, et al. Neuroblastoma involvement of the falx cerebri. Pediatr Blood Cancer. 2009;53:1337–9.
71. Vo KT, Matthay KK, Neuhaus J, et al. Clinical, biologic, and prognostic differences on the basis of primary tumor site in neuroblastoma: a report from the international neuroblastoma risk group project. J Clin Oncol. 2014;32:3169–76.
72. Adams GA, Shochat SJ, Smith EI, et al. Thoracic neuroblastoma: a Pediatric Oncology Group study. J Pediatr Surg. 1993;28:372–7; discussion 377–378.
73. Morris JA, Shcochat SJ, Smith EI, et al. Biological variables in thoracic neuroblastoma: a Pediatric Oncology Group study. J Pediatr Surg. 1995;30:296–302; discussion 302–293.
74. Haberle B, Hero B, Berthold F, von Schweinitz D. Characteristics and outcome of thoracic neuroblastoma. Eur J Pediatr Surg. 2002;12:145–50.
75. Cruccetti A, Kiely EM, Spitz L, et al. Pelvic neuroblastoma: low mortality and high morbidity. J Pediatr Surg. 2000;35:724–8.
76. Haase GM, O'Leary MC, Stram DO, et al. Pelvic neuroblastoma--implications for a new favorable subgroup: a Children's Cancer Group experience. Ann Surg Oncol. 1995;2:516–23.
77. Leclair MD, Hartmann O, Heloury Y, et al. Localized pelvic neuroblastoma: excellent survival and low morbidity with tailored therapy--the 10-year experience of the French Society of Pediatric Oncology. J Clin Oncol. 2004;22:1689–95.
78. Abramson SJ, Berdon WE, Ruzal-Shapiro C, et al. Cervical neuroblastoma in eleven infants--a tumor with favorable prognosis. Clinical and radiologic (US, CT, MRI) findings. Pediatr Radiol. 1993;23:253–7.
79. Moukheiber AK, Nicollas R, Roman S, et al. Primary pediatric neuroblastic tumors of the neck. Int J Pediatr Otorhinolaryngol. 2001;60:155–61.
80. Qureshi SS, Kembhavi S, Ramadwar M, et al. Outcome and morbidity of surgical resection of primary cervical and cervicothoracic neuroblastoma in children: a comparative analysis. Pediatr Surg Int. 2014;30:267–73.

81. Yoo SY, Kim JS, Sung KW, et al. The degree of tumor volume reduction during the early phase of induction chemotherapy is an independent prognostic factor in patients with high-risk neuroblastoma. Cancer. 2013;119:656–64.
82. Ladenstein R, Lambert B, Potschger U, et al. Validation of the mIBG skeletal SIOPEN scoring method in two independent high-risk neuroblastoma populations: the SIOPEN/HR-NBL1 and COG-A3973 trials. Eur J Nucl Med Mol Imaging. 2018;45:292–305.
83. Yanik GA, Parisi MT, Naranjo A, et al. Validation of post-induction Curie scores in high risk neuroblastoma. A Children's Oncology Group (COG) and SIOPEN group report on SIOPEN/HR-NBL1. J Nucl Med. 2018;59:502.
84. Therasse P, Arbuck SG, Eisenhauer EA, et al. New guidelines to evaluate the response to treatment in solid tumors. European Organization for Research and Treatment of Cancer, National Cancer Institute of the United States, National Cancer Institute of Canada. J Natl Cancer Inst. 2000;92:205–16.
85. Eisenhauer EA, Therasse P, Bogaerts J, et al. New response evaluation criteria in solid tumours: revised RECIST guideline (version 1.1). Eur J Cancer. 2009;45:228–47.
86. Trout AT, Towbin AJ, Klingbeil L, et al. Single and multidimensional measurements underestimate neuroblastoma response to therapy. Pediatr Blood Cancer. 2017;64:18–24.
87. Federico SM, Brady SL, Pappo A, et al. The role of chest computed tomography (CT) as a surveillance tool in children with high-risk neuroblastoma. Pediatr Blood Cancer. 2015;62:976–81.
88. Owens C, Li BK, Thomas KE, Irwin MS. Surveillance imaging and radiation exposure in the detection of relapsed neuroblastoma. Pediatr Blood Cancer. 2016;63:1786–93.

Image-Defined Risk Factors

6

Giovanni Cecchetto, Tom Monclair, and Hervé J. Brisse

6.1 Image-Defined Risk Factors (IDRFs): What They Are, and Why They Were Introduced

About one half of patients with neuroblastoma (NBL) present with disseminated disease for whom the currently recommended initial approach is limited to diagnostic biopsies. The other half of the patients have localized disease, and if complete excision of the tumor can be achieved at the time of diagnosis, the majority of these patients are cured by operation alone [1]. Accordingly, proper initial approach in NBL covers the range from percutaneous needle biopsies to complete excision of the primary tumor. However, bearing in mind that NBL is a chemosensitive tumor, the latter alternative should only be attempted if complete removal of the tumor can be achieved without mutilation of the patient. If this goal cannot be predicted with reasonable certainty, neoadjuvant chemotherapy is usually considered a better initial treatment alternative aiming at shrinkage of the tumor mass which may both facilitate surgical removal at a later stage and make the operation safer.

The choice between initial excision and biopsy in localized NBL has been based on several factors, among which imaging has a central position. Also the experience, ability, and attitude of the surgeons involved have played a key role. With successful initial tumor excision, the negative effects of chemotherapy are avoided, a fact which may have pushed surgeons to attempt initial operations in inappropriate

G. Cecchetto (✉)
Department of Woman's and Child's Health, Padova University Hospital, Padova, Italy
e-mail: giovanni.cecchetto@unipd.it

T. Monclair
Department of Hepatic, Gastrointestinal and Paediatric Surgery,
Oslo University Hospital – Rikshospitalet, Oslo, Norway
e-mail: tom.monclair@online.no

H. J. Brisse
Département d'Imagerie Médicale, Institut Curie, Paris, France
e-mail: herve.brisse@curie.fr

S. Sarnacki, L. Pio (eds.), *Neuroblastoma*,
https://doi.org/10.1007/978-3-030-18396-7_6

situations, with undue risks for the patient. For example, nephrectomy during surgery at diagnosis is today considered a too high price for obtaining complete tumor removal. With kidneys at risk, there are good reasons to believe that the chance of retaining two functioning kidneys increases when operations are done after neoadjuvant chemotherapy.

Taking into account that treatment decisions to a large extent were based on subjective considerations, it is not surprising that patients with similar clinical conditions have received different treatment depending on where they were treated. Obviously more precise definitions of the criteria of operability would be useful in order to choose the best treatment alternative and to discourage inappropriate operations with risks of morbidity or leaving gross residual disease. In addition, common terminology and definitions are considered prerequisites for conducting multicenter trials. With rare diseases like NBL, progress in treatment is highly dependent on multicenter studies.

In line with the considerations above, one of the objectives of the LNESG1 study on localized non-*MYCN*-amplified NBL, run by SIOPEN from 1995 to 1999, was the identification and evaluation of preoperative radiological features that could help the physicians in deciding whether initial safe, non-mutilating, and complete tumor excision was feasible or not [2]. In LNESG1 these features were called surgical risk factors (SRF). Later the major international cooperative children's cancer groups COG, GPOH, INRG, JNBSG, and SIOPEN have agreed to use the term image-defined risk factors (IDRFs) to emphasize that the assessment based on risk factors has to be taken on preoperative evaluation of imaging studies [3, 4]. The SRF/IDRFs (hereafter called IDRF only) describe the relationship between the primary tumor mass and the surrounding organs and structures. They are listed in Table 6.1. The LNESG1 study, with more than 700 evaluable patients undergoing surgical tumor excision at diagnosis, showed that presence of one or more of these factors was associated with higher frequencies of incomplete tumor excisions and surgery-related complications [2], as well as lower survival [5]. These findings have been confirmed by others [6, 7]. In recent years IDRFs have been shown to be equally well suited to predict success with operative treatment also when tumor excisions are done with minimal invasive surgery [8, 9] or after neoadjuvant chemotherapy [10, 11]. However, what applies to patients participating in trials does not necessarily apply to individual patients treated outside of a research protocol. In LNESG1 the differences in outcome were relatively small, and the possibility that patients *with* IDRF who underwent tumor excision at diagnosis in fact received the best treatment available cannot be excluded. An answer to that question would require a randomized study between two groups of patients with IDRF, one receiving neoadjuvant chemotherapy versus one treated with tumor excision at diagnosis; and this study we do not have. Therefore, in order not to inadvertently exaggerate the impact of IDRF, it is currently safe to consider presence of IDRF a warning sign justifying the term *advanced locoregional disease*. As a practical precaution, the presence of IDRFs should call for a more critical evaluation of the operative risks before embarking on surgery.

Table 6.1 Image-defined risk factors (IDRF) (from Monclair et al., JCO, 27; 298–303, 2009)

Image-defined risk factors in neuroblastic tumors
Ipsilateral tumor extension within two body compartments   Neck-chest, chest-abdomen, abdomen-pelvis

Neck
  Tumor encasing carotid and/or vertebral artery and/or internal jugular vein
  Tumor extending to the base of skull
  Tumor compressing the trachea

Cervicothoracic junction
  Tumor encasing brachial plexus roots
  Tumor encasing subclavian vessels and/or vertebral and/or carotid artery
  Tumor compressing the trachea

Thorax
  Tumor encasing the aorta and/or major branches
  Tumor compressing the trachea and/or principal bronchi
  Lower mediastinal tumor, infiltrating the costovertebral junction between T9 and T12

Thoracoabdominal   Tumor encasing the aorta and/or vena cava

Abdomen/pelvis
  Tumor infiltrating the porta hepatis and/or the hepatoduodenal ligament
  Tumor encasing branches of the superior mesenteric artery at the mesenteric root
  Tumor encasing the origin of the coeliac axis and/or the superior mesenteric artery
  Tumor invading one or both renal pedicles
  Tumor encasing the aorta and/or vena cava
  Tumor encasing the iliac vessels
  Pelvic tumor crossing the sciatic notch

Intraspinal tumor extension whatever the location provided that: More than one third of the spinal canal in the axial plane is invaded and/or the perimedullary leptomeningeal spaces are not visible and/or the spinal cord signal is abnormal
Infiltration of adjacent organs/structures   Pericardium, diaphragm, kidney, liver, duodeno-pancreatic block, and mesentery

Conditions to be recorded, but *not* considered IDRFs
  Multifocal primary tumors
  Pleural effusion, with or without malignant cells
  Ascites, with or without malignant cells

IDRFs image-defined risk factors

Another valuable asset with the concept of IDRF is that imaging investigations can be reviewed centrally, hereby allowing uniform evaluation of the preoperative condition of patients from different centers. Together with the use of common definitions and terminology, the latter issues support the use of IDRF in treatment planning.

In summary the concept of IDRF has been proven to be a valuable tool assisting in the decision on whether tumor excision can be considered safe and should be attempted or not; and evaluation of IDRF has currently become an integrated part of treatment planning.

6.2 The International Neuroblastoma Risk Group Staging System (INRGSS): A Clinical Classification Based on IDRF

Since Evans' staging in 1971 [12], several systems have been used for clinical classification of neuroblastoma. The International Neuroblastoma Staging System (INSS), which was introduced in 1988 [13] and revised in 1993 [14], had by the turn of the century become the most widely used classification (Table 6.2). The INSS is based on a combination of clinical, radiological, surgical, and pathologic findings, and patients with localized tumors have to be operated for proper staging (see below).

When introduced the INSS represented a major milestone in international cooperation, and it was anticipated that the system would constitute a foundation upon which future modifications and improvements could be based [13]. Maybe because it was tailored to the predominant treatment principle with operation at diagnosis (for biopsy or tumor excision) from the 1980s and onward, the INSS has functioned well for the vast majority of patients. However, INSS is a *postsurgical* staging system, and when the International Neuroblastoma Risk Group (INRG) project was initiated in 2004 (see below), the need for *pretreatment* staging was solved with the International Neuroblastoma Risk Group Staging System [4].

6.2.1 Staging Definitions of INRGSS

Stage L1: tumors are localized tumors that do not involve vital structures as defined by the list of IDRFs (Table 6.1). The tumor must be confined within one body compartment, neck, chest, abdomen, or pelvis. The isolated finding of intraspinal tumor

Table 6.2 The International Neuroblastoma Staging System (INSS) (from Brodeur et al., J Clin Oncol 11; 1466–1477, 1993)

Stage	Definition
1	Localized tumor with complete gross excision, with or without microscopic residual disease; representative ipsilateral lymph nodes negative for tumor microscopically (nodes attached to and removed with the primary tumor may be positive)
2A	Localized tumor with incomplete gross excision; representative ipsilateral nonadherent lymph nodes negative for tumor microscopically
2B	Localized tumor with or without complete gross excision, with ipsilateral nonadherent lymph nodes positive for tumor. Enlarged contralateral lymph nodes must be negative microscopically
3	Unresectable unilateral tumor infiltrating across the midline, with or without regional lymph node involvement; or localized unilateral tumor with contralateral regional lymph node involvement; or midline tumor with bilateral extension by infiltration (unresectable) or by lymph node involvement
4	Any primary tumor with dissemination to the distant lymph nodes, bone, bone marrow, liver, skin, and/or other organs (except as defined for stage 4S)
4S	Localized primary tumor (as defined for stage 1, 2A, or 2B), with dissemination limited to the skin, liver, and/or bone marrow (limited to infants <1 year of age)

extension that does not fulfill the criteria for an IDRF (Table 6.1) is consistent with stage L1.

Stage L2: tumors are locoregional tumors with one or more IDRFs. The tumor may be ipsilaterally continuous within body compartments (i.e., a left-sided abdominal tumor with left-sided chest involvement should be considered stage L2). However, a clearly left-sided abdominal tumor with right-sided chest (or vice versa) involvement is defined as metastatic disease.

Stage M is defined as distant metastatic disease (i.e., not contiguous with the primary tumor) except as defined for MS. Nonregional (distant) lymph node involvement is metastatic disease. However, an upper abdominal tumor with enlarged lower mediastinal nodes or a pelvic tumor with inguinal lymph node involvement is considered locoregional disease. Ascites and a pleural effusion, even with malignant cells, do not constitute metastatic disease unless they are remote from the body compartment of the primary tumor.

Stage MS is metastatic disease in patients younger than 18 months (547 days) with metastases confined to the skin, liver, and/or bone marrow. Bone marrow involvement should be limited to less than 10% of total nucleated cells on smears or biopsy. MIBG scintigraphy must be negative in the bone and bone marrow. Provided there is MIBG uptake in the primary tumor, bone scans or PET-CT are not required. The primary tumor can be L1 or L2, and there is no restriction regarding crossing or infiltration of the midline [4].

The short version of the four INRGSS stages is listed in Table 6.3 [4].

Since built on a similar template as the INSS (and Evans' staging), but limited to a specific description of the extent of disease based on imaging, the INRGSS can be considered a simplified modification of the older systems. However, whereas the INSS and Evans' staging also served as risk classifications, the INRGSS is restricted to constitute one of seven parameters used to define 16 pretreatment risk groups in the INRG system, the other six being age, histologic category, grade of tumor differentiation, *MYCN* status, aberration of chromosome 11q, and tumor DNA ploïdy [15] (see Chap. 15). If these parameters are included in the diagnostic workup, patients with neuroblastic diseases can be risk grouped according to INRG, not only prospectively at diagnosis but also retrospectively.

Table 6.3 The International Neuroblastoma Risk Group Staging System (INRGSS) (from Monclair et al., J Clin Oncol 27; 298–303, 2009)

International Neuroblastoma Risk Group Staging System	
Stage	Description
L1	Localized tumor not involving vital structures as defined by the list of image-defined risk factors and confined to one body compartment
L2	Locoregional tumor with presence of one or more image-defined risk factors
M	Distant metastatic disease (except stage MS)
MS	Metastatic disease in children younger than 18 months with metastases confined to the skin, liver, and/or bone marrow

Note: See text for detailed criteria. Patients with multifocal primary tumors should be staged according to the greatest extent of disease as defined in the table

The aim of the INRG project was to develop a classification system that would facilitate the comparison of risk-based clinical trials conducted in different regions of the world [15]. The INRG Task Force consisted of 52 investigators with expertise in neuroblastoma, and the Task Force members were appointed by the American, European, and Japanese cooperative children's cancer groups. The major goal of the project was to define homogenous pretreatment patient cohorts and to develop a consensus approach for pretreatment risk stratification of neuroblastoma based on statistical analyses of prognostic factors. The need for a pretreatment staging system precluded the postsurgical INSS, and the INRG Task Force designed the INRGSS for this purpose [4].

Since 1995 SIOPEN had classified locoregional tumors as *resectable* or *unresectable* dependent on the absence or presence of surgical risk factors (SRF) but independent of INSS stage [2]. The SIOPEN principle for stratifying patients with locoregional tumors by imaging features was adopted by the INRG Task Force. However, to avoid confusion with the INSS, the terms resectable and unresectable were not used in the INRG system. Further, the Task Force agreed upon using the SIOPEN list of SRF (with minor modifications), but preferred the term IDRF to SRF (Table 6.1). Detailed guidelines for imaging and description of the IDRF and staging of neuroblastic tumors were published in a consensus report from the INRG project in 2011 [3]. Whereas a patient's stage according to INRGSS is established once and for all at the time of diagnosis, his or her IDRF status can be reassessed throughout the course of the disease. A patient with INSS stage 1 must by definition have undergone "complete gross excision" of a localized tumor. Not only has a stage 1 patient been treated before staging, today we also know that 98% of patients with INSS stage 1 disease are cured by surgery alone [16]. This fact exemplifies that INSS and INRGSS are designed for different purposes and that direct comparison between the prognostic power of the two systems is not meaningful. A comparison between patients with INRGSS stage L1 and INSS stage 1 is in fact between untreated patients and patients who have already been cured. The more relevant counterpart to INSS within the INRG system is therefore not the INRGSS, but the INRG pretreatment risk classification; either the 16 risk groups (A–R) or the four lumped categories designated: very low risk (A, B, C), low risk (D, E, F), intermediate risk (G, H, I, J), or high risk (K, N, O, P, Q, R) [15] (see Chap. 15).

Since the turn of the century, an increasing number of patients that would have had INSS stage 1 disease (if properly staged by operation) are followed with a "wait and see" regimen of observation only [17, 18]. A substantial number of these patients have tumors that regress spontaneously, and most of them are cured without ever being operated upon and without ever having undergone proper INSS staging. Furthermore, the same localized tumor can be either stage 1 or 3 depending on the extent of surgical excision, a fact making direct comparison of clinical trials based on INSS difficult [19].

The INRGSS differs from INSS in five important ways. *First*, it is based on preoperative imaging and IDRFs, not surgicopathological findings. *Second*, whereas INSS has four stages (and Evans' three stages) of non-metastatic disease, the INRGSS has two. With time improved treatment had almost eliminated the differences in survival rates among the stages of localized disease. From the 1960s and until the turn of the century, survival in all stages of localized neuroblastoma had increased from 50% [12] to more than 90% [20–22]. Accordingly, for prediction of outcome in patients with localized neuroblastoma, the use of many clinical stages was no longer practical, and the INRG Task Force decided that the extent of localized disease was sufficiently described with two stages, *localized disease (L1)* and *advanced locoregional disease (L2)*. *Third*, the midline is not included in the staging criteria of the INRGSS. *Fourth*, lymph node status is not included in the staging of localized disease. *Fifth*, whereas INSS stage 4S has an upper age limit of 12 months, the Task Force decided to extend the age group for stage MS up to 18 months [15]. The extension to 18 months also made the clinical INRG staging and pretreatment risk grouping more in tune with the International Neuroblastoma Pathology Classification [23, 24].

Figure 6.1 shows the distribution of INRGSS stages L1 and L2 among the three INSS stages of localized disease. Four out of five patients with INSS stage 1 have INRGSS stage L1, and 19 out of 20 INSS stage 3 patients have INRGSS stage L2.

Since the INRGSS was not intended to substitute for the INSS, the INRG Task Force anticipated that most cooperative groups would continue to use INSS in parallel with INRGSS [4].

Finally, it must be emphasized that the INRGSS and the pretreatment risk grouping were developed by consensus among more than 50 international neuroblastoma experts on a background of statistical analyses of data from 8800 patients with neuroblastic diseases [15]. Obviously not everyone will find the list of IDRF and the INRG systems ideal. One must, however, keep in mind that consensus is never reached without compromises; and hitherto the systems seem to have been well received.

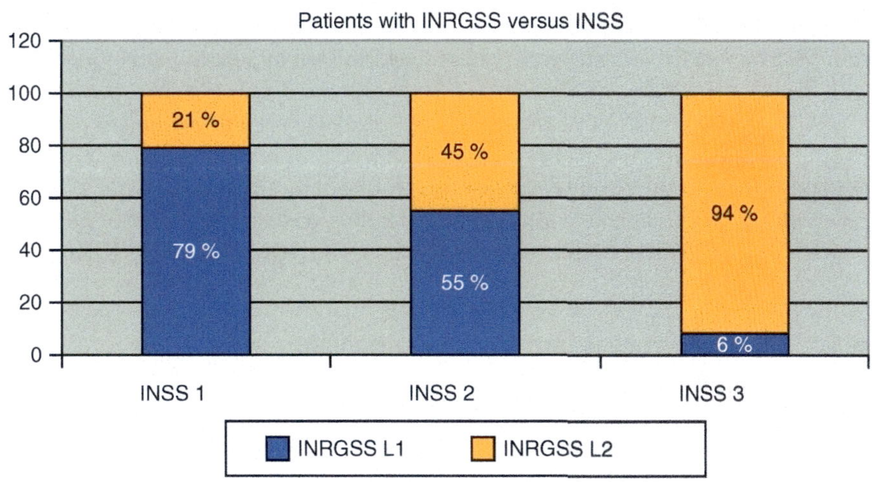

Fig. 6.1 Percentage distribution of 661 SIOPEN patients with locoregional neuroblastoma by INRGSS versus INSS. INSS 1, $n = 303$; INSS 2, $n = 147$; INSS 3, $n = 211$. Diagram based on data from Monclair et al., J Clin Oncol, 27; 298–303, 2009

6.3 Description of IDRF by Tumor Site and Relationship with Vital Structures

In the LNESG1 as well as in the SIOPEN High-Risk Neuroblastoma Studies 1–5, presence of IDRF contraindicated attempt at initial tumor excisions [2, 5, 16]. Other reports are in favor of this strategy [6, 7, 25, 26]. However, outside of a research protocol, the presence of IDRF itself does not imply that surgery is contraindicated. The concept of IDRF should rather be regarded as a way to facilitate a thorough assessment of the locoregional extent of the tumor prior to decision of the assumed best initial management. This is of special relevance for patients with non-metastatic tumors in order to choose between initial operation and secondary surgery after chemotherapy, as well as to evaluate the possibility of minimally invasive surgery [10]. Secondly, IDRFs are prognostic criteria significantly associated with survival [4, 5] and therefore included in the current INRG staging system. Moreover, recent studies have also demonstrated a significant link between the number of IDRF and the genomic profile of the tumors, i.e., the number of IDRF being significantly higher in MYCN-amplified NBL [27].

Local extension of neuroblastoma mainly consists of vascular involvement (mainly along arteries), infiltration of adjacent soft tissues and organs (mainly kidneys and liver), and infiltration of foramina and epidural space when NBL arise from paraspinal sympathetic chains. Accurate analysis and description of all vessels and adjacent organs or structures is therefore a critical part of the imaging report. However, numerous and variable terms are commonly used to describe the relationships between tumors and normal anatomic structures. Therefore and taking into account that few radiologists are specifically involved in pediatric oncology and aware of the most frequent complications associated with neuroblastoma surgery, in 2011 an international group of neuroblastoma experts published a special report [3] aiming to optimize imaging and uniform reporting, including specific definitions of terms recommended to be used as well as a checklist of all relevant structures to be assessed.

Although IDRFs were designed to be used at diagnosis, this method of detailed radiological assessment can also be used after neoadjuvant chemotherapy to preoperatively reassess the residual disease [8, 9]. Actually, in patients with initially "unresectable" NBL operated after chemoreduction, complete resection or minimal residual disease is more frequent among children who have reduction of IDRF [11].

6.3.1 Recommended Terms to Describe IDRFs in Imaging Reports

For adjacent organs and vessels, the terms "separation" and "contact" should be used according to the visibility or not of at least a thin fatty layer between the tumor and the adjacent structure. "Encasement" is the recommended term indicating that the neighboring structure is surrounded by the tumor. "Encasement" of a vessel was arbitrarily defined by a contact with the tumor of 50% or more of the vessel's circumference in a plane perpendicular to the long axis of the vessel (less than 50% should be called "contact" only). The term "flattened" is used for veins with reduced diameter but still partially visible lumen. When the lumen is no more visible, veins are also classified as "encased." The distinction by imaging between a simple contact and a true infiltration of an organ remains difficult. If the margins between the organ and the tumor are ill-defined, the term "infiltration" is used, whereas when margins are well delineated, the term "contact" is used. When a tumor is "separated" or "in contact" only with a vital structure or is "flattening" a vein without "encasement," an IDRF is *not* present. One exception is for renal vessels: a "contact" with the tumor is classified IDRF [3] since surgical dissection of the renal pedicle is particularly risky in neuroblastoma patients [2, 28]. "Encased" or "infiltrated" structures are classified as IDRF. The term "compression" is also used to describe relationships between cervicothoracic NBL and airways. When the short axis of the airways is reduced, IDRF is present. The term "invasion" is used for NBL extending into the epidural space of the spinal canal, mainly observed in paravertebral thoracic or lumbar "dumbbell" NBL. IDRF is present when the tumor invades more than one third of the spinal canal in the axial plane, when the leptomeningeal fluid spaces are no longer visible, or when the MR signal of the spinal cord is abnormal. NBL frequently involve two adjacent anatomical compartments (neck and chest, or abdomen and mediastinum, or abdomen and pelvis). This condition is also considered an IDRF.

6.3.2 IDRFs According to Anatomic Location of the Primary Tumor

According to the location of the primary tumor, radiologists should look carefully at specific anatomical structures [3]:

- In the neck (Fig. 6.2), NBL arise from the posterior carotid space. An IDRF is present when the internal carotid artery or internal jugular vein is encased, when the tumor reaches the skull base (along the carotid artery), or when it compresses the pharyngo-laryngeal lumen.
- Cervicothoracic NBL arises from the stellate ganglion above the subclavian artery at the level of the origin of the vertebral artery. IDRFs are present when the tumor encases the vertebral or carotid artery, the subclavian vessels, and the brachial plexus roots or when it compresses the trachea. Some of these tumors can also invade the spinal canal.
- In the chest (Figs. 6.3, 6.4, and 6.5), NBL usually arise from the paraspinal sympathetic chains in the posterior mediastinum and frequently invade one or more foramina or even epidural space in the spinal canal ("dumbbell" tumors) associated with the risk of spinal cord compression. IDRF is present when more than one third of the canal in the axial plane is invaded. Since mediastinal NBL located between T9 and T12 levels are associated with a theoretical risk of spinal cord ischemia during surgery, this situation is also considered an IDRF, although

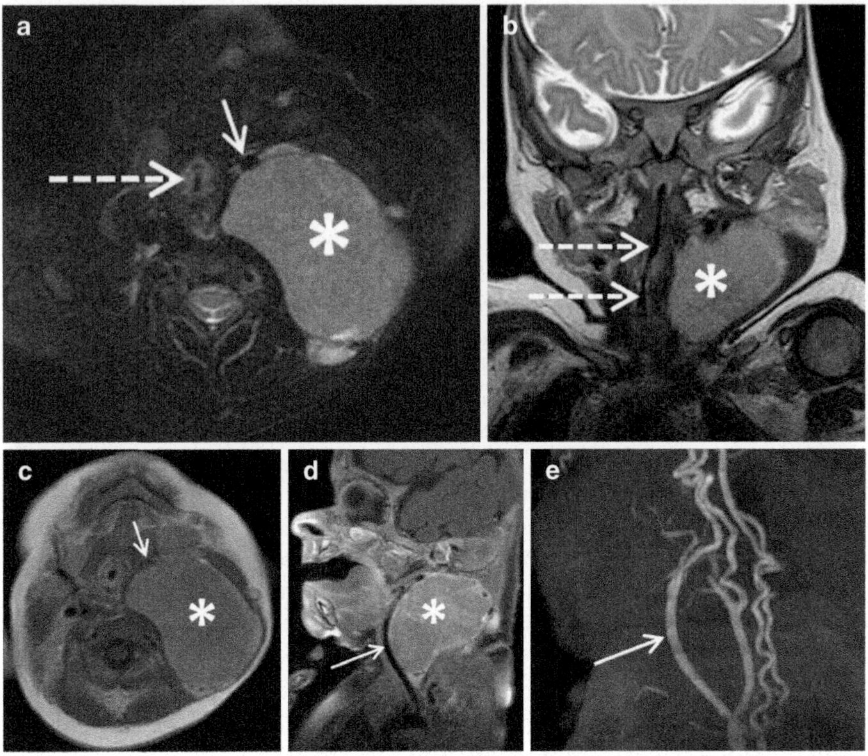

Fig. 6.2 A 5-month-old boy with nonsymptomatic localized left cervical neuroblastoma. MR transverse fat-saturated T2 (**a**) and coronal (**b**) T2-weighted sequences, enhanced transverse (**c**) and sagittal fat-saturated T1-weighted (**d**) sequences, and lateral MIP reconstruction of contrast-enhanced MR angiography. The tumor (asterisks) arises from the left posterior carotid space and displaces anteriorly the internal carotid artery (arrows), without encasement (not IDRF), and laterally the airways (dotted arrows) but without reduction of the laryngotracheal lumen (not IDRF)

the risk of injury to the spinal cord is regarded as very low in children. Encasement of the descending aorta, compression of the trachea or principal bronchi, and infiltration of the diaphragm or pleura are also considered IDRF.

– In the abdomen (Figs. 6.6, 6.7, 6.8, 6.9, 6.10, 6.11, and 6.12), NBL arise either from the adrenal gland or from sympathetic ganglia (celiac, superior, and inferior mesenteric ganglia) or from sympathetic fibers along the aorta and its branches. Main abdominal vessels (aorta, celiac axis, superior and inferior mesenteric arteries, portal vein, renal vessels, inferior vena cava, iliac vessels) must be assessed using the relevant terms. IDRFs are present when vessels are encased (or at least in contact for renal pedicles). IDRF is also present when the tumor infiltrates the porta hepatis (liver hilum) or directly the liver parenchyma, the diaphragm, the kidney, the duodeno-pancreatic block, or much less frequently the mesentery. Also paravertebral lumbar NBL (Figs. 6.11 and 6.12) are usually classified as "abdominal" NBL, the local extension is usually comparable to that

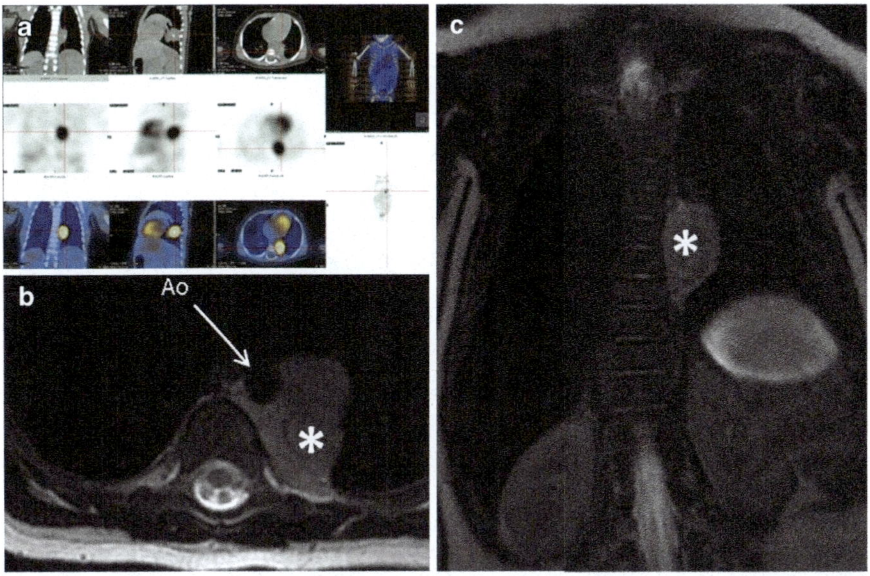

Fig. 6.3 A 5-month-old boy with nonsymptomatic localized left thoracic neuroblastoma. MIBG scan (SPECT-CT) (**a**) shows uptake of the primary tumor without distant metastasis. MR transverse (**b**) and coronal (**c**) T2-weighted sequences show the tumor (asterisks) in the posterior mediastinum encasing (curve arrow) the descending thoracic aorta over 180° (Ao, IDRF), but without infiltration of foramina or spinal canal

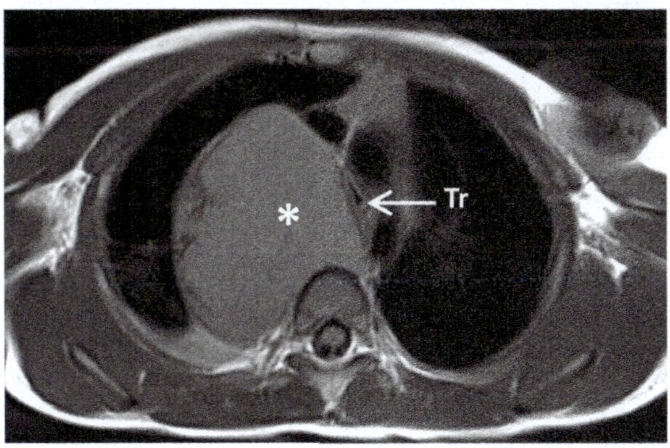

Fig. 6.4 A 15-month-old boy with nonsymptomatic localized right thoracic neuroblastoma. MR transverse T1-weighted sequence shows the tumor (asterisks) originating from the posterior mediastinum without infiltration of foramina or spinal canal but compressing the trachea (Tr, arrow) (IDRF)

of chest NBL with frequent spinal canal invasion, infiltration of the psoas muscle, and uncommonly the abdominal vessels.

- In the pelvis (Fig. 6.13), NBL arise from presacral sympathetic ganglia or along the lumbosacral junction (upper hypogastric sympathetic plexus). IDRF is present when the tumor encases the termination of the aorta, the origin of the inferior vena cava, or the iliac vessels. Lumbar or sacral foraminal extensions are not IDRF; intraspinal extension may also occur, but below the level of the L2, only

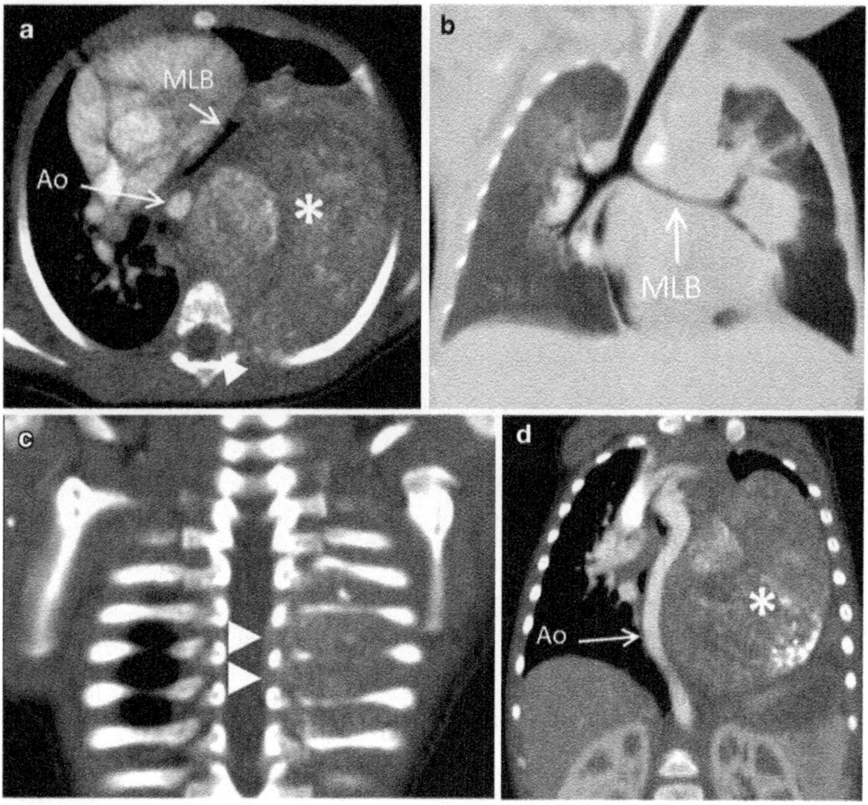

Fig. 6.5 An 11-month-old girl with symptomatic localized left thoracic neuroblastoma. Contrast-enhanced CT scan with transverse view (**a**) and coronal minimal intensity projection (**b**) and coronal MPR reconstruction (**c**, **d**). The calcified tumor (asterisks) arises from the lower posterior mediastinum (IDRF) and compresses the main left bronchus (MLB) (IDRF). The tumor displaced the descending thoracic aorta (Ao) without encasement (not IDRF) and invades the foramina (arrowheads) and the épidural space of the spinal canal but less than 30% in transverse plane (not IDRF)

radicular involvement can occur, and this condition is therefore not classified as IDRF. Tumors extending in the gluteal region through the greater sciatic foramen are also considered to be IDRF positive.

Since established by consensus and not by evidence-based rationale, the list of IDRFs and definition of terms recommended are arbitrary and of course debatable. Truly, neither the number of risk factors nor the type of IDRFs is taken into account in the INRGSS. New IDRFs have been suggested [29], and the guidelines [3] have also been accused of overestimating the surgical risks which "might lead to unnecessary chemotherapy" [30]. These criticisms are definitely valid, and the issue of overestimating surgical risks can be supported by data from the LNESG1 study: whereas patients with stage L1 disease had a 5-year EFS of 92% with primary

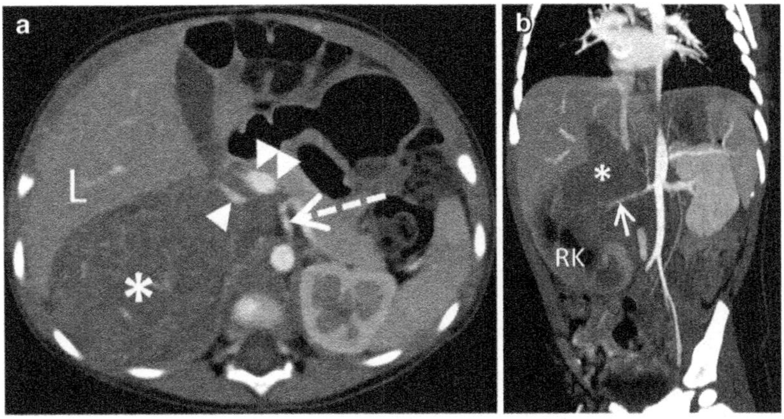

Fig. 6.6 A 12-month-old girl with localized (MYCN-amplified) right adrenal neuroblastoma (asterisks). Contrast-enhanced CT scan with transverse view (**a**) and coronal MIP reconstruction (**b**). IDRFs are present: encasement of the right renal artery (arrow), infiltration of the hilum of the right kidney (RK), and encasement of the inferior vena cava (arrowhead). Some relationships with adjacent organs are not IDRF: the liver (L) is displaced without direct infiltration; the celiac artery (dotted arrow) is separated from the tumor; the portal vein (double arrowhead) and the aorta are in contact with the tumor, without encasement

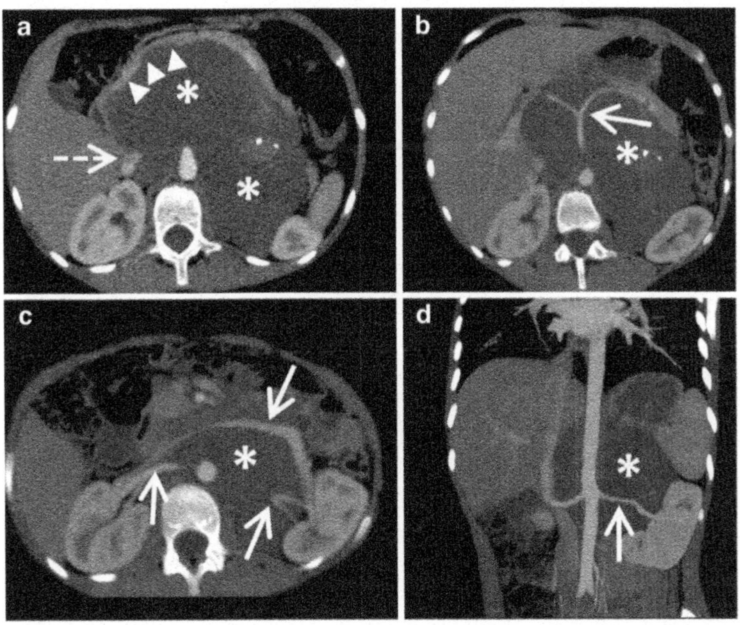

Fig. 6.7 A 9-month-old girl with localized left adrenal intermixed ganglioneuroblastoma (asterisks). Contrast-enhanced CT scan with transverse views (**a**, **b**) and axial (**c**) and coronal (**d**) MIP reconstructions. IDRFs are present (arrows): encasement of the aorta, the celiac, hepatic and splenic arteries, both renal arteries, and the left renal vein. The tumor is in contact with the IVC (dotted arrow), but its lumen is still visible (not IDRF). The duodeno-pancreatic bloc is invaded (arrowheads) (IDRF)

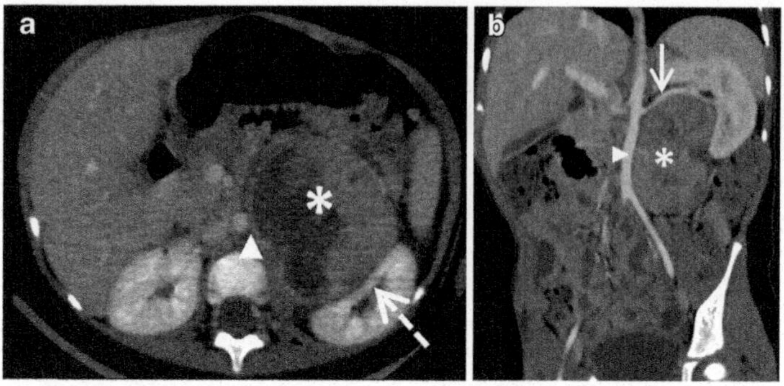

Fig. 6.8 A 3-year-old boy with localized left extra-adrenal retroperitoneal neuroblastoma (asterisks). Contrast-enhanced CT scan with transverse view (**a**) and coronal MIP reconstruction (**b**) show the displacement of the right kidney without infiltration (dotted arrow) (not IDRF), a contact with the aorta (arrowheads) without encasement (not IDRF), and a contact with the renal artery (arrow) (IDRF)

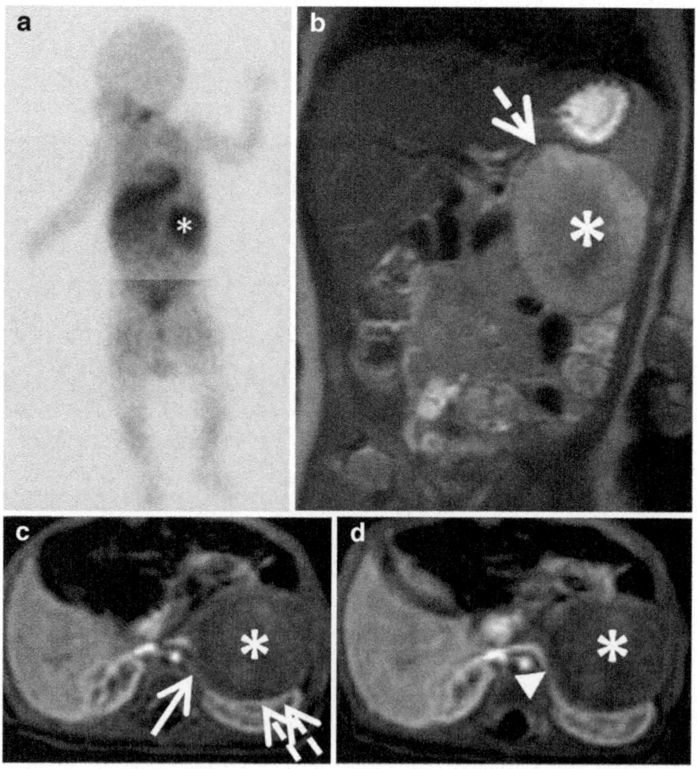

Fig. 6.9 A 2-month-old girl with localized left adrenal neuroblastoma. MIBG scan (anterior view) (**a**) shows uptake of the primary tumor (asterisk) without distant metastasis. MR coronal T2-weighted sequence (**b**) shows a contact (not IDRF) with the splenic artery (dotted arrow), and contrast-enhanced transverse fat-saturated T1-weighted sequences (**c**, **d**) show displacement of the right kidney without infiltration (double dotted arrow) (not IDRF) and a contact with the renal artery (arrow) and the renal vein (arrowhead) (IDRF)

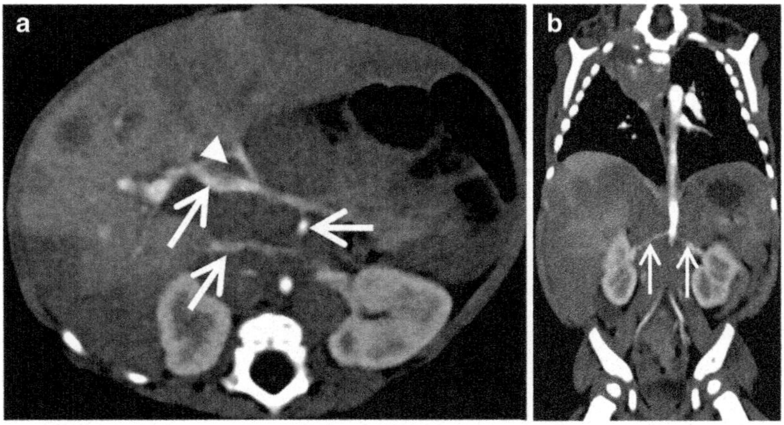

Fig. 6.10 A 3-month-old girl with multifocal neuroblastoma (chest and both adrenal glands) with distant metastases in the liver, pancreas, and bone marrow. Contrast-enhanced CT scan with transverse view (**a**) and coronal MPR reconstruction (**b**). IDRFs are present: infiltration of the liver hilum (arrowhead) and encasement of many vessels (arrows): the aorta, the mesenteric artery, both renal arteries, left renal vein, IVC, and portal vein

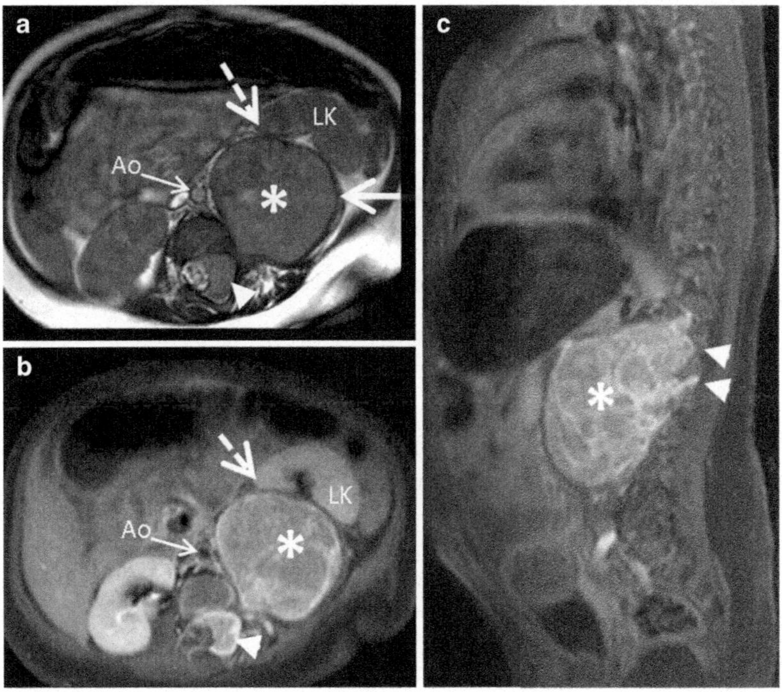

Fig. 6.11 A 6-month-old girl with localized left lumbar neuroblastoma. MR transverse T2-weighted (**a**) and enhanced fat-saturated T1-weighted transverse (**b**) and sagittal (**c**) sequences show the tumor (asterisks) infiltrating the psoas muscle (IDRF, arrow), infiltrating the foramina and the spinal canal (50% in axial plane, i.e., IDRF, arrowheads), displacing the left kidney (LK) (dotted arrow) without infiltration (not IDRF), and separated from the aorta (Ao)

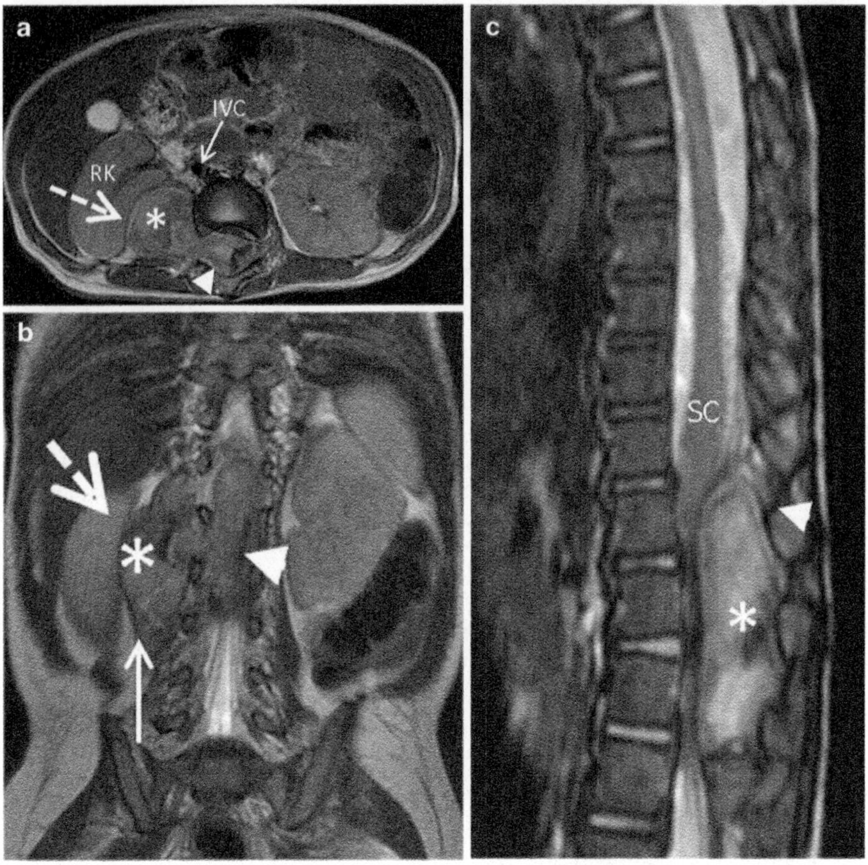

Fig. 6.12 A 10-month-old girl with paraplegia related to a localized right lumbar neuroblastoma. MR transverse (**a**), coronal (**b**), and sagittal (**c**) T2-weighted sequences show the tumor (asterisks) infiltrating the psoas muscle (IDRF, arrow), infiltrating the foramina and the spinal canal (75% in axial plane, i.e., IDRF, arrowheads), compressing the spinal cord (SC), displacing the right kidney (RK) (dotted arrow) without infiltration (not IDRF), and separated from the inferior vena cava (IVC, not IDRF)

tumor excision, the group of patients with stage L2 disease who (contrary to protocol recommendations) also underwent initial surgery had a 5-year EFS of 86% [5]. Evidently, a subset of patients with presence of IDRFs had almost equally good outcome with initial tumor excision as patients without IDRFs. In this setting it is therefore important to get rid of the misconception that presence of IDRFs is automatically linked to neoadjuvant chemotherapy. Rather it is important to keep in mind that the INRG concept was primarily designed to facilitate communication and comparisons between international clinical trials. It is anticipated that the list of IDRFs will be revised and further improved with time. However, matters like this must necessarily take time, and it is assumed that a future revision of the INRG concept will be better when more information on the impact on outcome of *individual* risk factors have been collected.

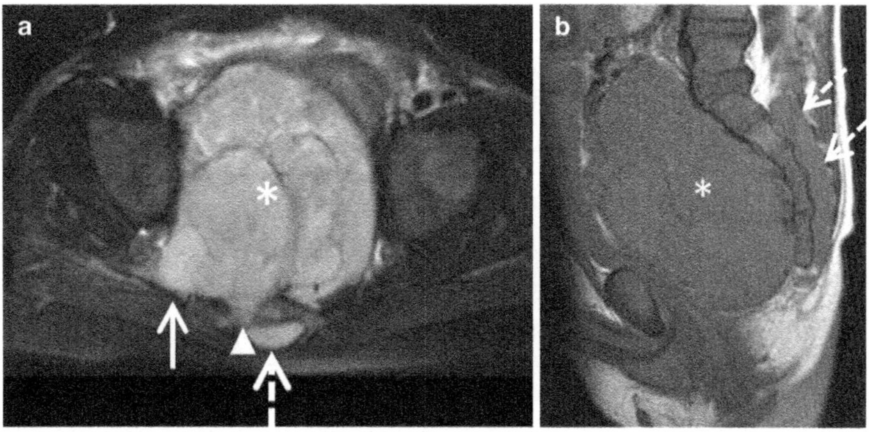

Fig. 6.13 A 1-year-old boy pelvic with presacral neuroblastoma. MR transverse FS T2-weighted (**a**) and sagittal T1-weighted (**b**) sequences show the tumor (asterisks) invading the sacral holes (arrowhead) and dural cul-de-sac (dotted arrows) (not an IDRF). Tumor extends into the gluteal region (arrow) through greater sciatic foramen (IDRF)

References

1. Pearson ADJ, Pinkerton R. Neuroblastoma. In: Pinkerton R, Plowman PN, Pieters R, editors. Paediatric oncology. 3rd ed. London: Arnold; 2004. p. 386–414.
2. Cecchetto G, Mosseri V, De Bernardi B, Helardot P, Monclair T, Costa E, et al. Surgical risk factors in primary surgery for localized neuroblastoma: the LNESG1 study of the European International Society of Pediatric Oncology Neuroblastoma Group. J Clin Oncol. 2005;23(33):8483–9.
3. Brisse HJ, McCarville MB, Granata C, Krug B, Wootton-Gorges SL, Kanegawa K, et al. Guidelines for imaging and staging of neuroblastic tumors: consensus report from the International Neuroblastoma Risk Group Project. Radiology. 2011;261:243–57.
4. Monclair T, Brodeur GM, Ambros P, Brisse HJ, Cecchetto G, Holmes K, et al. The International Neuroblastoma Risk Group (INRG) staging system: an INRG Task Force report. J Clin Oncol. 2009;27:298–303.
5. Monclair T, Mosseri V, Cecchetto G, De Bernardi B, Michon J, Holmes K. Influence of image-defined risk factors on the outcome of patients with localised neuroblastoma. A report from the LNESG1 study of the European International Society of Paediatric Oncology Neuroblastoma Group. Pediatr Blood Cancer. 2015;62(9):1536–42.
6. Pohl A, Erichsen M, Stehr M, Hubertus J, Bergmann F, Kammer B, et al. Image-defined risk factors correlate with surgical radicality and local recurrence in patients with neuroblastoma. Klin Padiatr. 2016;228(3):118–23.
7. Simon T, Hero B, Benz-Bohm G, von Schweinitz D, Berthold F. Review of image defined risk factors in localized neuroblastoma patients: results of the GPOH NB97 trial. Pediatr Blood Cancer. 2008;50(5):965–9.
8. Irtan S, Brisse HJ, Minard-Colin V, Schleiermacher G, Canale S, Sarnacki S. Minimally invasive surgery of neuroblastic tumors in children: indications depend on anatomical location and image-defined risk factors. Pediatr Blood Cancer. 2015a;62:257–61.
9. Tanaka Y, Kawashima H, Mori M, Fujiogi M, Suzuki K, Amano H, et al. Contraindications and image-defined risk factors in laparoscopic resection of abdominal neuroblastoma. Pediatr Surg Int. 2016;32(9):845–50.

10. Irtan S, Brisse HJ, Minard-Colin V, Schleiermacher G, Galmiche-Rolland L, Le Cossec C, et al. Image-Defined Risk Factor assessment of neurogenic tumors after neoadjuvant chemotherapy is useful for predicting intra-operative risk factors and the completeness of resection. Pediatr Blood Cancer. 2015b;62:1543–9.
11. Avanzini S, Pio L, Erminio G, Granata C, Holmes K, Gambart M, et al. Image-defined risk factors in unresectable neuroblastoma: SIOPEN study on incidence, chemotherapy-induced variation, and impact on surgical outcomes. Pediatr Blood Cancer. 2017;64(11):e26605.
12. Evans AE, D'Angio GJ, Randolph J. A proposed staging for children with neuroblastoma. Cancer. 1971;27:374–8.
13. Brodeur GM, Seeger RC, Barrett A, Berthold F, Castleberry RP, D'Angio G, et al. International criteria for diagnosis, staging, and response to treatment in patients with neuroblastoma. J Clin Oncol. 1988;6:1874–81.
14. Brodeur GM, Pritchard J, Berthold F, Carlsen NLT, Castel V, Castleberry RP, et al. Revisions of the international criteria for neuroblastoma diagnosis, staging and response to treatment. J Clin Oncol. 1993;11:1466–77.
15. Cohn SL, Pearson ADJ, London WB, Monclair T, Ambros PF, Brodeur GM, et al. The International Neuroblastoma Risk Group (INRG) classification system: an INRG Task Force report. J Clin Oncol. 2009;27:289–97.
16. De Bernardi B, Mosseri V, Rubie H, Castel V, Foot A, Ladenstein R, et al. Treatment of localized resectable neuroblastoma. Results of the LNESG1 study by the SIOP Europe Neuroblastoma Group. Br J Cancer. 2008;99:1027–33.
17. Hero B, Simon T, Spitz R, Ernestus K, Gnekow AK, Scheel-Walter H-G, et al. Localized infant neuroblastomas often show spontaneous regression: results of the prospective trials NB95-S and NB97. J Clin Oncol. 2008;26:1504–10.
18. Nuchtern JG, London WB, Barnewolt CE, Naranjo A, McGrady PW, Geiger JD, et al. A prospective study of expectant observation as primary therapy for neuroblastoma in young infants. Ann Surg. 2012;256:573–80.
19. Kushner BH, LaQuaglia MP, Kramer K. Cheung N-KV Radically different treatment recommendations for newly diagnosed neuroblastoma: pitfalls in assessment of risk. J Pediatr Hematol Oncol. 2004;26:35–9.
20. Baker DL, Schmidt ML, Cohn SL, Maris JM, London WB, Buxton A, et al. Outcome after reduced chemotherapy for intermediate-risk neuroblastoma. N Engl J Med. 2010;363:1313–23.
21. Ikeda H, Iehara T, Tsuchida Y, Kaneko M, Hata J, Naito H, et al. Experience with International Neuroblastoma Staging System and pathology classification. Br J Cancer. 2002;86:1110–6.
22. Matthay KK, Perez C, Seeger RC, Brodeur GM, Shimada H, Atkinson JB, et al. Successful treatment of Stage III neuroblastoma based on prospective biologic staging: a children's Cancer Group study. J Clin Oncol. 1998;16:1256–64.
23. Peuchmaur M, d'Amore ES, Joshi VV, Hata J, Roald B, Dehner LP, et al. Revision of the International Neuroblastoma Pathology Classification: confirmation of favorable and unfavorable prognostic subsets in ganglioneuroblastoma, nodular. Cancer. 2003;98:2274–81.
24. Shimada H, Ambros IM, Dehner LP, Hata J, Joshi VV, Roald B, et al. The International Neuroblastoma Pathology Classification (the Shimada system). Cancer. 1999;86:364–72.
25. Gunther P, Holland-Cunz S, Schupp CJ, Stockklausner C, Hinz U, Schenk JP. Significance of image-defined risk factors for surgical complications in patients with abdominal neuroblastoma. Eur J Pediatr Surg. 2011;21(5):314–7.
26. Yoneda A, Nishikawa M, Uehara S, Oue T, Usui N, Inoue M, et al. Can image-defined risk factors predict surgical complications in localized neuroblastoma? Eur J Pediatr Surg. 2016;26(1):117–22.
27. Brisse HJ, Blanc T, Schleiermacher G, Mosseri V, Philippe-Chomette P, Janoueix-Lerosey I, et al. Radiogenomics of neuroblastomas: relationships between imaging phenotypes, tumor genomic profile and survival. PLoS One. 2017;12(9):e0185190.

28. Shamberger RC, Smith EI, Joshi VV, Rao PV, Hayes FA, Bowman LC, et al. The risk of nephrectomy during local control in abdominal neuroblastoma. J Pediatr Surg. 1998;33(2):161–4.
29. Lim II, Goldman DA, Farber BA, Murphy JM, Abramson SJ, Basu E, et al. Image-defined risk factors for nephrectomy in patients undergoing neuroblastoma resection. J Pediatr Surg. 2016;51(6):975–80.
30. Fumino S, Kimura K, Iehara T, Nishimura M, Nakamura S, Souzaki R, et al. Validity of image-defined risk factors in localized neuroblastoma: a report from two centers in Western Japan. J Pediatr Surg. 2015;50(12):2102–6.

Nuclear Medicine Procedures in Neuroblastoma

7

Arnoldo Piccardo, Rita Castellani, Gianluca Bottoni, Michela Massollo, Giulia Anna Follacchio, and Egesta Lopci

7.1 Diagnostic Context

Neuroblastoma (NB) is an embryonic tumor deriving from the peripheral sympathetic nervous system [1]. It is the most frequent extra-cranial solid tumor in childhood, often presenting with large retroperitoneal masses detected on morphological imaging modalities, such as ultrasound, contrast-enhanced CT (ceCT), or magnetic resonance imaging (MRI).

Due to the heterogeneous profile of the disease, prognosis of NB patients is linked to several clinical and biological factors. In 2005, the International Neuroblastoma Risk Group (INRG) Task Force established criteria for an internationally risk group stratification system based on clinical factors (age, tumor stage) and genetic determinants (MYCN gene amplification, chromosome 1p36 abnormalities) [1, 2].

More recently, the INRG Task Force also released the consensus recommendations on molecular techniques, on the criteria of minimal residual disease, on neuroblastoma response criteria, and on radiographic techniques [2–6].

A. Piccardo (✉) · G. Bottoni · M. Massollo
Department of Nuclear Medicine, Ente Ospedaliero Ospedali Galliera, Genoa, Italy
e-mail: arnoldo.piccardo@galliera.it

R. Castellani
Nuclear Medicine Unit, Fondazione IRCCS Istituto Nazionale dei Tumori, Milan, Italy

G. A. Follacchio
Nuclear Medicine Unit, Policlinico Umberto I, Sapienza University of Rome, Rome, Italy

E. Lopci
Department of Nuclear Medicine, Humanitas Clinical and Research Center Rozzano, Milan, Italy

S. Sarnacki, L. Pio (eds.), *Neuroblastoma*,
https://doi.org/10.1007/978-3-030-18396-7_7

The high-risk phenotype, which affects nearly 50% of newly diagnosed patients and is related to poor long-term survival, is characterized by age >18 months on diagnosis, widespread disease dissemination, and MYCN amplification Conversely, patients with a low-risk phenotype (no MYCN amplification and age <18 months) have an excellent long-term survival [7–9].

Localized unresectable neuroblastoma in children >12 months and no MYC amplification constitute an intermediate-risk group [10].

Since risk group stratification is an essential step to select the most appropriate treatment option, diagnostic imaging is determinant in the initial assessment of disease extension.

Currently, no evidence-based criteria have defined the optimal imaging modality in evaluating the extent of NB disease. The recent INRG Consensus on imaging guidelines in neuroblastic tumors reported advantages and limitations of CT and MR imaging modalities in evaluating primary tumor and metastatic disease [6].

So far, contrast-enhanced CT (ceCT) represents the reference standard technique for the evaluation of primary tumor extent concerning eligibility to surgery, for the detection of residual disease after surgery, and to guide radiotherapeutic planning. Nevertheless, it may underestimate the extent of bone metastases and is unable to detect bone marrow involvement [11]. On the other side, magnetic resonance (MR) gained has been increasingly adopted in the last 20 years due to the high contrast resolution in evaluating soft tissue and bone marrow metastases and to the lack of ionizing radiation [12–15]. Furthermore, MR represents the recommended imaging modality for the study of spinal or paraspinal primary disease and metastases. Nevertheless, known limitations of MR are the limited field of view (FOV) and long acquisition time frequently requiring patient sedation.

The principal limitation of MRI, however, is related to treatment response evaluation, which is not well defined by this morphologic imaging modality especially when bone marrow involvement is considered in NB [16]. Indeed false-positive results have been described after treatment [16, 17].

In NB diagnostic setting, nuclear medicine procedures have demonstrated major accuracy for both staging and treatment response assessments, including the evaluation of bone and bone marrow involvement [18]. ^{123}I-MIBG scintigraphy has been extensively used in research and clinical practice for over 35 years, representing the most important functional imaging modality in NB assessment.

Furthermore, therapy with ^{131}I-MIBG has been extensively employed in neuroblastoma since the late 1980s, with a systematic review analyzing 1121 patients treated with ^{131}I-MIBG [19].

^{131}I-MIBG was used as single agent (monotherapy) in patients with a poor prognosis, in particular those with recurrent/refractory disease, as a palliative treatment. So far, ^{131}I-MIBG therapy is included in multicentric trials on high-risk neuroblastoma patients [20].

However, in recent years, different types of "new" PET tracers have been introduced in the diagnostic workup of NB showing very promising results [21, 22]. In this new diagnostic *scenario*, it seems important to identify strengths and limitation of each different functional diagnostic modality.

The aim of this chapter is to analyze, in terms of availability and accuracy, the principal nuclear medicine procedures used in NB. In addition, the prevalent or complementary role of each functional imaging method is highlighted.

7.2 MIBG Scintigraphy

Metaiodobenzylguanidine (MIBG) is a guanethidine derivative developed in the late 1970s as diagnostic agent for imaging of adrenal medulla [23]. Being chemically analogue to norepinephrine, MIBG is taken up by NB cells through type 1 active uptake and stored in cytoplasmic vesicles [24].

^{123}I- and ^{131}I -MIBG scintigraphy are both well-established diagnostic imaging modalities for diagnosis, staging, and restaging of NB. However, for clinical practice, the superiority of ^{123}I- over ^{131}I-labelled MIBG for the diagnosis of NB has been ascertained. Indeed, ^{123}I physical properties allow to perform planar, whole-body, and SPECT high-count scans providing better spatial resolution than ^{131}I-MIBG [25].

7.2.1 Staging

Owing to the high specificity and sensitivity in detecting primary NB and distant metastases, MIBG imaging is recommended as standard modality to assess disease extent at diagnosis in accordance with the International Neuroblastoma Risk Group (INRG) guidance [26].

Worthy to remember, in INRG recommendations, the presence of a single, unequivocal MIBG-positive lesion at a distant site is sufficient to define metastatic disease [5]. Consequently, since 1996, MIBG scan has been utilized to create a risk factor scoring system focusing on the extent and treatment response of bone disease [5, 27–31] [Fig. 7.1].

Considering the primary site of disease, it should be highlighted that MIBG imaging is not able to discriminate between well-differentiated ganglioneuroma from undifferentiated neuroblastoma or ganglioneuroblastoma [32]. These three histological types may all concentrate MIBG, even though the uptake pattern may differ on the basis of tumor cell differentiation [33]. An intense MIBG uptake is in fact observed in ganglioneuroblastoma, where ganglioneuroma elements are predominant, suggesting that the radiopharmaceutical uptake is influenced by tumor cell differentiation [21].

False-positive findings on MIBG scan can result from the misinterpretation of physiologic uptake foci, namely, distributed in the salivary glands, nasal mucosa, myocardium, liver, and bowel. Adrenal glands may also demonstrate MIBG uptake, especially after contralateral adrenalectomy. As a result, most of the false-positive

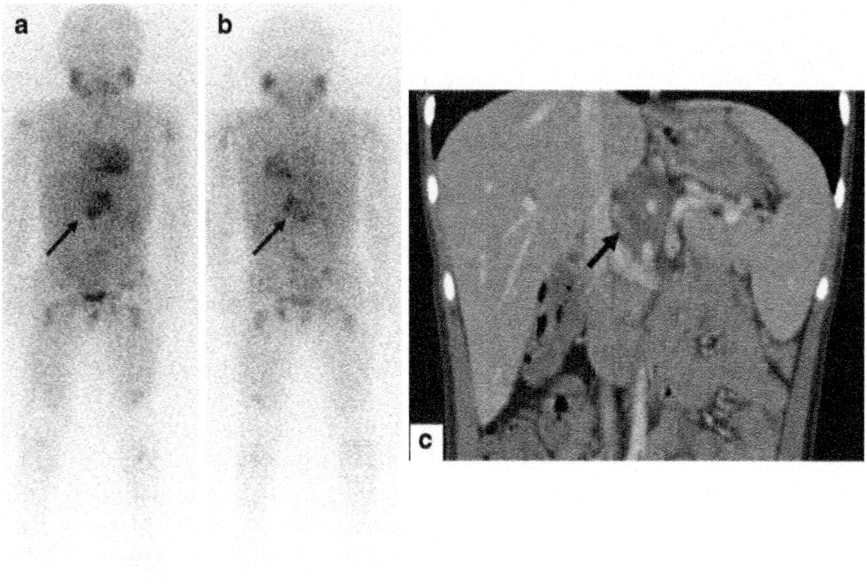

Fig. 7.1 A 6-year-old male affected by stage 4 NB. ^{123}I-MIBG scan at the time of first staging (**a**, **b**) identified primary tumor (arrows), well visualized by CT (coronal view, **c**), and bone-bone marrow metastases

MIBG findings are related to a nonspecific tracer accumulation in the urinary tract or gastrointestinal structures [34, 35]. Low-level uptake may also be seen in the lungs on 24-h images [36, 37]. Physiologic uptake in brown adipose tissue has also been described, most commonly leading to activity in the neck and supraclavicular regions [38, 39].

False-negative scans may occur in 10% of the cases [28] depending on several variables: (1) modifications of the active uptake mechanism due to the differentiation and maturation of tumor cells [40–42], (2) a prevalent necrotic component in primary tumor, (3) pharmacological interference [43, 44], and (4) low MIBG injected activity [45]. A further issue concerns the correct interpretation of the normal distribution pattern of MIBG in children. In these patients, the quality of MIBG scintigraphy may be conditioned by pathological changes in abdominal anatomy often caused by the disease [46].

^{123}I-MIBG scintigraphy commonly contemplates planar acquisitions, implying in most of the cases a difficult correlation with radiological examinations (i.e., ceCT or MRI). However, the wider use of SPECT or SPECT/CT imaging allows a greater accuracy, thanks to a more precise anatomical localization, avoiding false-positive findings and most importantly reducing false-negative findings both for visceral and bone metastases [47–49]. In this context, the essential intrinsic information provided by functional imaging (i.e., assessment of the viability of morphologically detectable lesions) may be associated with those of MRI such as high soft tissue resolution an definition of intraspinal tumor extension [50, 51].

7.2.2 Assessment of Treatment Response

Although primary staging is a "cornerstone" to correctly address the prognosis of children affected by NB, the assessment of treatment response after induction chemotherapy in high-risk NB patients is another important prognostic factor able to identify patients at higher risk of disease progression and death [12, 52]. Indeed, as mentioned before, the ability of MIBG scan in evaluating persistence of disease after therapy is higher than that of other imaging modalities (MRI and TC). Specifically, MIBG scan is particularly effective in the assessment of persistent bone marrow metastases [Figs. 7.2 and 7.3]. For this purpose, over time different skeletal scoring methods were developed based on MIBG scan images able to correctly address the skeletal tumor load at the time of first diagnosis and after treatment. The introduction of these criteria has improved the reproducibility with good concordance between readers and has allowed to distinguish a simple improvement from complete response [53, 54]. The most common scoring methods divide the skeleton into anatomical sectors and then give each sector an individual score for extension (quantity of metastases) and intensity (strength of uptake). The sum of the scores for each sector gives a separate MIBG score for extent and for intensity. The two principal scoring systems are the Curie score and SIOPEN score dividing the skeleton into 9 and 12 segments, respectively. The

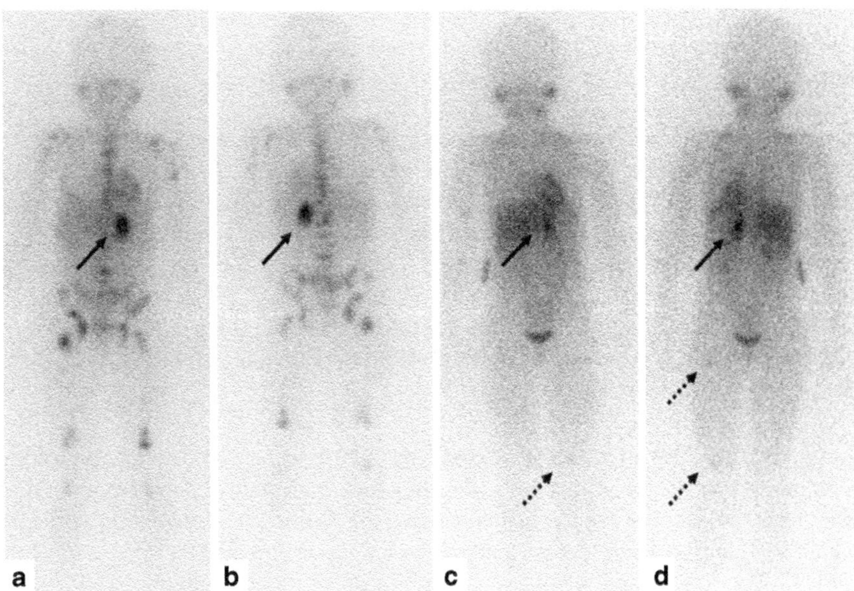

Fig. 7.2 A 4-year-old female affected by stage 4 NB. ^{123}I-MIBG scan at the time of first staging (**a**, **b**) identified primary tumor (arrows) and bone-bone marrow metastases. Partial but good response was observed after therapy (**c**, **d**). Primary tumor showed significant reduction in terms of MIBG uptake, and only two sites of bone marrow uptake were still detectable (dotted arrows)

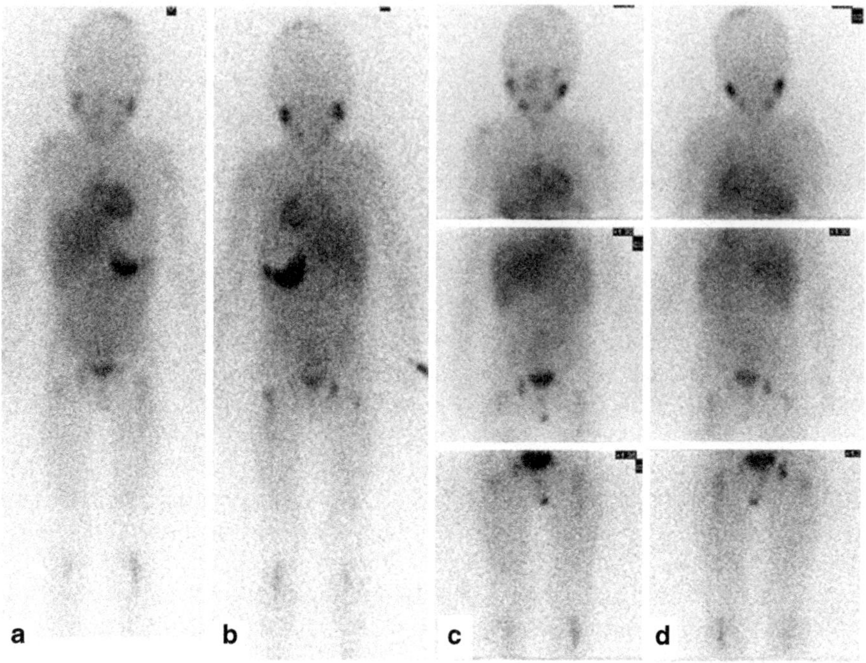

Fig. 7.3 A 5-year-old male affected by stage 4 NB. ^{123}I-MIBG scan at the time of first staging (**a**, **b**) identified primary tumor (arrows) and bone-bone marrow metastases. Incomplete response was observed after therapy (**c**, **d**). Primary tumor showed significant reduction in terms of MIBG uptake, but multiple sites of bone marrow uptake were still detectable

maximum score achievable for Curie score was 30, and that of SIOPEN was 70. These two scores have been tested and validated in large trials as independent NB risk factors. Indeed patients with Curie score >2 and SIOPEN score >3 after induction chemotherapy have extremely poor outcomes and should be considered for alternative strategies [12, 24, 28, 52].

7.2.3 ^{123}I-MIBG Scintigraphy for NB Surveillance During the Follow-Up

As more than 50% of patients affected by high-risk neuroblastoma (NB) may relapse after initial treatment [52], the long-term cure rate is low, ranging from 25% to 30% [53, 54]. The principal prognostic factor for post-relapse survival, which has recently been investigated, is the length of time to first relapse (TTFR) [55]. Although relapsing NB is often cause of death, it has been observed that an unsuspected and asymptomatic relapse with a smaller tumor load may be associated with a longer survival [56, 57]. On the contrary, prolonged survival and possibly effective treatment would be less likely if relapse involves extensive or bulky disease [56] [Fig. 7.4]. In this context, ^{123}I-MIBG scan is a sensitive biomarker able

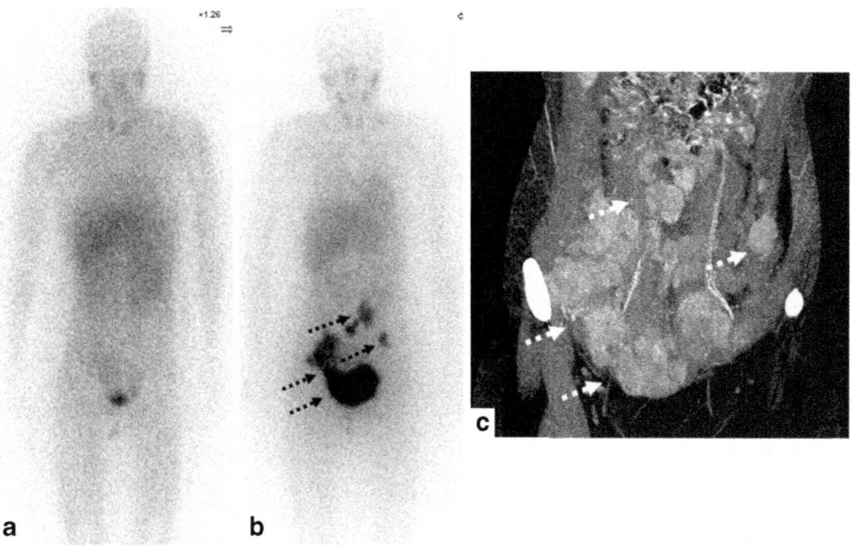

Fig. 7.4 A 15-year-old female affected by NB soft tissue relapse. The patient, after achieving complete remission (**a**), at 1 year follow-up, showed multiple peritoneal localizations detected by ^{123}I-MIBG scan (**b**) and CT (**c**)

to evaluate an early NB relapses (detection rate 82%), even when they are asymptomatic and unsuspected [56, 58]. In other words, ^{123}I-MIBG scan is able to correctly estimate the TTFR and at the same time to evaluate the tumor load at the time of recurrence. Indeed these two parameters are strictly related to disease progression and death [56, 57]. In addition, it was also reported that patients whose monitoring included ^{123}I-MIBG scan were significantly less likely to have an extensive osteomedullary relapse and had a significantly longer survival from relapse and from diagnosis [56].

7.3 ^{18}F-Fluorodihydroxyphenylalanine (^{18}F-DOPA)

On a functional point of view, NB cells display an increased metabolism of catecholamines, which determines their ability to produce biologically active hormones and some of their precursors [59, 60]. Dihydroxyphenylalanine (DOPA) and its Fluorine-18-labelled form (^{18}F-DOPA) are direct precursors of dopamine and catecholamine metabolism; therefore, they represent the potential PET substitute for ^{123}I-MIBG imaging. This radiopharmaceutical is actively transported into cells through the large amino acid transporter (LAT1) and then converted into dopamine by the amino acid decarboxylase (AADC) [61]. Subsequently, dopamine enters the vesicular storage system and is later on converted into norepinephrine and epinephrine [Fig. 7.5]. ^{18}F-DOPA PET is already regarded as a valuable tool for the assessment of neuroendocrine tumors, in particular pheochromocytoma, paraganglioma,

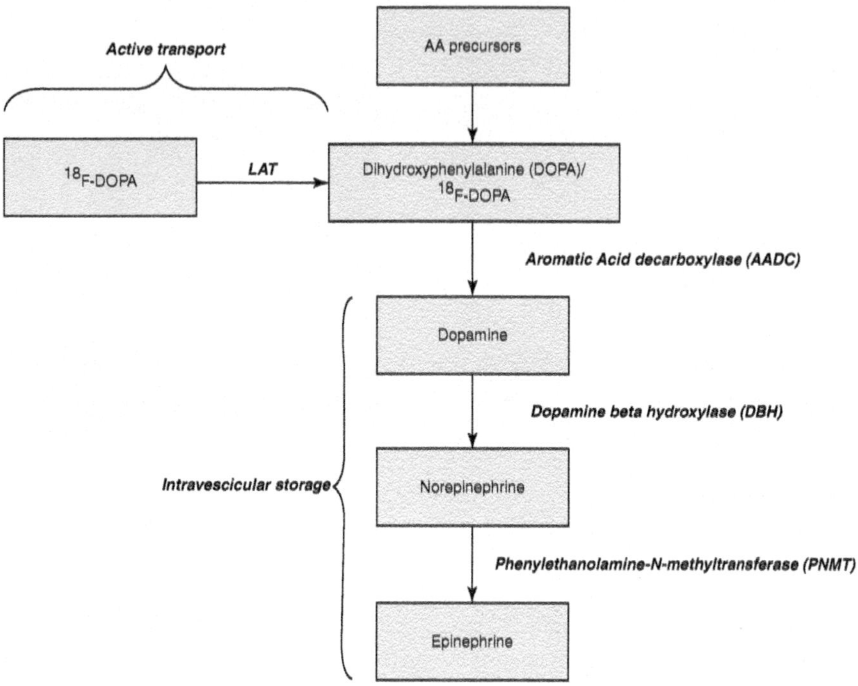

Fig. 7.5 Metabolic pathway of dihydroxyphenylalanine (DOPA) and ^{18}F-DOPA in tumor cells of neural crest origin; LAT = large amino acid transport; AA = amino acid

and medullary thyroid carcinoma [61–64]. In this context, the modality shows a better diagnostic performance compared to ^{123}I-MIBG scintigraphy and other conventional imaging modalities, such as CT and MRI, particularly in the case of tumors with high excretion of catecholamines [62–64].

^{18}F-DOPA PET has been recently enlisted in the recommended imaging techniques for NB assessment [http://www.eanm.org/publications/guidelines/], especially in the case of disease relapse and for the assessment of response to induction therapy [11, 22, 65–67]. Already during one of the first pilot studies conducted in primary/relapsed high-risk NB patients, ^{18}F-DOPA distribution in pathological sites resulted similar to that of ^{123}I-MIBG [66], but ^{18}F-DOPA PET displayed a higher accuracy than ^{123}I-MIBG scintigraphy, especially in smaller lesions (<1.5 cm). This influenced patient management and treatment decisions in 32% of the cases. In another publication from Lu et al. [68], on a retrospective analysis of 34 children with neuroblastic tumors (50 tumors: 26 neuroblastomas, 11 ganglioneuroblastomas, five ganglioneuromas, and eight lesions without viable tumor cells), ^{18}F-DOPA PET successfully detected viable tumors at a sensitivity of 97.6% (87.4–99.9%) and a specificity of 87.5% (47.3–99.7%) (Table 7.1). In the studies mentioned above [66, 68], ^{18}F-DOPA was injected at an activity of 4 MBq/kg, while image acquisitions were performed at different timings after tracer injection, more specifically 60 min for Piccardo et al. [66] and 90 min for Lu et al. [68]. Nevertheless, both

Table 7.1 Comparative studies in NB assessment of ^{18}F-DOPA and other imaging modalities

Study	Design	Number	Timing	Competitor	Purpose	^{18}F-DOPA Performance	Outcome
Piccardo et al. (2012), EJNMMI	Prospective	19 patients (28 paired scans)	At diagnosis ($n = 4$); at relapse ($n = 15$)	^{123}I-MIBG	Diagnostic performance	Sensitivity of 95%; accuracy of 96%	^{18}F-DOPA showed a sensitivity and accuracy higher than ^{123}I-MIBG ($p < 0.05$)
Lopci et al. (2012), CNM	Prospective	21 patients (37 paired scans; 139 sites)		CT/MRI	Diagnostic performance	Scan-based: Sensitivity 100%; Accuracy 97.3% Lesion-based: Sensitivity 90.6%; Accuracy 90.5%	^{18}F-DOPA showed a sensitivity and accuracy higher than CT/MRI on scan-based and lesion-based ($p = 0.014$ and $p < 0.001$ respectively)
Lu et al. (2013), JNM	Prospective	34 patients (50 tumors)	At diagnosis ($n = 19$); during chemotherapy ($n = 18$); at relapse ($n = 13$)	^{18}F-FDG and ^{123}I-MIBG	Diagnostic performance	Sensitivity 97.6% (range 87.4–99.9%); Specificity 87.5% (range 47.3–99.7%)	^{18}F-FDOPA demonstrated a higher sensitivity than ^{123}I-MIBG ($n = 18$; $P = 0.0455$) or ^{18}F-FDG ($n = 46$; $P = 0.0455$)

studies report a very high sensitivity and accuracy for ^{18}F-DOPA with respect to ^{123}I-MIBG scintigraphy, while there was no significant difference in terms of specificity, as a consequence of the ability of ^{18}F-DOPA to detect NB localizations [Figs. 7.6 and 7.7]. This fact is furthermore confirmed by an interesting case report from Piccardo et al. [68] illustrating the clear visualization of positive bone and nodal metastases on ^{18}F-DOPA PET and post-therapy ^{131}I-MIBG scan, which were completely undetectable on diagnostic ^{123}I-MIBG scintigraphy. In this case, the difference in injected dose between ^{131}I- and ^{123}I-MIBG can explain the gap in sensitivity [Fig. 7.8].

Also in comparison with morphological imaging, ^{18}F-DOPA PET outperformed CT/MRI in NB assessment [11]. In this later study, the authors prospectively enrolled 21 patients affected by high-risk NB, with overall 129 pathological sites involved. On a site-based analysis, sensitivity, specificity, and diagnostic accuracy for ^{18}F-DOPA PET resulted 90.6%, 90%, and 90.5%, respectively, while the same rates for CT/MRI were 47.5%, 27.5%, and 43%. In particular, the authors found that ^{18}F-DOPA PET had a significantly higher detection rate than CT/MRI in the bone

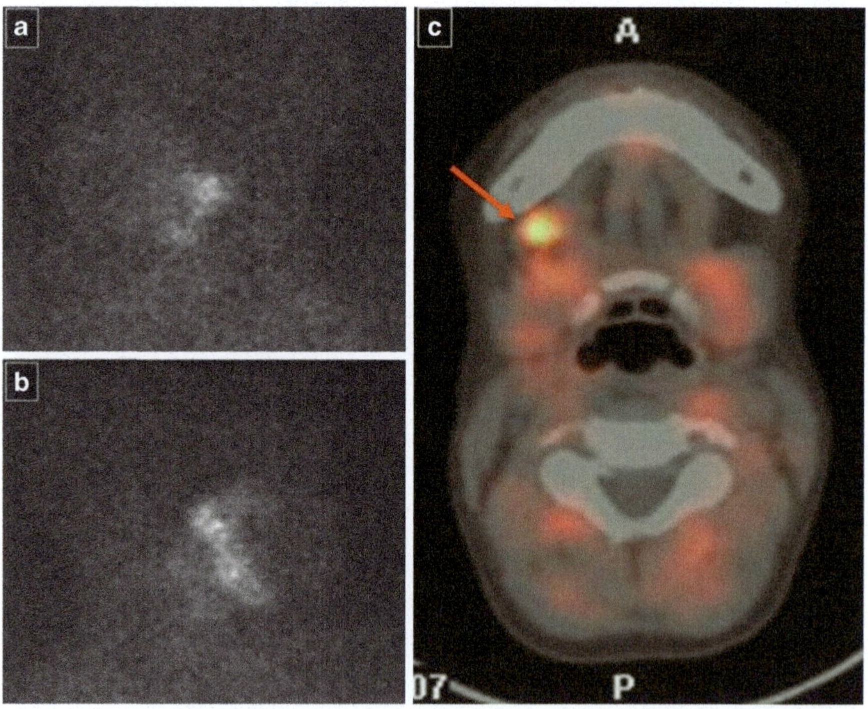

Fig. 7.6 Pictorial example of a patient with recurrent NB showing no pathological uptake in the ^{123}I-MIBG scintigraphy (**a**, **b** lateral views of the head); the same patient investigated with ^{18}F-DOPA PET/CT documented clear submandibular right node metastases (**c**, fused axial view; red arrow)

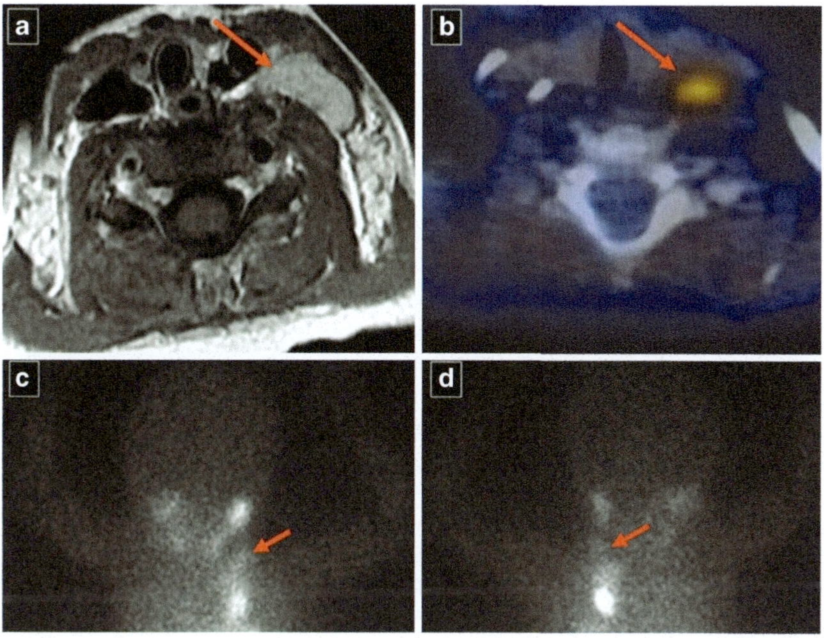

Fig. 7.7 Example of a patient with primary NB diagnosis showing an ancillary nodal involvement in the left supraclavicular region easily visualized with gadolinium-enhanced MRI (**a**) and ^{18}F-DOPA PET/CT (**b**); the corresponding lesion seen on ^{123}I-MIBG scintigraphy (**c**, **d**) is indicated with the red arrow

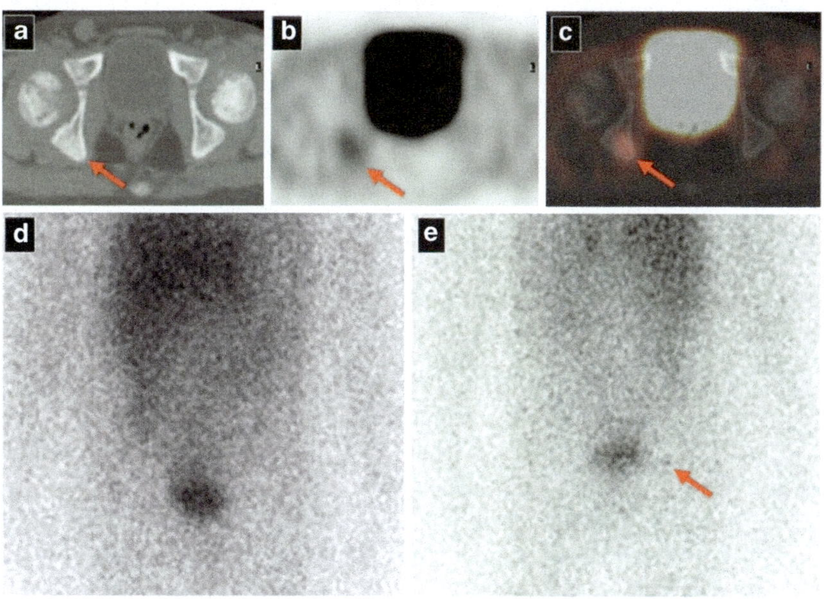

Fig. 7.8 Example of a patient with recurrent NB showing a clear pathological uptake on the right ischial bone on ^{18}F-DOPA PET/CT (**a**–**c**: red arrows); on counterpart, there is only a faint uptake visible in the posterior view (**e**) in the ^{123}I-MIBG scintigraphy while undetectable on anterior projection (**d**)

and bone marrow (90%), in lymph nodes (94%), and in soft tissue lesions (100%) [11, 22]. There were anyhow some false-positive cases (four lesions), all attributed to biliary stasis mimicking liver lesions. These cases were better characterized by morphological imaging, although the overall accuracy of ^{18}F-DOPA PET in either site-based or lesion-based analysis was superior [11].

Comparison with ^{18}F-FDG PET has been also performed, but the experience is limited to the paper from Lu et al. in 46 NB lesions [68]. In this report, ^{18}F-DOPA PET shows an overall better sensitivity (97.4% vs. 86.6%), specificity (87.5% vs. 62.5%), and diagnostic accuracy (95.6% vs. 82.6%), in detecting neuroblastic tumors. Another specific advantage reported is the better detection of skull and brain lesions, much is more difficult with ^{18}F-FDG PET due to the physiologic tracer uptake in the gray matter. With this regard, it is important to know that brain metastases are a real pitfall also for ^{123}I-MIBG scintigraphy, while ^{18}F-DOPA is already reported to detect brain metastases in a previously treated high-risk NB patient [69].

At the time of recurrence, ^{18}F-DOPA PET demonstrates a similar prognostic potential to that of ^{123}I-MIBG scintigraphy [58], which is well known as an unfavorable prognostic factor after induction therapy in case of scan positivity. In particular, patients with a score >3 at post-induction scintigraphy are reported to have a significantly worse event-free survival (EFS) [70]. The group from Piccardo et al. [58] investigated this prognostic potential in 24 relapsed NB patients. The authors at first found that patients with ^{123}I-MIBG score >3 had a significantly higher risk of disease progression and death. In the meantime, also patients with a ^{18}F-DOPA whole-body metabolic burden (WBMB) >7.5 presented a significantly higher risk of disease progression and death. Both cutoffs were significantly associated with progression-free survival (PFS), but ^{18}F-DOPA PET was better related to PFS than ^{123}I-MIBG scan (HR 37 vs. HR 17), and its score could better stratify patients based on risk of progression or death. These very results get even more promising if we consider that ^{18}F-DOPA PET can be used also in response assessment after induction therapy. So far, however, only one case report has described the application [71], and clearly the data need to be confirmed in larger series and possibly in multicentric studies.

All the abovementioned diagnostic and prognostic advantages for ^{18}F-DOPA PET in NB compared to other imaging modalities are strengthened also by the fact that this modality is patient-friendly, requires no specific preparation except few hours of fasting, and can be performed in the majority of the cases without patient sedation. There is one limited evidence that carbidopa premedication might improve image quality [72], but today this preparation is not routinely used nor is it recommended [http://www.eanm.org/publications/guidelines/]. On the other side, potential limitations and technical issues related to ^{18}F-DOPA application in NB exist. At first, the overall radiation exposure is higher when compared to the diagnostic ^{123}I-MIBG scintigraphy [73, 74]. The radiopharmaceutical is moreover costly, and some attention must be paid to its electrophilic synthesis, since residual ^{18}F-fluoride levels can lead to false-positive skeletal uptake mimicking metastases [75].

7.4 ^{18}F-FDG PET/CT

The current standard imaging studies for the staging and follow-up of neuroblastic tumors include CT/MR imaging and ^{123}I-MIBG scintigraphy [25]. Indeed, ^{123}I-MIBG scintigraphy is also a well-established diagnostic method to assess response to treatment [7]. However, the assessment of MIBG scans presents some difficulties. False-negative MIBG scans were reported as early as 1990 [76, 77], and false-negative ^{123}I-MIBG scintigraphy is still a problem and may lead to an incorrect downstaging [7, 77].

Other disadvantages of this modality such as limited spatial resolution, limited sensitivity in small lesions, and the logistic need of two or—in the case of SPECT—even more acquisition sessions should be also considered. Furthermore, in most of the cases, MIBG imaging is not sufficient for operative or biopsy planning.

Most of these disadvantages can potentially be overcome by PET/CT imaging, which is performed by using a glucose analogue PET tracer (i.e., ^{18}F-FDG) widely available in clinical practice. Indeed, cancer cells avidly take up glucose and metabolize it to lactate even when oxygen is abundantly present. This glucose metabolism in cancer cells enables specific detection by PET with the glucose analogue FDG.

The principal advantages of PET/CT images over planar and SPECT images are higher spatial resolution and the possibility to perform whole-body acquisitions in shorter time. Indeed, high-resolution images of ^{18}F-FDG PET/CT have excellent anatomical delineation comparable to that of CT and MRI. In addition, the limited scanning time of PET has the potential for reducing the number of sedations.

As for other malignancies, NB is often characterized by a high ^{18}F-FDG. Although data about the role of ^{18}F-FDG in NB are limited and no prospective multicentric studies have been conducted, ^{18}F-FDG PET/CT represents an important and widely available alternative to ^{123}I-MIBG scan, especially in case of non-MIBG-concentrating NB.

As described in the literature, in about 10% of patients with histologically proven NB, the primary tumor does not accumulate ^{123}I-MIBG (false-negative results) [46, 78, 79]. For these patients, it is advisable to perform additional tests especially at the time of first staging.

Although there is no evidence to support the routine use of ^{18}F-FDG PET/CT in the initial diagnosis and staging of NB, it was found that ^{18}F-FDG PET identified disease sites in stage 1 and 2 NB better than ^{123}I-MIBG and detected more sites of primary tumors or loco-regional metastases [20, 80]. Moreover, ^{18}F-FDG PET/CT better detected sites of disease in stages 3 and 4 when tumors did not accumulate ^{123}I-MIBG or did so only weakly. In addition, ^{18}F-FDG PET/CT could provide important information about disease extension in the chest, abdomen, and pelvis and should be used when CT or MRI seems to show more extensive disease than that revealed by ^{123}I-MIBG scan [80].

However, ^{123}I-MIBG seems to be superior to ^{18}F-FDG PET/CT in staging high-risk NB (i.e., stage 4), owing to its better accuracy in detecting bone and bone marrow metastases, which are the most frequent sites of disease progression [80, 81]. This situation may be particularly evident during induction chemotherapy or under granulocyte colony-stimulating factor, when bone marrow FDG uptake may mask or mimic metastatic disease, thus reducing the sensitivity of ^{18}F-FDG PET techniques [80, 81]. Another limitation of ^{18}F-FDG PET/CT is the normal high uptake of FDG in the brain, which makes this technique less effective for imaging cranial vault lesions [81].

Another issue is that MIBG imaging was overall considered more specific and superior to FDG-PET, particularly in the delineation of residual disease. Indeed, NB avidly concentrate ^{18}F-FDG before cytoreductive therapy, but the intra- and post-therapeutic uptake is variable [20, 80].

When detection of NB relapse is considered, ^{123}I-MIBG proved superior to ^{18}F-FDG in depicting the bone-bone marrow component of disease [81, 82]. In this field, ^{18}F-FDG can sometimes play a complementary role, particularly in soft tissue lesions. Indeed, it has been hypothesized that ^{18}F-FDG might be better in detecting liver lesions, due to the high physiologic liver uptake of ^{123}I-MIBG [83].

Which is the best tracer during the follow-up surveillance of NB is still under debate. Indeed, in the same cases, the behavior of NB is difficult to predict. There are reports of lesions that had been ^{123}I-MIBG-positive at the initial diagnosis, which became negative when the disease relapsed or vice versa [56, 83–85].

Some authors suggested that, in the absence of cranial vault disease, ^{18}F-FDG PET and bone marrow biopsy might be sufficient for follow-up [86]. However, no data are still available to support this conclusion, and in the follow-up, it is prudent to repeat ^{123}I-MIBG scans in patients deemed to be at high risk of relapse, especially those with previous cranial bone involvement. ^{18}F-FDG PET/CT has also been recommended during follow-up as an additional imaging modality (Fig. 7.9) in the event of discrepancies between ^{123}I-MIBG scan and morphological imaging [77].

^{18}F-FDG PET/CT imaging is able to monitor treatment response, especially in patients with ^{123}I-MIBG-negative tumors [87]. In this setting, it has been demonstrated that the majority of NB are able to concentrate ^{18}F-FDG both before and after cytoreductive therapy [88].

The principal limitation of ^{18}F-FDG PET/CT remains the nonspecific bone marrow uptake during chemotherapy or administration of granulocyte colony-stimulating factor. This problem can be avoided by scheduling ^{18}F-FDG PET just before the scheduled course of chemotherapy.

In this context, it is important to determine the prognostic implications of ^{123}I-MIBG-positive residual NB tumors. If ^{18}F-FDG PET/CT is negative but ^{123}I-MIBG scan is still positive, biopsy might confirm whether the tumor has matured or has only been temporarily stunned in terms of metabolic activity [81]. The combined use of ^{18}F-FDG PET/CT and ^{123}I-MIBG scintigraphy might better depict residual disease in this clinical scenario, thus adding important information, especially before stem cell transplantation.

Beyond disease detection, it is not known whether ^{18}F-FDG PET is able to provide prognostic information or whether the imaging results correlate with survival; similarly, it is unclear whether, within this cohort of patients with high-risk, aggressive tumors, ^{18}F-FDG PET can identify those who are likely to fail multimodality treatment.

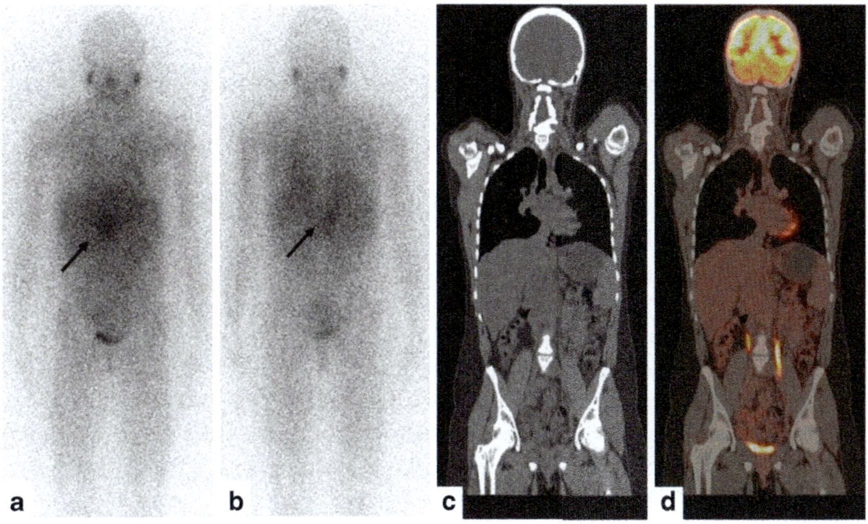

Fig. 7.9 A 16-year-old female affected by stage 3 poorly differentiated abdominal NB. Residual and unresectable abdominal mass remained stable over time after treatment (chemotherapy and ^{131}I-MIBG therapy). ^{123}I-MIBG scintigraphy (planar anterior and posterior images **a**, **b**) showed inhomogeneous uptake correspondent to the big abdominal mass (arrows). The absence of ^{18}F-FDG uptake shown by coronal PET/CT images (dotted arrows) confirmed the suspected progressive maturation of this neuroblastic tumor (**c**, **d**)

Some studies have shown that ^{18}F-FDG PET/CT would seem to have significant prognostic implications in high-risk NB patients undergoing ^{131}I-MIBG treatment. Tumoral metabolic activity (SUVmax) and extent of ^{18}F-FDG-avid bone-bone marrow disease (^{18}F-FDG skeletal scores) were identified as poor prognostic factors associated with decreased survival [82]. A pattern of increased ^{18}F-FDG activity, surpassing tumoral avidity for ^{123}I-MIBG, corresponded to more aggressive disease and worse outcome [82]. It is unknown whether this pattern mirrors NB cell dedifferentiation. In a significant number of preclinical and clinical studies, ^{18}F-FDG uptake was found to correlate with high proliferative activity, cellular dedifferentiation, and aggressive behavior of neuroendocrine tumors [82, 89, 90]. However, preclinical models have failed to verify any association between ^{18}F-FDG and NB proliferation [91].

The practical incorporation of ^{18}F-FDG-PET/CT in treatment decision-making would require the development of novel effective treatments [82, 92]. In such a setting, ^{18}F-FDG-PET/CT could aid in identifying patients for whom a more aggressive treatment strategy would be required.

In conclusion, any fixed scheme regarding the use of ^{123}I-MIBG scintigraphy and ^{18}F-FDG-PET in NB will have frequent exceptions. ^{18}F-FDG imaging is a not specific tracer for NB, but it is an important diagnostic resource especially in challenging diagnostic contexts.

7.5 Somatostatin Analogues

Five different types of somatostatin receptors (SSTR) have been discovered so far, and radiolabelled somatostatin analogues have been introduced as imaging agents for neuroendocrine tumors in the last decade, starting with ^{123}I-Tyr3-octreotide and ^{111}In-pentetreotide [93].

Somatostatin derivatives bind to SSTR, and then, they are internalized via endocytosis in endosomes/lysosomes [20].

Like other neuroendocrine tumors, NB can be also characterized by an overexpression of somatostatin receptors, more precisely SSTR types 1 and 2 [94, 95]. For this reason, ^{111}In-pentetreotide scintigraphy or somatostatin receptor scintigraphy (SRS) has been investigated in the past for the assessment of NB [96, 97], and the same concept has been readopted recently with the PET technology.

SSTR imaging can now be performed with positron emission tomography/computed tomography (PET/CT) by using -68-radiolabelled somatostatin analogues. PET provides superior imaging resolution and speed, as well as multislice CT for anatomic correlation.

In addition, more effective somatostatin analogues, characterized by a higher affinity for SSTR subtype 2 (SSTR 2), have been introduced in the last years (e.g., ^{68}Ga DOTATATE) [98]. Some clinical studies reported discordant findings between MIBG scans and somatostatin analogue imaging in NB tumors. However, SRS has not proven to be superior to ^{123}I-MIBG, but SRS has been considered as a complementary method of ^{123}I-MIBG scintigraphy [19].

Indeed, Kroiss et al. [99], in a small group of patients (n = 4), compared the accuracy of ^{123}I-MIBG scintigraphy with that of ^{68}Ga DOTATOC PET/CT in the diagnosis and staging of metastatic NB. On per-lesion-based analysis, ^{68}Ga DOTATOC PET/CT was able to detect additional sites of NB in two patients.

More recently, Kong and colleagues confirmed that ^{68}Ga-somatostatin analogues are able to identify additional sites of disease when compared with MIBG scan. In addition, ^{68}Ga DOTATATE PET/CT demonstrated high tumor-to-background uptake at all known disease sites paving the way for peptide receptor radionuclide therapy (PRRT) [100]. The theranostic implications of the somatostatin analogue imaging seem to be very promising especially for NB at very high risk not responding to conventional treatments.

In this context, Gains and colleagues demonstrated that ^{68}Ga DOTATATE PET could be used to image children with relapsed or primary refractory high-risk NB and ^{68}Ga DOTATATE PET could be used to identify potential candidates for ^{177}Lu-DOTA-TATE treatment [101]. In this study, six out of eight children demonstrated high uptake of ^{68}Ga DOTATATE and proceeded to treatment. Patients received two or three administrations of ^{177}Lu-DOTA-TATE (0.3 GBq/kg; 8.1 mCi/kg per dose) at a median interval of 9 weeks and a median administered activity of 7.3 GBq. Five of these patients had stable disease as assessed using the Response Evaluation Criteria in Solid Tumors (RECIST). This study, while limited in the number of patients studied, provided proof of principle that children with NB can be imaged and treated with somatostatin receptor-targeted agents.

In the same field, Kong et al. treated six patients with palliative intent by using PRRT. They did not find significant toxicity attributed to PRRT, and they reported that all patients achieved early symptomatic and partial imaging response [100].

7.6 Other PET Tracers

In the last 10 years, at least other three PET tracers have been tested in children affected by neuroblastoma. However, limited data are available to support or not their use in clinical practice.

7.6.1 ^{11}C-Hydroxyephedrine

The first pioneering experience was that of ^{11}C-hydroxyephedrine (HED). ^{11}C-Hydroxyephedrine (HED) is a catecholamine analogue whose uptake reflects the catecholamine transport, storage, and recycling. Biodistribution studies in experimental animal and human studies have demonstrated selective uptake in organs with rich sympathetic innervation, including the heart and adrenal medulla. Shulkin and colleagues [102] investigated the feasibility and role of ^{11}C-HED PET in localizing NB in humans. The authors showed that HED was promptly accumulated by NB and, in all patients investigated, HED was able to identify NB lesions. In comparison to ^{123}I-MIBG requiring at least 18–24 h for adequate tumor-to-nontumor ratios, early HED tumor uptake was relatively high, and, thus, NB can be imaged within minutes. Whole-body exposure to radiation, and especially thyroid exposure, was considerably lower on ^{11}C-HED PET as compared to ^{123}I-MIBG. A drawback reported by these authors, however, was that hepatic and renal uptake were prominent and liver uptake often exceeded tumor concentration [102]. In two patients, tumor deposits in the abdomen were better visualized with MIBG scintigraphy due to a relatively lower hepatic accumulation of MIBG than HED. One other group [103] compared ^{11}C-HED PET/CT with ^{123}I-MIBG SPECT/CT in NB, and they found that both tracers were able to identify NB lesions with a high sensitivity (96% and 100%, respectively). However, in one patient, ^{11}C-HED PET/CT missed a large abdominal recurrence, which was confirmed on histopathology. Moreover, MIBG uptake proved to be more intense than HED uptake in 10 out of 14 soft tissue metastases.

In conclusion, despite the higher spatial resolution of PET, ^{11}C-HED PET/CT has some disadvantages in comparison to ^{123}I-MIBG scan. Indeed, the high renal excretion of the HED can reduce the possibility to localize tumor close the urinary tract. Moreover, the high physiologic liver uptake may hinder the detection of small liver metastases [103]. Indeed same false-negative results have been reported [102, 103]. Finally, another important limitation is related to the short half-life of ^{11}C, which requires an on-site cyclotron and a rigid time schedule.

7.6.2 ^{124}I-MIBG PET/CT

No clinical pilot studies on the diagnostic role of ^{124}I-MIBG PET/CT in NB are available, but one case study was published on this issue [104]. Cistaro et al. reported two interesting cases of children affected by metastatic NB scheduled for ^{131}I-MIBG therapy who underwent ^{124}I-MIBG PET/CT before MIBG treatment. In this series, ^{124}I-MIBG PET/CT identified the same NB lesions detected by high-dose post-therapy ^{131}I-MIBG scan. In addition, ^{124}I-MIBG PET/CT provided more accurate evaluation of disease extension in one patient affected by spine metastases with intraspinal and extraspinal involvement. The authors suggested performing ^{124}I-MIBG PET/CT as a pre-therapy examination, given the high diagnostic accuracy. Indeed it should be useful in case of suspected NB relapse, with doubtful findings on ^{123}I-MIBG scan [104].

Beyond this very limited clinical experience, ^{124}I-MIBG represents several advantages in image quantification, radionuclide characteristics (^{124}I half-life of 4.2 days, that is, more similar to the 8.02-day half-life of ^{131}I), and whole-body PET acquisition [105], which can be exploited for both diagnostic imaging and dosimetry.

In the clinical setting, ^{124}I-MIBG has been used for dosimetric purposes [106, 107]. When radiation dose exposure is considered, Lee et al. [107] reported that ^{124}I-MIBG is significantly more advantageous than other ^{124}I compounds, especially ^{124}I-NaI, and that the estimated effective dose of ^{124}I-MIBG is more than ten times lower than that of ^{124}I-NaI (0.25 mSv/MBq radiation dose estimated for ^{124}I-MIBG vs. 6.5 mSv/MBq for ^{124}I-NaI). However, these effective dose values are tenfold higher than those obtained with ^{123}I-MIBG (0.019 mSv/MBq) [105, 107]. Therefore, some authors recommend administering of low doses, especially in small children, and suggested that the best indication for ^{124}I-MIBG PET is pre-therapy dosimetric study before ^{131}I-MIBG treatment [105]. However, the additional dose can be considered negligible when ^{124}I-MIBG is performed as a pre-therapy evaluation tool before ^{131}I-MIBG treatment.

In conclusion, more extensive investigation of ^{124}I-MIBG is needed before defining the correct use of this tracer in NB patient. An ongoing phase I/II trial of ^{124}I-MIBG in NB, supported by the Cancer Research UK's Centre for Drug Development (CDD), was implemented to compare this PET imaging with ^{123}I-MIBG scan. The results are expected to validate the role of this interesting procedure. Indeed, this tracer seems to be very promising considering that is able to provide important implicit theranostic implication.

7.7 Conclusions

In the current era of a growing number of available PET tracers, pediatric imaging may benefit from the combined use of different metabolic and receptor-specific tracer. However, in children, the selective and conscious use of tracers based on the evidence of specific cost-effective analyses is highly suggested to reduce futile radiation exposure. Planar and SPECT imaging with ^{123}I-MIBG remains the first step procedure to evaluate NB. PET/CT imaging by using ^{18}F-FDG may be useful especially in case of suspected MIBG-negative NB component at the time of first staging. The uptake mechanism and the physiologic distribution of ^{18}F-DOPA seem in favor of its use in NB. Indeed, DOPA and MIBG have very similar uptake mechanisms, and they show the same pathological distribution in soft tissue and bone/bone marrow metastases. Its principal application seems to be very promising to evaluate disease persistence after chemotherapy and to detect NB relapse. Among the other PET tracers available, the somatostatin analogues seem to be very promising in NB imaging. Indeed ^{68}Ga-somatostatin analogues are able to detect more sites of disease when compared with MIBG scan and to select patients for PRRT.

References

1. Monclair T, Brodeur GM, Ambros PF, Brisse HJ, Cecchetto G, Holmes K, et al. The International Neuroblastoma Risk Group (INRG) staging system: an INRG Task Force report. J Clin Oncol. 2009;27:298–303.
2. Cohn SL, Pearson AD, London WB, Monclair T, Ambros PF, Brodeur GM, et al. The International Neuroblastoma Risk Group (INRG) classification system: an INRG Task Force report. J Clin Oncol. 2009;27:289–97.
3. Beiske K, Burchill SA, Cheung IY, Hiyama E, Seeger RC, Cohn SL, et al. Consensus criteria for sensitive detection of minimal neuroblastoma cells in bone marrow, blood and stem cell preparations by immunocytology and QRT-PCR: recommendations by the International Neuroblastoma Risk Group Task Force. Br J Cancer. 2009;100:1627–37.
4. Ambros PF, Ambros IM, Brodeur GM, Haber M, Khan J, Nakagawara A, et al. International consensus for neuroblastoma molecular diagnostics: report from the International Neuroblastoma Risk Group (INRG) Biology Committee. Br J Cancer. 2009;100:1471–82.
5. Matthay KK, Shulkin B, Ladenstein R, Michon J, Giammarile F, Lewington V, et al. Criteria for evaluation of disease extent by (123)I-metaiodobenzylguanidine scans in neuroblastoma: a report for the International Neuroblastoma Risk Group (INRG) Task Force. Br J Cancer. 2010;102:1319–26.
6. Brisse HJ, McCarville MB, Granata C, Krug KB, Wootton-Gorges SL, Kanegawa K, et al. Guidelines for imaging and staging of neuroblastic tumors: consensus report from the International Neuroblastoma Risk Group project. Radiology. 2011;261:243–57.
7. Maris JM. Recent advances in neuroblastoma. N Engl J Med. 2010;362:2202–11.
8. Pinto NR, Applebaum MA, Volchenboum SL, Matthay KK, London WB, Ambros PF, et al. Advances in risk classification and treatment strategies for neuroblastoma. J Clin Oncol. 2015;33:3008–17.
9. Canete A, Gerrard M, Rubie H, Castel V, Di Cataldo A, Munzer C, et al. Poor survival for infants with MYCN-amplified metastatic neuroblastoma despite intensified treatment: the International Society of Paediatric Oncology European Neuroblastoma Experience. J Clin Oncol. 2009;27:1014–9.
10. Garaventa A, Boni L, Lo Piccolo MS, Tonini GP, Gambini C, Mancini A, et al. Localized unresectable neuroblastoma: results of treatment based on clinical prognostic factors. Ann Oncol. 2002;13:956–64.
11. Lopci E, Piccardo A, Nanni C, Altrinetti V, Garaventa A, Pession A, et al. 18F-DOPA PET/CT in neuroblastoma comparison of conventional imaging with CT/MR. Clin Nucl Med. 2012;37:e71–8.
12. Sofka CM, Semelka RC, Kelekis NL, Worawattanakul S, Chung CJ, Gold S, et al. Magnetic resonance imaging of neuroblastoma using current techniques. Magn Reson Imaging. 1999;17:193–8.

13. Pfluger T, Schmied C, Porn U, Leinsinger G, Vollmar C, Dresel S, et al. Integrated imaging using MRI and 123I metaiodobenzylguanidine scintigraphy to improve sensitivity and specificity in the diagnosis of pediatric neuroblastoma. Am J Roentgenol. 2002;181:1115–24.
14. Siegel MJ, Jaju A. MR imaging of neuroblastic masses. Magn Reson Imaging Clin N Am. 2008;16(3):499–513.
15. Hiorns MP, Owens CM. Radiology of neuroblastoma in children. Eur Radiol. 2001;11(10):2071–81.
16. Lebtahi N, Gudinchet F, Nenadov-Beck M, et al. Evaluating bone marrow metastasis of neuroblastoma with iodine-123- MIBG scintigraphy and MRI. J Nucl Med. 1997;38:1389–92.
17. Tanabe M, Takahashi H, Ohnuma N, Iwai J, Yoshida H. Evaluation of bone marrow metastasis of neuroblastoma and changes after chemotherapy by MRI. Med Pediatr Oncol. 1993;21:54–9.
18. Bleeker G, Tytgat GA, Adam JA, Caron HN, Kremer LC, Hooft L, van Dalen EC. 123I-MIBG scintigraphy and 18F-FDG-PET imaging for diagnosing neuroblastoma. Cochrane Database Syst Rev. 2015;29(9):CD009263. https://doi.org/10.1002/14651858.CD009263.pub2.
19. Bleeker G, Tytgat GA, Adam JA, Caron HN, Kremer LC, Hooft L, et al. 123I-MIBG scintigraphy and 18F-FDG-PET imaging for diagnosing neuroblastoma. Cochrane Database Syst Rev. 2015;(9):CD009263. https://doi.org/10.1002/14651858.CD009263.pub2.
20. Wilson JS, Gains JE, Moroz V, Wheatley K, Gaze MN. A systematic review of 131I-meta iodobenzylguanidine molecular radiotherapy for neuroblastoma. Eur J Cancer. 2014;50:801–15.
21. Castellani MR, Scarale A, Lorenzoni A, Maccauro M, Balaguer Guill J, Luksch R. Treatment with 131I-MIBG (indications, procedures and results). Chapter 19. In: Bombardieri E, editor. Clinical applications of nuclear medicine targeted therapy. Cham: Springer Nature; 2018.
22. Pfluger T, Piccardo A. Neuroblastoma: MIBG imaging and new tracers. Semin Nucl Med. 2017;47(2):143–57.
23. Piccardo A, Lopci E, Conte M, Foppiani L, Garaventa A, Cabria M, et al. PET/CT imaging in neuroblastoma. Q J Nucl Med Mol Imaging. 2013;57:29–39.
24. Wieland DM, Wu J, Brown LE, Mangner TJ, Swanson DP, Beierwaltes WH. Radiolabeled adrenergic neuron-blocking agents: adrenomedullary imaging with [131I]iodobenzylguanidine. J Nucl Med. 1980;21:349–53.
25. Sharp SE, Parisi MT, Gelfand MJ, Yanik GA, Shulkin BL. Functional-metabolic imaging of neuroblastoma. Q J Nucl Med Mol Imaging. 2013;57:6–20.
26. Shulkin BL, Shapiro B, Francis IR, et al. Primary extra-adrenal pheochromocytoma: positive I-123 MIBG imaging with negative I-131 MIBG imaging. Clin Nucl Med. 1986;11:851–4.
27. Brodeur GM, Pritchard J, Berthold F, Carlsen NL, Castel V, Castelberry RP, et al. Revisions of the international criteria for neuroblastoma diagnosis, staging, and response to treatment. J Clin Oncol. 1993;11:1466–77.
28. Schmidt M, Simon T, Hero B, et al. The prognostic impact of functional imaging with (123) ImIBG in patients with stage 4 neuroblastoma. 1 year of age on a high-risk treatment protocol: results of the German neuroblastoma trial NB97. Eur J Cancer. 2008;44:1552–8.
29. Boubaker A, Bischof DA. MIBG scintigraphy for the diagnosis and follow-up of children with neuroblastoma. Q J Nucl Med Mol Imaging. 2008;52:388–402.
30. Kushner BH, Yeh SD, Kramer K, et al. Impact of metaiodobenzylguanidine scintigraphy on assessing response of high-risk neuroblastoma to dose-intensive induction chemotherapy. J Clin Oncol. 2003;21:1082–6.
31. Matthay KK, Edeline V, Lumbroso J, et al. Correlation of early metastatic response by 123I-metaiodobenzylguanidine scintigraphy with overall response and event-free survival in stage IV neuroblastoma. J Clin Oncol. 2003;21:2486–91.
32. Ady N, Zucker JM, Asselain B, et al. A new 123I-MIBG whole body scan scoring method: application to the prediction of the response of metastases to induction chemotherapy in stage IV neuroblastoma. Eur J Cancer. 1995;31A:256–61.
33. Lonergan GJ, Schwab CM, Suarez ES, Carlson CL. Neuroblastoma, ganglioneuroblastoma, and ganglioneuroma: radiologic-pathologic correlation. Radiographics. 2002;22:911–34.

34. Bonnin F, Lumbroso J, Tenenbaum F, Hartmann O, Parmentier C. Refining interpretation of MIBG scans in children. J Nucl Med. 1994;35:803–10.
35. Geatti O, Shapiro B, Shulkin B, et al. Gastrointestinal iodine-131-metaiodobenzylguanidine activity. Am J Physiol Imaging. 1988;3:188–91.
36. Pfluger T, Schmied C, Porn U, et al. Integrated imaging using MRI and 123I metaiodobenzylguanidine scintigraphy to improve sensitivity and specificity in the diagnosis of pediatric neuroblastoma. AJR Am J Roentgenol. 2003;181:1115–24.
37. Granata C, Carlini C, Conte M, et al. False positive MIBG scan due to accessory spleen. Med Pediatr Oncol. 2001;37:138–9.
38. Paltiel HJ, Gelfand MJ, Elgazzar AH, et al. Neural crest tumors: I-123 MIBG imaging in children. Radiology. 1994;190:117–21.
39. Okuyama C, Sakane N, Yoshida T, et al. (123)I- or (125)I-metaiodobenzylguanidine visualization of brown adipose tissue. J Nucl Med. 2002;3:1234–40.
40. Okuyama C, Ushijima Y, Kubota T, et al. 123I-metaiodobenzylguanidine uptake in the nape of the neck of children: likely visualization of brown adipose tissue. J Nucl Med. 2003;44:1421–5.
41. Piccardo A, Lopci E. Potential role of 18F-DOPA PET in neuroblastoma. Clin Transl Imag. 2016;4:79–86.
42. Moyes JSE, Babich JW, Carter R, Meller ST, Agrawal M, McElwain TJ. Quantitative study of radioiodinated metaiodobenzylguanidine uptake in children with neuroblastoma: correlation with tumor histopathology. J Nucl Med. 1989;30:474–80.
43. Lebtahi Hadj-Djilani N, Lebtahi NE, Bischof Delaloye A, Laurini R, Beck D. Diagnosis and follow-up of neuroblastoma by means of iodine-123 metaiodobenzylguanidine scintigraphy and bone scan, and the influence of histology. Eur J Nucl Med. 1995;22:322–9.
44. Geatti O, Shapiro B, Sisson JC, Hutchinson RJ, Mallette S, Eyre P, et al. Iodine-131 metaiodobenzylguanidine scintigraphy for the location of neuroblastoma: preliminary experience in ten cases. J Nucl Med. 1985;26:736–42.
45. Khafagi FA, Shapiro B, Fig LM, Mallette S, Sisson JC. Labetalol reduces iodine-131 MIBG uptake by pheochromocytoma and normal tissues. J Nucl Med. 1989;30:481–9.
46. Biasotti S, Garaventa A, Villavecchia GP, Cabria M, Nantron M, De Bernardi B. False-negative metaiodobenzylguanidine scintigraphy at diagnosis of neuroblastoma. Med Pediatr Oncol. 2000;35:153–5.
47. Sharp SE, Gelfand MJ, Shulkin BL. Pediatrics: diagnosis of neuroblastoma. Semin Nucl Med. 2011;41:345–53.
48. Rufini V, Fisher GA, Shulkin BL, et al. Iodine-123-MIBG imaging of neuroblastoma: utility of SPECT and delayed imaging. J Nucl Med. 1996;37:1464–8.
49. Černý I, Prášek J, Kašpárková H. Superiority of SPECT/CT over planar 123ImIBG images in neuroblastoma patients with impact on Curie and SIOPEN score values. Nuklearmedizin. 2016;55:151–7.
50. Gelfand MJ, Elgazzar AH, Kriss VM, et al. Iodine-123-MIBG SPECT versus planar imaging in children with neural crest tumors. J Nucl Med. 1994;35:1753–7.
51. Hugosson C, Nyman R, Jorulf H, et al. Imaging of abdominal neuroblastoma in children. Acta Radiol. 1999;40:534–42.
52. Yanik GA, Parisi MT, Shulkin BL, Naranjo A, Kreissman SG, London WB, et al. Semiquantitative mIBG scoring as a prognostic indicator in patients with stage 4 neuroblastoma: a report from the Children's oncology group. J Nucl Med. 2013;54:541–8.
53. Ladenstein R, Lambert B, Pötschger U, Castellani MR, Lewington V, Bar-Sever Z, et al. Validation of the mIBG skeletal SIOPEN scoring method in two independent high-risk neuroblastoma populations: the SIOPEN/HR-NBL1 and COG-A3973 trials. Eur J Nucl Med Mol Imaging. 2018;45:292.
54. Matthay KK, Villablanca JG, Seeger RC, Stram DO, Harris RE, Ramsay NK, et al. Treatment of high-risk Neuroblastoma with intensive chemotherapy, radiotherapy, autologous bone marrow transplantation, and 13-cis-retinoic acid. Children's Cancer Group. N Engl J Med. 1999;341:1165–73.

55. Pearson AD, Pinkerton CR, Lewis IJ, Imeson J, Ellershaw C, Machin D. High-dose rapid and standard induction chemotherapy for patients aged over 1 year with stage 4 neuroblastoma: a randomised trial. Lancet Oncol. 2008;9:247–56.
56. Zage PE, Kletzel M, Murray K, Marcus R, Castleberry R, Zhang Y, et al. Outcomes of the POG 9340/9341/9342trials for children with high-risk neuroblastoma: a report from the Children's Oncology Group. Pediatr Blood Cancer. 2008;51:747–53.
57. London WB, Castel V, Monclair T, Ambros PF, Pearson AD, Cohn SL, et al. Clinical and biologic features predictive of survival after relapse of neuroblastoma: a report from the International Neuroblastoma Risk Group project. J Clin Oncol. 2011;29:3286–92.
58. Kushner BH, Kramer K, Modak S, Cheung NK. Sensitivity of surveillance studies for detecting asymptomatic and unsuspected relapse of high-risk neuroblastoma. J Clin Oncol. 2009;27:1041–6.
59. Piccardo A, Puntoni M, Lopci E, Conte M, Foppiani L, Sorrentino S, et al. Prognostic value of ^{18}F-DOPA PET/CT at the time of recurrence in patients affected by neuroblastoma. Eur J Nucl Med Mol Imaging. 2014;41:1046–56.
60. LaBrosse EH, Comoy E, Bohuon C, Zucker JM, Schweisguth O. Catecholamine metabolism in neuroblastoma. J Natl Cancer Inst. 1976;57:633–8.
61. Brodeur GM. Neuroblastoma and other peripheral neuroectodermal tumors. In: Fernbach DJ, Vietti TJ, editors. Clinical pediatric oncology. 4th ed. St. Louis, MO: CV Mosby; 1991. p. 337.
62. Jager PL, Chirakal R, Marriott CJ, Brouwers AH, Koopmans KP, Gulenchyn KY, et al. 6-L-18F-fluorodihydroxyphenylalanine PET in neuroendocrine tumors: basic aspects and emerging clinical applications. J Nucl Med. 2008;49:573–86.
63. Timmers AJLM, Chen CC, Carrasquillo JA, Whatley M, Ling A, Havekes B, et al. Comparison of 18F-fluoro-L-DOPA, 18F-fluoro-deoxyglucose and 18F-fluorodopamine PET and 123I-MIBG scintigraphy in the localization of phaeochromocytoma and paraganglioma. J Clin Endocrinol Metab. 2009;94:4757–67.
64. Fiebrich H, Brouwers AH, Kerstens MN, Pijl ME, Kema IP, de Jong JR, et al. 6-[F-18]Fluoro-L-dihydroxyphenylalanine positron emission tomography is superior to conventional imaging with 123I-metaiodobenzylguanidine scintigraphy, computer tomography, and magnetic resonance imaging in localizing tumours causing catecholamine excess. J Clin Endocrinol Metab. 2009;94:3922–30.
65. Treglia G, Castaldi P, Villani MF, Perotti G, de Waure C, Filice A, et al. Comparison of 18F-DOPA, 18F-FDG and 68Ga-somatostatin analogue PET/CT in patients with recurrent medullary thyroid carcinoma. Eur J Nucl Med Mol Imaging. 2012;39:569–80.
66. Piccardo A, Lopci E, Conte M, Garaventa A, Foppiani L, Altrinetti V, et al. Comparison of (18)F-dopa PET/CT and (123)I-MIBG scintigraphy in stage 3 and 4 neuroblastoma: a pilot study. Eur J Nucl Med Mol Imaging. 2012;39:57–61.
67. Piccardo A, Lopci E, Conte M, Cabria M, Cistaro A, Garaventa A, Villavecchia G. al. Bone and lymph node metastases from neuroblastoma detected by 18F-DOPA-PET/CT and confirmed by posttherapy 131I-MIBG but negative on diagnostic 123I-MIBG. Clin Nucl Med. 2014;39(1):e80–3.
68. Lu MY, Liu YL, Chang HH, et al. Characterization of Neuroblastic Tumors Using 18F-FDOPA PET. J Nucl Med. 2013;54:42–9.
69. Piccardo A, Morana G, Massollo M, Pescetto M, Conte M, Garaventa A. Brain metastasis from neuroblastoma depicted by (18)F-DOPA PET/CT. Nucl Med Mol Imaging. 2015;49(3):241–2.
70. Lewington V, Bar Sever Z, Lynch T, Giammarile F, McEwan A, Shulkin B, et al. Development of a semi-quantitative I-123 mIBG reporting method in high risk neuroblastoma. J Nucl Med. 2009;36:334.
71. Piccardo A, Lopci E, Foppiani L, Morana G. Conte M (18)F-DOPA PET/CT for assessment of response to induction chemotherapy in a child with high-risk neuroblastoma. Pediatr Radiol. 2014;44:355–61.

72. Lopci E, D'Ambrosio D, Nanni C, Chiti A, Pession A, Marengo M, et al. Feasibility of carbidopa premedication in pediatric patients: a pilot study. Cancer Biother Radiopharm. 2012;27:729–33.
73. ICRP. Radiation dose to patients from radiopharmaceuticals - addendum 3 to ICRP Publication 53. ICRP Publication 106. Ann ICRP. 2008;38(1-2)
74. ICRP. Radiation Dose to Patients from Radiopharmaceuticals (Addendum to ICRP Publication 53). ICRP Publication 80. Ann ICRP. 1998;28(3)
75. Huang YY, Tzen KY, Liu YL, Chiu CH, Tsai CL, Wen HP, et al. Impact of residual 18F-fluoride in 18F-FDOPA for the diagnosis of neuroblastoma. Ann Nucl Med. 2015;29:489–98.
76. Gordon I, Peters AM, Gutman A, Morony S, Dicks-Mireaux C, Pritchard J. Skeletal assessment in neuroblastoma – the pitfalls of iodine-123-MIBG scans. J Nucl Med. 1990;31:129–34.
77. Melzer HI, Coppenrath E, Schmid I, Albert MH, von Schweinitz D, Tudball C, et al. ^{123}I-MIBG scintigraphy/SPECT versus ^{18}F-FDG PET in paediatric neuroblastoma. Eur J Nucl Med Mol Imaging. 2011;38:1648–58.
78. Lebtahi Hadj-Djilani N, Lebtahi NE, Delaloye AB, Laurini R, Beck D, et al. Diagnosis and follow-up of neuroblastoma by means of iodine-123 metaiodobenzylguanidine scintigraphy and bone scan, and the influence of histology. Eur J Nucl Med. 1995;22:322–9.
79. Giammarile F, Lumbroso J, Ricard M, Aubert B, Hartmann O, Schlumberger M, et al. Radioiodinated metaiodobenzylguanidine in neuroblastoma: influence of high dose on tumour site detection. Eur J Nucl Med. 1995;22:1180–3.
80. Sharp SE, Shulkin BL, Gelfand MJ, Salisbury S, Furman WL. 123IMIBG scintigraphy and 18F-FDG PET in neuroblastoma. J Nucl Med. 2009;50:1237–43.
81. Taggart DR, Han MM, Quach A, Groshen S, Ye W, Villablanca JG, et al. Comparison of iodine-123 metaiodobenzylguanidine (MIBG) scan and [18F] fluorodeoxyglucose positron emission tomography to evaluate response after iodine-131 MIBG therapy for relapsed neuroblastoma. J Clin Oncol. 2009;27:5343–9.
82. Papathanasiou ND, Gaze MN, Sullivan K, Aldridge M, Waddington W, Almuhaideb A, et al. 18F-FDG PET/CT and 123I-metaiodobenzylguanidine imaging in high-risk neuroblastoma: diagnostic comparison and survival analysis. J Nucl Med. 2011;52:519–25.
83. Colavolpe C, Guedj E, Cammilleri S, Taïeb D, Mundler O, Coze C. Utility of FDG-PET/CT in the follow-up of neuroblastoma which became MIBG-negative. Pediatr Blood Cancer. 2008;51:828–31.
84. Mc Dowell H, Losty P, Barnes N, Kokai G. Utility of FDG-PET/CT in the follow-up of neuroblastoma which became MIBG negative. Pediatr Blood Cancer. 2009;52:552.
85. Schwarz KB, Driver I, Lewis IJ, Taylor RE. Positive MIBG scanning at the time of relapse in neuroblastoma which was MIBG negative at diagnosis. Br J Radiol. 1997;70:90–2.
86. Kushner BH, Yeung HW, Larson SM, Kramer K, Cheung NK. Extending positron emission tomography scan utility to high-risk neuroblastoma: fluorine-18 fluorodeoxyglucose positron emission tomography as sole imaging modality in follow-up of patients. J Clin Oncol. 2001;219:3397–405.
87. Kushner BH. Neuroblastoma: a disease requiring a multitude of imaging studies. J Nucl Med. 2004;45:1172–88.
88. Shulkin BL, Hutchinson RJ, Castle VP, Yanik GA, Shapiro B, Sisson JC, et al. Neuroblastoma: positron emission tomography with 2-[fluorine-18]-fluoro-2-deoxy-D-glucose compared with metaiodobenzylguanidine scintigraphy. Radiology. 1996;199:743–50.
89. Adams S, Baum RP, Hertel A, Schumm-Dräger PM, Usadel KH, Hör G. Metabolic (PET) and receptor (SPET) imaging of well- and less well-differentiated tumours: comparison with the expression of the Ki-67 antigen. Nucl Med Commun. 1998;19:641–7.
90. Kayani I, Bomanji JB, Groves A, Conway G, Gacinovic S, Win T, et al. Functional imaging of neuroendocrine tumors with combined PET/CT using 68Ga-DOTATATE (DOTA-DPhe1,Tyr3-octreotate) and 18F-FDG. Cancer. 2008;112:2447–55.
91. Krieger-Hinck N, Gustke H, Valentiner U, Mikecz P, Buchert R, Mester J, et al. Visualisation of neuroblastoma growth in a Scid mouse model using [18F]FDG and [18F]FLT-PET. Anticancer Res. 2006;26:3467–72.

92. Wagner LM, Danks MK. New therapeutic targets for the treatment of high-risk neuroblastoma. J Cell Biochem. 2009;107:46–57.
93. Krenning EP, Kwekkeboom DJ, Bakker WH, Breeman WA, Kooij PP, Oei HY, et al. Somatostatin receptor scintigraphy with [111In-DTPA-D-Phe1]- and [123I-Tyr3]-octreotide: the Rotterdam experience with more than 1000 patients. Eur J Nucl Med. 1993;20:716–31.
94. O'Dorisio MS, Chen F, O'Dorisio TM, Wray D, Qualman SJ. Characterization of somatostatin receptors on human neuroblastoma tumors. Cell Growth Differ. 1994;5:1–8.
95. Albers AR, O'Dorisio MS, Balster DA, Caprara M, Gosh P, Chen F, et al. Somatostatin receptor gene expression in neuroblastoma. Regul Pept. 2000;88:61–73.
96. Kropp J, Hofmann M, Bihl H. Comparison of MIBG and pentetreotide scintigraphy in children with neuroblastoma. Is the expression of somatostatin receptors a prognostic factor? Anticancer Res. 1997;17:1583–8.
97. Shalaby-Rana E, Majd M, Andrich MP, Movassaghi N. In-111 pentetreotide scintigraphy in patients with neuroblastoma. Comparison with I-131 MIBG, N-MYC oncogene amplification, and patient outcome. Clin Nucl Med. 1997;22:315–9.
98. Storch D, Béhé M, Walter MA, Chen J, Powell P, Mikolajczak R, et al. Evaluation of [99mTc/EDDA/HYNIC0]octreotide derivatives compared with [111In- DOTA0,Tyr3, Thr8]octreotide and [111In-DTPA0]octreotide: does tumor or pancreas uptake correlate with the rate of internalization? J Nucl Med. 2005;46:1561–9.
99. Kroiss A, Putzer D, Uprimny C, Decristoforo C, Gabriel M, Santner W, et al. Functional imaging in phaeochromocytoma and neuroblastoma with 68Ga-DOTATyr3-octreotide positron emission tomography and 123I metaiodobenzylguanidine. Eur J Nucl Med Mol Imaging. 2011;38:865–73.
100. Kong G, Hofman MS, Murray WK, Wilson S, Wood P, Downie P, et al. Initial experience with gallium-68 DOTA-octreotate PET/CT and peptide receptor radionuclide therapy for pediatric patients with refractory metastatic neuroblastoma. J Pediatr Hematol Oncol. 2016;38:87–96.
101. Gains JE, Bomanji JB, Fersht NL, Sullivan T, D'Souza D, Sullivan KP, et al. 177Lu-DOTATATE molecular radiotherapy for childhood neuroblastoma. J Nucl Med. 2011;52(7):1041–7.
102. Shulkin BL, Wieland DM, Baro ME, Ungar DR, Mitchell DS, Dole MG, et al. PET hydroxyephedrine imaging of neuroblastoma. J Nucl Med. 1996;37:16–21.
103. Franzius C, Hermann K, Weckesser M, Kopka K, Juergens KU, Vormoor J, et al. Whole-body PET/CT with 11C-meta-hydroxyephedrine in tumors of the sympathetic nervous system: feasibility study and comparison with 123I-MIBG SPECT/CT. J Nucl Med. 2006;47:1635–42.
104. Cistaro A, Quartuccio N, Caobelli F, Piccardo A, Paratore R, Coppolino P, et al. 124I-MIBG: a new promising positron-emitting radiopharmaceutical for the evaluation of neuroblastoma. Nucl Med Rev Cent East Eur. 2015;18:102–6.
105. Lopci E, Chiti A, Castellani MR, Pepe G, Antunovic L, Fanti S, et al. Matched pairs dosimetry: 124I/131I metaiodobenzylguanidine and 124I/131I and 14 T. 86Y/90Y antibodies. Eur J Nucl Med Mol Imaging. 2011;38:S28–40.
106. Herzog H, Tellmann L, Scholten B, Coenen HH, Qaim SM. PET imaging problems with the non-standard positron emitters Yttrium-86 and Iodine-124. Q J Nucl Med Mol Imaging. 2008;52:159–65.
107. Lee CL, Wahnishe H, Sayre GA, Cho HM, Kim HJ, Hernandez-Pampaloni M, et al. Radiation dose estimation using preclinical imaging with 124I-metaiodobenzylguanidine (MIBG) PET. Med Phys. 2010;37:4861–7.

Radiotherapy for Neuroblastoma

8

Tom Boterberg

8.1 Introduction

Radiotherapy has a long history of use in neuroblastoma treatment protocols, especially in high-risk disease. However, most evidence is biological or indirect as there are almost no randomised trials specifically addressing the role of radiotherapy in neuroblastoma.

Neuroblastoma originates from the adrenergic neuroblasts in neural crest and sympathetic nervous system tissue. The cells of this tissue are usually very radiosensitive. In addition, radiotherapy reduces local failure in almost any cancer type. This is also the case in neuroblastoma, with even rather low doses compared to other diseases like sarcoma. Finally, molecular radiotherapy with ^{131}I-mIBG (metaiodobenzylguanidine) has also shown to be beneficial in neuroblastoma. mIBG is concentrated by neurosecretory granules of cells originating from the neural crest. Radio-labelled ^{131}I-mIBG is also taken up by the tumour cells, resulting in efficient killing of these cells by radiation originating from ^{131}I coupled to mIBG.

However, convincing randomised evidence for the use of radiotherapy in the treatment of neuroblastoma is not available. Comparing the results of the different reports on the role of radiotherapy is challenging as well. Several trials and collaborative groups used different end points and different staging systems over time, multiple stages were grouped in a single trial or study, and different target volumes and multiple radiotherapy schedules were used, even within the same trial or study. Despite this lack of randomised evidence, radiotherapy is an important part of multimodality treatment schedules. Moreover, as treatment results have improved significantly over the past decades, local control may even become more important since metastatic disease can be cleared better by more appropriate systemic and immunological therapy.

T. Boterberg (✉)
Department of Radiation Oncology, Ghent University Hospital, Ghent, Belgium
e-mail: tom.boterberg@ugent.be

S. Sarnacki, L. Pio (eds.), *Neuroblastoma*,
https://doi.org/10.1007/978-3-030-18396-7_8

As neuroblastoma is commonly subdivided in low-, intermediate- and high-risk disease, the use of radiotherapy in these risk categories will be discussed separately.

8.2 Radiotherapy for Low-Risk Disease

Patients with low-risk disease have an excellent prognosis after surgery alone, and some patients don't even need surgery at all, but just careful observation. Adjuvant chemotherapy or radiotherapy does not improve the outcome in these patients. Some tumours may need chemotherapy or very occasionally radiotherapy to make them resectable or to stabilise them.

8.3 Radiotherapy for Intermediate-Risk Disease

Most patients with intermediate-risk disease can be managed with chemotherapy and/or surgery. However, some patients clearly benefit from radiotherapy, like those with unfavourable histology. Castleberry et al. [1] published the only randomised radiotherapy trial in neuroblastoma so far. In patients older than 1 year with positive lymph nodes, post-operative chemotherapy alone was compared with post-operative chemotherapy, followed by radiotherapy. The EFS at 5 years was 32% and 59% ($p = 0.009$), respectively, clearly demonstrating the benefit of radiotherapy in these patients. This was also demonstrated in OS at 5 years with 41% and 73%, respectively ($p = 0.008$). Radiotherapy at a dose of 21 Gy is currently recommended in patients over 18 months and with poorly or undifferentiated histology. The ongoing SIOPEN LINES trial investigates if intensified treatment (including radiotherapy) can improve the treatment results in these patients.

Patients with spinal cord compression pose a separate problem in this patient category and were historically treated with laminectomy with or without radiotherapy and chemotherapy. However, the morbidity (especially spine deformities) of this strategy may be significant, and currently most patients are treated with upfront chemotherapy [2, 3]. Although the optimal treatment strategy for these patients is still unclear, the role of radiotherapy is usually limited, but should not be forgotten if other treatment modalities fail.

8.4 Radiotherapy for High-Risk Disease

Despite the lack of convincing randomised treatment data of radiotherapy versus no radiotherapy, this treatment modality now has an established role in the management of high-risk neuroblastoma, mainly based on indirect, but substantial clinical evidence. Over the past decades, several international groups have used several treatment strategies. These include radiotherapy in all patients, total body irradiation (TBI) in addition to local irradiation, intraoperative radiotherapy and local radiotherapy in case of residual disease only. The most optimal treatment strategy is still unclear.

In the CCG-321P3 study, Matthay et al. [4] used a rather low dose of 10–20 Gy only if disease was present immediately prior to bone marrow transplantation (BMT). This resulted in a quite high reported relapse rate at the primary site in 32 of 68 (47%) patients with disease progression following BMT. Kremens et al. [5] used chemotherapy and BMT and systematically increased the dose to 21 Gy to the primary site of all 26 patients investigated. They observed (only) 4/14 (29%) relapses involving the primary site. Kushner et al. [6] investigated 25 patients treated with myeloablative combination chemotherapy and surgery without total body irradiation but local irradiation up to 21 Gy. Ten relapses of any kind occurred, but only one of these ten relapses involved the primary site, again suggesting a beneficial effect of local radiation. A Japanese study [7] in 36 patients examined the role of intraoperative radiotherapy and did not find any relapse at the primary site after surgery and intraoperative radiotherapy.

In addition to local radiotherapy, TBI has also been used in the treatment of neuroblastoma. Twelve gray TBI followed or not by a 8–24 Gy local boost resulted in a PFS at 5 years of 68% versus 33% in case 12 Gy TBI was not followed by a boost [8]. However, with a p-value of 0.24, the difference was only marginally significant. One of the largest series (on 539 patients) investigated the sequence of chemotherapy, surgery and 10 Gy local radiotherapy in case of residual disease followed by further chemotherapy, or followed by 10 Gy TBI as part of the conditioning regimen for an autologous bone marrow transplantation [9]. Addition of TBI resulted in a 5-year local recurrence rate of 22%, while patients treated with further chemotherapy had a local recurrence rate of 52% ($p = 0.022$). It is obviously impossible to separate the effect of radiotherapy from the effect of the more intensified systemic treatment patients received in the transplantation arm, but these results suggest once more that a dose around 20 Gy is needed to obtain an effect on neuroblastoma. However, despite its beneficial effect on local control, acute and especially long-term complications of TBI in the treatment of neuroblastoma turned out to be significant. TBI resulted in endocrine deficiencies, hearing and visual disturbances, lung toxicity, height deficiency and an almost threefold increase in secondary tumours [10]. This was even more pronounced in very young children. Therefore, this strategy has now been abandoned.

Local radiotherapy on the primary tumour may not only improve local control but also have an impact on overall survival, which may obviously be even more important. A retrospective analysis on 44 patients by Pai Panandiker et al. [11] showed that locoregional tumour control may impact the overall survival in high-risk neuroblastoma. The influence of locoregional control reached borderline statistical significance ($p = 0.06$). The overall survival at 5 years was 48.3 ± 14.2% for patients without locoregional failure versus 21.8 ± 19.3% for patients with locoregional failure.

Currently, different treatment strategies for radiotherapy are or have been followed by different international groups.

In the USA, the Children's Oncology Group (COG) ANBL0532 trial (which closed in 2012) prescribed 21.6 Gy in 12 fractions of 1.8 Gy to the pre-surgical primary tumour bed, after chemotherapy, surgery and high-dose chemotherapy, followed by autologous stem cell transplantation. In case of incomplete resection, a boost of 14.4 Gy in 8 fractions of 1.8 Gy (resulting in a cumulative dose of 36 Gy) was given to the residual tumour. The systematic use of ^{131}I-mIBG treatment in addition to local external beam radiotherapy is currently under investigation.

The recently closed SIOPEN High-Risk Neuroblastoma Study 1 prescribed a dose of 21 Gy in 14 fractions of 1.5 Gy to the pre-surgical primary tumour volume, including regional lymph nodes if invaded, for all patients. Treatment consisted first of chemotherapy, surgery and high-dose chemotherapy, followed by autologous stem cell transplantation. A compromise to dose or volume was allowed to respect normal tissue tolerance in case of very large volumes. This dose was given regardless of the disease extent and the extent of surgery. Preliminary retrospective results presented at ASCO 2018 [12] showed that the 5-year EFS for patients with complete macroscopic excision who received radiotherapy was 44 ± 2%, but 31 ± 6% without radiotherapy ($p = 0.013$), again pointing towards an important role for radiotherapy in local control. However, some bias may play a role as delivery of radiotherapy or not was not randomised. Reasons not to give radiotherapy included very young age and very large primary tumours.

In Germany, it has been standard practice to give radiotherapy only in patients above 1 year old with local mIBG-positive residual disease after induction chemotherapy, surgery and high-dose chemotherapy, followed by stem cell transplantation. Thirty-six Gy is administered post-operatively to the residual tumour volume. A retrospective analysis [13] on 110 patients showed that 13 patients who received EBRT for local residual disease had a similar outcome (3-year EFS 85 ± 10%, 3-year OS 92 ± 7%) as 74 patients without any mIBG-positive residual (3-year EFS 61 ± 6%, 3-year OS 75 ± 6%). The outcome was worse in 23 children without EBRT to the residual primary (3-year EFS 25 ± 10%, 3-year OS 51 ± 11%). However, once more, the omission of radiotherapy was not randomised and results could be biased by unknown factors.

Based on these results and the previous SIOPEN experience, the SIOPEN High-Risk Neuroblastoma Study 2 (SIOPEN/HR-NBL2, due to open in 2019) will investigate if dose escalation beyond 21 Gy would translate into better outcomes in terms of local control and survival for patients with residual disease. This randomised question (21 Gy to the preoperative tumour bed only versus 21 Gy to the preoperative tumour bed + a 15 Gy boost to the residual tumour) will be asked for patients with macroscopic residual disease after induction chemotherapy, surgery and high-dose chemotherapy, followed by autologous stem cell rescue.

In addition to irradiation of the primary tumour site, radiotherapy with curative intent to (a limited number of) metastatic sites is still controversial as no solid data are available. A recent single institution study by Casey et al. [14] retrospectively analysed 159 patients with 244 metastatic sites irradiated. The dose ranged between

10 and 36 Gy. Metastatic sites that cleared with induction chemotherapy had improved local control (LC) compared with sites with persistent uptake on mIBG scans (LC rate, 92% vs. 67%; $p < 0.0001$). Patients who had LC at irradiated metastatic sites had improved overall survival compared with those who did not (overall survival rate, 71% vs. 50%; $p < 0.0001$). The authors concluded that response to chemotherapy is an important prognostic factor for LC at irradiated metastatic sites in neuroblastoma. An earlier retrospective study by Polishchuk et al. [15] on 43 patients showed that metastatic bone relapse in neuroblastoma usually occurs at anatomic sites of previous disease. Metastatic sites identified at diagnosis that did not receive radiation appeared to have a higher risk of involvement at first relapse relative to previously irradiated metastatic sites. Currently, the SIOPEN strategy is not to irradiate metastatic disease, as this approach has not been studied systematically, while this is more common in the USA and actually recommended in COG trials. Based on these findings, randomised trials seem to be needed to more accurately define the role of radiotherapy with curative intent for metastatic sites in neuroblastoma.

Radiotherapy also provides excellent palliation for symptomatic metastatic sites like bone or brain metastases, even at low doses and using convenient hypofractionated schedules with minimal burden for the patient [16]. Symptomatic visceral metastases (like liver or lung) have also been successfully palliated with radiotherapy.

8.5 Radiotherapy Techniques

Specific technical details on radiotherapy are beyond the scope of this book. However, it is important to know that radiotherapy has evolved significantly since the 1990s and now allows to deliver a highly conformal dose, clearly reducing side effects to surrounding organs. Traditional techniques with parallel-opposed anteroposterior and postero-anterior fields (commonly known as "APPA") sometimes irradiated more normal tissue than actual tumour volume. Modern techniques like intensity-modulated radiotherapy (IMRT), intensity-modulated arc therapy (IMAT) or proton therapy allow to increase the dose to the target volume and decrease acute and long-term side effects [17–19].

However, these new techniques also pose other and new challenges like dealing with fluctuating air cavities or organ motion in proton therapy. While an APPA technique inherently resulted in homogeneous irradiation of vertebrae (and hence avoided asymmetrical growth), more conformal techniques need to reconsider how to deal with the dose or dose gradients to certain normal tissues [20].

Quality assurance is an important issue that may impact local control and even survival. In a retrospective analysis of patients treated in the SIOPEN High-Risk Neuroblastoma Study 1, Gaze et al. [21] found 17% unjustified deviations, with a risk of an adverse outcome. Therefore, the SIOPEN/HR-NBL2 study will implement prospective radiotherapy quality assurance using the SIOPE/EORTC QUARTET platform.

8.6 Side Effects of Radiotherapy

Taking into account the rather low dose that is commonly used for radiotherapy in neuroblastoma, the short-term side effects are usually mild. However, when higher boost doses are applied, toxicity may also increase. In most cases gastrointestinal toxicity can easily be dealt with using standard anti-emetics like setrons. In case of irradiation of large volumes, haematological toxicity (or slower recovery after stem cell transplantation) may occur. Irradiation of large liver volumes may be accompanied by sinusoidal obstruction syndrome (SOS, formerly called veno-occlusive disease, VOD), especially if busulfan has been used earlier in treatment.

Long-term side effects depend on several factors: total dose, dose per fraction, location, volume, concomitant chemotherapy and age. Spinal deformities like kyphosis or scoliosis may occur, but can usually be prevented by use of an appropriate technique avoiding an inhomogeneous dose distribution over the vertebrae. Reduced height is more difficult to avoid if a large volume (including several vertebrae) has to be irradiated. Kidney failure and hypertension may develop and can be aggravated by the chemotherapy used [22]. A more recently recognised long-term side effect of especially abdominal radiotherapy is the metabolic syndrome. It is characterised by higher blood pressure, increased levels of triglycerides, cholesterol and free fatty acids and increased adiposity [23].

Although the acute side effects of radiotherapy for neuroblastoma are usually mild, taken together with the effects of chemotherapy and surgery, long-term side effects may be an issue in neuroblastoma survivors. Those patients should be offered a careful long-term follow-up programme.

References

1. Castleberry RP, Kun LE, Shuster JJ, Altshuler G, Smith IE, Nitschke R, et al. Radiotherapy improves the outlook for patients older than 1 year with Pediatric Oncology Group stage C neuroblastoma. J Clin Oncol. 1991;9(5):789–95.
2. Angelini P, Plantaz D, De Bernardi B, Passagia JG, Rubie H, Pastore G. Late sequelae of symptomatic epidural compression in children with localized neuroblastoma. Pediatr Blood Cancer. 2011;57(3):473–80. https://doi.org/10.1002/pbc.23037.
3. Kraal K, Blom T, van Noesel M, Kremer L, Caron H, Tytgat G, van der Pal H. Treatment and outcome of neuroblastoma with intraspinal extension: a systematic review. Pediatr Blood Cancer. 2017;64(8):e26451. https://doi.org/10.1002/pbc.26451.
4. Matthay KK, O'Leary MC, Ramsay NK, Villablanca J, Reynolds CP, Atkinson JB, et al. Role of myeloablative therapy in improved outcome for high risk neuroblastoma: review of recent Children's Cancer Group results. Eur J Cancer. 1995;31A(4):572–5.
5. Kremens B, Klingebiel T, Herrmann F, Bender-Götze C, Burdach S, Ebell W, et al. High-dose consolidation with local radiation and bone marrow rescue in patients with advanced neuroblastoma. Med Pediatr Oncol. 1994;23(6):470–5.
6. Kushner BH, O'Reilly RJ, Mandell LR, Gulati SC, LaQuaglia M, Cheung NK. Myeloablative combination chemotherapy without total body irradiation for neuroblastoma. J Clin Oncol. 1991;9(2):274–9.

7. Mugishima H, Harada K, Suzuki T, Chin M, Shimada T, Takamura M, et al. Comprehensive treatment of advanced neuroblastoma involving autologous bone marrow transplant. Acta Paediatr Jpn. 1995;37(4):493–9.
8. Sibley GS, Mundt AJ, Goldman S, Nachman J, Reft C, Weichselbaum RR, et al. Patterns of failure following total body irradiation and bone marrow transplantation with or without a radiotherapy boost for advanced neuroblastoma. Int J Radiat Oncol Biol Phys. 1995;32(4):1127–35.
9. Haas-Kogan DA, Swift PS, Selch M, Haase GM, Seeger RC, Gerbing RB, et al. Impact of radiotherapy for high-risk neuroblastoma: a Children's Cancer Group study. Int J Radiat Oncol Biol Phys. 2003;56(1):28–39.
10. Flandin I, Hartmann O, Michon J, Pinkerton R, Coze C, Stephan JL, et al. Impact of TBI on late effects in children treated by megatherapy for Stage IV neuroblastoma. A study of the French Society of Pediatric oncology. Int J Radiat Oncol Biol Phys. 2006;64(5):1424–31.
11. Pai Panandiker AS, McGregor L, Krasin MJ, Wu S, Xiong X, Merchant TE. Locoregional tumor progression after radiation therapy influences overall survival in pediatric patients with neuroblastoma. Int J Radiat Oncol Biol Phys. 2010;76(4):1161–5. https://doi.org/10.1016/j.ijrobp.2009.03.068.
12. Holmes K, Poetschger U, Sarnacki S, Monclair T, Cecchetto G, Gomez Chacon J, et al. The influence of surgical excision on survival in high-risk neuroblastoma revisited after introduction of ch14.18/CHO immunotherapy in the HR-NBL1/SIOPEN trial. J Clin Oncol. 2018;36:10521. Poster discussion session. https://meetinglibrary.asco.org/record/160218/abstract.
13. Simon T, Hero B, Bongartz R, Schmidt M, Müller RP, Berthold F. Intensified external-beam radiation therapy improves the outcome of stage 4 neuroblastoma in children >1 year with residual local disease. Strahlenther Onkol. 2006;182(7):389–94.
14. Casey DL, Pitter KL, Kushner BH, Cheung NV, Modak S, LaQuaglia MP, Wolden SL. Radiation therapy to sites of metastatic disease as part of consolidation in high-risk neuroblastoma: can long-term control be achieved? Int J Radiat Oncol Biol Phys. 2018;100(5):1204–9. https://doi.org/10.1016/j.ijrobp.2018.01.008.
15. Polishchuk AL, Li R, Hill-Kayser C, Little A, Hawkins RA, Hamilton J, et al. Likelihood of bone recurrence in prior sites of metastasis in patients with high-risk neuroblastoma. Int J Radiat Oncol Biol Phys. 2014;89(4):839–45. https://doi.org/10.1016/j.ijrobp.2014.04.004.
16. Lazarev S, Kushner BH, Wolden SL. Short hypofractionated radiotherapy in palliation of pediatric malignancies: outcomes and toxicities. Int J Radiat Oncol Biol Phys. 2018; https://doi.org/10.1016/j.ijrobp.2018.07.2012. pii: S0360-3016(18)33470-9.
17. Gains JE, Stacey C, Rosenberg I, Mandeville HC, Chang YC, D'Souza D, Moroz V, Wheatley K, Gaze MN. Intensity-modulated arc therapy to improve radiation dose delivery in the treatment of abdominal neuroblastoma. Future Oncol. 2013;9(3):439–49.
18. Hill-Kayser C, Tochner Z, Both S, Lustig R, Reilly A, Balamuth N, et al. Proton versus photon radiation therapy for patients with high-risk neuroblastoma: the need for a customized approach. Pediatr Blood Cancer. 2013;60(10):1606–11. https://doi.org/10.1002/pbc.24606.
19. Pai Panandiker AS, Beltran C, Billups CA, McGregor LM, Furman WL, Davidoff AM. Intensity modulated radiation therapy provides excellent local control in high-risk abdominal neuroblastoma. Pediatr Blood Cancer. 2013;60(5):761–5.
20. Kandula S, Sutter A, Prabhu RS, Jegadeesh N, Esiashvili N. Reassessing dose constraints of organs at risk in children with abdominal neuroblastoma treated with definitive radiation therapy: a correlation with late toxicity. Pediatr Blood Cancer. 2015;62(6):970–5. https://doi.org/10.1002/pbc.25372.
21. Gaze MN, Boterberg T, Dieckmann K, Hörmann M, Gains JE, Sullivan KP, Ladenstein R. Results of a quality assurance review of external beam radiation therapy in the International Society of Paediatric Oncology (Europe) Neuroblastoma Group's High-risk Neuroblastoma Trial: a SIOPEN study. Int J Radiat Oncol Biol Phys. 2013;85(1):170–4. https://doi.org/10.1016/j.ijrobp.2012.05.004.

22. Ducassou A, Gambart M, Munzer C, Padovani L, Carrie C, Haas-Kogan D, et al. Neuroblastoma study group and radiotherapy group of the French Society of Children with Cancer (SFCE). Long-term side effects of radiotherapy for pediatric localized neuroblastoma: results from clinical trials NB90 and NB94. Strahlenther Onkol. 2015;191(7):604–12.
23. van Waas M, Neggers SJCMM, Raat H, van Rij CM, Pieters R, van den Heuvel-Eibrink MM. Abdominal radiotherapy: a major determinant of metabolic syndrome in nephroblastoma and neuroblastoma survivors. PLoS One. 2012;7(12):e52237. https://doi.org/10.1371/journal.pone.0052237.

Part III

Clinical Management

9 Spinal Canal Involvement in Peripheral Neuroblastic Tumors

Shifra Ash, Stefania Sorrentino, Kathelijne Kraal, and Bruno De Bernardi

Abbreviations

MRI	Magnetic resonance imaging
NB	Neuroblastoma
PNT	Peripheral neuroblastic tumor
SCI	Spinal canal invasion
SDI	Symptom-diagnosis interval
SIOPEN	International Society of Paediatric Oncology Europe Neuroblastoma

9.1 Introduction

Peripheral neuroblastic tumors (PNTs) represent a family of tumors mostly of early childhood originating from cells of the primitive neural crest that migrate to eventually populate the paravertebral, celiac, and mesenteric sympathetic ganglia and the inner adrenal gland [1]. PNTs arising in the sympathetic ganglia are anatomically connected with the spinal cord (Fig. 9.1). By growing along this connection, the

S. Ash
Schneider Children's Medical Center of Israel, Sackler Faculty of Medicine, Tel Aviv University, Petach Tikvah, Israel
e-mail: n-ash@zahav.net.il

S. Sorrentino · B. De Bernardi (✉)
Paediatric Oncology, IRCCS Istituto Giannina Gaslini, Genova, Italy
e-mail: brunodebernardi@gaslini.org

K. Kraal
Emma Children's Hospital/Academic Medical Centre (EKZ/AMC), Amsterdam, The Netherlands

Princess Máxima Centre, Utrecht, The Netherlands

S. Sarnacki, L. Pio (eds.), *Neuroblastoma*,
https://doi.org/10.1007/978-3-030-18396-7_9

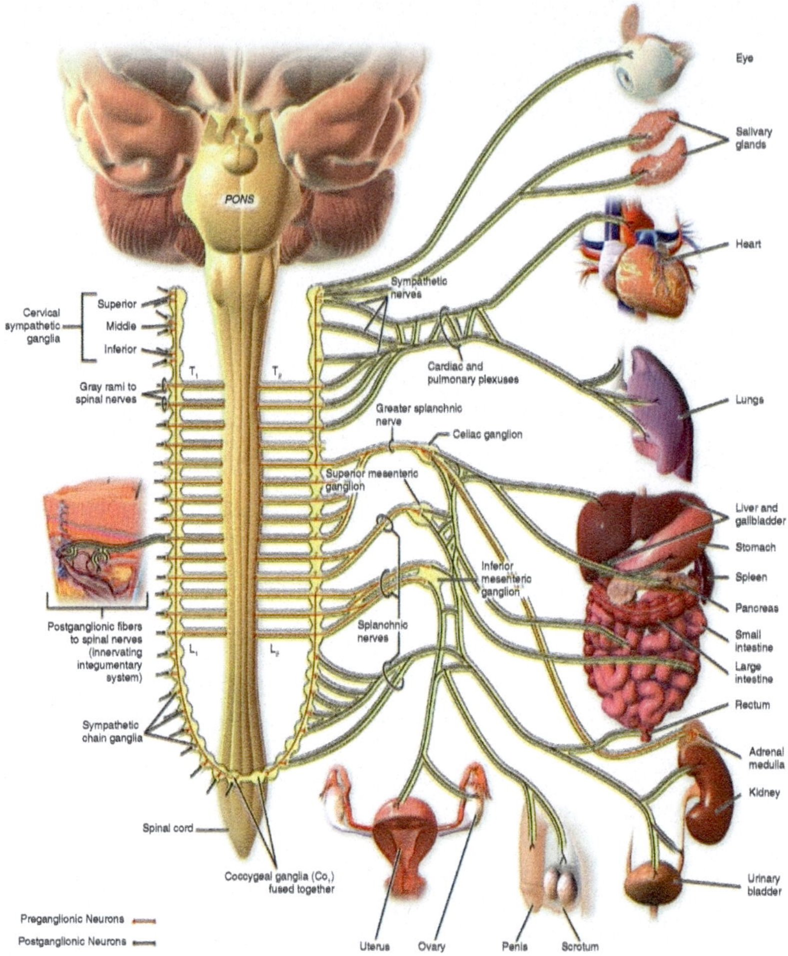

Fig. 9.1 Schematic representation of sympathetic nervous system

tumor may infiltrate the adjacent intervertebral foramina and enter the spinal canal. Despite the fact that tumor growth remains extradural, it may eventually compress the spinal cord and/or the intraspinal part of the spinal nerves [2, 3]. About 15% of all PNT patients develop spinal canal involvement (SCI) (Fig. 9.2). The majority of them have favorable clinical features, i.e., are diagnosed during infancy (0–11 months) and have the primary tumor more often in the thorax. In addition, the histologic and main biologic features of tumor cells (involving, in particular, *MYCN* gene status, chromosome 1p, and DNA content) are usually in the normal range. Approximately half of these patients are symptomatic at time of diagnosis [4–6] and present with one or more of the following: pain and irritability, bowel and bladder dysfunction, and neurologic and motor deficits (weakness, loss of sensibility, gait disturbances, paralysis) that may progressively aggravate, ending sometimes in the

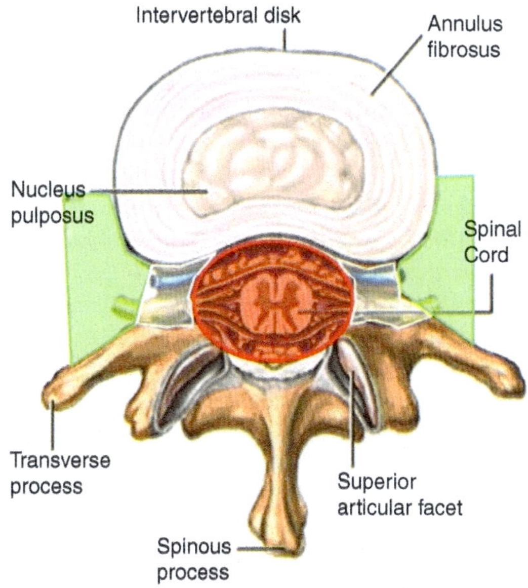

Fig. 9.2 Spinal canal involvement (SCI) is defined when, referring to an axial plane of the spinal cord MRI scan, the tumour extends into the vertebral canal and goes beyond a mentally drown ellipsoid (red circle) passing through the cortical bone of both anterior and posterior arches of the vertebra

potentially irreversible pattern of transverse myelopathy (quadriplegia or paraplegia). PNT patients with SCI are highly susceptible to develop late health problems, which may significantly alter the quality of life [7–10].

Both symptomatic and asymptomatic PNT patients presenting with SCI documented by imaging must be promptly investigated in adequate medical structures and properly managed to avoid the establishment of permanent sequelae. While SCI in asymptomatic patients may sometimes require only careful observation, symptomatic SCI must be treated on an emergency basis. Specific therapeutic measures include neurosurgical decompression, chemotherapy, and radiation therapy. However, the optimal treatment to relieve epidural compression remains a controversial issue. In particular, there are remarkably different opinions on which therapeutic modality should be preferred in a given situation [11]. This is reflected in the limited number of series regarding PNT children diagnosed with SCI.

9.1.1 Review of Series of Children with PNT and SCI

In 1980, ***Punt et al.*** *[2] described 21 PNT patients with symptomatic SCI diagnosed in a 17-year period. Thirteen (61%) survived disease-free. Eleven/21 were infants. Late morbidity affected 6/13 evaluable patients, mostly diagnosed early in life. All patients underwent laminectomy, and 12 received also chemotherapy and 17 radiotherapy. AA concluded that decompressive neurosurgery was essential part of therapeutic approach, while chemotherapy was indicated in case of metastases and unresectable primary tumor. Radiation therapy was recommended in case of known residual disease. In 1984,* ***Hayes et al.*** *[3] described 14 patients with small* *blue-round cells (of which nine PNTs) with intraspinal extension of the tumor. Five underwent laminectomy with neurologic recovery in only one. Other nine patients were given chemotherapy without radiotherapy, and all recovered. For the AA, chemotherapy was a feasible alternative to laminectomy and radiation therapy in the management of epidural disease. In 1996,* **Plantaz et al.** *[4] reported a series of 42 French PNT patients with SCI diagnosed between 1990 and 1994. There were 27 symptomatic (64%) and 15 asymptomatic patients. Thirty-two received chemotherapy as first-line treatment with complete regression in 13/15 asymptomatic and partial regression in 5/27 symptomatic. In 2001,* **De Bernardi et al.** *[5] described 76 Italian PNT cases with symptomatic SCI diagnosed between 1979 and 1998 (5.2% of the total PNTs), of whom 33 underwent chemotherapy first, 32 laminectomy, and 11 radiation therapy. Neurosurgery was preferred in patients with severe motor deficit and chemotherapy in those with advanced disease. Full recovery was achieved in 33 patients and partial recovery in 14, while 22 remained stable and eight did worse. None of the ten paraplegic patients recovered or improved. In the other 66, response to therapy was comparable for the three treatment modalities. Of 76 patients, 54 survived. Twenty-six of 54 survivors (44%) developed sequelae, mainly scoliosis and sphincter deficits. In the same year,* **Katzenstein et al.** *[6] described 83 Pediatric Oncology Group PNT patients with intraspinal extension diagnosed between 1990 and 1998, of whom 43 (52%) had neurologic symptoms at diagnosis. Six/15 severely affected patients fully recovered vs. 2/5 with moderate deficits and 17/22 with mild symptoms. Seven/24 who underwent laminectomy developed scoliosis vs. 1/49 managed without laminectomy. AA concluded that severity of presenting symptoms correlated with quality of recovery, with similar results for chemotherapy and laminectomy. The latter was definitely associated with more orthopedic sequelae. In 2003,* **Sandberg et al.** *[12] described 46 patients diagnosed between 1987 and 1998. Thirteen high-risk (HR = stage 4) patients were asymptomatic, of whom 12 were treated by chemotherapy (one worsened). Of 18 HR symptomatic patients, 7/10 treated with chemotherapy and 6/6 treated by operation improved or remained stable. Nine low-risk (LR = <stage 4) asymptomatic patients remained neurologically intact, independently of the treatment given. In the AA's opinion, both asymptomatic and symptomatic HR patients should be offered chemotherapy, with some of the latter not responding and thus requiring laminectomy. Chemotherapy should be avoided in favor of laminectomy in LR patients, although some of them may develop spinal deformities. In 2003,* **Yiin et al.** *[13] described 13 Chinese PNT patients with symptomatic SCI diagnosed between 1985 and 2000. All received chemotherapy first, of whom three recovered, four improved, and six aggravated. Of the last six, two were operated and recovered. AA recommends neurologic decompression for patients who develop neurologic deterioration during chemotherapy. In 2005,* **De Bernardi et al.** *[11] wrote a mini-review of a 2004 Workshop on PNTs with SCI held in Genova, at the 2005 ANR. A number of experts from France, Italy, United Kingdom, Japan, Poland, and Memorial Sloan Kettering and Children Oncology Group from the United States reported their own experience. Remarkable discrepancies emerged regarding several important issues, i.e., terminology of neurologic deficits, optimal imaging, role and efficacy of the various therapeutic modalities,*

and follow-up strategies to pick up and manage late complications. The participants agreed to create "an International Registry to collect a complete and uniform set of data which would hopefully lead to the development of an evidence-based approach" to SCI in children with PNT. In 2014, **De Bernardi et al.** *[14] described 34 infants with PNT and SCI, all symptomatic, diagnosed between 2000 and 2011. Symptom-diagnosis interval was 12 days (IQR, 7–34) with frequency of grade 3 motor deficit and bladder dysfunction increasing with the increase of the interval. First treatment for SCI was neurosurgery in 14 patients and chemotherapy in 20. Symptoms regressed in 11 patients, improved in nine, and remained stable in 14 without difference in relation to the treatment administered. At last visit, 11 patients were sequelae-free, while 23 had sequelae, including motor deficit (56%), bladder dysfunction (50%), bowel dysfunction (28%), and spinal deformities (28%). Sequelae were severe in 50% of patients and prevailed in those presenting with SCI >66% and grade 3 motor deficit. AA stated that both neurosurgery and chemotherapy were ineffective when paraplegia had established. In 2015,* ***Fawzy et al.*** *[15] described 51 Egyptian patients diagnosed between 2007 and 2012, of whom 34 symptomatic, the majority for >4 weeks. Complete recovery occurred in 16 and partial in 11, while seven did not improve. Patients with short interval from diagnosis to therapy did better. Response was not influenced by the type of therapy, patient age, and tumor site. AA concluded that SCI can be effectively managed by upfront chemotherapy and that surgical decompression should be reserved for benign variants.*

This body of information clearly demonstrates the uncertainty existing regarding time and modality of diagnosis, therapeutic strategy, and long-term follow-up of children with PNT who present or develop SCI. Herewith we will analyze the status of the art of these issues.

9.1.1.1 Recognition of Symptoms of SCI

The interval between appearance of symptoms and diagnosis (SDI) varied remarkably from one patient to another and from one series to another. Infants (about half of these patients) more easily escaped recognition with delay of diagnostic work-up and initiation of therapy. In the early **Punt et al.** paper [2], the SDI ranged from 1 day to 36 months (median, 6 weeks). In the 2001 series, **De Bernardi et al.** [5] reported that the SDI was less than 2 weeks in 54% of patients, between 2 weeks and 2 months in 18% and >2 months in 28%. In the recent **Kraal et al.** series [10], SDI ranged from 1.5 to 12 weeks (median, 6). None of these AA clearly stated that a longer SDI corresponded to more severe presenting symptoms, poor response to therapy, and worse outcome. However, in the **2012 Simon et al.** paper [9], where the SDI was highly variable (0–1838 days; median, 12), the length of SDI had no clear impact on likelihood of recovery. In synthesis, the published papers provide contrasting data on the effect of a short SDI over efficacy of treatment and establishment of late effects. Despite that, it seems reasonable that children with symptoms of epidural compression secondary to tumors should benefit from timely recognition and prompt referral to a physician. We suggest that widespread information at public level and greater awareness by pediatricians regarding this rare but important clinical pattern could translate into shortening of the SDI and better functional outcome [16].

9.1.1.2 Patient Referral to Medical Institutions

Once symptoms of SCI have been recognized, patient should be considered as a true emergency and addressed to an "expert" pediatric institution. Ideally, a center taking care of these patients should have a multidisciplinary team, composed of expert neurosurgeons, neuroradiologists, and pediatric oncologists, capable to meet in few hours to organize the appropriate imaging studies and define treatment strategy.

9.1.1.3 Imaging of SCI

At the present, myelography and lumbar puncture are considered risky and poorly informative and are thus contraindicated. Computed tomography does not provide optimal imaging. Instead, magnetic resonance imaging (MRI) represents the gold standard technique to document SCI [17] (Figs. 9.3 and 9.4). At the best, MRI should include sagittal and transverse T1-weighted imaging (Sag&Tra T1WI), three planar T2WI, and three planar contrast-enhanced T1WI (three planar CET1WI). The field of view (FOV) of the scan should cover the whole extent of the backbone, from the cervical vertebrae to coccyx, in order to detect multiple levels of

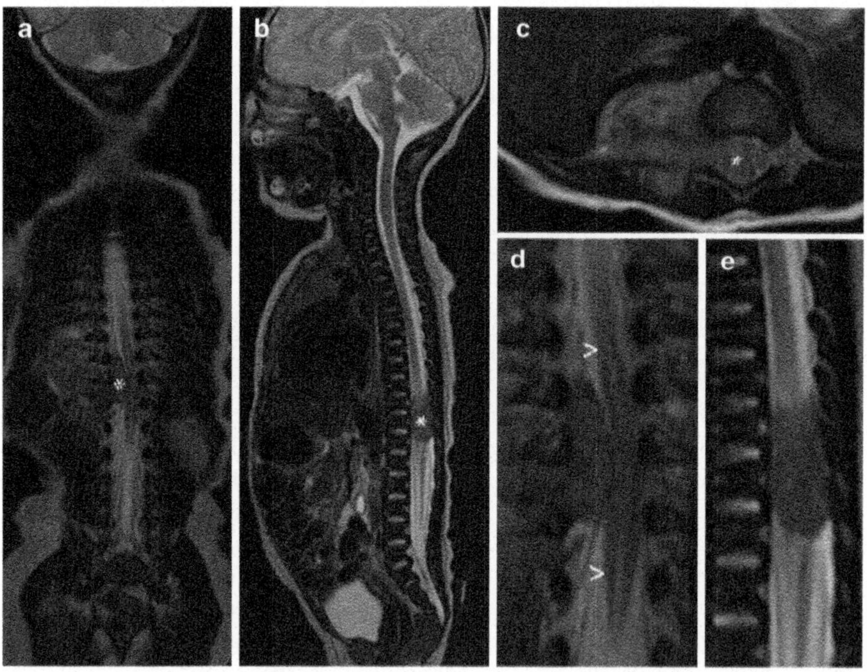

Fig. 9.3 Complete MRI scan in a baby harbouring a PNT with evidence of SCI. A reliable three planar T2WI sequence should avoid 3D acquisition with postprocessing reconstruction; native coronal (**a**), sagittal (**b**) and tranverse (**c**) sequences have to cover the whole length of the backbone in order to depict multiple levels of invasion and coexisting abnormalities. A typical dumbbell appearance of PNT invasion is shown (asterisk), passing trough the enlarged foramina and dislocating/compressing the spinal cord. Magnification views (**d, e**) show the normal appearance of the central canal (less than sign), often misread as T2WI hyperintensity of the spinal cord

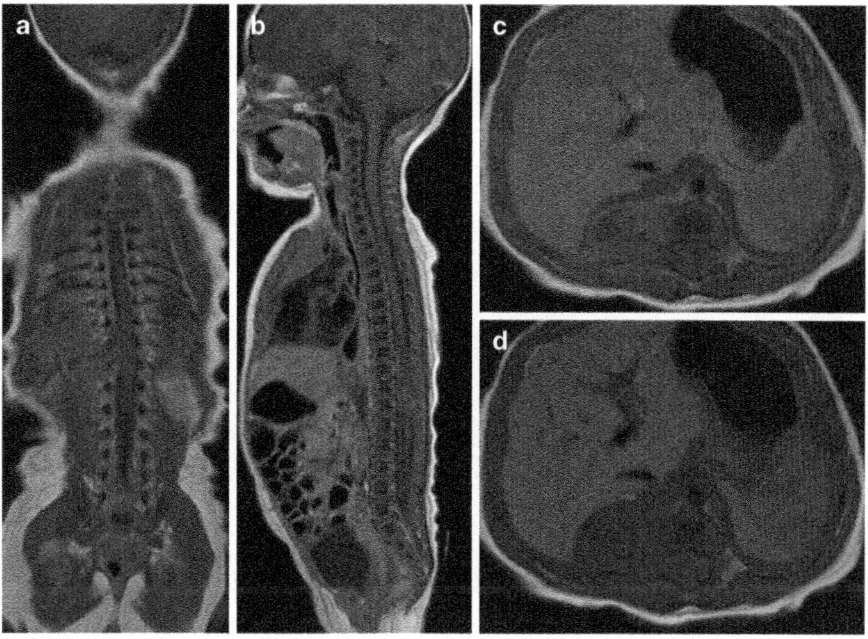

Fig. 9.4 A three planar T1WI acquisition after gadolinium injection completes the basic MRI scan (**a–c**) and shows a mild contrast-enhancing (CE) of the tumour, compared to not-enhanced T1WI (**d**)

involvement as well as other coexisting abnormalities. However, even a well-done MRI may fail to accurately assess the volume of the intraspinal tumor component due to its half-moon configuration. As indicated in the Imaging Guidelines in the SIOP Europe LINES protocol, "… it is suggested to consider the ratio between the maximum axial diameter of the tumour within the spinal canal and the diameter of the spinal canal itself. When more than a third of the spinal canal is invaded by the tumor, an *Image Defined Risk Factor* (IDRF) is present. The cranio-caudal extent of the intraspinal component is measured in relation to the number of the involved vertebrae. The subdural space (between the compressed dura mater and neuraxis) must be assessed by T2WI sequences in order to determine the relationship of the tumor with the spinal cord/cauda equina. The spinal cord MRI signal has to be evaluated as an off-midline T2WI hyperintensity is likely to express a poorer prognostic value, regardless of other MRI scan features." In selected cases, notably PNT with SCI at medium-low thoracic level, angiography can be useful to depict the origin of the Adamkiewicz artery, major responsible of blood supply to the anterior spinal artery [18] (Fig. 9.5). Although normally arising from the IX, X, or XI left intercostal vessels, the Adamkiewicz artery shows a wide anatomical variability and must be detected as its damage occurring at surgery may lead to an anterior spinal artery syndrome [19].

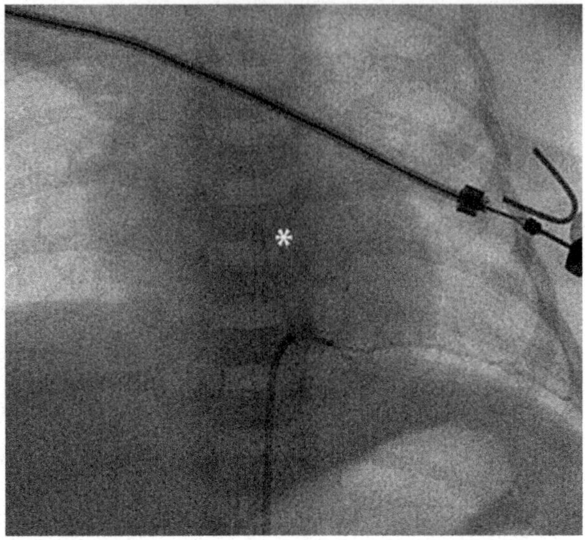

Fig. 9.5 Angiographic study to identify the origin of the Adamkiewicz artery. Selective trans-aortic catheterization of the X left intercostal artery shows the classical hairpin appearance of the great anterior radiculomedullary artery, that contraindicates a surgical approach at that level

9.1.1.4 Treatment

Asymptomatic SCI not always require specific treatment besides that planned for the tumor itself. However, according to the LINES protocol, if the spinal cord component occupies greater than 33% of the spinal canal, recommendation is given to treat these patients with chemotherapy even in the absence of symptoms of SCI. The therapeutic approach includes neurosurgical decompression, chemotherapy, and radiation therapy.

1. *Neurosurgical decompression*. The only therapeutic approach before the advent of radiation therapy and chemotherapy, neurosurgery may rapidly relieve the symptoms of SCI. In addition, it allows the removal of almost all the intraspinal tumor and provides tissue material suitable for diagnostic histology and biologic investigations [20, 21]. The operation consists of either laminectomy or laminotomy (laminoplasty). Technically, laminectomy (Fig. 9.6) is based on the removal of the lamina, i.e., the posterior component of the vertebra covering the spinal canal. Laminotomy (Fig. 9.7) represents a less invasive approach, as the removed bone is repositioned after tumor removal, thus restoring the original vertebral anatomy [22]. In expert hands and proper environments, both techniques are presently considered devoid of major risks [23]. However, both seem to imply greater risk of late spinal deformities, especially in infants, perhaps less with laminotomy [24].
2. *Chemotherapy*. The first evidence that chemotherapy may effectively relieve the symptoms of SCI and substitute for neurosurgery goes back to 1984 [3] and then confirmed by others. A number of chemotherapeutic agents have been used over time, in particular the association of vincristine and cyclophosphamide with or without the complement of doxorubicin. Since at least a decade, the pre-

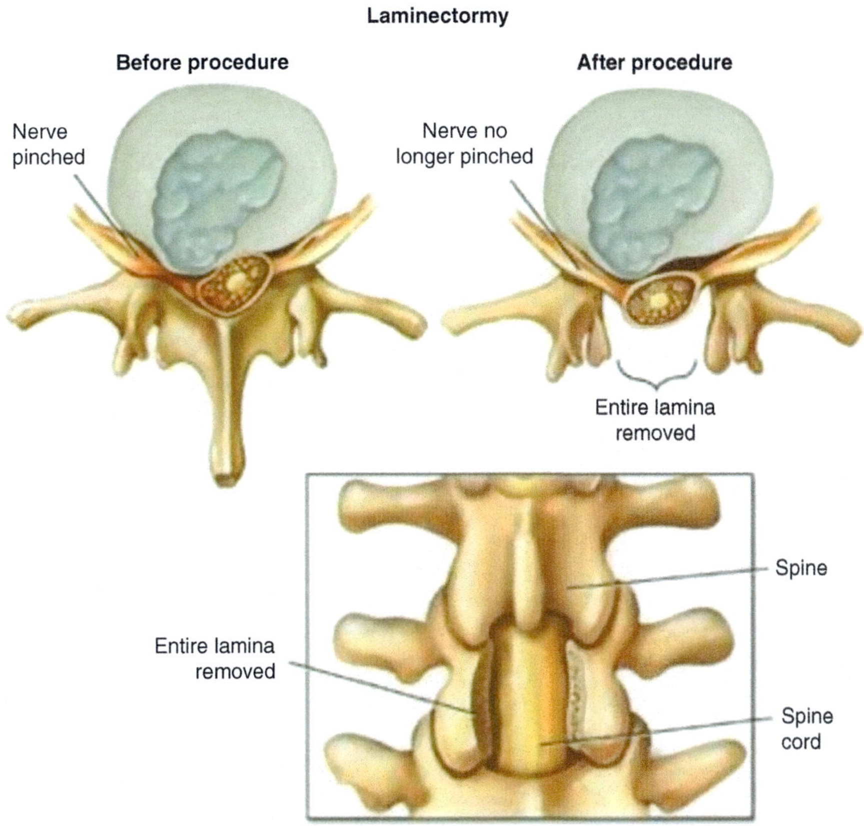

Fig. 9.6 Laminectomy: it is based on the removal of the lamina, i.e., the posterior component of the vertebra covering the spinal canal

ferred combination is carboplatin and etoposide, easy to administer and less toxic than other combinations [4–6]. In the past, the administration of chemotherapy had to be delayed until histologic diagnosis, considered a prerequisite to start therapy. However, the time lapse could be of several days, during which a significant worsening of symptoms could occur. In the early 2000, an international agreement was reached to allow initiation of treatment in absence of histologic report. On this basis, a patient showing progressive symptoms of SCI may undergo positioning of a central catheter and start chemotherapy. Clearly, parents must be fully informed and give their consent before any chemotherapeutic drug be injected. At the present, the chance that a provisional diagnosis of PNT, or other small blue cell tumor, finds no histologic confirmation is very uncommon.

3. *Radiation therapy*. The irradiation of a small paravertebral tumor with intraspinal extension can be delivered easily and promptly through the use of a single posterior field. A straightforward technique is to deliver 300 cGy to the target on each

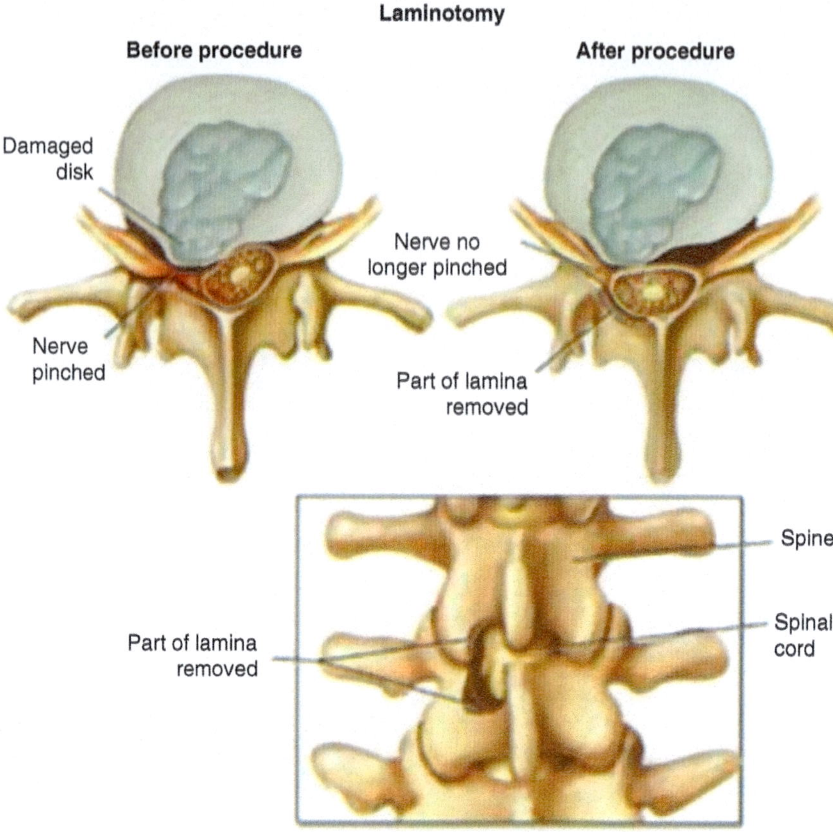

Fig. 9.7 Laminotomy: the removed bone is repositioned after tumour removal

of 3 successive days. The effect on normal growth and development after such a dose is given to field 3–5 vertebral bodies in length is negligible even in babies (***D'Angio***, in [11]). Perhaps 3 cm of shortening in total height at maturity can be expected after such irradiation is given to an infant. Late effects on the thyroid are of major concern when the neck or upper thoracic spine is treated. This is because even very low scattered doses of radiation can cause trouble with function, and/or give rise to growths, both benign and malignant. More modern techniques are available that localize the radiation therapy very precisely to the tumor volume. However, these methods require more elaborate planning, which may take days, and longer time the child must lie still on the table. In addition, thyroid problems after upper spine irradiation are not obviated, because the gland receives scattered radiation even under the most stringent limitations of filed edges. On balance, simpler field arrangements are quicker and easier to do (**D'Angio** in [11]).

4. *Steroid treatment*. Although no solid prove exists that corticosteroids exert a significant antitumor effect, nor improve the long-term outcome, their use is widespread and recommended, as they rapidly alleviate pain and reduce peri-tumor

inflammation. Dexamethasone is commonly used as an initial intravenous bolus of 0.5 mg/kg followed by 0.2 mg/kg/day in three divided daily doses for 4–7 days (SIOPEN LINES protocol).

In summary, a child who presents clear symptoms of SCI requires immediate and accurate imaging studies and therapeutic decisions in a matter of 1–2 days. The choice whether to operate or administer chemotherapy should be taken after urgent discussion between oncologist, neurosurgeon, and radiation therapist in front of imaging. A neurosurgical approach should be preferred only in infants showing very rapid neurologic deterioration. This however occurs infrequently. If chemotherapy is considered necessary, it should be initiated with/without performing tumor biopsy. There is no urgent indication to remove the extraspinal tumor (which is likely to be unresectable, and such an operation runs the risk to worsen the neurologic deficit). The tumor can be biopsied (by Tru-Cut, fine needle, or open biopsy) when patient has improved under effect of chemotherapy. Initial chemotherapy in this situation should never be postponed in order to obtain a biopsy.

9.2 SCI at Birth and in the Neonate

The occurrence of PNTs with symptoms of SCI at birth and in the neonate (0–28 days) is rare but requires even greater attention and prompt care to limit severe late complications. However, no established guidelines are available regarding the management of these patients.

9.2.1 Review of the Literature on Neonatal and Congenital PNTs Presenting with SCI

In 2012, ***Fischer and Tweddle*** *[25], in an UKCCSG Registry Study of neonatal PNTs, showed that 6 of 33 neonates (18%) had symptomatic SCI. The overall survival of the group was 91%. Long-term complications occurred in ten children including all six presenting with SCI.*

In 1997, ***Asabe et al.*** *[26] described a case of a paraplegic newborn with congenital intraspinal neuroblastoma and reviewed the related literature. They collected 38 such cases, of whom 26 underwent laminectomy and 12 did not. Treatment with or without laminectomy was associated with a poor neurologic recovery, suggesting that irreversible damage occur antenatally. The AA concluded that laminectomy is not indicated for these patients. In 2008, Blackman et al. [27] and Walter et al. [28]. independently described the only two cases with congenital PNT and SCI who survived without sequelae being delivered prematurely, following detection by ultrasound (US) of an extraspinal tumor mass in late pregnancy. The AA suggested that prenatal detection of a tumor mass entering the spinal canal might induce anticipation of delivery and timely treatment may lead to good functional* *outcome. However, Suffia et al. described in 2016 [29] a female born by caesarian section at the 36th week following discovery by US of oligohydramnios. At birth patient had motor deficit and urine incontinence secondary to a PNT not picked up at US. Tumor responded to therapy, but no neurologic improvement occurred, suggesting that anticipation of delivery is not always sufficient to prohibit the development of late sequelae. Again in 2016, Gigliotti et al. [30] reported three newborns with PNT and motor deficit for whom prenatal US had failed to detect any tumor mass and were delivered at term of pregnancy. Tumors responded well to chemotherapy, but all patients developed severe motor deficit and bladder dysfunction. Scoliosis developed in the case with longest follow-up.*

Despite the above reports appear contradictory, the importance of early diagnosis of a tumor mass in late pregnancy must be stressed. Neonatologists should be aware of this rare clinical entity and take it into account in the differential diagnosis with other conditions, including early-onset hypotonia. On the other hand, obstetric sonologists should be aware of the possibility to detect such rare tumors in late pregnancy, as anticipation of delivery might reduce the risk of late sequelae. In the case symptomatic SCI is evident at birth, initiation of chemotherapy on an emergency basis even in the absence of histologic diagnosis may translate into lesser risk of long-term sequelae and better quality of life for some of these patients.

9.3 Late Sequelae

Children with PNTs and SCI are susceptible to develop long-term sequelae caused both by epidural compression and treatment. The most common sequelae include motor impairment, spasticity, kyphoscoliosis (Fig. 9.8), and bladder and bowel dysfunction. There are difficulties in comparing long-term side effects of different treatment modalities because neurosurgical decompression is more likely to be used in severely symptomatic patients and long-term outcome reflects both the severity of functional impairment at presentation and treatment modalities. Few papers have focused on the late functional outcome of PNT patients with SCI at diagnosis.

9.3.1 Review of the Literature Concerning Late Sequelae in Children with PNT Presenting with SCI

In 1999, ***Hoover et al.*** *[7] reported on long-term outcome of 26 children with intraspinal PNTs diagnosed between 1967 and 1994. Twenty-four/26 patients survived with a follow-up of 2–29 years. A low incidence of neurologic recovery was seen in patients with long-standing severe epidural compression regardless of treatment modality. In case of partial neurologic deficit, recovery was seen in most patients following chemotherapy or neurosurgical intervention. Eleven/15 patients who underwent laminectomy developed mild to severe spinal deformities. Four of 11 patients with intraspinal tumor who did not undergo laminectomy have mild to severe scoliosis. A higher incidence of spinal deformities was seen in patients*

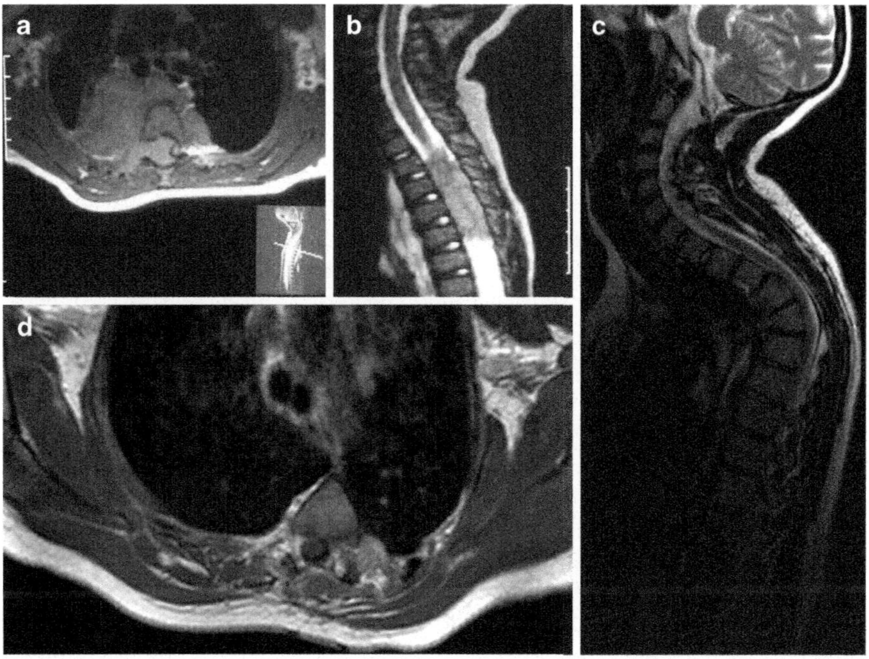

Fig. 9.8 Left thoracic neuroblastoma with spinal canal invasion in a 3-years old girl diagnosed in 1998 (**a**, **b**). Treated by initial laminectomy and chemotherapy. Severe kyphoscoliosis and thoracic asymmetry at 22 years, after 19 years follow-up (**c**, **d**).

treated with laminectomy. In 2011, ***Angelini et al.*** *[8] described late sequelae and their correlations with presenting clinical features and tumor treatment in 98 children with symptomatic SCI. Initial treatment was chemotherapy in 66 (especially younger patients and stage 3 disease), neurosurgery in 29, and radiotherapy in three. After a median follow-up of 7 years, 57 children (58.2%) had one or more sequelae, with motor deficit involving 50 of them, correlated with young age, severe motor deficit, and neurosurgical operation at onset. Spine deformities involved 20/57, more frequent in those presenting with severe motor deficit and treated with neurosurgery or radiotherapy. Sphincter dysfunctions involved 31/57 children, more often in those with sphincter symptoms and severe motor deficit at diagnosis. AA concluded that late sequelae occurred in more than half of their patients with severe motor deficit at diagnosis being the main risk factor. In 2012,* ***Simon et al.*** *[9] described 122 PNT patients who had symptoms of epidural compression, of whom 99 were included in the final analysis. AA noticed better survival in these patients compared to other PNTs. The main presenting symptoms were motor deficit (95%), impaired cutaneous sensibility (58%), neuropathic pain (56%), and bladder and bowel dysfunctions (44% and 34%). Symptoms improved after upfront neurosurgery in 36/52 patients and after chemotherapy in 30/47 (not significant). After a median observation of 8 years, the large majority of patients (71/99) still had residual impairment: motor deficit (43%), impaired sensibility (31%), scoliosis (31%),* *bladder dysfunction (26%), constipation (19%), growth delay (14%), and neuropathic pain (5%). AA concluded that the initial treatment had no clear impact on frequency of late effects. In 2016,* ***Kraal et al.*** *[10] published the results of a Dutch retrospective single-center study that evaluated the prevalence of health problems (HPs) in 5-year survivors of PNT patients with SCI diagnosed between 1980 and 2007. The cohort study involved 19 such patients, of whom seven had no neurologic symptoms at diagnosis, median age 1.2 years, median follow-up 16 years. Ninety-five percent of survivors had at least one HP with a mean of four HPs per survivor. Fifty-three percent of survivors had at least one severe HP, the three most prevalent being kyphosis and/or scoliosis (68%), motor deficit (32%), and sensory neuropathy (26%). Of 13 who underwent laminotomy, seven (54%) developed grade 4 HP. Among six patients who avoided neurosurgery, one developed grade 3 and one grade 4 HP. AA concluded that grade 3 and 4 HPs prevail in the laminectomy group and emphasize the importance of specialized long-term multidisciplinary follow-up for these patients.*

From the above publications, it appears evident that children diagnosed with a PNT presenting with SCI have a concrete risk of developing permanent severe sequelae. The risk appears greater for younger patients and in case of prolonged SDI. Neurosurgical interventions may increase the risk of spine deformities, but this has not been exactly quantified. In addition, improved surgical techniques could limit the damaging potential of operating on the spine. Finally, careful multidisciplinary follow-up may be effective in significantly reducing the occurrence and entity of sequelae.

9.4 Multidisciplinary Follow-Up of Patients with Intraspinal PNT

The optimal follow-up of children diagnosed with intraspinal PNT has not been defined so far. Given the complexity of problems these children offer, the establishment of a specific *multidisciplinary outpatient clinic and follow-up* is seen with great favor by all subjects involved, including parents and patients themselves. The aim of this clinic is to develop and propose to the pediatric oncology community a common strategy for children who survive after treatment for a PNT presenting with SCI, focused on both short-term results (tumor reduction) and prevention of late HPs, in particular neurologic and musculoskeletal. By actively following these subjects, a better insight in their quality of life would possibly be achieved. To this purpose, the definition of shared guidelines for follow-up of patients and survivors with intraspinal PNT is in progress based on the indications derived from SIOPEN LINES protocol, the DCOG 2009 treatment protocol, and COG guidelines.

A model of *multidisciplinary clinic for patients with intraspinal PNT* has been established 3 years ago at the Princess Maxima Centre (PMC) for Pediatric Oncology in Utrecht. This institution is the unique center in the Netherlands treating patients with PNTs (and other pediatric tumors of the chest/abdomen). This outpatient clinic is currently taking place monthly under the coordination of one of the

AA of this chapter (KK) in the context of a multidisciplinary outpatient clinic for patients/survivors. This multidisciplinary team dedicated to patients who have been treated for an intraspinal PNT consists of pediatric medical oncologists, orthopedics, neurosurgeons, psychologists, rehabilitation medicine physicians, and physiotherapists. The goals of this clinic are to report symptoms/HPs uniformly and ultimately develop targeted follow-up programs for patients treated for an intraspinal PNT that could translate into a better defined treatment strategy. Patients are seen at least once at diagnosis and after 5 years of follow-up. Depending on the peculiarity and severity of symptoms, visits can be intensified. The clinic visit is started with a presentation of the medical history of the patient, for the involved health professionals, and then each member of the multidisciplinary team sees the patient. The findings/HPs (if any) are discussed at the end of the clinic, and appropriate course of action is then taken.

9.5 The SIOPEN NB-SCI Study Registry

The SIOPEN (International Society of Paediatric Oncology Europe Neuroblastoma) is coordinating an international, observational, prospective study registry for data collection regarding children with PNT presenting with symptomatic and asymptomatic SCI (NB-SCI Study Registry). The Study, opened on June 2014, aims to collect data at minimum of 150 patients by June 2020. In this Study, management is not indicated but will be decided by individual clinicians and institutions.

The NB-SCI Study Registry primary aims are to describe the natural history of PNTs presenting with SCI and evaluate the combined effects of different risk factors on neurologic and orthopedic outcomes. Secondary aims are to (1) describe the diagnostic and therapeutic approaches adopted in participating centers; (2) correlate pathologic and biologic characteristics with clinical features, response to therapy, and sequelae; (3) develop common guidelines for management of children with any PNTs presenting with SCI; and (4) increase the awareness regarding symptoms indicative of SCI.

To this purpose, patient data at the time of diagnosis will be collected from centers of both SIOPEN and non-SIOPEN National Neuroblastoma Groups. Data will include patient demographics, clinical features, and length of SDI. Disease characteristics include pathology, biology (*MYCN* gene status and segmental chromosome aberrations), and stage and level of tumor intraspinal invasion. Imaging studies at the time of diagnosis and of best response will also be evaluated by a panel of expert neuroradiologists. Information will also be collected on (1) initial treatment (observation, chemotherapy, neurosurgery, and/or radiation therapy) and (2) symptoms/signs of SCI including neurologic and orthopedic dysfunctions and neuroradiologic findings. Age-related, standardized tools for symptom grading and functional impacts are being used, including the Common Toxicity Criteria for Adverse Events (CTCAE), FLACC (Face, Legs, Activity, Cry, Consolability) pain scores, and American Spinal Injury Association (ASIA) impairment scales. The early response following treatment decision will be documented at 72 h, 1 week, 2 weeks, 4 weeks, and 2 months. A management summary will be collected including all SCI treatment(s), the evolution of SCI symptoms/signs, and the best clinical and neuroradiologic responses.

Prospective, detailed clinical follow-up data will be collected at standardized intervals (6 months from diagnosis, annually up to 10 years from diagnosis) to document long-term functional outcomes. It is expected that prospective collection of standardized data on PNTs and SCI, and that correlation of clinical, pathologic, biologic features with response to therapy and sequelae, will generate an improved evidence base to evaluate the impact of different risk factors on long-term outcome including neurologic functioning and orthopedic consequences. The ultimate goal is to develop better evidence-based guidelines for the management of PNTs and SCI to improve early management of epidural compression and reduce the incidence and severity of long-term disabilities.

References

1. Luksch R, Castellani MR, Collini P, et al. Neuroblastoma (Peripheral neuroblastic tumors). Crit Rev Oncol Hematol. 2016;107:106–81.
2. Punt J, Pritchard J, Pincott JR, Till K. Neuroblastoma: a review of 21 cases presenting with spinal cord compression. Cancer. 1980;45:3095–101.
3. Hayes FA, Thompson EI, Hvizdala E, O'Connor D, Green AA. Chemotherapy as an alternative to laminectomy and radiation in the management of epidural tumor. J Pediatr. 1984;104:221–4.
4. Plantaz D, Rubie H, Michon J, et al. The treatment of neuroblastoma with intraspinal extension with chemotherapy followed by surgical removal of residual disease: A prospective study of 42 patients—Results of the NBL 90 study of the French Society of Pediatric Oncology. Cancer. 1996;78:311–319.
5. De Bernardi B, Pianca C, Pistamiglio P, et al. Neuroblastoma with symptomatic spinal cord compression at diagnosis: treatment and results with 76 cases. J Clin Oncol. 2001;19:183–90.
6. Katzenstein HM, Kent PM, London WB, Cohn SL. Treatment and outcome of 83 children with intraspinal neuroblastoma: the Pediatric Oncology Group experience. J Clin Oncol. 2001;19:1047–55.
7. Hoover M, Bowman LC, Crawford SE, et al. Long-term outcome of patients with intraspinal neuroblastoma. Med Pediatr Oncol. 1999;32:353–9.
8. Angelini P, Plantaz D, De Bernardi B, et al. Late sequelae of symptomatic epidural compression in children with localized neuroblastoma. Pediatr Blood Cancer. 2011;57:473–80.
9. Simon T, Niemann CA, Hero B, et al. Short- and long-term outcome of patients with symptoms of spinal cord compression by neuroblastoma. Dev Med Child Neurol. 2012;54:347–52.
10. Kraal K, Blom T, Tytgat L, et al. Neuroblastoma with intraspinal extension: health problems in long-term survivors. Pediatr Blood Cancer. 2016;63:990–6.
11. De Bernardi B, Balwierz W, Bejent J, et al. Epidural compression in neuroblastoma: diagnostic and therapeutic aspects. Cancer Lett. 2005;228:283–99.
12. Sandberg DI, Bilsky MH, Kushner BH, et al. Treatment of spinal involvement in neuroblastoma patients. Pediatr Neurosurg. 2003;39:291–8.
13. Yiin JJ, Chang CS, Jan YJ, Wang YC. Treatment of neuroblastoma with intraspinal extensions. J Clin Neurosci. 2003;10:579–83.
14. De Bernardi B, Quaglietta L, Haupt R, et al. Neuroblastoma with symptomatic epidural compression in the infant: the AIEOP experience. Pediatr Blood Cancer. 2014;61:1369–75.
15. Fawzy M, El-Beltagy M, Shafei ME, et al. Intraspinal neuroblastoma: treatment options and neurological outcome of spinal cord compression. Oncol Lett. 2015;9:907–11.

16. Trahair T, Sorrentino S, Russell SJ, et al. Spinal canal involvement in neuroblastoma. J Pediatr. 2017;188:294–8.
17. Hoffer FA. Magnetic resonance imaging of abdominal masses in the pediatric patient. Semin Ultrasound CT MR. 2005;26:212–23.
18. Yoshioka K, Tanaka R, Takagi H, et al. Ultra-high-resolution CT angiography of the artery of Adamkiewicz: a feasibility study. Neuroradiology. 2018;60:109–15.
19. Boglino C, Martins AG, Ciprandi G, Sousinha M, Inserra A. Spinal cord vascular injuries following surgery and advanced thoracic neuroblastoma: an unusual catastrophic complication. Med Pediatr Oncol. 1999;35:349–52.
20. Sainte-Rose C, Roux FX, Pierre-Kahn A, Renier D, Hirsch JF. Congenital intraspinal neuroblastomas. A propos of 7 cases treated surgically. Neurochirurgie. 1982;28:409–15.
21. Sundaresan N, Sachdev VP, Holland JF, et al. Surgical treatment of spinal cord compression from epidural metastasis. J Clin Oncol. 1995;13:2330–5.
22. Meyer NJ, Flatley TJ, Dunn DK. Superiorly based laminoplasty in children. J Spin Disor Techn. 2003;16:156–62.
23. Ozerov SS, Samarin AE, Andreev ES, et al. Neurosurgical aspects of the treatment of neuroblastoma patients. Zh Vopr Neirokhir Im N N Burdenko. 2016;80:50–7.
24. McGirt MJ, Chaichana KL, Atiba A, et al. Incidence of spinal deformity after resection of intramedullary spinal cord tumors in children who underwent laminectomy compared with laminoplasty. J Neurosurg Pediatr. 2008;1:57–62.
25. Fischer JP, Tweddle DA. Neonatal neuroblastoma. Semin Fetal Neonatal Med. 2012;17:207–15.
26. Asabe K, Handa N, Tamai Y, Kajiwara M, Hide T. A case of congenital intraspinal neuroblastoma. J Pediatr Surg. 1997;32:1371–6.
27. Blackman SC, Evenson A, Voss SD, et al. Prenatal diagnosis and subsequent treatment of an intermediate-risk paraspinal neuroblastoma: case report and review of the literature. Fetal Diagn Ther. 2008;24:119–25.
28. Walter KN, Kratz C, Uhl M, Niemeyer C. Chemotherapy as a therapeutic option for congenital neuroblastoma complicated by paraplegia. Klin Padiatr. 2008;220:175–7.
29. Suffia C, Sorrentino S, Vetrella S, et al. Neuroblastoma presenting with symptoms of epidural compression at birth: a case report. Ital J Pediatr. 2016;42:52.
30. Gigliotti AR, De Ioris MA, De Grandis E, et al. Congenital neuroblastoma with symptoms of epidural compression at birth. Pediatr Hematol Oncol. 2016;33:94–101.

Neonatal Neuroblastoma 10

Dominique Plantaz and Claire Freycon

10.1 Introduction

Neuroblastoma is the most common solid extra-cranial malignant tumor in childhood and infants, with an overall incidence of 1 case per 100,000 children in Europe and in the United States [1]. The french of childhood cancer registry estimates that neonatal neuroblastoma, defined as neuroblastoma diagnosed prenatally or within 28 days after birth, accounts for approximately 5% of all cases of the diseases (E. Desandes, RNTE, personal communication).

Overall, the 5-year survival for children with neuroblastoma is 72% [2], while patients younger than 1 year of age have a 5-year survival of around 90% [3–5].

Neuroblastoma accounts for approximately 8% of all malignancies diagnosed in children. However, it is a very heterogeneous disease with some tumors spontaneously regressing or maturing, while others are aggressive with a malignant phenotype and poor response to therapy. Several important clinical factors are associated with prognosis such as stage and age at diagnosis [6]. Biologic factors such as *MYCN* status and pathologic classification are also strong prognostic factors [7, 8]. On the basis of these factors, patients with neuroblastoma can be stratified into groups that have been shown to have different risks of recurrence and can be treated according to these risk groups from simple observation to heavy multimodal combined therapy. Age at diagnosis is one of the most powerful risk factors in such risk group stratifications, with age less than 18 months generally associated with better prognosis [9]. In this review, we discuss the clinical presentation, staging, screening, biology of regression, and treatment options and risks of sequelae for neonates with neuroblastoma.

D. Plantaz (✉) · C. Freycon
Department of Pediatrics, Hôpital Couple Enfant, University Hospital Centre of Grenoble-Alpes, Grenoble Cedex, France
e-mail: Dplantaz@chu-grenoble.fr

S. Sarnacki, L. Pio (eds.), *Neuroblastoma*,
https://doi.org/10.1007/978-3-030-18396-7_10

10.2 Clinical Presentation

Neonatal neuroblastomas can be diagnosed in the prenatal or postnatal period, although more than 70% are first noted in the postnatal period [10]. Regarding the prenatal diagnosis, antenatal suprarenal masses can be identified as incidental solid, cystic, or mixed adrenal masses on 20-week or later screening ultrasounds [11, 12]. There are also cases of maternal or fetal symptoms of neuroblastoma (e.g., catecholamine surge, spinal cord compression) which serve as the initial presentation [13–15]. The increased use of fetal ultrasonography has led to an increase of the suprarenal masses [11], which can be localized neuroblastomas but also other diagnoses which can present similarly such as adrenal hemorrhage, extrapulmonary sequestration, bronchogenic cyst, and urologic abnormalities [12].

Localized neuroblastomas in neonates not diagnosed prenatally by imaging are usually found incidentally when obtaining an imaging study for other medical issues. These are asymptomatic masses arising from the adrenal gland or the sympathetic chain [16]. Paravertebral tumors presenting with spinal cord compression with the possibility of flaccid leg paralysis and bladder or bowel dysfunction were reported in more than 13% of neonates with localized neuroblastoma [10]. Lastly, although very uncommon, neonatal patients can also present with paraneoplastic syndromes such as opsoclonus-ataxia syndrome [17].

10.3 Staging

The current staging system for neuroblastoma is based on the International Neuroblastoma Staging System (INSS). The INSS is a surgical-pathologic staging system that takes into account several variables including completeness of resection of the primary tumor, ipsilateral and contralateral involvement of lymph nodes, and tumor location in relation to the midline [18]. Complete evaluation for metastatic disease must also be undertaken for accurate staging. The extent of metastatic disease can be measured by a methyliodobenzylguanidine (MIBG) scan positive for approximately 90% of neuroblastomas. MIBG scan measures the uptake of catecholamine precursors by these tumors, both at the primary site and in metastatic sites such as the bone, bone marrow, and lymph nodes. The presence of metastatic disease can also be assessed by performing bone marrow aspiration and by assessing lymph nodes through imaging studies, including computed tomography (CT) or magnetic imaging scans (PRI), or surgical exploration. Table 10.1 summarizes the overall distribution of stage by patient age (less than 30 days versus more than or equal to 30 days in the Children Oncology Group experience) [19]: patients younger than 30 days present more less with metastatic disease (12% with stage 4 and 25% with stage 4s) than children over 30 days of age (46% with stage 4 and 4% with stage 4s) (Table 10.1); more than 30% of the neonates are with stage 1 disease. Of particular interest are patients younger than 1 year of age with metastatic disease who have a localized primary tumor with tumor dissemination limited to the skin and liver and/or less than 10% of neuroblastoma cells in the bone marrow (stage 4s) with generally an excellent prognosis with the exception of those harboring a tumor

Table 10.1 Distribution of neonatal patients versus patients older than 30 days by the International Neuroblastoma Staging System from a total of 7217 patients

INSS staging	Age <30 days (%)	Age <30 days (%)
Stage 1	32%	20%
Stage 2A	6%	6%
Stage 2B	9%	9%
Stage 3	16%	15%
Stage 4	12%	46%
Stage 4s	25%	4%
Total	5%	95%

Adapted from RB Interiano (reference [19])

Table 10.2 International Neuroblastoma Risk Group staging system (reference [43])

Stage	Description
L1	Localized tumor not involving vital structures as defined by the list of image-defined risk factors and confined to one body compartment
L2	Locoregional tumor with presence of one or more image-defined risk factors
M	Distant metastatic disease (except stage Ms)
MS	Metastatic disease in children younger than 18 months with metastases confined to the skin, liver and/or bone marrow

with *MYCN* amplification. Of patients with stage 4s disease, 20% are younger than 30 days at diagnosis.

More recently, other staging systems have sought to stage patients before treatment: the International Neuroblastoma Risk Group (INRG) (Table 10.2) task force proposed a staging system that included the absence (L1) or the presence (L2) of one or more of 20 image-defined risk factors (IDRFs) [20]. This staging system was initially designed to enable comparison of risk-based clinical trials worldwide and allows for the staging on the basis of tumor imaging rather than the extent of surgical resection. Table 10.3 details the IDRFs that use preoperative, diagnostic images to stratify patients on the basis of these imaging features [20].

Finally, SIOPEN introduced the notion of life-threatening symptoms in order to choose the adequate treatment for patients with "unresectable" tumors (L2), particularly for those who should receive emergent chemotherapy, rather than those who can be closely observed without any treatment for spontaneous regression (Table 10.4).

The stratification for the risk of disease relapse is shown in Table 10.5. Patients are stratified in low, intermediate, and high risk, with the probability of disease-free survival being >95%, >90%, and <30%, respectively. Recently, the concepts of very low risk have been defined for neonatal adrenal masses less than 5 cm diameter, without lymph node involvement which can be observed without any treatment with a 3-year disease-free survival of >80% (ref). It is important to observe that although low- and intermediate-risk patients account for approximately 36% and 21%, respectively, of patients of all stages, neonatal patient presents with low- and intermediate-risk disease in 58% and 40% of cases, respectively [19]. Patients younger than 28 days, as patients younger than 365 days are at low risk of relapse if histologic INSS stage 1, non-*MYCN*-amplified stage 2A/2B, or non-*MYCN*-amplified favorable histology aneuploid stage 4s disease.

Table 10.3 Image-defined risk factors (IDRFs) in neuroblastic tumors [20]

Neck	Tumor encasing carotid and/or vertebral artery and/or internal jugular vena cava
	Tumor extending to the base of the skull
	Tumor compressing the trachea
Cervico-thoracic junction	Tumor encasing brachial plexus roots
	Tumor encasing subclavian vessels and/or vertebral and/or carotid artery
	Tumor compressing the trachea
Thorax	Tumor encasing aorta and/or major branches
	Tumor compressing the trachea and/or principal bronchi
	Lower mediastinal tumor, infiltrating the costo-vertebral junction between T9 and T12
Thoraco-abdominal	Tumor encasing the aorta and/or vena cava
Abdomen/pelvis	Tumor infiltrating the porta hepatis and/or the hepatoduodenal ligament
	Tumor encasing branches of the superior mesenteric artery at the mesenteric root
	Tumor encasing the origin of the coeliac axis and/or the superior mesenteric artery
	Tumor invading one or both renal pedicles
	Tumor encasing the aorta and/or vena cava
	Tumor encasing the iliac vessels
	Pelvic tumor crossing the sciatic notch
Intraspinal tumor extension	Whatever the location, provided that more than one third of the spinal canal is invaded and/or the perimedullary leptomeningeal spaces are not visible and/or the spinal cord signal is abnormal
Infiltration of adjacent organs/structures	For example, pericardium, diaphragm, kidney, liver, duodeno-pancreatic block, and mesentery

Table 10.4 List of life-threatening symptoms (LTS)

Respiratory	Not infectious distress
	Polypnea superior in 60/mn
	Oxygen requirement
	Assisted ventilation
Cardiovascular	Arterial high blood pressure
	Superior cava syndrome
(Gastro)intestinal	Food intolerance
	Needs enteral or parenteral nutritional support
Renal	Oliguria
	Uretero-hydronephrosis
Sphincter dysfunction	Anorectal
	Vesical
Dumbbell neuroblastoma	Motor deficit
	Tumor occupying more of 1/3 of the width of the canal in the axial plan
	Not visible lepto-meningeal spaces
	Abnormal spinal signal

Table 10.5 The International Neuroblastoma Risk Group (INRG) pretreatment classification schema (adapted from reference [44])

INRG stage	Age (months)	Histology	Grade of tumor differentiation	*MYCN*	11 q aberration	Ploidy	Pretreatment risk group
Neonatal suprarenal masses <5 cm	<90 days	NA					Very low
L1/L2		GN maturing Or GNB intermixed					Very low
L1		Any except GN maturing Or GNB intermixed		Non-amplified Amplified	No Yes		Low High
L2	<18 months	Any except GN maturing Or GNB intermixed		Non-amplified Non-amplified			Low Intermediate
L2	>18 months	GNB nodular neuroblastoma	Differentiating Differentiating Poorly differentiated or undifferentiated	Non-amplified Non-amplified Non-amplified Amplified	No Yes		Low Intermediate Intermediate High
M	<18 months <12 months 12– 18 months <18 months >18 months			Non-amplified Non-amplified Non-amplified Amplified Amplified		Hyperdiploid Diploid Diploid	Low Intermediate Intermediate High High
MS	<18 months			Non-amplified Non-amplified Amplified	No Yes		Very low High High

10.4 Screening

The prognosis of patients with neuroblastoma depends considerably on patient age and stage at diagnosis, with younger patients having the best prognosis. Therefore, several groups hypothesized that early screening for neuroblastoma would improve the survival of children with this disease by detecting the presence of neuroblastoma in patients at an earlier stage. Thus, several trials conducted mass population screening for neuroblastoma by evaluating urinary catecholamine level [21]. These studies were performed in Japan and later in Germany and North America. These studies reported an increase in the incidence of lower-stage neuroblastoma, but they were discontinued because they did not provide any survival benefit for the patient population [22, 23]. These findings implied that if younger patients with non-high-risk disease have been identified, many of them have had never been detected, because of spontaneous regression.

10.5 Spontaneous Regression

Spontaneous regression of "in situ neuroblastoma" was first hypothesized by Beckwith et al. when they reported necropsies on infants younger than 3 months of age who died from other causes [24]; they encountered incidental adrenal tumors that were histologically identical to malignant neuroblastoma without any evidence of metastases; they observed a higher incidence (1 in 200) of these "in situ neuroblastomas" that would have been predicted from the known clinical incidence of neuroblastoma (1 in 8000 live births), suggesting that the natural history of these lesions may often involve spontaneous regression. Moreover, the Children Oncology Group study conducted a prospective trial of the expectant observation of infants with small adrenal tumors identified either prenatally or within the first 6 months of life [25]; the vast majority of the patients who completed the observation arm had a decrease in the volume of the adrenal mass: among 56 patients, 27 (48%) had no residual mass, 13 (23%) had a mass larger than 0 but 1 mL or less, 8 (14%) had a mass larger than 1 but 2 mL or less, and 8 (14%) had a mass larger than 2 mL. The 3-year survival was 100%. In Germany, a prospective cooperative trial on observation of unresectable localized neuroblastoma was conducted without cytotoxic treatment [26]; of 93 patients with unresected tumors, spontaneous regression was seen in 44; time to regression was variable with first signs of regression noted 1–18 months after diagnosis. The idea that many of these incidentally and some of the clinically detected neuroblastomas in neonates tend to spontaneously regress and are likely to have a favorable prognosis has been the premise for current treatment options for the management of neonatal neuroblastoma.

10.6 Biology

Three major genetic 1, 2A, and 2B subtypes can be designed in neuroblastoma tumors on the basis of cytogenetic abnormalities detected by comparative genomic hybridization profiles [27]. Neuroblastomas of subtype 1 are characterized by numeric chromosome alterations but no or few segmental abnormalities (SCAs), and patients with these tumors have favorable features and prognosis. Neuroblastomas of subtypes 2A and 2B are characterized by near diploid with recurrent SCAs and occur in patients of older age, advanced tumor stage, and poor clinical outcome. These genomic profiles can be now determined by circulating free tumor DNA analysis (liquid biopsies) avoiding a tumor biopsy which can be difficult or impossible or dangerous in fragile patients, such as neonates [28].

10.7 Biology of Spontaneous Regression

There is evidence to support several possible mechanisms of spontaneous regression in neuroblastoma [29]. The developmental program in sympathetic neuronal precursor is primarily regulated by the TrkA neurotrophin receptor and the limiting availability of its ligand, nerve growth factor (NGF), at their target site; the neuronal precursor survives, migrates, and proliferates in the absence of NGF during early embryogenesis followed by a putative developmental switch from an NGF-independent to an NGF-dependent state. Tumors of infants generally have a high level of TrkA expression. Taken together with the pivotal role of TrkA and NGF of the sympathetic system, tumors undergo neuronal differentiation to a ganglioneuroma, or they undergo spontaneous regression (apoptosis), depending on the presence or the absence, respectively, in the microenvironment. Loss of telomerase activity and telomerase shortening has been proposed as another possible mechanism for spontaneous regression of neuroblastoma. Another potential explanation of spontaneous regression is tumor destruction mediated by an anti-tumor immune response. Epigenetic regulation (promoter methylation, histone modification, and chromatin remodeling) may affect neuroblastoma cell survival or differentiation.

10.8 Treatment

10.8.1 Low-Risk Disease

Neonatal patients with INSS stage 1, 2A, and 2B non-*MYCN*-amplified favorable histology neuroblastoma account for more than 50% of neonatal neuroblastoma and have a favorable prognosis after surgical resection [30]. However if surgical resection has been the mainstay of therapy for patients with low-risk disease, these procedures may be associated with significant morbidity in neonates, including major vascular injuries, raising the question as to whether surgery is really indicated in low-risk patients [31]. Image-defined risk factor helped to define patients (L2) for which chemotherapy or observation should be considered first [32], with an excellent outcome in the SIOPEN experience [33]. Chemotherapy based on low doses of vincristine and cyclophosphamide or carboplatin-vepesid may allow to switch for resectable tumor [33] or serve as a trigger for the tumor regression [34]. However, chemotherapy should be administered very cautiously in newborns with reduction

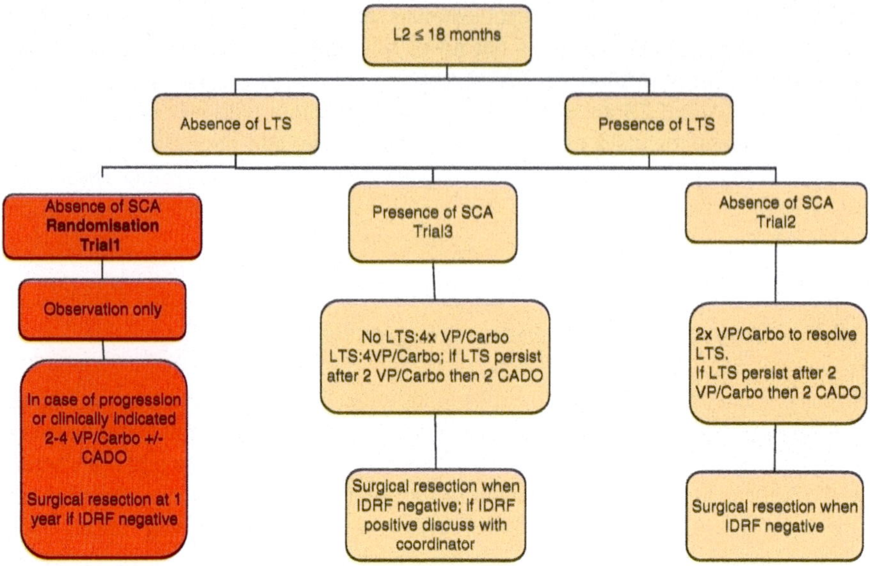

Fig. 10.1 Response and biology-based risk factor-guided therapy in treating younger patients with non-high risk neuroblastoma

dose (33% of normal dose) and adaptation by weight [33]. Currently, SIOPEN LINES protocol recommends observation for patients with unresectable (L2) tumor harboring only numerical chromosomal abnormalities (Fig. 10.1).

10.8.2 Very Low-Risk Disease

Based on previous studies showing that tumor of small size and with a cystic component shows spontaneous regression, Holgersen et al. found that the expectant observation of four patients with adrenal masses revealed that all tumors spontaneously resolved with no recurrence [35]. With these previous findings, a prospective protocol was developed to expectantly observe infants with small adrenal masses that were clinically consistent with neuroblastoma [25]. This study evaluated observation alone in infants less than 6 months of age who had a sonography that identified adrenal mass of 16 mL or less in volume if solid, or 65 mL or less if the mass was at least 25% cystic, and did not cross the midline with a disease limited to the adrenal gland as shown by imaging work-up. Follow-up investigations included measurement of urinary catecholamine levels and serial abdominal ultrasound studies. Infants with an increase of 50% in tumor volume were referred for surgery. Of the 87 patients of this study, 83 were enrolled in the observation arm, of whom 56 completed the observation; 16 patients underwent surgical resection after observation; 67 out of 83 patients were spared surgery.

A prospective SIOPEN study of patients <90 days, with suprarenal masses <5 cm, no midline extension, nor lymph node/distant spreading, was performed within the LINES protocol (data unpublished). Initial evaluation included sonography, MRI,

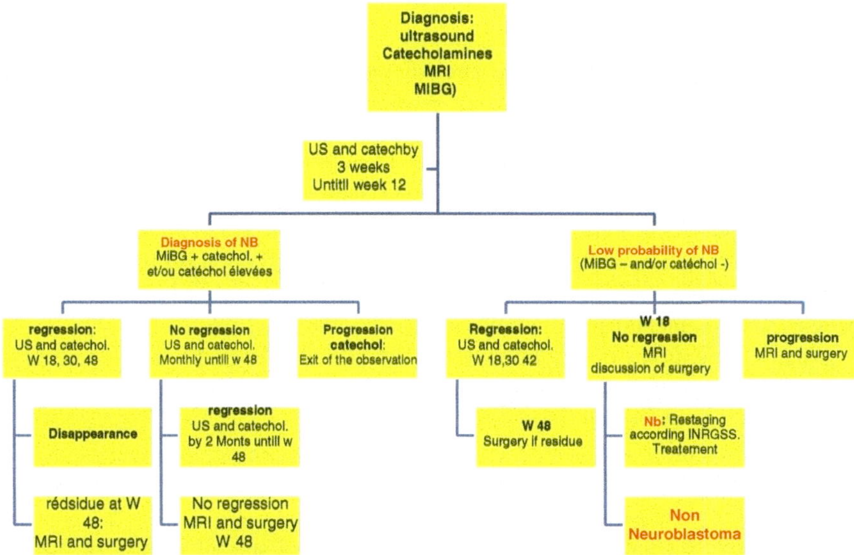

Fig. 10.2 Work-up and surveillance of antenatal supra-renal masses

urinary catecholamines, and MIBG scintigraphy. Sera were collected for MYCN analysis. Observation with US and urine catecholamines (if elevated at diagnosis) during a 48-week period was suggested. Infants experiencing >40% volume increase, L2 progression, or metastases were considered events and were fully restaged for appropriate treatment (Fig. 10.2). Surgical resection was performed for patients with >40% volume increase remaining resectable or for patients with residual mass at week 48. One hundred twenty-six infants were registered by 2012 and 2017. Masses were described as cystic (28%), solid (37%), or mixed (35%). Antenatal diagnosis was evident in 54 cases. Of 119 patients, 36 (28%) underwent resection, 17 during observation and 19 at the end of the observation period, and 25 proved neuroblastomas (73%). Ninety-seven sera were collected and analyzed, and all were negative for MYCN amplification, although one tumor at excision after 1 year observation was found MYCN amplified. The 1- and 3-year EFS was 89% and 86%, respectively, and OS was 100%, with a median follow-up of 27 months. Sixteen events were observed: progression to MS ($n = 6$) or L1/L2 tumors ($n = 10$). In conclusion, expectant observation for infants <90 days with diagnosed localized suprarenal masses <5 cm discovered antenatally or postnatal proved safe. The value of MYCN serum analyses is not definable. Close monitoring is effective, without jeopardizing overall outcome, and most patients can avoid surgery.

10.8.3 Intermediate-Risk Disease

Infants younger than 1 year of age with INSS stage 3, stage 4, or stage 4s disease with non-*MYCN*-amplified tumors are designated as intermediate-risk patients and make up 40% of neonatal neuroblastomas. Infants with 4s non-*MYCN*-amplified disease are also considered intermediate risk if they are either symptomatic or have unfavorable histology. The use of chemotherapy for all infants with stage 3 disease is not uniform as already mentioned: several prospective studies have reported excellent outcome for infants with nonresectable non-*MYCN*-amplified neuroblastoma, who received chemotherapy [33, 36]. Hero et al. [26] reported observing 93 infants with non-*MYCN*-amplified unresected neuroblastoma: 44 (47%) exhibited regression and 35 (38%) progressed locally or to stage 4s or 4 (4%) requiring high-risk therapy. Schleiermacher et al. demonstrated that regression is mainly observed in tumors with favorable biology and SIOPEL LINES protocol recommends to treat patients with segmental abnormalities with chemotherapy [27].

Finally, patients with stage 4 non-*MYCN*-amplified tumors also have a favorable outcome with chemotherapy and surgery [37].

10.8.4 Stage 4S Disease

Stage 4s is a "special" group of patients who have a special pattern of diffuse involvement and carry a good prognosis [38]. Infants younger than 1 year with dissemination limited to the skin or liver or less than 10% of neuroblasts in the bone marrow, without bone metastases, are considered to have a stage 4s disease. Gigliotti et al. reported 45 of 134 newborns (33%) having stage 4s disease [4]. Although these patients have extensive metastatic disease, these tumors generally undergo spontaneous regression even without treatment. Therefore, patients are generally treated with supportive therapy only and have excellent outcome [39]. However, this disease can cause significant life-threatening complications, particularly in the neonatal period [40]. The signs and symptoms of organ distress caused by hepatomegaly can occur in the lungs, the kidneys, the gastrointestinal tract, the inferior vena cava, and the liver [41]. A scoring scale reflecting organ compromise was developed, the scores ranging from 0 to 10. Scores were derived for 32 of 35 patients; 13 were neonates when first seen, and 19 were infants aged 1–12 months. Neonates were more likely than infants to develop increasing symptomatology (50% versus 25%) and were more likely to die when a score of 2 or more developed. None of the six neonates who did so survived despite treatment, compared with three of four infants. Early intervention is recommended for 4s neonates who develop a score of 1.

10.8.5 High-Risk Disease

Infants younger than 1 year of age with stage 2, 3, 4, or 4s disease with *MYCN* amplification are considered to be at high risk and so are treated with a combination of chemotherapy, surgical resection, high-dose chemotherapy with autologous hematopoietic stem cell transplantation, radiation therapy, and immunotherapy with anti-GD2. This group however accounts for less than 2% of neonatal neuroblastoma [19]. Neonates with high-risk disease have a 2-year overall survival of only 30% despite the treatment regimen [42].

10.9 Conclusion

Neonatal neuroblastoma accounts for less than 5% of all neuroblastoma and carries a favorable prognosis with more than 98% of patients having a low or intermediate risk of tumor recurrence and an overall survival over than 95%. Low-risk neonatal patients can most often be observed expectantly without further exposure to surgery or chemotherapy. Ongoing studies are aiming to reduce the therapy given to the non-high-risk patients. Further studies will help to dictate the careful selection of patients for observation as well as for aggressive therapy. Long-term follow-up is needed for these patients.

References

1. Georgakis MK, Dessypris N, Baka M, Moschovi M, Papadakis V, Polychronopoulou S, Kourti M, Hatzipantelis E, Stiakaki E, Dana H, Bouka E, Antunes L, Bastos J, Coza D, Demetriou A, Agius D, Eser S, Gheorghiu R, Sekerija M, Trojanowski M, Zagar T, Zborovskaya A, Ryzhov A, Tragiannidis A, Panagopoulou P, Steliarova-Foucher E, Petridou ET. Neuroblastoma among children in Southern and Eastern European cancer registries: variations in incidence and temporal trends compared to US. Int J Cancer. 2018;142:1985.
2. Gatta G, Botta L, Rossi S, Aareleid T, Bielska-Lasota M, Clavel J, Dimitrova N, Jakab Z, Kaatsch P, Lacour B, Mallone S, Marcos-Gragera R, Minicozzi P, Sánchez-Pérez MJ, Sant M, Santaquilani M, Stiller C, Tavilla A, Trama A, Visser O, Peris-Bonet R, EUROCARE Working Group. Childhood cancer survival in Europe 1999-2007: results of EUROCARE-5--a population-based study. Lancet Oncol. 2014;15:35–47.
3. Koh V, Soh SY, Chan MY, Tan AM. Neuroblastoma in children under 12 months in singapore-15-year experience and outcomes from KKH. Fetal Pediatr Pathol. 2015;34:155–61.
4. Gigliotti AR, Di Cataldo A, Sorrentino S, Parodi S, Rizzo A, Buffa P, Granata C, Sementa AR, Fagnani AM, Provenzi M, Prete A, D'Ippolito C, Clerico A, Castellano A, Tonini GP, Conte M, Garaventa A, De Bernardi B. Neuroblastoma in the newborn. A study of the Italian Neuroblastoma Registry. Eur J Cancer. 2009;45:3220–7.
5. Zhou Y, Li K, Zheng S, Chen L. Retrospective study of neuroblastoma in Chinese neonates from 1994 to 2011: an evaluation of diagnosis, treatments, and prognosis: a 10-year retrospective study of neonatal neuroblastoma. J Cancer Res Clin Oncol. 2014;140:83–7.
6. Evans AE, D'Angio GJ, Propert K, Anderson J, Hann HW. Prognostic factor in neuroblastoma. Cancer. 1987;59:1853–9.
7. Seeger RC, Brodeur GM, Sather H, Dalton A, Siegel SE, Wong KY, Hammond D. Association of multiple copies of the N-myc oncogene with rapid progression of neuroblastomas. N Engl J Med. 1985;313(18):1111–6.
8. Goto S, Umehara S, Gerbing RB, Stram DO, Brodeur GM, Seeger RC, Lukens JN, Matthay KK, Shimada H. Histopathology (International Neuroblastoma Pathology Classification) and MYCN status in patients with peripheral neuroblastic tumors: a report from the Children's Cancer Group. Cancer. 2001;92:2699–708.
9. London WB, Castleberry RP, Matthay KK, Look AT, Seeger RC, Shimada H, Thorner P, Brodeur G, Maris JM, Reynolds CP, Cohn SL. Evidence for an age cutoff greater than 365 days for neuroblastoma risk group stratification in the Children's Oncology Group. J Clin Oncol. 2005;23:6459–65.
10. Michalowski MB, Rubie H, Michon J, Montamat S, Bergeron C, Coze C, Perel Y, Valteau-Couanet D, Guitard J, Guys JM, Piolat C, Munzer C. Plantaz D; Neonatal localized neuroblastoma: 52 cases treated from 1990 to 1999. Arch Pediatr. 2004;11:782–8.

11. Acharya S, Jayabose S, Kogan SJ, Tugal O, Beneck D, Leslie D, Slim M. Prenatally diagnosed neuroblastoma. Cancer. 1997;80:304–10.
12. Sauvat F, Sarnacki S, Brisse H, Medioni J, Rubie H, Aigrain Y, Gauthier F, Audry G, Helardot P, Landais P, Michon J, Hartmann O, Nihoul-Fékété C. Outcome of suprarenal localized masses diagnosed during the perinatal period: a retrospective multicenter study. Cancer. 2002;94:2474–80.
13. Voûte PA Jr, Wadman SK, van Putten WJ. Congenital neuroblastoma. Symptoms in the mother during pregnancy. Clin Pediatr. 1970;9:206–7.
14. Newton ER, Louis F, Dalton ME, Feingold M. Fetal neuroblastoma and catecholamine-induced maternal hypertension. Obstet Gynecol. 1985;65:49S–52S.
15. Delahaye S, Doz F, Sonigo P, Saada J, Mitanchez D, Sarnacki S, Benachi A. Prenatal diagnosis of dumbbell neuroblastoma. Ultrasound Obstet Gynecol. 2008;3:92–5.
16. Dhir S, Wheeler K. Neonatal neuroblastoma. Early Hum Dev. 2010;86:601–5.
17. Fisher JP, Tweddle DA. Neonatal neuroblastoma. Semin Fetal Neonatal Med. 2012;17:207–15.
18. Brodeur GM, Pritchard J, Berthold F, Carlsen NL, Castel V, Castelberry RP, De Bernardi B, Evans AE, Favrot M, Hedborg F, et al. Revisions of the international criteria for neuroblastoma diagnosis, staging, and response to treatment. J Clin Oncol. 1993;11:1466–77.
19. Interiano RB, Davidoff AM. Current Management of Neonatal Neuroblastoma. Curr Pediatr Rev. 2015;11:179–87.
20. Brisse HJ, McCarville MB, Granata C, Krug KB, Wootton-Gorges SL, Kanegawa K, Giammarile F, Schmidt M, Shulkin BL, Matthay KK, Lewington VJ, Sarnacki S, Hero B, Kaneko M, London WB, Pearson AD, Cohn SL, Monclair T. International Neuroblastoma Risk Group Project. Guidelines for imaging and staging of neuroblastic tumors: consensus report from the International Neuroblastoma Risk Group Project. Radiology. 2011;261:243–57.
21. Schilling FH, Oberrauch W, Schanz F, Treuner J. Evaluation of a rapid and reliable method for mass screening for neuroblastoma in onfants. Prog Clin Biol Res. 1991;366:579–83.
22. Schilling FH, Spix C, Berthold F, Erttmann R, Fehse N, Hero B, Klein G, Sander J, Schwarz K, Treuner J, Zorn U, Michaelis J. Neuroblastoma screening at one year of age. N Engl J Med. 2002;346:1047–53.
23. Shinagawa T, Kitamura T, Katanoda K, Matsuda T, Ito Y, Sobue T. The incidence and mortality rates of neuroblastoma cases before and after the cessation of the mass screening program in Japan: a descriptive study. Int J Cancer. 2017;140:618–25.
24. Beckwith JB, Perrin EV. In situ neuroblastoma: a contribution to the natural history of neural crest tumors. Am J Pathol. 1963;43:1089–104.
25. Nuchtern JG, London WB, Barnewolt CE, Naranjo A, McGrady PW, Geiger JD, Diller L, Schmidt ML, Maris JM, Cohn SL, Shamberger RC. A prospective study of expectant observation as primary therapy for neuroblastoma in young infants: a Children's Oncology Group study. Ann Surg. 2012;256:573–80.
26. Hero B, Simon T, Spitz R, Ernestus K, Gnekow AK, Scheel-Walter HG, Schwabe D, Schilling FH, Benz-Bohm G, Berthold F. Localized infant neuroblastomas often show spontaneous regression: results of the prospective trials NB95-S and NB97. J Clin Oncol. 2008;26:1504–10.
27. Schleiermacher G, Michon J, Ribeiro A, Pierron G, Mosseri V, Rubie H, Munzer C, Bénard J, Auger N, Combaret V, Janoueix-Lerosey I, Pearson A, Tweddle DA, Bown N, Gerrard M, Wheeler K, Noguera R, Villamon E, Cañete A, Castel V, Marques B, de Lacerda A, Tonini GP, Mazzocco K, Defferrari R, de Bernardi B, di Cataldo A, van Roy N, Brichard B, Ladenstein R, Ambros I, Ambros P, Beiske K, Delattre O, Couturier J. Segmental chromosomal alterations lead to a higher risk of relapse in infants with MYCN-non-amplified localised unresectable/disseminated neuroblastoma (a SIOPEN collaborative study). Br J Cancer. 2011;105:1940–8.
28. Chicard M, Boyault S, Colmet Daage L, Richer W, Gentien D, Pierron G, Lapouble E, Bellini A, Clement N, Iacono I, Bréjon S, Carrere M, Reyes C, Hocking T, Bernard V, Peuchmaur M, Corradini N, Faure-Conter C, Coze C, Plantaz D, Defachelles AS, Thebaud E, Gambart M, Millot F, Valteau-Couanet D, Michon J, Puisieux A, Delattre O, Combaret V, Schleiermacher G. Genomic copy number profiling using circulating free tumor DNA highlights heterogeneity in neuroblastoma. Clin Cancer Res. 2016;22:5564–73.

29. Brodeur GM. Spontaneous regression of neuroblastoma. Cell Tissue Res. 2018;372:277. https://doi.org/10.1007/s00441-017-2761-2.
30. De Bernardi B, Mosseri V, Rubie H, Castel V, Foot A, Ladenstein R, Laureys G, Beck-Popovic M, de Lacerda AF, Pearson AD, De Kraker J, Ambros PF, de Rycke Y, Conte M, Bruzzi P, Michon J, SIOP Europe Neuroblastoma Group. Treatment of localised resectable neuroblastoma. Results of the LNESG1 study by the SIOP Europe Neuroblastoma Group. Br J Cancer. 2008;99:1027–33.
31. Ikeda H, Suzuki N, Takahashi A, Kuroiwa M, Nagashima K, Tsuchida Y, Matsuyama S. Surgical treatment of neuroblastomas in infants under 12 months of age. J Pediatr Surg. 1998;33:1246–50.
32. Cecchetto G, Mosseri V, De Bernardi B, Helardot P, Monclair T, Costa E, Horcher E, Neuenschwander S, Tomà P, Rizzo A, Michon J, Holmes K. Surgical risk factors in primary surgery for localized neuroblastoma: the LNESG1 study of the European International Society of Pediatric Oncology Neuroblastoma Group. J Clin Oncol. 2005;23:8483–9.
33. Rubie H, De Bernardi B, Gerrard M, Canete A, Ladenstein R, Couturier J, Ambros P, Munzer C, Pearson AD, Garaventa A, Brock P, Castel V, Valteau-Couanet D, Holmes K, Di Cataldo A, Brichard B, Mosseri V, Marquez C, Plantaz D, Boni L, Michon J. Excellent outcome with reduced treatment in infants with nonmetastatic and unresectable neuroblastoma without MYCN amplification: results of the prospective INES 99.1. J Clin Oncol. 2011;29:449–55.
34. Owens C, Irwin M. Neuroblastoma: the impact of biology and cooperation leading to personalized treatments. Crit Rev Clin Lab Sci. 2012;49:85–115.
35. Holgersen LO, Subramanian S, Kirpekar M, Mootabar H, Marcus JR. Spontaneous resolution of antenatally diagnosed adrenal masses. J Pediatr Surg. 1996;31:153–5.
36. Baker DL, Schmidt ML, Cohn SL, Maris JM, London WB, Buxton A, Stram D, Castleberry RP, Shimada H, Sandler A, Shamberger RC, Look AT, Reynolds CP, Seeger RC, Matthay KK, Children's Oncology Group. Outcome after reduced chemotherapy for intermediate-risk neuroblastoma. N Engl J Med. 2010;363:1313–23.
37. De Bernardi B, Gerrard M, Boni L, Rubie H, Cañete A, Di Cataldo A, Castel V, Forjaz de Lacerda A, Ladenstein R, Ruud E, Brichard B, Couturier J, Ellershaw C, Munzer C, Bruzzi P, Michon J, Pearson AD. Excellent outcome with reduced treatment for infants with disseminated neuroblastoma without MYCN gene amplification. J Clin Oncol. 2009;27:1034–40.
38. D'Angio GJ, Evans AE, Koop CE. Special pattern of widespread neuroblastoma with a favourable prognosis. Lancet. 1971;1:1046–9.
39. Nickerson HJ, Matthay KK, Seeger RC, Brodeur GM, Shimada H, Perez C, Atkinson JB, Selch M, Gerbing RB, Stram DO, Lukens J. Favorable biology and outcome of stage IV-S neuroblastoma with supportive care or minimal therapy: a Children's Cancer Group study. J Clin Oncol. 2000;18:477–86.
40. Moppett J, Haddadin I, Foot AB. Neonatal neuroblastoma. Arch Dis Child Fetal Neonatal Ed. 1999;81:F134–7.
41. Hsu LL, Evans AE, D'Angio GJ. Hepatomegaly in neuroblastoma stage 4s: criteria for treatment of the vulnerable neonate. Med Pediatr Oncol. 1996;27:521–8.
42. Canete A, Gerrard M, Rubie H, Castel V, Di Cataldo A, Munzer C, Ladenstein R, Brichard B, Bermúdez JD, Couturier J, de Bernardi B, Pearson AJ, Michon J. Poor survival for infants with MYCN-amplified metastatic neuroblastoma despite intensified treatment: the International Society of Paediatric Oncology European Neuroblastoma Experience. J Clin Oncol. 2009;27:1014–9.
43. Monclair T, Brodeur GM, Ambros PF, Brisse HJ, Cecchetto G, Holmes K, Kaneko M, London WB, Matthay KK, Nuchtern JG, von Schweinitz D, Simon T, Cohn SL, Pearson AD, INRG Task Force. The International Neuroblastoma Risk Group (INRG) staging system: an INRG Task Force report. J Clin Oncol. 2009;2:298–303.
44. Cohn SL, Pearson AD, London WB, Monclair T, Ambros PF, Brodeur GM, Faldum A, Hero B, Iehara T, Machin D, Mosseri V, Simon T, Garaventa A, Castel V, Matthay KK, INRG Task Force. The International Neuroblastoma Risk Group (INRG) classification system: an INRG Task Force report. J Clin Oncol. 2009;27:289–97.

Low- and Intermediate-Risk Neuroblastoma

11

Vanessa Segura and Adela Cañete

11.1 Introduction

The new International Neuroblastoma Risk Group (INRG) classification system takes into account the clinical heterogeneity of this disease and provides the clinicians with a powerful and robust tool for treatment stratification. This tool combines clinical parameters such as age and INRG staging as well as the data obtained by the analysis of tumour tissue (histology, molecular data such as *MYCN* oncogene status, DNA ploidy and 11q deletion). Based on these features, the system defines 16 pretreatment groups stratified (labelled A to R) [1].

According to this classification, 28.2% of the patients are considered very low risk with an estimated 5-year EFS of more than 85%, 26.8% are considered low risk with an estimated 5-year EFS >75% to ≤85% whereas 9% are classified as intermediate risk with an estimated 5-year EFS ≥50% to ≤75% [1]. The INRG classification has been valuable, guiding systematic therapy decisions suggested by international cooperative groups [2]. In this review, we compare the past and current therapeutic strategies for low- and intermediate-risk populations based on this tool.

Strictly speaking, low-risk patients are INRG pretreatment risk groups D, E and F and intermediate-risk patients are groups G, H, I and J. For most clinicians from the International Society of Paediatric Oncology European Neuroblastoma (SIOPEN), "low risk" refers to patients of any age that have L1 tumours and can be treated only with surgery but also children younger than 18 months with stage L2 and MS without *MYCN* amplification (no-*MNA*). On the other hand, intermediate-risk patients are those children over 18 months with no-*MNA* stage L2. Besides, the SIOPEN group includes also in this risk category infants with no-*MNA* M disease.

V. Segura · A. Cañete (✉)
Unidad de Oncohematología Pediátrica, Hospital Infantil La Fe and GICT-Cáncer IIS La Fe, Valencia, Spain
e-mail: segura_van@gva.es; canyete_ade@gva.es

S. Sarnacki, L. Pio (eds.), *Neuroblastoma*,
https://doi.org/10.1007/978-3-030-18396-7_11

11.1.1 Low Risk

11.1.1.1 Children with L1 Tumours (Equivalent to INRG Pretreatment Risk Group A and B): «High Survival Rates in This Population Were Reached with Surgery Alone in All Cooperative Groups in the Last Decades»

The LNESG1 trial, which ran from 1995 to 1999, was the first European multicentre study that confirmed a 5-year EFS of 94.3% and an excellent OS of 98.9% in 288 INSS stage 1 patients with surgery alone. Likewise, for the 123 INSS stage 2 patients, the 5-year EFS and OS was 82.8% and 93.2%, respectively [3]. It was followed by a confirmation trial (LNESG2) run by SIOPEN group with 380 patients (manuscript in preparation). In the low-risk COG P9641 study (Children's Oncology Group P9641; ClinicalTrials.gov identifier NCT00003119), a 5-year OS rate (±standard deviation [SD]) of 96 ± 1% was achieved with surgery alone for patients with asymptomatic INSS stage 2a or 2b tumours [4]. Other studies have demonstrated that subsets of infants with localised tumours can be cured without any treatment, including surgery [5, 6].

The INRG database showed less favourable EFS and OS in patients with *MNA* INSS stage 1 and 2 tumours than in patients with non-amplified tumours (53% ± 8% and 72% ± 7% vs. 90% ± 1% and 98% ± 1%, $p < 0.0001$, respectively) [7]. The question regarding this very scarce group of patients with L1 neuroblastoma tumours with *MNA* remains to be solved [8].

11.1.1.2 Infants and Children Aged 12–18 Months with Neuroblastoma (Equivalent to INRG Pretreatment Risk Group C, D, G and Q)

The age cut-off in INRG is referred to 547 days (18 months), but all the former published experiences refer mostly to infants, that stand for the largest number of patients in this age group. The current ongoing trials such as SIOPEN LINES study (ClinicalTrials.gov Identifier NCT01728155) in Europe will show the real impact of age as a continuous variable in prognosis.

Here, we summarise the former SIOPEN experience described in two out of four trials devoted to infants with low-risk neuroblastoma:

- *Infants with localised unresectable disease without MYCN amplification* were eligible for SIOPEN INES99.1 study and represent INRG pretreatment risk group D and G. In INES99.1 study, they received upfront chemotherapy in order to achieve surgery of the primary tumour. Five-year OS and EFS were excellent, and in 61% of the cases, anthracyclines were avoided [9]. These excellent results were the basis to propose a randomised study in the SIOPEN low-risk trial (LINES, Group 1), which is still ongoing.
- *Infants with disseminated neuroblastoma without MYCN amplification* are equivalent to INRG pretreatment risk group C and Q, and historically, it is well-known that they are a "special cohort" with an excellent prognosis. INES 99.2

trial dealt with 4 s patients that received chemotherapy or not according to the presence or absence of life-threatening symptoms (LTS). Surgery was to be performed only in the absence of surgical risk factors. The 125 infants treated on INES99.2 study had a 2-year overall survival (OS) of 97.6% with no difference between asymptomatic and symptomatic patients (97.7% vs. 97.3%), patients with or without unresectable primary tumours (96.8% vs. 100%) and patients with or without positive skeletal scintigraphy without radiologic abnormalities (97.2% vs. 100%). No patients died of surgery- or chemotherapy-related complications. Infants with disseminated disease without *MYCN* amplification have excellent survival with minimal or no treatment. Asymptomatic infants with an unresectable primary tumour or positive skeletal scintigraphy without radiologic abnormalities may undergo observation alone [10]. Special features of infants and neonates with 4s disease have already been described in other parts of this chapter.

The International SIOPEN study LINES (Low and Intermediate Risk Neuroblastoma European Study; Eudract number:2010-021396-81) groups together in a single protocol the treatment of all patients with "non-high-risk" neuroblastoma. Image-defined risk factors, the presence or absence of symptoms and the presence or absence of segmental chromosome aberrations are being used in the decision-making process to stratify treatment. It is an "umbrella" type of trial that consists in 11 different studies, six of them related to "low-risk" patients. Low-risk patients are included after informed consent, diagnostic evaluation, stage assignment and centrally reviewed biological studies, whose results drive "patients' road" to inclusion in one of the six low-risk groups. Treatment by protocol oscillates between a "wait and watch approach" and mild chemotherapy either to resolve LTS or to prevent relapses (as per LINES group 2 [L2] and 6 [Ms], both tumours with segmental chromosomal abnormalities [SCA], corresponding to INRG pretreatment risk group G and Q [Fig. 11.1]).

Finally, if successful, the low-risk LINES study will demonstrate the following:

- It is feasible to minimise the amount of treatment (chemotherapy and surgery) for all appropriate low-risk patients (by clinical and pangenomic data), who in previous studies have been shown to have an excellent long-term outcome (as in the SIOPEN INES99.1 study). This treatment reduction is supported by the previous INES trial and the excellent results reported from the German group who in a non-randomised study reduced chemotherapy in certain situations, thus showing that these selected patients do not require chemotherapy [5].
- Survival in L2 and Ms patients who have segmental chromosomal changes in their tumour genomic profile is improved by electively treating these patients with chemotherapy despite the absence of symptoms [11].

While SIOPEN is recruiting low-risk patients in the LINES trial, other cooperative groups are following their own trials. For instance, the German group will

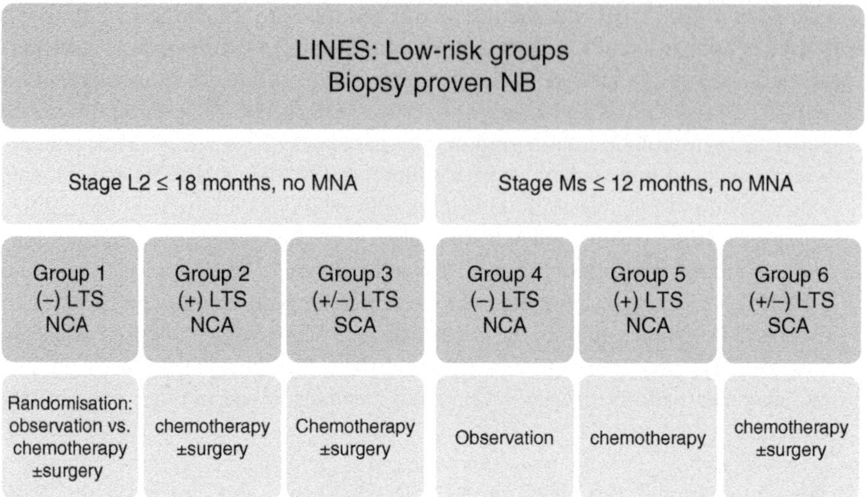

Fig. 11.1 Treatment stratification overview for low-risk neuroblastoma in LINES study. *LTS* life-threatening symptoms, *NCA* numerical chromosomal abnormalities, *SCA* segmental chromosomal abnormalities, – absence, + presence

implement a new neuroblastoma treatment stratification system that integrates gene expression-based classification and established prognostic markers in prospective clinical trials, in a very similar way as SIOPEN [12].

11.1.2 Intermediate Risk

This is a very heterogenous population that represents 9% of the total neuroblastoma patients, with an expected 5-year EFS over 50% and below 75%. Here, we review only the patients with neuroblastoma that are considered intermediate risk by the SIOPEN group.

11.1.2.1 Children Aged 18 Months or Older with L2-Stage Neuroblastoma or Nodular Ganglioneuroblastoma, Poorly Differentiated/Undifferentiated or Differentiating, 11qdeleted No-NMA (Equivalent to INRG Pretreatment Risk Group H)

Patients with these features are in the "border" between being treated either with high-intensity multimodal or intermediate treatment strategies. So far, there have not been randomised trials trying to answer this question: which is the best approach for these patients? The answer still remains unknown, and the different groups follow different strategies. In the past, the intermediate-risk COG A3961 study demonstrated a 3-year OS rate of 96% ± 1% with substantial reductions in the duration of treatment and dose of chemotherapeutic agents compared with regimens used in earlier American clinical trials [13]. The impact of additional decreases in therapy intensity for specific subsets of patients is being evaluated in the current COG study for non-high-risk disease. The SIOPEN European Unresectable Neuroblastoma Study (EUNS) (2001–2006) recruited 164 eligible patients aged more than 12 months with *MYCN* non-amplified unresectable NB [14]. After biopsy, patients received six courses of chemotherapy (three of carboplatin–etoposide and three of CADO) and a surgical resection of the primary tumour, without further treatment (no radiotherapy). Five-year OS and EFS were not satisfactory (79% and 68%, respectively) although age was the most important prognostic factor, significantly improved in younger patients (age 12–18 months) vs. older patients (OS 100% vs. 70%, $p = 0.006$, and EFS 78% vs. 62%, $p = 0.001$). Histology (central review in 127/164 cases) also proved to be of significant prognostic value. OS in the "differentiating" histology group (46% of patients) reached 100% vs. 63% in the "poorly differentiated or undifferentiated" cases ($p = 0.004$), and EFS was 91% vs. 62% ($p = 0.002$). Local relapses were worrisome, reporting 28 cases (19 isolated and 9 combined with metastatic sites) involving primary site. This indicates that a more intensive regimen including radiotherapy is warranted for older patients with unresectable tumours of unfavourable histology, although in previous studies radiotherapy has not consistently demonstrated a clear improvement in survival. These results comply with the INRG conclusions and were taken into account while designing the following SIOPEN trial. Given the fact that there are not enough patients to do a randomised study unless all cooperative groups join in a global trial, the SIOPEN group considers radiotherapy as part of the scheduled regimen for patients with poorly differentiated or undifferentiated histotypes. Although not many, there were nine metastatic relapses, and that prompted the SIOPEN group to add 13-cis retinoic acid (13-cis-RA) to the strategy while preserving high-dose treatment (HDT) as rescue therapy. Although mortality related to HDT has decreased enormously, this procedure is not exempt of severe acute and long-term effects and its role is not so clearly demonstrated for stage 3 patients [15, 16]. The fact that 11 out of the 30 relapses were metastatic (2 isolated and 9 both local and metastatic) could mean that there is a need not only to intensify local treatment but also to introduce a maintenance treatment for minimal residual disease that could persist after chemotherapy, surgery and radiotherapy. Our hypothesis is that 13-cis-RA could prevent metastatic relapses, avoiding the intensity and toxicity of megatherapy in a non-amplified *MYCN* non-metastatic population [17]. At the time of LINES design (Fig. 11.2), no other minimal residual disease (MRD) treatments were approved and available in Europe [18, 19].

Therefore, groups 7 and 8 of LINES trial are those devoted to these IR patients and are proposed in order to

- Reduce the amount of chemotherapy for differentiating histology INRG stage L2 NB and ganglioneuroblastoma nodular patients who have been shown to have an excellent long-term outcome.
- Increase the amount of treatment (radiotherapy and 13-cis-RA) for poorly differentiated or undifferentiated histology INRG stage L2 NB or ganglioneuroblastoma nodular patients in order to improve the EFS.

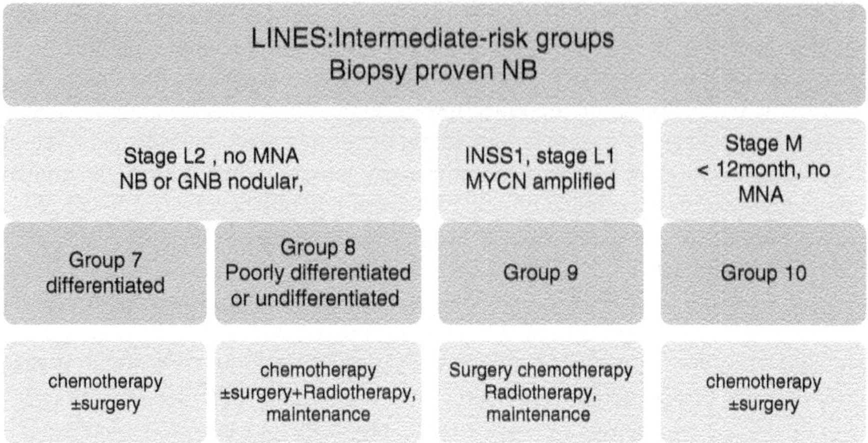

Fig. 11.2 Treatment stratification overview for intermediate-risk neuroblastoma in LINES study

11.1.2.2 Patients Younger Than 12 Months with M Stage Tumour, Diploid, No-NMA (Equivalent to INRG Pretreatment Risk Group I)

This group includes in SIOPEN those infants with overt metastases to skeleton, lung, or central nervous system (CNS) and no-NMA tumours. SIOPEN trial INES99.3 was designed to treat them with chemotherapy until complete metastatic response was obtained followed by surgery only in the absence of surgical risk factors [10]. The 45 infants treated on this trial had a 2-year OS of 95.6%. No patients died of surgery- or chemotherapy-related complications. Infants with disseminated disease without *MYCN* amplification have excellent survival with a moderate-intensity chemotherapy and surgery alone, without high-dose chemotherapy. The current group 10 in LINES will confirm these results.

In conclusion, collaborative efforts of international cooperative groups have led to refinements in risk classification to guide therapies, resulting in improved outcome in neuroblastoma, although further work is needed to continue this progress.

References

1. Cohn SL, Pearson AD, London WB, Monclair T, Ambros PF, Brodeur GM, Faldum A, Hero B, Iehara T, Machin D, Mosseri V, Simon T, Garaventa A, Castel V, Matthay KK, INRG Task Force. The International Neuroblastoma Risk Group (INRG) classification system: an INRG Task Force report. J Clin Oncol. 2009;27:289–97.
2. Tolbert VP, Matthay KK. Neuroblastoma: clinical and biological approach to risk stratification and treatment. Cell Tissue Res. 2018;372(2):195–209.
3. De Bernardi B, Mosseri V, Rubie H, Castel V, Foot A, Ladenstein R, Laureys G, Beck-Popovic M, de Lacerda AF, Pearson AD, De Kraker J, Ambros PF, de Rycke Y, Conte M, Bruzzi P, Michon J, SIOP Europe Neuroblastoma Group. Treatment of localized resectable neuroblastoma. Results of the LNESG1 study by the SIOP Europe Neuroblastoma Group. Br J Cancer. 2008;99:1027–33.

4. Strother DR, London WB, Schmidt ML, Brodeur GM, Shimada H, Thorner P, Collins MH, Tagge E, Adkins S, Reynolds CP, Murray K, Lavey RS, Matthay KK, Castleberry R, Maris JM, Cohn SL. Outcome after surgery alone or with restricted use of chemotherapy for patients with low-risk neuroblastoma: results of Children's Oncology Group study P9641. J Clin Oncol. 2012;30(15):1842–8.
5. Hero B, Simon T, Spitz R, Ernestus K, Gnekow AK, Scheel-Walter HG, Schwabe D, Schilling FH, Benz-Bohm G, Berthold F. Localized infant neuroblastomas often show spontaneous regression: results of the prospective trials NB95-S and NB97. J Clin Oncol. 2008;26:1504–10.
6. Nuchtern JG, London WB, Barnewolt CE, Naranjo A, McGrady PW, Geiger JD, Diller L, Schmidt ML, Maris JM, Cohn SL, Shamberger RC. A prospective study of expectant observation as primary therapy for neuroblastoma in young infants: a Children's Oncology Group study. Ann Surg. 2012;256(4):573–80.
7. Bagatell R, Beck-Popovic M, London WB, Zhang Y, Pearson AD, Matthay KK, Monclair T, Ambros PF, Cohn SL, International Neuroblastoma Risk Group. Significance of MYCN amplification in international neuroblastoma staging system stage 1 and 2 neuroblastoma: a report from the International Neuroblastoma Risk Group database. J Clin Oncol. 2009;27(3):365–70.
8. Pinto NR, Applebaum MA, Volchenboum SL, Matthay KK, London WB, Ambros PF, Nakagawara A, Berthold F, Schleiermacher G, Park JR, Valteau-Couanet D, Pearson AD, Cohn SL. Advances in risk classification and treatment strategies for neuroblastoma. J Clin Oncol. 2015;33(27):3008–17.
9. Rubie H, De Bernardi B, Gerrard M, Canete A, Ladenstein R, Couturier J, Ambros P, Munzer C, Pearson AD, Garaventa A, Brock P, Castel V, Valteau-Couanet D, Holmes K, Di Cataldo A, Brichard B, Mosseri V, Marquez C, Plantaz D, Boni L, Michon J. Excellent outcome with reduced treatment in infants with nonmetastatic and unresectable neuroblastoma without MYCN amplification: results of the prospective INES 99.1. J Clin Oncol. 2011;29:449–55.
10. De Bernardi B, Gerrard M, Boni L, Rubie H, Cañete A, Di Cataldo A, Castel V, Forjaz de Lacerda A, Ladenstein R, Ruud E, Brichard B, Couturier J, Ellershaw C, Munzer C, Bruzzi P, Michon J, Pearson AD. Excellent outcome with reduced treatment for infants with disseminated neuroblastoma without MYCN gene amplification. J Clin Oncol. 2009;27:1034–40.
11. Schleiermacher G, Michon J, Ribeiro A, Pierron G, Mosseri V, Rubie H, Munzer C, Bénard J, Auger N, Combaret V, Janoueix-Lerosey I, Pearson A, Tweddle DA, Bown N, Gerrard M, Wheeler K, Noguera R, Villamon E, Cañete A, Castel V, Marques B, de Lacerda A, Tonini GP, Mazzocco K, Defferrari R, de Bernardi B, di Cataldo A, van Roy N, Brichard B, Ladenstein R, Ambros I, Ambros P, Beiske K, Delattre O, Couturier J. Segmental chromosomal alterations lead to a higher risk of relapse in infants with MYCN-non-amplified localised unresectable/disseminated neuroblastoma (a SIOPEN collaborative study). Br J Cancer. 2011;105:1940–8.
12. Oberthuer A, Juraeva D, Hero B, Volland R, Sterz C, Schmidt R, Faldum A, Kahlert Y, Engesser A, Asgharzadeh S, Seeger R, Ohira M, Nakagawara A, Scaruffi P, Tonini GP, Janoueix-Lerosey I, Delattre O, Schleiermacher G, Vandesompele J, Speleman F, Noguera R, Piqueras M, Bénard J, Valent A, Avigad S, Yaniv I, Grundy RG, Ortmann M, Shao C, Schwab M, Eils R, Simon T, Theissen J, Berthold F, Westermann F, Brors B, Fischer M. Revised risk estimation and treatment stratification of low- and intermediate-risk neuroblastoma patients by integrating clinical and molecular prognostic markers. Clin Cancer Res. 2015;21(8):1904–15.
13. Baker DL, Schmidt ML, Cohn SL, Maris JM, London WB, Buxton A, Stram D, Castleberry RP, Shimada H, Sandler A, Shamberger RC, Look AT, Reynolds CP, Seeger RC, Matthay KK, Children's Oncology Group. Outcome after reduced chemotherapy for intermediate-risk neuroblastoma. N Engl J Med. 2010;363(14):1313–23.
14. Kohler JA, Rubie H, Castel V, Beiske K, Holmes K, Gambini C, Casale F, Munzer C, Erminio G, Parodi S, Navarro S, Marquez C, Peuchmaur M, Cullinane C, Brock P, Valteau-Couanet D, Garaventa A, Haupt R. Treatment of children over the age of one year with unresectable localised neuroblastoma without MYCN amplification: results of the SIOPEN study. Eur J Cancer. 2013;49(17):3671–9.
15. Park JR, Villablanca JG, London WB, Gerbing RB, Haas-Kogan D, Adkins ES, Attiyeh EF, Maris JM, Seeger RC, Reynolds CP, Matthay KK, Children's Oncology Group. Outcome of

high-risk stage 3 neuroblastoma with myeloablative therapy and 13-cis-retinoic acid: a report from the Children's Oncology Group. Pediatr Blood Cancer. 2009;52(1):44–50.
16. Matthay KK, Villablanca JG, Seeger RC, Stram DO, Harris RE, Ramsay NK, Swift P, Shimada H, Black CT, Brodeur GM, Gerbing RB, Reynolds CP. Treatment of high-risk neuroblastoma with intensive chemotherapy, radiotherapy, autologous bone marrow transplantation, and 13-cis-retinoic acid. Children's Cancer Group. N Engl J Med. 1999;341(16):1165–73.
17. Ladenstein R, Pötschger U, ADJ P, Brock P, Luksch R, Castel V, Yaniv I, Papadakis V, Laureys G, Malis J, Balwierz W, Ruud E, Kogner P, Schroeder H, de Lacerda AF, Beck-Popovic M, Bician P, Garami M, Trahair T, Canete A, Ambros PF, Holmes K, Gaze M, Schreier G, Garaventa A, Vassal G, Michon J, Valteau-Couanet D, SIOP Europe Neuroblastoma Group (SIOPEN). Busulfan and melphalan versus carboplatin, etoposide, and melphalan as high-dose chemotherapy for high-risk neuroblastoma (HR-NBL1/SIOPEN): an international, randomised, multi-arm, open-label, phase 3 trial. Lancet Oncol. 2017 Apr;18(4):500–14.
18. Ladenstein R, Weixler S, Baykan B, Bleeke M, Kunert R, Katinger D, Pribill I, Glander P, Bauer S, Pistoia V, Michon J, Garaventa A, Lode HN. Ch14.18 antibody produced in CHO cells in relapsed or refractory Stage 4 neuroblastoma patients: a SIOPEN Phase 1 study. MAbs. 2013;5(5):801–9.
19. Castel V, Segura V, Cañete A. Treatment of high-risk neuroblastoma with anti-GD2 antibodies. Clin Transl Oncol. 2010;12(12):788–93.

High-Risk Neuroblastoma and Current Protocols

12

Katherine K. Matthay and Dominique Valteau-Couanet

12.1 Definition of High-Risk Neuroblastoma

12.1.1 COG

High-risk neuroblastoma comprises nearly half of all neuroblastoma and continues to have a long-term survival of <50%. The first classification of high-risk neuroblastoma defined in North America in the 1980s included children >1 year of age at diagnosis with metastatic neuroblastoma or invasive unresectable tumor crossing the midline [1] with unfavorable histology [2] or elevated ferritin [3]. Similar systems with minor variation were used by the Children's Oncology Group, by St. Jude [4], and by the Pediatric Oncology Group. An international group of clinical and translational investigators then convened to more precisely define stage and response as the International Neuroblastoma Staging System (INSS) [5]. Finally, in a second iteration of international consensus, the International Neuroblastoma Risk Group (INRG) workforce replaced the surgical staging with a system based upon radiological risk factors rather than surgical resectability since surgical resection at diagnosis is rarely used in high-risk neuroblastoma [6]. The combination of INRG staging with age, histological risk factors [7], and molecular features (*MYCN* gene amplification, ploidy, segmental chromosome aberrations) was then analyzed to define subgroups of patients with differing prognoses [8–10]. Thus, the exact definition of high risk has evolved over the past four decades, and the details of risk classification should be kept in mind in any comparison of outcomes in various trials.

K. K. Matthay (✉)
Pediatric Hematology-Oncology, University of California San Francisco School of Medicine and UCSF Benioff Children's Hospital, San Francisco, CA, USA
e-mail: Kate.Matthay@ucsf.edu

D. Valteau-Couanet (✉)
Children and Adolescent Oncology Department, Gustave Roussy, Villejuif Cedex, France
e-mail: Dominique.VALTEAU@gustaveroussy.fr

S. Sarnacki, L. Pio (eds.), *Neuroblastoma*,
https://doi.org/10.1007/978-3-030-18396-7_12

Major factors continue to be metastatic disease (INSS 4; INRG, M) in patients >547 days (18 months), although an intermediate-risk group age 12–18 months with metastatic disease but non-amplified *MYCN* tumors has been identified who should not be included in the high-risk protocols. Any patient with *MYCN* amplified tumors and stage L2, M, or MS regardless of age is high risk [11]. Thus, for current North American cooperative trials in high-risk neuroblastoma, eligibility usually includes (1) all patients with INRG stage M disease and age >547 days or stage M <547 days with tumor *MYCN* amplification (>4 copies relative to reference signal); (2) INRG stage MS with tumor *MYCN* amplification; (3) INRG L2 with *MYCN* amplification; (4) patients >547 days of age initially diagnosed with INRG L1, L2, or MS who progress to stage M without chemotherapy; and (5) patients ≥365 days of age initially diagnosed with *MYCN* amplified INRG stage L1 disease who progress to stage M without systemic therapy (may enroll within 4 weeks of progression to stage M). In prior trials, patients with L2 tumors >547 days and unfavorable histology were also considered high risk, but the current active trial excludes L2 without *MYCN* amplification.

12.1.2 SIOPEN

12.1.2.1 Difference Between North American and SIOPEN Criteria for HR Treatment at Diagnosis and During Treatment

The definition of high-risk patients is based on the rationale described in the North American approach but is slightly different between COG and SIOPEN.

Patients >18 months with INSS stage 4 disease and those with a tumor INSS >1 with *MYCN* amplification are considered as patients with a high-risk disease in both groups. Patients with a stage 4 disease between 12 and 18 months are considered to have a high-risk disease in the SIOPEN group only if segmental abnormalies are displayed in their tumor. In addition, patients with a localized disease are included in high-risk protocols only in case of *MYCN* amplification. Presently, based on the results of the different studies performed during the past 3 decades, the HR-NBL treatment strategy combines four treatment phases: induction chemotherapy aiming to decrease the tumor burden, local treatment combining surgery of the primary tumor and radiotherapy of the primary tumor site, a consolidation phase with high-dose chemotherapy (HDC) ± other myeloablative treatments and autologous stem cell rescue (ASCR), and a maintenance treatment.

The metastatic response evaluated at the end of the induction treatment with a scoring method of the ^{123}I metaiodobenzylguanidine (MIBG) scans has been identified as a pronostic factor on both groups whatever the scoring methods, Curie score, or SIOPEN score used [12, 13].

When in North America, only patients with progressive disease were excluded from the different protocols, in the SIOPEN group, patients had to reach at least a partial response (PR) and less than three skeleton spots on the MIBG scans to receive the HDC and ASCR planned in the HR-NBL1 protocol [14]. In the next HR-NBL2/SIOPEN protocol, the criterium will be metastatic PR and SIOPEN score ≤ 3 on MIBG scans. Patients failing to reach this criterium are currently included either in innovative treatments or treated according to a "very-high-risk protocol."

In the future, one of the tasks of the INRG workforce will be to define additional criteria to identify specific risks that will allow testing early innovative adapted treatments. These criteria could be additonal biological risk criteria identified at diagnosis such as 6q loss [15], ATRX, and TERT [16, 17]. In addition, the best response criteria using MRD (Burchill), and MIBG score will have to be defined as well as the right timing to use them to propose a modified therapeutic approach.

12.2 Evolution of High-Risk Neuroblastoma Therapy

12.2.1 COG

12.2.1.1 Intensive Combination Chemotherapy and Myeloablative Therapy

The 5-year overall survival (OS) probability for patients 0–30 years of age with high-risk neuroblastoma in the era prior to myeloablative therapy was well below 15%. In more recent eras, the 5-year OS has been estimated as 29% (patients diagnosed between 1990 and 1994; n = 356), 34% (patients diagnosed between 1995 and 1999; n = 497), 47% (patients diagnosed between 2000 and 2004; n = 1015), and 50% (patients diagnosed between 2005 and 2010; n = 1484). This increase in overall survival has been attributed to the addition of induction chemotherapy and local control, and the introduction of myeloablative therapy, differentiation therapy, and immunotherapy [18–20].

Most patients presented in the late 1970s with inoperable or metastatic disease, which was uniformly fatal. Cyclophosphamide and vincristine were evaluated, but neither improved survival [21]. Other agents available during the 1970s, including doxorubicin, DTIC, and peptichemio improved the outcome of metastatic disease only in infants <1 year of age, while epipodophyllotoxins and CDDP were shown to produce tumor responses in patients with neuroblastoma [22, 23]. By the early 1990s, the role of combination chemotherapy with increasing dose intensity came into use, yielding response rates after 5–6 months of induction of 70–80% [24–28]. The COG initially adopted the intensive induction chemotherapy N7 piloted at Memorial Sloan Kettering [29], but then piloted the substitution of two cycles of pharmacokinetically guided topotecan/cyclophosphamide which was more tolerable than the very-high-dose cyclophosphamide with continuous vincristine and one of the cisplatin cycles, and incorporated this into the ANBL0532 phase III study [30]. Local control was generally achieved during or at the end of induction therapy with delayed surgical resection and radiation of the tumor bed, shown to decrease local relapse [31, 32].

In order to further increase dose intensity, the concept of very-high-dose chemotherapy or chemoradiotherapy was proposed, with hematopoietic cell reconstitution, either with autologous or allogeneic bone marrow or later with autologous peripheral blood stem cells. Therefore, initially, three pilot single arm trials were done in North America Children's Cancer Group suggesting feasibility of both allogeneic bone marrow transplant and autologous bone marrow transplant with conditioning with etoposide, cisplatin, melphalan, and total body radiation. The autologous bone marrow had reduction of potential residual tumor with immunomagnetic purging [33]. Relapse rate was actually apparently higher for the allogeneic group, and there was greater toxicity, leading to a general disinterest in allogeneic approach. A comparison was then done between two concurrent CCG studies using identical induction therapy and different consolidations: one with autologous purged bone marrow transplant (321P3) and the other with continuation of standard dose chemotherapy (321P2). Using Cox regression analysis, the relative risk (RR) of an event after chemoradiotherapy/ABMT was estimated to be 58% of that for patients who continued chemotherapy ($p = 0.01$). Similarly, Kaplan–Meier analysis estimated EFS at 4 years for the chemoradiotherapy/ABMT and chemotherapy groups to be 40% and 19%, respectively ($p = 0.019$) [34].

Based on these pilot trials showing apparent improvement in EFS with the use of myeloablative therapy, the CCG undertook a randomized trial comparing myeloablative therapy with carboplatin, etoposide, melphalan, and TBI to an intensive non-myeloablative consolidation with cisplatin, doxorubicin, ifosfamide, and etoposide. Both the early and 5-year follow-up showed a significantly higher EFS with the autologous transplant arm but no significant difference in OS. The superiority of myeloablative therapy to standard chemotherapy was further validated by two European randomized trials [35, 36]. To further capitalize on this advantage, and to eliminate the TBI portion of the conditioning, known to be associated with acute and late toxicity, a pilot trial showed a similar disease outcome using higher doses of carboplatin, etoposide, and melphalan (CEM) without the TBI [37]. Therefore, the COG undertook a randomized trial that eliminated TBI and tested whether the use of purged PBSC would improve outcome [38]. The results showed no improvement with purging of PBSC and showed a similar outcome to prior trials with TBI.

Therefore, the next group of trials proceeded to further test myeloablative therapy by using a tandem ASCT. Pilot trials both separately and in the COG showed the feasibility and favorable outcomes [25, 39–41], so a randomized trial comparing tandem transplant with thiotepa/cyclophosphamide followed 6 weeks later by CEM was compared to a single CEM transplant. The results showed a significant improvement in 3-year EFS and OS, as reported at the ASCO meeting in 2016 (Table 12.1) [42].

Due to the results of the SIOPEN trial which showed a significantly better outcome for patients randomized to conditioning with busulfan and melphalan (Bu-Mel) compared to CEM [14], a COG pilot trial was recently completed to gain further results in North America with this regimen (ANBL12P1, Table 12.1). This trial also showed the ability to test for tumor ALK mutations and amplifications in real time, in order to later incorporate ALK inhibitors into therapy of newly diagnosed patients. The COG also decided to try to improve the response to induction by testing the addition of a targeted radiotherapy with ^{131}I-metaiodobenzylguandine (^{131}I-MIBG). Despite intensification of induction chemotherapy for metastatic

Table 12.1 Completed cooperative group trials in North America for newly diagnosed high-risk neuroblastoma

Trial/Ref.	Group	Years	Primary aim	EFS (years)	OS (years)
321P1/P2/P3 [33, 34]	CCG	1985–1994	Comparison of allogeneic to autologous BMT and to chemotherapy	25/40/19% 4-year	NR
P9341/41/42 [28]	POG	1993–1995	Phase II window, multi-agent induction, myeloablative therapy	27% 7-year	29%
3891 [27]	CCG	1991–1996	Randomized trial of autologous BMT vs. chemotherapy	30 vs. 19% 5-year	39 vs. 30% 5-year
3891 [27, 50]	CCG	1991–1996	Randomized trial of MRD therapy with 13-cis-RA vs. none	42 vs. 31% 5-year	50 vs. 39% 5-year
A3973 [38]	COG	2001–2006	Randomized trial of purged vs. unpurged ASCT	40 vs. 36% 5-year	50 vs. 51% 5-year
ANBL00P1 [41]	COG	2001–2004	Pilot study of tandem ASCT	45% 3-year	59% 3-year
ANBL0032 [56]	COG	2001–2009	Randomized trial of MRD therapy with 13-cis-RA vs. ch14.18 + cytokines	66 vs. 46% 2-year	86 vs. 75% 2-year
ANBL0931	COG	2009–2011	Further safety study of ch14.18 + cytokines	NR	NR
ANBL09P1	COG	2010–2016	Feasibility trial of adding ^{131}I-MIBG at end of induction prior to ASCT	74% 1-year	NR
ANBL12P1	COG	2013–2015	Pilot trial of induction + Bu–Mel ASCT	NR	NR
ANBL0532 [42]	COG	2007–2012	Randomized trial of tandem vs. single ASCT	62 vs. 49% 3-year	74 vs. 69% 3-year

Abbreviations: *BMT* bone marrow transplant, *MRD* minimal residual disease, *13-cis-RA* 13-cis-retinoic acid (isotretinoin), *NR* not yet reported, *ASCT* autologous stem cell transplant, *Bu–Mel* busulfan–melphalan conditioning

high-risk neuroblastoma over the past three decades, 15–20% of patients will not achieve a complete or partial response. ^{131}I-MIBG has shown promise in the treatment of relapsed and refractory neuroblastoma, with 30–40% responses [43, 44]. Therefore, another pilot trial, ANBL09P1, tested the addition of ^{131}I-MIBG therapy at the end of induction followed by consolidation with Bu–Mel. This trial showed that incorporating ^{131}I-MIBG therapy into a multi-institution induction regimen was feasible and tolerable in preparation for a phase III randomized trial, ANBL1531.

The new ANBL1531 trial activated in May 2018 has the aims of testing in a randomized trial whether ^{131}I-MIBG given after cycle 3 of an induction that includes five cycles of chemotherapy will improve outcome in patients compared to chemotherapy induction without ^{131}I-MIBG. Patients on both arms will receive consolidation with tandem transplant, followed by standard maintenance with immunotherapy and isotretinoin. A third arm will incorporate the ^{131}I-MIBG into induction but use a single Bu–Mel transplant as consolidation followed by standard maintenance as above. There will be two non-randomized arms, one for patients with ALK aberration who will receive crizotinib throughout the therapy and otherwise receive the standard five-cycle induction chemotherapy, and tandem myeloablative consolidation and maintenance. The other non-randomized arm is for patients whose tumors do not take up MIBG and who do not have an ALK aberration. They will receive standard induction, tandem consolidation, and maintenance. A pilot trial in newly diagnosed patients with high-risk neuroblastoma combining anti-GD2 antibody with induction chemotherapy is planned to open this year, based upon data from a St. Jude clinical trial [45].

12.2.1.2 Therapy for Minimal Residual Disease

Approximately 30–50% of patients will relapse despite induction chemotherapy, surgery, radiation, and myeloablative therapy. Therefore, investigations have increasingly focused on detection of minimal residual disease and on ways to eliminate minimal residual disease (MRD). Currently, MRD testing in the COG uses both pathology of bilateral bone marrow and is studying bone marrow and blood samples with a 5-gene TaqMan low-density array, shown to correlate with outcome in relapsed patients [46]. ^{123}I-MIBG scans are another important test for MRD, as any positivity on an MIBG scan at the end of induction or after myeloablative therapy portends a worse outcome [47].

One of the early attempts to treat MRD involved the use of isotretinoin, a drug known to induce differentiation of neuroblastoma cells in vitro. Since this is a relatively non-toxic oral drug with established in vitro activity at concentrations >5–10 μM, the CCG tested isotretinoin in a high-dose interrupted schedule of 160 mg/m^2/day for 14 days followed by a 14-day rest for six cycles [48, 49]. Patients who were progression-free after myeloablative therapy or after intensive chemotherapy consolidation on the CCG-3891 trial were randomized to receive isotretinoin or no further therapy. The EFS for the isotretinoin arm was significantly better than no further therapy, and a post hoc analysis also showed the greatest benefit was seen in patients who received isotretinoin after myeloablative therapy (Table 12.1) [27, 50]. The small number of patients who had measurable disease at the time of randomization did not benefit, suggesting that this agent was only effective in MRD.

Meanwhile, phase I and II studies with anti-GD2 antibodies showed promising activity in relapsed neuroblastoma, since the GD2 ganglioside is widely expressed on the surface of most neuroblastoma tumors [51–54]. The next phase III study to test an MRD agent, therefore, added the chimeric form of the anti-GD2 monoclonal antibody (ch14.18) along with two cytokines to improve the ADCC response (GM-CSF) and stimulate natural killer cells (IL-2) [55]. The study randomized patients with evidence of progressive disease after myeloablative therapy and local radiation to receive isotretinoin alone or isotretinoin interspersed with five cycles of ch14.18 with GM-CSF or IL-2 alternating with each antibody course (Table 12.1) [56]. The study was closed earlier than planned, as the results were highly significant after 2 years favoring the antibody arm. The 2-year EFS for the ch14.18/cytokine arm was 66% compared to 46% for the isotretinoin alone ($p = 0{,}01$), and the OS was 86% vs. 75% ($p = 0.02$) [56]. Further studies are ongoing to investigate the safety of this agent, recently approved for neuroblastoma by the FDA.

12.2.1.3 Relapse Therapy

Table 12.2 details the phase II studies of particular interest for neuroblastoma since the 1990s in cooperative groups in North America, which tested newer chemotherapy, radiopharmaceutical therapy with MIBG, immunotherapy, and small-molecule inhibitors. The chemotherapy trials showed the activity of camptothecins alone and topotecan combined with cyclophosphamide [57], and irinotecan combined with temozolomide [58], although for the latter it has not been shown whether the irinotecan adds activity to the combination, since a small phase II study of temozolomide alone in Europe showed a 20% response rate [59]. Nonetheless, the combination of irinotecan with temozolomide and the combination of topotecan with cyclophosphamide has become the backbone for addition of other agents to enhance response. Multiple other COG phase II novel chemotherapy trials for solid tumors have not shown significant single activity in neuroblastoma to date, including paclitaxel, ABT-751 [60], rebeccamycin [61], oxaliplatin [62], navelbine [63], taxotere [64], pemetrexed [65], and ixabepilone [66].

^{131}I-MIBG has been a long-standing active therapy for relapsed neuroblastoma with 30–40% responses in single institution and in NANT consortium trials, alone and in combination [43, 44]. However, only recently, the increasing number of institutions capable of safely administering and monitoring this radioactive drug to young children has been brought into up-front trials, as discussed above. A phase II trial in NANT (N1101) has focused on testing in a randomized "pick-the-winner" strategy on testing two combination therapies, vorinostat (HDAC inhibitor) vs. irinotecan (radiosensitizer) that were promising in phase I setting and comparing these to MIBG alone [67–69]. An upcoming NANT trial will test the combination of dinutuximab with MIBG.

Targeted inhibitors of interest in neuroblastoma have also been tested as single agents in phase II COG trials. Two of particular interest targeting pathways in neuroblastoma were the aurora kinase A inhibitor, MLN8237 (alisertib), and the *ALK* inhibitor crizotinib. Aurora kinase A stabilizes *MYCN*, and therefore, inhibition increases degradation of *MYCN*, an important oncogene amplified in 30–40% of high-risk neuroblastoma. Although no responses were seen with a single agent, a combination of alisertib with irinotecan and temozolomide in preclinical studies and a phase I and phase II New Approaches to Neuroblastoma Therapy (NANT) trial elicited a significant number of responses [70, 71]. Crizotinib targets *ALK* mutations, found in up to 15% of neuroblastoma. In a phase I trial, this was very active against anaplastic large cell lymphoma (ALCL) and IMRT, where there is a translocation, but showed one response in neuroblastoma, with a phase II trial ongoing as a single agent and combined with chemotherapy [72]. Newer *ALK* inhibitors

Table 12.2 Recent cooperative phase II single agent studies in relapsed and refractory neuroblastoma

Trial	Group	Years	Drug	Target/mechanism	Responses in NB (CR + PR)
P9340 [26]	POG	1993–1995	Paclitaxel, topo, topo/cyclo in up-front phase II window	Mitotic inhibitor topoisomerase I Alkylation	Topo, 67%; topo-cyclo, 76%; paclitaxel, 25%
P9462 [57]	POG/ CCG	1996–2001	Topotecan vs. topo/cyclo	Topoisomerase I	Topo/cyclo, 32% Cyclo, 19%
9962 [64]	CCG	1997–2001	Taxotere	Inhibits microtubule polymerization	0/9
A09705 [63]	CCG	1998–2001	Navelbine	Inhibits microtubule polymerization	0/6
P9963 [61]	POG	2000–2004	Rebeccamycin	Topoisomerase I and II	1/8
ANBL0321 [78]	COG	2003–2004	Capsular fenretinide	Retinoic acid receptors; apoptotic properties	1/62 (SD, 13/62)
ADVL0421 [62]	COG	2004–2005	Oxaliplatin	DNA adducts block replication	0/10
ANBL0322 [75]	COG	2005–2007	Hu14.18-IL2 immunocytokine	GD2 and NK cells	5/36 (all responses in pts. with bone/BM only)
N2004-04 [74]	NANT	2005–2014	Fenretinide (4HPR-LXS) lipid complex	Retinoic acid receptors; apoptotic properties	Phase I: 4/29 (in BM only) Phase II NR
ANBL0421 [58]	COG	2006–2008	Irinotecan + temozolomide	Topoisomerase I DNA hypermethylation, alkylating agent	8/55
ADVL0524 [66]	COG	2006–2007	Ixabepilone	Microtubule stabilizing agent	0/10
ANBL0621 [60]	COG	2007–2009	ABT-751	Binds the colchicine site of beta-tubulin, inhibits microtubule polymerization	6/91 (TTP 42 days, similar to control)

Trial	Group	Years	Drug	Target/mechanism	Responses in NB (CR + PR)
ADVL0525 [65]	COG	2007–2009	Pemetrexed	Folate antimetabolite	0/10
ADVL0821 [79]	COG	2009–2012	IMC-A12 (cixutumumab)	IGFR-1	4/30 (all in BM/bone)
ADVL0921 [71]	COG	2011–2013	MLN8237 (alisertib)	Aurora kinase A	Phase I: 0/11 Phase II NR
ADVL0912 [80]	COG	2009–2015	Crizotinib	ALK mutations and translocations	Phase I: 1/11 Phase II: NR
ANBL1021	COG	2011–2012	Hu14.18-IL2 + isotretinoin	GD2, NK, retinoic acid receptor	Feasibility trial; NR
ADVL1522	COG	2015–2016	Lorvotuzumab	CD56 antibody linked to maytansinoid (DMI)	NR

Abbreviations used: *POG* Pediatric Oncology Group, *COG* Children's Oncology Group, *CCG* Children's Cancer Group, *NANT* New Approaches to Neuroblastoma Therapy consortium, *topo* topotecan, *cyclo* cyclophosphamide, *PR* partial response, *CR* complete response, *BM* bone marrow, *TTP* time to progression, *NR* not reported may be more effective in overcoming resistant mutations, with ongoing phase I trials [73]. Fenretinide was also of interest from preclinical studies and the MRD success of isotretinoin. Although the results with the capsular formulation were disappointing, much higher plasma levels and some bone marrow responses were seen in a NANT trial with a new oral suspension of a lipid complex formulation, 4HPR-LXS [74]. However, to date, this agent does not have a clear path to approval. Future investigations will test combinations of inhibitors targeting molecular pathways in neuroblastoma as well as combinations with chemotherapy.

Immunotherapy trials based on targeting the GD2 ganglioside have been a major focus to capitalize on the prior phase I and II trials of ch14.18 and the positive results in MRD on ANBL0032. There have been responses using an immunocytokine, Hu14.18-IL2, although mainly in bone and bone marrow sites, rather than bulky soft tissue measurable disease [75]. The most impressive results to date in relapsed neuroblastoma have been with the combination of ch14.18 (dinutuximab) with irinotecan and temozolomide in the recent phase II randomized trial of this combination compared to irinotecan/temozolomide with temsirolimus (an mTOR inhibitor) [76]. In this phase II randomized trial, 9/17 patients on the arm with dinutuximab had CR or PR, including some with prior exposure to dinutuximab or to the same chemotherapy. Only 1/18 on the temsirolimus arm responded. As reported by abstract this year (ANR2018; abstract #339), in the expansion of the phase II study, the impressive response rate of 40% continues to be seen in patients with first relapse/refractory neuroblastoma, although the mechanism of this synergy has not been elucidated. This success has led to the incorporation of dinutuximab into induction therapy in a new pilot COG trial opening this year. There are also ongoing phase I and II investigations into GD2 vaccine therapy for neuroblastoma [77], NK cell infusions, and COG trials testing the PD1/PDL1 inhibitors, but these are too early for definitive results.

12.2.2 SIOPEN

12.2.2.1 HR-NBL1 Rationale and Different Steps

The first SIOPEN/HR-NBL protocol opened in 2002 and was designed taking into account the national expertise of the 18 participating countries.

Different questions have been sequentially asked.

Induction Chemotherapy

The first randomized study conducted by the European Neuroblastoma Study Group (ENSG), between 1990 and 1999 (ENSG5), investigated the effect of dose intensity of induction therapy on EFS in patients over the age of 1 year with metastatic disease. Patients ($n = 262$) were randomized to receive either COJEC (rapid) or OPEC/OJEC (standard) induction regimens [81]. Each regimen utilized the same drugs—cisplatin, carboplatin, etoposide, cyclophosphamide, and vincristine—at the same dose, but the dose intensity (in mg/m^2 per week) of COJEC was 1.8-fold higher. Therapy in the COJEC arm was administered every 10 days, regardless of hematological recovery, while it was delivered every 21 days in the OPEC/OJEC arm, dependent on hematological recovery. Complete (CR) and very good partial (VGPR) responses were achieved in 53% patients assigned to standard treatment and in 74% patients assigned to COJEC treatment ($p = 0.002$).

The intensified regimen (RAPID COJEC) was therefore adopted as the "standard" induction regimen for the SIOPEN/HR-NBL1 trial and was administered to all patients recruited to the trial between 2002 and 2013. The addition of granulocyte colony–stimulating factor (G-CSF) to COJEC induction was randomized (R0), showing a significantly reduced toxicity profile when G-CSF was used [82].

From April 2007 to October 2009, 65 patients with metastatic HR-NBL who had not achieved the SIOPEN criteria for HDC after induction received two courses of topotecan 1.5 mg/m^2/day for 5 days, followed by a 48-h infusion of vincristine, 2 mg/m^2, and doxorubicin, 45 mg/m^2 (TVD). Following two courses of TVD, four (6.4%) patients had an overall CR, while 23 patients achieved the metastatic criteria to receive HDC [83]. Two courses of TVD were then proposed for patients with an insufficient metastatic response.

In 2013, a randomization (R3) was introduced to compare the standard SIOPEN induction regimen RAPID COJEC with the modified N7 regimen [29, 84, 85], developed in North America. This intensive induction chemotherapy regimen combined initially seven courses and then five courses of two putatively non-cross-resistant drug combinations: high-dose cyclophosphamide plus doxorubicin/vincristine (CAV) and high-dose cisplatin/etoposide (P/E). The initial results reported by the Memorial Sloan Kettering Cancer Center (MSKCC) (overall CR/VGPR of 83%) have not been replicated by two randomized studies conducted by the French (SFOP) and Austrian neuroblastoma groups, although both groups reported that patients achieving CR have higher long-term EFS [86–88]. The primary aim of the R3 randomization was to compare metastatic response rates and event-free survival (EFS) of both arms. The results of this randomization showed no difference in terms of survival and metastatic response rates between the two arms (Garaventa, ANR 2018). RAPID COJEC having less acute toxicity than the modified N7 has been selected to be the SIOPEN reference induction regimen.

Consolidation Phase

HDC followed by ASCR has improved outcomes in patients with HR-NBL in European and North America randomized trials, becoming the standard of care for these patients [27, 35, 36].

Busulfan–melphalan (Bu-Mel) was the conditioning regimen mainly used in Europe basing on results showing a significant advantage of Bu-Mel in patients with high-risk neuroblastoma [89]. The long-term results of this single institution cohort of patients with HR-NBL treated with HD Bu-containing regimens confirmed the good results of this regimen, with 5-year EFS and OS rates of 35% and 40%, respectively [90].

These data provided the rationale to widely implement the use of Bu-Mel, which was then compared with CEM in the HR-NBL1/SIOPEN randomized trial (R1). Of the 1577 patients with HR-NBL, 563 were randomly assigned in a 1:1 ratio to either Bu-Mel or CEM following rapid induction therapy with COJEC. The trial was stopped because a prespecified interim analysis showed a 49% EFS rate with Bu-Mel vs 33% for CEM ($p < 0.001$) [14]. The 3-year OS was 60% with Bu-Mel vs 48% for CEM ($p = 0.003$), and the rate of relapse or progression was significantly lower in the Bu-Mel group (47% vs 60%; $p < 0.001$). The rate of acute toxic death was 3% for Bu-Mel and 5% for CEM, and severe toxicity was not significantly different in the two arms. Therefore, HD Bu-Mel has now become the standard HD regimen in the SIOPEN HR strategy.

Local Treatment

Surgery aimed to achieve complete primary tumor excision, to improve local control as shown in the analysis of the SIOPEN cohort (K Holmes submitted). Usually performed prior to HDC, it could be postponed in case of surgical risk factors. Radiotherapy was performed at the dose of 21-Gy radiotherapy on the presurgical primary tumor volume to all patients as a standard dose regardless of the disease extent and the quality of surgery.

Maintenance

Based on the CCG results [27], retinoic acid (13-cis-RA) maintenance was administered with the same dose and schedule in HR-NBL1. In addition, SIOPEN developed dinutuximab beta, the ch14/18/CHO antibody, in several successive trials since 2009. The benefit of IL-2 given in addition to dinutuximab beta was investigated in a prospective phase III trial [91]. Four hundred and six patients were randomized (R2) to receive five cycles of dinutuximab beta (100 mg/m^2/cycle as five daily 8-h infusions) or in combination with IL-2 (6×10^6 IU/m^2 on days 1–5 and 8–12 of each cycle). Outcomes were favorable compared to historical controls (13-cis-RA alone as maintenance treatment), but no survival benefit was found with the addition of IL-2 with a significantly increased toxicity in the combination arm. The long-term infusion (LTI) study was designed as a phase I/II dose-finding study administering continuous infusion dinutuximab beta over 10 days (100 mg/m^2/cycle) in patients with relapsed/refractory neuroblastoma with the objective of determining a tolerable treatment schedule, while maintaining satisfactory immunomodulatory efficacy. The 10-day continuous infusion schedule combined with IL-2 at a dose of 6×10^6 IU/m^2/day was found to be tolerable (HN [92]). The protocol met the primary efficacy endpoint. With the improved tolerance and favorable immunomodulatory effects of the LTI schedule demonstrated in the LTI study, SIOPEN elected to adopt the LTI schedule into the HR-NBL1 trial and to randomize a decreased dose of IL-2 (R4) to clarify whether there is a benefit to adding IL-2 to dinutuximab beta.

12.2.2.2 Very-High-Risk (VHR) Strategy: Veritas

A SIOPEN protocol, Veritas (EudraCT N°: 2015-003130-27), has been designed for patients with a poor response at the end of induction, defined as less of metastatic PR or a MIBG SIOPEN score >3, identified to have a low survival with a 3-year survival of 15% with the ongoing HR protocols. Tandem HDC with thiotepa and Bu-Mel has been demonstrated in a single institution cohort of 26 VHR patients to improve the survival with a 3-year EFS of 36% [93]. Topotecan is a topoisomerase I inhibitor which has activity against neuroblastoma and it is a radiosensitizer. There is evidence from laboratory studies that the combination of ^{131}I-mIBG and topotecan is synergistic when topotecan is given simultaneously or secondarily to ^{131}I-mIBG [94].The combination of topotecan with ^{131}I-mIBG, secondarily supported by peripheral blood stem cell transplantation, has been demonstrated to be a feasible treatment in both patients with relapsed, heavily pretreated neuroblastoma, and also in patients with primary refractory high-risk disease [94, 95]. The toxicity of a second course of Bu-Mel administered 2 months after a first course of topotecan-^{131}I-mIBG and ASCR is acceptable [96].

The main objective of the Veritas randomized study is to evaluate the efficacy of two intensified consolidation strategies, a tandem HDC with a first course of thiotepa (900 mg/m^2) or topotecan/^{131}I-mIBG followed by ASCR. In both arms, in the absence of disease progression, patients will receive a second course of Bu-Mel with ASCR.

GPOH

From the very first GPOH NB79 trial on high-risk neuroblastoma that was initiated in 1979, multiple chemotherapy regimens have been evaluated by the German cooperative group. The NB79 induction chemotherapy consisted of three ACVD cycles (doxorubicin, cyclophosphamide, vincristine, and dacarbazine) followed by 5 AC cycles (doxorubicin and cyclophosphamide). In the subsequent NB82 trial, a total number of ten alternating chemotherapy cycles, ACVD and PCVm (cisplatin, cyclophosphamide, and etoposide), was scheduled. In the NB85 trial, the combination of ifosfamide and etoposide was introduced (IVp). It consisted of nine chemotherapy cycles by repeating the sequence IVp, ACVD, PCVm three times. After three chemotherapy cycles, the objective response rate was 89% (12% complete response, 77% partial response) but with an increased toxic death rate of 8.6%. The 5-year EFS rate of the NB85 trial was 14% [97, 98]. In the NB90 trial, short infusions of cytotoxic drugs were substituted by continuous infusions aiming to increase efficacy. Further, the cytotoxic drugs were rearranged into two different cycles referred to as N1 (cisplatin, etoposide, and vindesine) and N2 (ifosfamide, vincristine, dacarbazine, and doxorubicin). Among the 230 evaluable patients, the complete and partial remission rate was 31% and 44% after four cycles, and 58% and 11% after eight cycles, respectively. The toxic death rate was 5.1%. The 5-year EFS rate of all patients treated in NB90 was 27% [98]. The improvement of the outcome of patients with HR-NBL was mostly related to the evolution of induction chemotherapy since only a limited number of patients underwent consolidation by HDC and ASCR. In the NB97 trial, the NB90 induction chemotherapy was modified to decrease toxicity, with lower etoposide dose, shorter doxorubicin infusion time, and reduced number of chemotherapy cycles from 8 to 6. The modified chemotherapy cycles were referred to as N5 (cisplatin, etoposide, and vindesine) and N6 (ifosfamide, vincristine, dacarbazine, and doxorubicin). The response rate at the end of the NB97 induction chemotherapy was maintained and the toxic death rate during induction chemotherapy decreased to 0.6% [35].

The GPOH NB2004-HR trial was opened between 2004 and 2016. Patients with HR-NBL were either randomized for standard induction chemotherapy identical to the NB97 trial or experimental induction chemotherapy having two additional topotecan-containing cycles (cyclophosphamide, topotecan, and etoposide—N8). Topotecan-containing chemotherapy was chosen because of its proven efficacy in previous phase II trials [26, 99, 100]. Preliminary data from NB2004-HR trial were extracted for the design of HR-NBL2 trial. In this data cutoff (October 2017), complete metastatic response rate at the end of induction was 40% and 3-year EFS was 36%. Of note, most of the patients received HD melphalan–etoposide–carboplatin (MEC) and had no immunotherapy.

12.2.2.3 Next Steps

HR-NBL2/SIOPEN

GPOH has joined SIOPEN. The design of the next SIOPEN study aims to answer three questions on the induction chemotherapy, the consolidation phase, and the local treatment. Patients will receive a maintenance treatment with six courses of retinoic acid and five courses of dinutuximab beta. The combination with IL2 will depend on the HR-NBL1/R4 results. As the metastatic response has been identified as a major prognostic factor, the first randomization will compare the response rate and 3-year EFS of two induction protocols, rapid COJEC, and the GPOH one. The second randomization will evaluate the impact of an intensified consolidation in standard HR neuroblastoma comparing Bu-Mel with the tandem HDC, thiotepa/Bu-Mel. In case of persistent macroscopic residual primary tumor, the dose of radiotherapy on the tumor bed will be randomized (R-RTx) between 21 Gy and 21 Gy plus a boost of 15 Gy on the residual disease (up to 36 Gy). In case of no macroscopic residual tumor, radiotherapy at 21 Gy will be performed at the preoperative tumor bed.

The tumor ALK status will be evaluated prospectively but no specific treatment will be added in case of ALK aberration.

Pilot Studies

Evidence of the feasibility and the efficacy of the combination of immunotherapy with chemotherapy has been demonstrated both in relapse patients [76] and at diagnosis [101]. SIOPEN is currently designing pilot studies to define the best schedule to combine long-term infusion of dinutuximab beta with the two regimens used in the SIOPEN group, the GPOH, and the rapid COJEC induction chemotherapies. The defined schedule will be compared in the future with chemotherapy alone to evaluate the impact of a combined immunotherapy on the metastatic response rate and survival.

12.2.2.4 Relapse Strategy

Based on the results of a phase I study on the combination of topotecan and temozolomide (TOTEM) in pediatric tumors [102] ITCC (Innovative Therapies for Children with Cancer) conducted a single arm phase II trial of TOTEM in patients with a refractory or relapsed neuroblastoma, the response rate was 24% with a 12-month progression free survival of 45% with an acceptable toxicity profile [103].

A phase II COG study displayed a 19% objective response in 55 patients with a relapsed or refractory neuroblastoma [58]. Bevacizumab improved delivery and efficacy of chemotherapy in neuroblastoma models and treatment with bevacizumab alone [104] or combined with topotecan decreased tumor growth in neuroblastoma xenografts [105]. The combination of bevacizumab and topotecan showed enhanced preclinical activity.

Based on these results, ITCC designed an ongoing randomized study with six arms, the BEACON protocol comparing the efficacy of temozolomide, TOTEM, and irinotecan–temozolomide alone or in combination with bevacizumab. The next step will compare the best arm to the combination of the best chemotherapy with dinutuximab beta.

The GPOH is currently conducting a randomized study in refractory/relapsed neuroblastoma patients comparing the combination of irinotecan–temozolomide with or without dasatinib and rapamycin (RIST-rNB 2011 trial) [106].

Different programs of precision medicine are currently conducted in the ITCC centers—MAPPYACTS in France, Italy, Spain, and Israel, INFORM in Germany, and iTHER in the Netherlands. A tumor biopsy is performed at relapse with a genetic analysis (whole exome sequencing, RNA sequencing). Data interpretation is discussed in a molecular tumor board between biologists, bio-informaticians, and pediatric oncologists to identify actionable targets. The treatment is then discussed in a clinical molecular board to define a treatment according to the identified targets with access to either phase I/II protocols or linked in the MAPPYACTS program to the ESMART (European Proof-of-Concept Therapeutic Stratification of Molecular Anomalies in Relapsed Refractory Tumors in children) multi-arm trial with currently eight and soon ten arms combining either targeted drugs, immunotherapy, or chemotherapy.

The Neuroblastoma New Drug Development Strategy (NDDS) has established a group with expertise in drug development, prioritized targets, and drugs according to tumor biology (target expression, dependency, preclinical data; potential combinations; biomarkers), identifying as priority targets ALK, MEK, CDK4/6, MDM2, MYCN (druggable by BET bromodomain, aurora kinase, mTORC1/2), BIRC5, and checkpoint kinase 1 and promoted clinical trials with target-prioritized drugs. Drugs showing activity can be rapidly transitioned via parallel randomized trials into frontline studies. The objective of this approach is to accelerate development of neuroblastoma drugs [107].

The potential benefits of haploidentical stem cell transplantation has been explored in Germany in refractory relapsed patients with a disease controlled by a previous relapse treatment [108].

A phase I study of ^{131}I MIBG followed by nivolumab and dinutuximab beta antibody in children with relapsed/refractory neuroblastoma is proposed in some European centers (MiNiVan study). The rationale is to combine the direct cytotoxic effect of the anti-GD2 antibody with immunomodulatory effects of anti-PD1 in addition to the depletion of T regulator lymphocytes and direct tumor cell killing by

^{131}I MIBG. GD2-targeting CAR T cells is evaluated in preclinical models and early development trials [109].

A working group linking representatives from SIOPEN, NDDSand ITCC) is working to identify new drugs to be administered in very-high-risk patients and to define the best strategy that could allow to cure high-risk neuroblastoma patients after relapse.

12.3 Conclusion

In summary, the current standard North American and European approach to therapy of high-risk neuroblastoma involves an intensive induction therapy with local control using surgery and radiation, a consolidation phase with single or tandem HDC and autologous transplant, and differentiating and immunotherapy for MRD. Future improvements will depend on more extensive tumor molecular profiling at diagnosis and relapse, improvement of the quality of response using immunotherapy or other targeted therapy such as tyrosine kinase inhibitors or ^{131}I-MIBG, and further improvements of the MRD therapy with more targeted small molecules, guided by more precise methods of ascertaining the patients at higher risk of relapse with MRD assays and their molecular profile. Complementary approaches are currently developed and shared to improve survival of these patients with HR neuroblastoma.

References

1. Evans AE, D'Angio GJ, Randolph J. A proposed staging for children with neuroblastoma. Children's Cancer Study Group A. Cancer. 1971;27:374–8.
2. Shimada H, Chatten J, Newton WA Jr, Sachs N, Hamoudi AB, Chiba T, Marsden HB, Misugi K. Histopathologic prognostic factors in neuroblastic tumors: definition of subtypes of ganglioneuroblastoma and an age-linked classification of neuroblastomas. J Natl Cancer Inst. 1984;73:405–16.
3. Hann HW, Evans AE, Siegel SE, Wong KY, Sather H, Dalton A, Hammond D, Seeger RC. Prognostic importance of serum ferritin in patients with stages III and IV neuroblastoma: the Childrens Cancer Study Group experience. Cancer Res. 1985;45:2843–8.
4. Evans AE, D'Angio GJ, Sather HN, de Lorimier AA, Dalton A, Ungerleider RS, Finklestein JZ, Hammond GD. A comparison of four staging systems for localized and regional neuroblastoma: a report from the Childrens Cancer Study Group. J Clin Oncol. 1990;8:678–88.
5. Brodeur GM, Pritchard J, Berthold F, Carlsen NL, Castel V, Castelberry RP, De Bernardi B, Evans AE, Favrot M, Hedborg F, et al. Revisions of the international criteria for neuroblastoma diagnosis, staging, and response to treatment [see comments]. J Clin Oncol. 1993;11:1466–77.
6. Monclair T, Brodeur GM, Ambros PF, Brisse HJ, Cecchetto G, Holmes K, Kaneko M, London WB, Matthay KK, Nuchtern JG, et al. The International Neuroblastoma Risk Group (INRG) staging system: an INRG Task Force report. J Clin Oncol. 2009;27:298–303.
7. Shimada H, Ambros IM, Dehner LP, Hata J, Joshi VV, Roald B, Stram DO, Gerbing RB, Lukens JN, Matthay KK, et al. The International Neuroblastoma Pathology Classification (the Shimada system). Cancer. 1999;86:364–72.
8. Ambros PF, Ambros IM, Brodeur GM, Haber M, Khan J, Nakagawara A, Schleiermacher G, Speleman F, Spitz R, London WB, et al. International consensus for neuroblastoma

molecular diagnostics: report from the International Neuroblastoma Risk Group (INRG) Biology Committee. Br J Cancer. 2009;100:1471–82.
9. Cohn SL, Pearson AD, London WB, Monclair T, Ambros PF, Brodeur GM, Faldum A, Hero B, Iehara T, Machin D, et al. The International Neuroblastoma Risk Group (INRG) classification system: an INRG Task Force report. J Clin Oncol. 2009;27:289–97.
10. Schleiermacher G, Janoueix-Lerosey I, Ribeiro A, Klijanienko J, Couturier J, Pierron G, Mosseri V, Valent A, Auger N, Plantaz D, et al. Accumulation of segmental alterations determines progression in neuroblastoma. J Clin Oncol. 2010;28:3122–30.
11. Seeger RC, Brodeur GM, Sather H, Dalton A, Siegel SE, Wong KY, Hammond D. Association of multiple copies of the N-myc oncogene with rapid progression of neuroblastomas. N Engl J Med. 1985;313:1111–6.
12. Ladenstein R, Lambert B, Pötschger U, Castellani M-R, Lewington V, Bar-Sever Z, Oudoux A, Śliwińska A, Taborska K, Biassoni L, et al. Validation of the mIBG skeletal SIOPEN scoring method in two independent high-risk neuroblastoma populations: the SIOPEN/HR-NBL1 and COG-A3973 trials. Eur J Nucl Med Mol Imaging. 2018;45:292–305.
13. Yanik GA, Parisi MT, Naranjo A, Nadel H, Gelfand MJ, Park JR, Ladenstein RL, Poetschger U, Boubaker A, Valteau-Couanet D, et al. Validation of postinduction curie scores in high-risk neuroblastoma: a Children's Oncology Group and SIOPEN Group Report on SIOPEN/HR-NBL1. J Nucl Med. 2018;59:502–8.
14. Ladenstein R, Pötschger U, Pearson ADJ, Brock P, Luksch R, Castel V, et al. Busulfan and melphalan versus carboplatin, etoposide, and melphalan as high-dose chemotherapy for high-risk neuroblastoma (HR-NBL1/SIOPEN): an international, randomised, multi-arm, open-label, phase 3 trial. Lancet Oncol. 2017;18:500–14.
15. Depuydt P, Boeva V, Hocking TD, Cannoodt R, Ambros IM, Ambros PF, Asgharzadeh S, Attiyeh EF, Combaret V, Defferrari R, et al. Genomic amplifications and distal 6q loss: novel markers for poor survival in high-risk neuroblastoma patients. J Natl Cancer Inst. 2018;110(10):1084–93.
16. Cheung N-KV, Zhang J, Lu C, Parker M, Bahrami A, Tickoo SK, Heguy A, Pappo AS, Federico S, Dalton J, et al. Association of age at diagnosis and genetic mutations in patients with neuroblastoma. JAMA. 2012;307:1062–71.
17. Valentijn LJ, Koster J, Zwijnenburg DA, Hasselt NE, van Sluis P, Volckmann R, van Noesel MM, George RE, Tytgat GAM, Molenaar JJ, et al. TERT rearrangements are frequent in neuroblastoma and identify aggressive tumors. Nat Genet. 2015;47:1411–4.
18. Green DM, Kun LE, Matthay KK, Meadows AT, Meyer WH, Meyers PA, Spunt SL, Robison LL, Hudson MM. Relevance of historical therapeutic approaches to the contemporary treatment of pediatric solid tumors. Pediatr Blood Cancer. 2013;60:1083–94.
19. Matthay KK, Maris JM, Schleiermacher G, Nakagawara A, Mackall CL, Diller L, Weiss WA. Neuroblastoma. Nat Rev Dis Primers. 2016;2:16078.
20. Pinto NR, Applebaum MA, Volchenboum SL, Matthay KK, London WB, Ambros PF, Nakagawara A, Berthold F, Schleiermacher G, Park JR, et al. Advances in risk classification and treatment strategies for neuroblastoma. J Clin Oncol Off J Am Soc Clin Oncol. 2015;33:3008–17.
21. Finklestein JZ, Hittle RE, Hammond GD. Evaluation of a high dose cyclophosphamide regimen in childhood tumors. Cancer. 1969;23:1239–42.
22. Nitschke R, Starling KA, Vats T, Bryan H. Cis-diamminedichloroplatinum (NSC-119875) in childhood malignancies: a Southwest Oncology Group study. Med Pediatr Oncol. 1978;4:127–32.
23. Rivera G, Green A, Hayes A, Avery T, Pratt C. Epipodophyllotoxin VM-26 in the treatment of childhood neuroblastoma. Cancer Treat Rep. 1977;61:1243–8.
24. Cheung NV, Heller G. Chemotherapy dose intensity correlates strongly with response, median survival, and median progression-free survival in metastatic neuroblastoma [see comments]. J Clin Oncol. 1991;9:1050–8.
25. George RE, Li S, Medeiros-Nancarrow C, Neuberg D, Marcus K, Shamberger RC, Pulsipher M, Grupp SA, Diller L. High-risk neuroblastoma treated with tandem autologous peripheral-blood

stem cell-supported transplantation: long-term survival update. J Clin Oncol Off J Am Soc Clin Oncol. 2006;24:2891–6.

26. Kretschmar CS, Kletzel M, Murray K, Thorner P, Joshi V, Marcus R, Smith EI, London WB, Castleberry R. Response to paclitaxel, topotecan, and topotecan-cyclophosphamide in children with untreated disseminated neuroblastoma treated in an upfront phase II investigational window: a pediatric oncology group study. J Clin Oncol Off J Am Soc Clin Oncol. 2004;22:4119–26.
27. Matthay KK, Villablanca JG, Seeger RC, Stram DO, Harris RE, Ramsay NK, Swift P, Shimada H, Black CT, Brodeur GM, et al. Treatment of high-risk neuroblastoma with intensive chemotherapy, radiotherapy, autologous bone marrow transplantation, and 13-cis-retinoic acid. Children's Cancer Group. N Engl J Med. 1999;341:1165–73.
28. Zage PE, Kletzel M, Murray K, Marcus R, Castleberry R, Zhang Y, London WB, Kretschmar C. Outcomes of the POG 9340/9341/9342 trials for children with high-risk neuroblastoma: a report from the Children's Oncology Group. Pediatr Blood Cancer. 2008;51:747–53.
29. Kushner BH, Kramer K, LaQuaglia MP, Modak S, Yataghene K, Cheung N-KV. Reduction from seven to five cycles of intensive induction chemotherapy in children with high-risk neuroblastoma. J Clin Oncol Off J Am Soc Clin Oncol. 2004;22:4888–92.
30. Park JR, Scott JR, Stewart CF, London WB, Naranjo A, Santana VM, Shaw PJ, Cohn SL, Matthay KK. Pilot induction regimen incorporating pharmacokinetically guided topotecan for treatment of newly diagnosed high-risk neuroblastoma: a Children's Oncology Group study. J Clin Oncol Off J Am Soc Clin Oncol. 2011;29:4351–7.
31. Haas-Kogan DA, Swift PS, Selch M, Haase GM, Seeger RC, Gerbing RB, Stram DO, Matthay KK. Impact of radiotherapy for high-risk neuroblastoma: a Children's Cancer Group study. Int J Radiat Oncol Biol Phys. 2003;56:28–39.
32. Wolden SL, Gollamudi SV, Kushner BH, LaQuaglia M, Kramer K, Rosen N, Abramson S, Cheung NV. Local control with multimodality therapy for Stage 4 neuroblastoma. Int J Radiat Oncol Biol Phys. 2000;46:969–74.
33. Matthay KK, Seeger RC, Reynolds CP, Stram DO, O'Leary MC, Harris RE, Selch M, Atkinson JB, Haase GM, Ramsay NK. Allogeneic versus autologous purged bone marrow transplantation for neuroblastoma: a report from the Childrens Cancer Group. J Clin Oncol. 1994;12:2382–9.
34. Stram DO, Matthay KK, O'Leary M, Reynolds CP, Haase GM, Atkinson JB, Brodeur GM, Seeger RC. Consolidation chemoradiotherapy and autologous bone marrow transplantation versus continued chemotherapy for metastatic neuroblastoma: a report of two concurrent Children's Cancer Group studies [see comments]. J Clin Oncol. 1996;14:2417–26.
35. Berthold F, Boos J, Burdach S, Erttmann R, Henze G, Hermann J, Klingebiel T, Kremens B, Schilling FH, Schrappe M, et al. Myeloablative megatherapy with autologous stem-cell rescue versus oral maintenance chemotherapy as consolidation treatment in patients with high-risk neuroblastoma: a randomised controlled trial. Lancet Oncol. 2005;6:649–58.
36. Pritchard J, Cotterill SJ, Germond SM, Imeson J, de Kraker J, Jones DR. High dose melphalan in the treatment of advanced neuroblastoma: results of a randomised trial (ENSG-1) by the European Neuroblastoma Study Group. Pediatr Blood Cancer. 2005;44:348–57.
37. Villablanca JG, Matthay KK, Swift PS, Harris RE, Ramsay NK, Brodeur GM, Sondel PM, Stram D, Reynolds CP, Seeger RC. Phase I trial of carboplatin, etoposide, melphalan and local irradiation (CEM-LI) with purged autologous bone marrow transplantation for children with high risk neuroblastoma. Med Pediatr Oncol. 1999;33:170.
38. Kreissman SG, Seeger RC, Matthay KK, London WB, Sposto R, Grupp SA, Haas-Kogan DA, Laquaglia MP, Yu AL, Diller L, et al. Purged versus non-purged peripheral blood stem-cell transplantation for high-risk neuroblastoma (COG A3973): a randomised phase 3 trial. Lancet Oncol. 2013;14:999–1008.
39. Bensimhon P, Villablanca JG, Sender LS, Matthay KK, Park JR, Seeger R, London WB, Yap JS, Kreissman SG. Peripheral blood stem cell support for multiple cycles of dose intensive induction therapy is feasible with little risk of tumor contamination in advanced stage neuroblastoma: a report from the Childrens Oncology Group. Pediatr Blood Cancer. 2010;54:596–602.

40. Grupp SA, Stern JW, Bunin N, Nancarrow C, Ross AA, Mogul M, Adams R, Grier HE, Gorlin JB, Shamberger R, et al. Tandem high-dose therapy in rapid sequence for children with high-risk neuroblastoma. J Clin Oncol Off J Am Soc Clin Oncol. 2000;18:2567–75.
41. Seif AE, Naranjo A, Baker DL, Bunin NJ, Kletzel M, Kretschmar CS, Maris JM, McGrady PW, von Allmen D, Cohn SL, et al. A pilot study of tandem high-dose chemotherapy with stem cell rescue as consolidation for high-risk neuroblastoma: Children's Oncology Group study ANBL00P1. Bone Marrow Transplant. 2013;48:947–52.
42. Park JR, Kreissman SG, London WB, Naranjo A, Cohn SL, Hogarty MD, Tenney SC, Haas-Kogan D, Shaw PJ, Geiger JD, et al. A phase 3 randomized clinical trial (RCT) of tandem myeloablative autologous stem cell transplant (ASCT) using peripheral blood stem cell (PBSC) as consolidation therapy for high-risk neuroblastoma (HR-NB): a Children's Oncology group (COG) study. J Clin Oncol. 2016;34 https://doi.org/10.1200/JCO.2016.34.15_suppl.LBA3.
43. Matthay KK, Yanik G, Messina J, Quach A, Huberty J, Cheng SC, Veatch J, Goldsby R, Brophy P, Kersun LS, et al. Phase II study on the effect of disease sites, age, and prior therapy on response to iodine-131-metaiodobenzylguanidine therapy in refractory neuroblastoma. J Clin Oncol. 2007;25:1054–60.
44. Wilson JS, Gains JE, Moroz V, Wheatley K, Gaze MN. A systematic review of 131I-meta iodobenzylguanidine molecular radiotherapy for neuroblastoma. Eur J Cancer. 2014;50:801–15.
45. Federico SM, McCarville MB, Shulkin BL, Sondel PM, Hank JA, Hutson P, Meagher M, Shafer A, Ng CY, Leung W, et al. A pilot trial of humanized anti-GD2 monoclonal antibody (hu14.18K322A) with chemotherapy and natural killer cells in children with recurrent/refractory neuroblastoma. Clin Cancer Res. 2017;23:6441–9.
46. Marachelian A, Villablanca JG, Liu CW, Liu B, Goodarzian F, Lai HA, Shimada H, Tran HC, Parra JA, Gallego R, et al. Expression of five neuroblastoma genes in bone marrow or blood of patients with relapsed/refractory neuroblastoma provides a new biomarker for disease and prognosis. Clin Cancer Res. 2017;23:5374–83.
47. Yanik GA, Parisi MT, Shulkin BL, Naranjo A, Kreissman SG, London WB, Villablanca JG, Maris JM, Park JR, Cohn SL, et al. Semiquantitative mIBG scoring as a prognostic indicator in patients with stage 4 neuroblastoma: a report from the Children's oncology group. J Nucl Med. 2013;54:541–8.
48. Matthay KK. Targeted isotretinoin in neuroblastoma: kinetics, genetics, or absorption. Clin Cancer Res. 2013;19:311–3.
49. Veal GJ, Cole M, Errington J, Pearson AD, Foot AB, Whyman G, Boddy AV. Pharmacokinetics and metabolism of 13-cis-retinoic acid (isotretinoin) in children with high-risk neuroblastoma – a study of the United Kingdom Children's Cancer Study group. Br J Cancer. 2007;96:424–31.
50. Matthay K, Reynolds C, Seeger R, Shimada H, Adkins E, Haas-Kogan D, et al. Long-term results for children with high-risk neuroblastoma treated on a randomized trial of myeloablative therapy followed by 13-cis-retinoic acid: a Children's Oncology Group study. J Clin Oncol. 2009;27:1007–13.
51. Gilman AL, Ozkaynak MF, Matthay KK, Krailo M, Yu AL, Gan J, Sternberg A, Hank JA, Seeger R, Reaman GH, et al. Phase I study of ch14.18 with granulocyte-macrophage colony-stimulating factor and interleukin-2 in children with neuroblastoma after autologous bone marrow transplantation or stem-cell rescue: a report from the Children's Oncology Group. J Clin Oncol Off J Am Soc Clin Oncol. 2009;27:85–91.
52. Ozkaynak MF, Sondel PM, Krailo MD, Gan J, Javorsky B, Reisfeld RA, Matthay KK, Reaman GH, Seeger RC. Phase I study of chimeric human/murine anti-ganglioside G(D2) monoclonal antibody (ch14.18) with granulocyte-macrophage colony-stimulating factor in children with neuroblastoma immediately after hematopoietic stem-cell transplantation: a Children's Cancer Group study. J Clin Oncol. 2000;18:4077–85.
53. Uttenreuther-Fischer MM, Huang CS, Reisfeld RA, Yu AL. Pharmacokinetics of anti-ganglioside GD2 mAb 14G2a in a phase I trial in pediatric cancer patients. Cancer Immunol Immunother. 1995;41:29–36.

54. Yu AL, Uttenreuther MM, Kamps A, Batova A, Reisfeld RA. Combined use of a human-mouse chimeric anti-GD2 (ch14.18) and GM-CSF in the treatment of refractory neuroblastoma. Antib Immunoconjug Radiopharm. 1995;8:12.
55. Hank JA, Robinson RR, Surfus J, Mueller BM, Reisfeld RA, Cheung NK, Sondel PM. Augmentation of antibody dependent cell mediated cytotoxicity following in vivo therapy with recombinant interleukin 2. Cancer Res. 1990;50:5234–9.
56. Yu AL, Gilman AL, Ozkaynak MF, London WB, Kreissman SG, Chen HX, Smith M, Anderson B, Villablanca JG, Matthay KK, et al. Anti-GD2 antibody with GM-CSF, interleukin-2, and isotretinoin for neuroblastoma. N Engl J Med. 2010;363:1324–34.
57. London WB, Frantz CN, Campbell LA, Seeger RC, Brumback BA, Cohn SL, Matthay KK, Castleberry RP, Diller L. Phase II randomized comparison of topotecan plus cyclophosphamide versus topotecan alone in children with recurrent or refractory neuroblastoma: a Children's Oncology Group study. J Clin Oncol Off J Am Soc Clin Oncol. 2010;28:3808–15.
58. Bagatell R, London WB, Wagner LM, Voss SD, Stewart CF, Maris JM, Kretschmar C, Cohn SL. Phase II study of irinotecan and temozolomide in children with relapsed or refractory neuroblastoma: a Children's Oncology Group study. J Clin Oncol Off J Am Soc Clin Oncol. 2011;29:208–13.
59. Rubie H, Chisholm J, Defachelles AS, Morland B, Munzer C, Valteau-Couanet D, Mosseri V, Bergeron C, Weston C, Coze C, et al. Phase II study of temozolomide in relapsed or refractory high-risk neuroblastoma: a joint Societe Francaise des Cancers de l'Enfant and United Kingdom Children Cancer Study Group-New Agents Group Study. J Clin Oncol. 2006;24:5259–64.
60. Fox E, Mosse YP, Meany HM, Gurney JG, Khanna G, Jackson HA, Gordon G, Shusterman S, Park JR, Cohn SL, et al. Time to disease progression in children with relapsed or refractory neuroblastoma treated with ABT-751: a report from the Children's Oncology Group (ANBL0621). Pediatr Blood Cancer. 2014;61:990–6.
61. Langevin AM, Bernstein M, Kuhn JG, Blaney SM, Ivy P, Sun J, Chen Z, Adamson PC. A phase II trial of rebeccamycin analogue (NSC #655649) in children with solid tumors: a Children's Oncology Group study. Pediatr Blood Cancer. 2008;50:577–80.
62. Beaty O 3rd, Berg S, Blaney S, Malogolowkin M, Krailo M, Knight R, Schaiquevich P, Stewart C, Chen Z, Nelson M, et al. A phase II trial and pharmacokinetic study of oxaliplatin in children with refractory solid tumors: a Children's Oncology Group study. Pediatr Blood Cancer. 2010;55:440–5.
63. Kuttesch JF Jr, Krailo MD, Madden T, Johansen M, Bleyer A, Children's Oncology Group. Phase II evaluation of intravenous vinorelbine (Navelbine) in recurrent or refractory pediatric malignancies: a Children's Oncology Group study. Pediatr Blood Cancer. 2009;53:590–3.
64. Zwerdling T, Krailo M, Monteleone P, Byrd R, Sato J, Dunaway R, Seibel N, Chen Z, Strain J, Reaman G, et al. Phase II investigation of docetaxel in pediatric patients with recurrent solid tumors: a report from the Children's Oncology Group. Cancer. 2006;106:1821–8.
65. Warwick AB, Malempati S, Krailo M, Melemed A, Gorlick R, Ames MM, Safgren SL, Adamson PC, Blaney SM. Phase 2 trial of pemetrexed in children and adolescents with refractory solid tumors: a Children's Oncology Group study. Pediatr Blood Cancer. 2013;60:237–41.
66. Jacobs S, Fox E, Krailo M, Hartley G, Navid F, Wexler L, Blaney SM, Goodwin A, Goodspeed W, Balis FM, et al. Phase II trial of ixabepilone administered daily for five days in children and young adults with refractory solid tumors: a report from the children's oncology group. Clin Cancer Res. 2010;16:750–4.
67. DuBois SG, Chesler L, Groshen S, Hawkins R, Goodarzian F, Shimada H, Yanik G, Tagen M, Stewart C, Mosse YP, et al. Phase I study of vincristine, irinotecan, and ^{131}I-metaiodobenzylguanidine for patients with relapsed or refractory neuroblastoma: a new approaches to neuroblastoma therapy trial. Clin Cancer Res. 2012;18:2679–86.
68. DuBois SG, Allen S, Bent M, Hilton JF, Hollinger F, Hawkins R, Courtier J, Mosse YP, Matthay KK. Phase I/II study of (131)I-MIBG with vincristine and 5 days of irinotecan for advanced neuroblastoma. Br J Cancer. 2015a;112:644–9.

69. DuBois SG, Groshen S, Park JR, Haas-Kogan DA, Yang X, Geier E, Chen E, Giacomini K, Weiss B, Cohn SL, et al. Phase I study of vorinostat as a radiation sensitizer with 131I-metaiodobenzylguanidine (131I-MIBG) for patients with relapsed or refractory neuroblastoma. Clin Cancer Res. 2015b;21:2715–21.
70. DuBois SG, Marachelian A, Fox E, Kudgus RA, Reid JM, Groshen S, Malvar J, Bagatell R, Wagner L, Maris JM, et al. Phase I study of the aurora a kinase inhibitor alisertib in combination with irinotecan and temozolomide for patients with relapsed or refractory neuroblastoma: a NANT (new approaches to neuroblastoma therapy) trial. J Clin Oncol. 2016;34(12):1368–75.
71. Mosse YP, Lipsitz E, Fox E, Teachey DT, Maris JM, Weigel B, Adamson PC, Ingle MA, Ahern CH, Blaney SM. Pediatric phase I trial and pharmacokinetic study of MLN8237, an investigational oral selective small-molecule inhibitor of Aurora kinase A: a Children's Oncology Group Phase I Consortium study. Clin Cancer Res. 2012;18:6058–64.
72. Mosse YP, Voss SD, Lim MS, Rolland D, Minard CG, Fox E, Adamson P, Wilner K, Blaney SM, Weigel BJ. Targeting ALK with crizotinib in pediatric anaplastic large cell lymphoma and inflammatory myofibroblastic tumor: a Children's Oncology Group study. J Clin Oncol. 2017;35:3215–21.
73. Infarinato NR, Park JH, Krytska K, Ryles HT, Sano R, Szigety KM, Li Y, Zou HY, Lee NV, Smeal T, et al. The ALK/ROS1 inhibitor PF-06463922 overcomes primary resistance to crizotinib in ALK-driven neuroblastoma. Cancer Discov. 2015;6(1):96–107.
74. Maurer BJ, Kang MH, Villablanca JG, Janeba J, Groshen S, Matthay KK, Sondel PM, Maris JM, Jackson HA, Goodarzian F, et al. Phase I trial of fenretinide delivered orally in a novel organized lipid complex in patients with relapsed/refractory neuroblastoma: a report from the new approaches to neuroblastoma therapy (NANT) consortium. Pediatr Blood Cancer. 2013;60:1801–8.
75. Shusterman S, London WB, Gillies SD, Hank JA, Voss SD, Seeger RC, Reynolds CP, Kimball J, Albertini MR, Wagner B, et al. Antitumor activity of hu14.18-IL2 in patients with relapsed/refractory neuroblastoma: a Children's Oncology Group (COG) phase II study. J Clin Oncol. 2010;28:4969–75.
76. Mody R, Naranjo A, Van Ryn C, Yu AL, London WB, Shulkin BL, Parisi MT, Servaes S-E-N, Diccianni MB, Sondel PM, et al. Irinotecan-temozolomide with temsirolimus or dinutuximab in children with refractory or relapsed neuroblastoma (COG ANBL1221): an open-label, randomised, phase 2 trial. Lancet Oncol. 2017;18:946–57.
77. Kushner BH, Cheung IY, Modak S, Kramer K, Ragupathi G, Cheung NK. Phase I trial of a bivalent gangliosides vaccine in combination with beta-glucan for high-risk neuroblastoma in second or later remission. Clin Cancer Res. 2014;20:1375–82.
78. Villablanca JG, London WB, Naranjo A, McGrady P, Ames MM, Reid JM, McGovern RM, Buhrow SA, Jackson H, Stranzinger E, et al. Phase II study of oral capsular 4-hydroxyphenylretinamide (4-HPR/fenretinide) in pediatric patients with refractory or recurrent neuroblastoma: a report from the Children's Oncology Group. Clin Cancer Res. 2011;17:6858–66.
79. Weigel B, Malempati S, Reid JM, Voss SD, Cho SY, Chen HX, Krailo M, Villaluna D, Adamson PC, Blaney SM. Phase 2 trial of cixutumumab in children, adolescents, and young adults with refractory solid tumors: a report from the Children's Oncology Group. Pediatr Blood Cancer. 2014;61:452–6.
80. Mosse YP, Lim MS, Voss SD, Wilner K, Ruffner K, Laliberte J, Rolland D, Balis FM, Maris JM, Weigel BJ, et al. Safety and activity of crizotinib for paediatric patients with refractory solid tumours or anaplastic large-cell lymphoma: a Children's Oncology Group phase 1 consortium study. Lancet Oncol. 2013;14:472–80.
81. Pearson ADJ, Pinkerton CR, Lewis IJ, Imeson J, Ellershaw C, Machin D. High-dose rapid and standard induction chemotherapy for patients aged over 1 year with stage 4 neuroblastoma: a randomised trial. Lancet Oncol. 2008;9:247–56.
82. Ladenstein R, Valteau-Couanet D, Brock P, Yaniv I, Castel V, Laureys G, Malis J, Papadakis V, Lacerda A, Ruud E, et al. Randomized trial of prophylactic granulocyte colony-stimulating

factor during rapid COJEC induction in pediatric patients with high-risk neuroblastoma: the European HR-NBL1/SIOPEN study. J Clin Oncol Off J Am Soc Clin Oncol. 2010;28:3516–24.
83. Amoroso L, Erminio G, Makin G, Pearson ADJ, Brock P, Valteau-Couanet D, Castel V, Pasquet M, Laureys G, Thomas C, et al. Topotecan-vincristine-doxorubicin in stage 4 high-risk neuroblastoma patients failing to achieve a complete metastatic response to rapid COJEC: a SIOPEN study. Cancer Res Treat. 2018;50:148–55.
84. Cheung NK, Kushner BH, LaQuaglia M, Kramer K, Gollamudi S, Heller G, Gerald W, Yeh S, Finn R, Larson SM, et al. N7: a novel multi-modality therapy of high risk neuroblastoma (NB) in children diagnosed over 1 year of age. Med Pediatr Oncol. 2001;36:227–30.
85. Mora J, Cruz O, Lavarino C, Rios J, Vancells M, Parareda A, Salvador H, Suñol M, Carrasco R, Guillen A, et al. Results of induction chemotherapy in children older than 18 months with stage-4 neuroblastoma treated with an adaptive-to-response modified N7 protocol (mN7). Clin Transl Oncol. 2015;17:521–9.
86. Kohler JA, Ellershaw C, Machin D, Neuroblastoma Working Group of the Children's Cancer and Leukaemia Group. Response to N7 induction chemotherapy in children more than one year of age diagnosed with metastatic neuroblastoma treated in UKCCSG centers. Pediatr Blood Cancer. 2007;49:234–9.
87. Valteau-Couanet D, Michon J, Boneu A, Rodary C, Perel Y, Bergeron C, Rubie H, Coze C, Plantaz D, Bernard F, et al. Results of induction chemotherapy in children older than 1 year with a stage 4 neuroblastoma treated with the NB 97 French Society of Pediatric Oncology (SFOP) protocol. J Clin Oncol Off J Am Soc Clin Oncol. 2005;23:532–40.
88. Valteau-Couanet D, Le Deley M-C, Bergeron C, Ducassou S, Michon J, Rubie H, Le Teuff G, Coze C, Plantaz D, Sirvent N, et al. Long-term results of the combination of the N7 induction chemotherapy and the busulfan-melphalan high dose chemotherapy. Pediatr Blood Cancer. 2014;61:977–81.
89. Hartmann O, Valteau-Couanet D, Vassal G, Lapierre V, Brugières L, Delgado R, Couanet D, Lumbroso J, Benhamou E. Prognostic factors in metastatic neuroblastoma in patients over 1 year of age treated with high-dose chemotherapy and stem cell transplantation: a multivariate analysis in 218 patients treated in a single institution. Bone Marrow Transplant. 1999;23:789–95.
90. Proust-Houdemont S, Pasqualini C, Blanchard P, Dufour C, Benhamou E, Goma G, Semeraro M, Raquin M-A, Hartmann O, Valteau-Couanet D. Busulfan-melphalan in high-risk neuroblastoma: the 30-year experience of a single institution. Bone Marrow Transplant. 2016;51:1076–81.
91. Ladenstein R, Poetschger U, Gray J, Valteau-Couanet D, Luksch R, Castel V, et al. Toxicity and outcome of anti-GD2 antibody ch14.18/CHO in front-line, high-risk patients with neuroblastoma: Final results of the phase III immunotherapy randomisation (HR-NBL1/SIOPEN trial). J Clin Oncol. 2016;34:10500.
92. Lode HN, Valteau-Couanet D, Garaventa A, Gray J, Castel V, Yaniv I, et al. Long-term infusion of anti-GD2 antibody ch14.18/CHO in combination with interleukin-2 (IL2) activity and efficacy in high-risk relapsed/refractory neuroblastoma patients. J Clin Oncol. 2015;33:10080.
93. Pasqualini C, Dufour C, Goma G, Raquin M-A, Lapierre V, Valteau-Couanet D. Tandem high-dose chemotherapy with thiotepa and busulfan-melphalan and autologous stem cell transplantation in very high-risk neuroblastoma patients. Bone Marrow Transplant. 2016;51:227–31.
94. Gaze MN, Chang Y-C 'i, Flux GD, Mairs RJ, Saran FH, Meller ST. Feasibility of dosimetry-based high-dose 131I-meta-iodobenzylguanidine with topotecan as a radiosensitizer in children with metastatic neuroblastoma. Cancer Biother Radiopharm. 2005;20:195–9.
95. Gaze MN, Bomanji JB, Lacerda A, Saran FH, Brock PR, Uyttebroeck A, et al. Long-term outcome of MATIN, a schedule of high-administered activity iodine 131 metaiodobenzylguanidine and topotecan in neuroblastoma: a SIOPEN study. Toronto: ANR; 2012.
96. Ferry I, Kolesnikov-Gauthier H, Oudoux A, Cougnenc O, Schleiermacher G, Michon J, Bogart E, Chastagner P, Proust S, Valteau-Couanet D, et al. Feasibility of busulfan melphalan

and stem cell rescue after 131I-MIBG and topotecan therapy for refractory or relapsed metastatic neuroblastoma: the French experience. J Pediatr Hematol Oncol. 2018;40(6):426–32.

97. Berthold F, Burdach S, Kremens B, Lampert F, Niethammer D, Riehm H, Ritter J, Treuner J, Utsch S, Zieschang J. The role of chemotherapy in the treatment of children with neuroblastoma stage IV: the GPO (German Pediatric Oncology Society) experience. Klin Padiatr. 1990;202:262–9.
98. Berthold F, Hero B, Kremens B, Handgretinger R, Henze G, Schilling FH, Schrappe M, Simon T, Spix C. Long-term results and risk profiles of patients in five consecutive trials (1979–1997) with stage 4 neuroblastoma over 1 year of age. Cancer Lett. 2003;197:11–7.
99. Park JR, Slattery J, Gooley T, Hawkins D, Lindsley K, Villablanca JG, et al. Phase I topotecan preparative regimen for high-risk neuroblastoma, high-grade glioma, and refractory/recurrent pediatric solid tumors. Med Pediatr Oncol. 2000;35:719–23.
100. Längler A, Christaras A, Abshagen K, Krauth K, Hero B, Berthold F. Topotecan in the treatment of refractory neuroblastoma and other malignant tumors in childhood – a phase-II-study. Klin Padiatr. 2002;214:153–6.
101. Furman WL, Shulkin BL, SA F, MB M, AM D, MJ K, et al. Early response rates and Curie scores at end of induction: an update from a phase II study of an anti-GD2 monoclonal antibody (mAb) with chemotherapy (CT) in newly diagnosed patients (pts) with high-risk (HR) neuroblastoma (NB). J Clin Oncol. 2017;35(Suppl):10534.
102. Rubie H, Geoerger B, Frappaz D, Schmitt A, Leblond P, Ndiaye A, Aerts I, Le Deley M-C, Gentet J-C, Paci A, et al. Phase I study of topotecan in combination with temozolomide (TOTEM) in relapsed or refractory paediatric solid tumours. Eur J Cancer. 2010;1990(46):2763–70.
103. Di Giannatale A, Dias-Gastellier N, Devos A, Mc Hugh K, Boubaker A, Courbon F, Verschuur A, Ducassoul S, Malekzadeh K, Casanova M, et al. Phase II study of temozolomide in combination with topotecan (TOTEM) in relapsed or refractory neuroblastoma: a European Innovative Therapies for Children with Cancer-SIOP-European Neuroblastoma study. Eur J Cancer. 2014;50:170–7.
104. Segerström L, Fuchs D, Bäckman U, Holmquist K, Christofferson R, Azarbayjani F. The anti-VEGF antibody bevacizumab potently reduces the growth rate of high-risk neuroblastoma xenografts. Pediatr Res. 2006;60:576–81.
105. Dickson PV, Hamner JB, Sims TL, Fraga CH, Ng CYC, Rajasekeran S, Hagedorn NL, McCarville MB, Stewart CF, Davidoff AM. Bevacizumab-induced transient remodeling of the vasculature in neuroblastoma xenografts results in improved delivery and efficacy of systemically administered chemotherapy. Clin Cancer Res. 2007;13:3942–50.
106. Corbacioglu S, Steinbach D, Lode HN, Gruhn B, Fruehwald M, Broeckelmann M, Suttorp M, Escherich G, Cario G, Ehlert K, et al. The RIST design: a molecularly targeted multimodal approach for the treatment of patients with relapsed and refractory neuroblastoma. J Clin Oncol. 2013;31:-10017.
107. Moreno L, Caron H, Geoerger B, Eggert A, Schleiermacher G, Brock P, Valteau-Couanet D, Chesler L, Schulte JH, De Preter K, et al. Accelerating drug development for neuroblastoma – new drug development strategy: an innovative therapies for children with cancer, European Network for Cancer Research in Children and Adolescents and International Society of Paediatric Oncology Europe Neuroblastoma project. Expert Opin Drug Discov. 2017;12:801–11.
108. Illhardt T, Toporski J, Feuchtinger T, Turkiewicz D, Teltschik H-M, Ebinger M, Schwarze C-P, Holzer U, Lode HN, Albert MH, et al. Haploidentical stem cell transplantation for refractory/relapsed neuroblastoma. Biol Blood Marrow Transplant. 2018;24:1005–12.
109. Thomas S, Straathof K, Himoudi N, Anderson J, Pule M. An optimized GD2-targeting retroviral cassette for more potent and safer cellular therapy of neuroblastoma and other cancers. PLoS One. 2016;11:e0152196.

Immunotherapy

13

Francesca del Bufalo and Franco Locatelli

13.1 Neuroblastoma Immunology

The role played by the immune system in the biological behavior of neuroblastoma (NBL) has been long postulated, especially in consideration of some peculiar features of this tumor: the well-known phenomenon of spontaneous regression of widespread lesions; the wide age-related and stage-related differences in outcome; and the association with paraneoplastic syndromes.

Spontaneous regression of cancer occurs when either a primary tumor or metastatic disease undergoes a decrease in size, until disappearance, without therapeutic intervention. It has been described for few other tumors, such as carcinoma of the kidney, malignant melanoma, choriocarcinoma, and some lymphoid malignancies [1–3].

The prevalence of this phenomenon in NBL is very hard to define precisely and remains largely unknown. However, a more detailed insight into its magnitude was recently provided by large studies conducted in Europe, Canada, and Japan on wide mass screening of infants by measuring urine catecholamines (homovanillic acid—HVA—and vanillylmandelic acid—VMA) [4–7]. These studies revealed a substantial increase in the prevalence of neuroblastoma in the screened population, reaching 1:2000 live births, as compared with the unscreened population (1:7000 live births). Despite these results, overall mortality remained unchanged. These data strongly suggest that spontaneous regression of neuroblastoma without clinical detection of the disease occurs even more frequently than the clinically detected neuroblastoma.

F. del Bufalo · F. Locatelli (✉)
Department of Paediatric Haematology, Oncology and Cell and Gene Therapy, IRCCS Bambino Gesù Children's Hospital, Rome, Italy

Department of Gynecology/Obstetrics and Pediatrics, Sapienza University of Rome, Rome, Italy
e-mail: franco.locatelli@opbg.net

S. Sarnacki, L. Pio (eds.), *Neuroblastoma*,
https://doi.org/10.1007/978-3-030-18396-7_13

Although several mechanisms take place in this complex phenomenon, a large body of evidence for the involvement of the immune system has been published to date [8]. It has been reported that spontaneous regression of cancer is sometimes observed after an acute infection [1, 9, 10]. This association has been described in several different cancers and has been the basis for the work of Dr. Coley who began, in the late nineteenth century, to treat cancer patients with bacterial vaccines, obtaining 5-year survival rates that were considered impressive for the time [11]. It has been, subsequently, shown that the interactions between the pathogen-associated molecular patterns (PAMP) and the Toll-like receptors (TLR) on various immune cells, including T cells and dendritic cells, result in the production of pro-inflammatory cytokines that, in turn, activate the cytotoxic T-cell response [12]. Similarly, several reports showed the induction of the regression of experimental tumor metastases by immunomodulatory cytokines [13–15]. It is, therefore, plausible that spontaneous regression could be mediated by the host immune response (Fig. 13.1).

The involvement of the immune system has been implicated also in the different age-related and stage-related outcomes of NBL, revealing that the inflammatory response and the immunosuppressive tumor microenvironment might have important effects on the natural history of the disease. It has been shown that patients older than

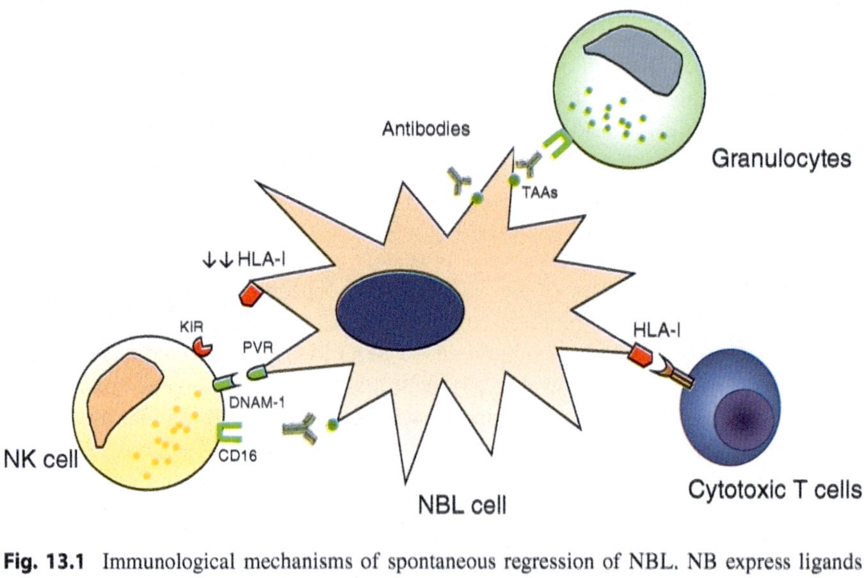

Fig. 13.1 Immunological mechanisms of spontaneous regression of NBL. NB express ligands that are recognized by several players of the immune system which are thought to have a relevant role in the spontaneous regression of the tumor. NK receptors can have activating or inhibitory function and DNAM-1/PVR interactions, together with the binding of CD16 to the FC fragment of the opsonizing antibodies, play a pivotal role in triggering NK cell-mediated killing, HLA-I recognition through KIR dampens NK cell function. NB usually lack or express low, non-protective levels of HLA class I molecules. However, these molecules might be recognized by cytotoxic T cells, important in mediating the NBL cell lysis and controlling tumor growth. Lastly, antibody-dependent cell-mediated cytotoxicity involves also macrophages and granulocytes. The concert between innate and adaptive immunity is therefore essential in inducing NBL regression

18 months of age presenting with MYCN non-amplified metastatic disease display a higher expression of tumor-associated macrophage (TAM) genes in the tumor (IL6R, IL10, CD16, CD33, FCGR3) than those younger than 18 months of age, this signature correlating with a worse outcome [16]. The same study also revealed that, regardless of patient age, there is a significantly higher infiltration of CD163+ M2 cells in stage 4 NBL biopsies than in those patients with stage 1–3 and stage 4s disease. Another study revealed that high-risk, MYCN non-amplified NBL with 11q deletions represents an inflammatory subset of tumor with increased levels of the prostaglandin E_2 (PGE_2) compared with low-risk tumors, suggesting also an implication of the cancer-associated fibroblasts (CAF) as mediators of this process [17]. PGE_2 has an important role in favoring tumor progression since it enhances neuroblast growth and chemoresistance and recruits additional suppressive myeloid populations [18].

The very well-known role of MYCN amplification as prognostic predictor for NBL has also important correlation with the tumor immunology. The group of Metelitsa clearly showed that non-amplified MYCN high-risk tumors produce the chemoattractant CCL2, which acts on invariant natural killer T (iNKT) cells, an evolutionary conserved subset of T cells recognizing glycolipids presented by the HLA class I molecule CD1d, whereas MYCN pos tumors did not, and, therefore, were not infiltrated by iNKT cells [19]. Subsequently, MYCN was found to downregulate CCL2 expression, providing the explanation for the different compositions of tumor-infiltrating lymphocytes observed in MYCN amplified (lower numbers of NKT, T cells, and monocytes) versus non-amplified high-risk NBL [20]. Another important role of MYCN in the modulation of the immunogenicity of NBL cells is mediated through the downregulation of the major histocompatibility complex class I (MHC I) molecules, by transcriptional inhibition of the p50 subunit of the NF-kB transcription factor [21, 22]. NBL cells from patients with high-risk disease have been shown to evade immune recognition through this mechanism, whereas most tumors from patients with 4s NBL express normal levels of MHC I [23, 24]. It must be noted, however, that a study on human NBL cell lines questioned the direct role of MYCN expression in MHC I downregulation, revealing a complex interplay between a low transcriptional availability of NF-kB and the imbalance in the expression of both MHC I and two antigen-processing gene products (the endoplasmic reticulum aminopeptidases ERAP 1 and ERAP2) [25]. On the other side, several defects in multiple antigen-processing machinery (APM) components, the molecular complex responsible for the conversion of the protein antigens into short peptides that are then presented by MHC I, have been involved in the process of impaired antigen presentation [23]. If, on one hand, downregulation of MHC I hampers the recognition of NBL cells by cytotoxic T cells, on the other hand, it might render tumor cells highly susceptible to natural killer (NK)-mediated cytolysis, as they do not express the class I ligand of NK-cell killer inhibitory receptors (KIR) [26]. This evidence needs to be carefully evaluated in planning approaches of immunotherapy of NBL. Downregulation of MHC I was, in fact, shown to be reversed, in vitro, by treatment of the cells with interferon (IFN)-γ, this finding providing the rationale for improving T-cell clearance of the tumor in vivo [27]. However, although T cells can mediate potent and, most of all, long-lasting antitumor immunity, the role of NK cells in immune-surveillance of these tumors must not be underestimated. For example, the combination of IL-2 and anti-GD2 monoclonal antibody (mAb) in NBL immunotherapy clinical trials has been shown to potentiate NK-cell-mediated antibody-dependent cell-mediated cytotoxicity (ADCC) [28].

In a study by Venstrom et al., patients with relapsed/refractory NB were genotyped for KIR and HLA alleles, in order to identify the potential correlation between the KIR–HLA genotype and the response to autologous hematopoietic stem cell transplantation (HSCT). Interestingly, they showed that the response to treatment was correlated with autologous KIR/KIR-ligand mismatch, this finding supporting a role played by NK cells in NB-cell elimination [29].

Finally, another relevant immunosuppressive mechanism associated with MYCN amplification has very recently been demonstrated: the oncogene acts by negatively regulating the expression of relevant ligands of NK-cell activating receptors, such as NKG2D and DNAM1, lessening tumor recognition by NK cells [30, 31].

Further evidence for the strict correlation between NBL and immune-surveillance arises from the association of this tumor with paraneoplastic syndromes, such as opsoclonus-myoclonus syndrome (OMS) or anti-ANNA-1 (anti-Hu) syndrome. OMS is the only commonly recognized paraneoplastic syndrome in pediatrics and is present at diagnosis in 1:200 children with NBL. Multiple authors reported that NBL and ganglioneuroblastoma in children with OMS have unique histopathological and biological features: these tumors are typically extensively infiltrated by lymphocytes and show a benign behavior, being often very small, minimally active, and without high rate of catecholamine secretion [32–34]. The clinical presentation of OMS includes various combinations of opsoclonus, ataxia, myoclonic movements, marked irritability, regression of speech and language, and sleep disturbances. The autoimmune nature of the syndrome is sustained by the findings of pro-inflammatory, predominantly Th2, cytokines and chemokines patterns in both serum and cerebrospinal fluid (CSF) of these patients, and by the clinical response after administration of immunosuppressive treatments. Typically, the CSF of these patients display a high percentage of B-lymphocytes and oligoclonal bands [35]. Moreover, several autoantibodies against intracellular and surface structures of the brain and NBL tissue are often detected in patients with OMS [36–41]. Taken together, these findings suggest that OMS is mainly mediated by an abnormal humoral autoimmunity.

Anti-Hu1 syndrome is characterized more frequently by limbic encephalitis but can present with brainstem encephalitis or posterior cord syndrome [42–44]. As reported for OMS, NBL associated with this syndrome is usually not very aggressive and frequently is small in size. Autoantibody titers in these patients are usually high in both serum and CSF, but, since anti-Hu antibodies are directed against intracellular antigens, they are unlikely to be pathogenic. These syndromes are in fact mainly T-cell mediated [45].

The observation of the peculiar, benign, behavior of NBL in children with paraneoplastic syndrome suggests that, in these cases, NBL cells have been recognized by the immune system and eliminated, on one side, whereas, on the other side, they induced the production of cross-reactive antibodies and/or T cells, responsible for the clinical autoimmune manifestations.

Interestingly, NBL shows, in general, high lymphocytic infiltration, with variable distribution and characteristics, the most striking infiltration being observed, as mentioned, in OMS-associated tumors [31]. The presence of tumor-infiltrating lymphocytes (TILs) in tumor masses represents a favorable prognostic factor in NBL, as for many other cancers, indicating tumor recognition by cells involved in immune-surveillance. Characterization of the NBL-associated TILs is difficult, considering the low frequency of these cells. However, Facchetti and colleagues have been able to investigate immunophenotypic and functional features of these cells, documenting the presence of CD4 and CD8 T cells, with a polyclonal Vß gene expression repertoire, as well as CD56+ NK cells [46]. In OMS-associated NBL, TILs not only are overall more abundant but also frequently organize in complex structures resembling follicles of lymphoid organs, with germinal center, follicular mantle, and follicular dendritic cells [47].

Another subset of tumor-infiltrating immune cells with particular relevance is represented by NKT cells, whose infiltration of primary tumors has been shown to predict a better prognosis for NBL patients, as mentioned previously [19]. These cells are thought to provide very early signals, through cytokines production, for other cells of the immune system to initiate innate and adaptive responses [48]. The role of NKT cells in NBL is complex and not yet fully understood. It is, in fact, known that these cells mediate the tumor immune-surveillance indirectly via activation of NK cell cytotoxicity [49]. However, the extremely low levels of NK cell infiltrates in primary NBL suggest that other mechanisms mediate NKT cell function in established tumors. An interesting insight into these mechanisms has been provided by Song et al. who demonstrate that NKT cells mediate killing of $CD68^+$ tumor-associated monocytes/macrophages (TAMs), a subset of cells expressing CD1d in primary NBL tumors and known to promote the emergence of a tumor-induced immune-suppressive microenvironment [50]. The authors suggested that this mechanism might explain the association between NKT-cell infiltration of the tumor and a more favorable patient outcome.

13.2 Rationale for Immunotherapy

Notwithstanding more risk-refined treatment of children with NBL, the prognosis for patients belonging to the high-risk group (i.e., children older than 18 months with metastatic diseases—stage IV—at diagnosis or with MYCN amplification) remains grim, their 5-year probability of disease-free survival (DFS) still being 35–40% [51–53]. Disease recurrence remains the main cause of treatment failure, despite the integrated use of chemotherapy, including myeloablative therapy with autologous HSCT, surgery, and radiotherapy, followed by differentiation therapy with isotretinoin [54].

In light of these observations, there is an urgent need to implement and develop novel therapeutic approaches able to change this poor outcome, possibly sparing the relevant long-term toxicities associated with conventional treatments. Taken together all the evidences for the interactions between NBL cells and the immune system, immunotherapy represents a promising opportunity for advancement in the field.

The concept of treating tumors by harnessing the immune system finds its basis in the physiological, complex phenomenon known as *cancer immunoediting* [55]. Physiologically, the immune system has the potential to recognize and eliminate malignant cells by inducing their apoptosis. The innate and adaptive mechanisms taking place in this cancer immune-surveillance cooperate synergistically in the first phase of the process, namely the *elimination phase*. During this phase, tumor cells are eliminated because transformed cells often co-express both ligands for activating receptors present on cells of innate immunity and antigens recognized by lymphocyte of adaptive immunity (Fig. 13.2). A fundamental basis of immunosurveillance is that, in order for a cancer cell to be immunogenic, it must express antigens that differ from the non-transformed counterparts. Such antigens, known as tumor-associated antigens (TAAs), can derive from different mechanisms active during the malignant transformation of the cell. In particular, they can be mutational antigens,

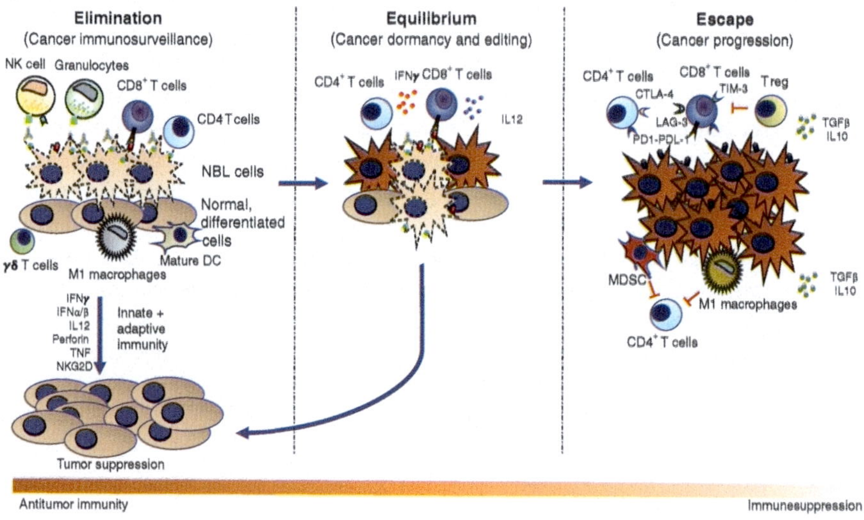

Fig. 13.2 The phases of cancer immunoediting: elimination, equilibrium, and escape. Cancer immunoediting is a dynamic process encompassing three different phases. In the first phase, the concerted action of the innate and adaptive immunity efficiently eliminates the newly formed cancer cells in a sophisticated cancer immunosurveillance mechanism restoring the normal tissue (*elimination*). If rare cancer cells variants are not destroyed, however, the second phase starts, and there is a fine balance between the tumor persistence and the prevention of the tumor overgrowth mediated mainly by the adaptive immune system (*equilibrium*). This phase might represent the end stage of the immunoediting process, with the cancer maintaining an occult status for the lifetime of the host; it might also revert to the elimination phase and lead to the spontaneous regression of the tumor, as observed for NBL. Lastly, the constant pressure of the immune system might induce the editing of the tumor cells, which might develop mechanisms of resistance to the immunosurveillance, and select genetic variants that can evade the elimination. The tumor cells themselves can therefore induce an immunosuppressive state in concert with the microenvironment and favor the tumor overgrowth, entering the third phase (*escape*)

originated from the acquisition of new genetic aberrations, or be overexpressed cellular antigens or viral antigens. Alternatively, they can be embryonal antigens that persist, instead of being silenced after birth, with the exception of the germ cells of the testis and ovary (the "cancer/testis antigens"—CTAs). In NBL, some TAAs have been described, such as the CTAs of the antigen families of the melanoma antigen–encoding gene (MAGE) transcripts or NY-ESO1, the diasialoganglioside GD2, or the tumor-promoting B7-H3 molecule [56–59].

In this phase of cancer immunoediting, several immune cells and soluble factors interact to control the tumor growth, including macrophages, dendritic cells (DC), NK cells, CD4 and CD8 T cells, NKT cells, and IFN-γ, IFN-aß, IL12, and TNF [60].

For mechanisms not completely understood, however, in certain subjects, cancer cells can enter an immune-mediated dormancy, which defines the *equilibrium phase*. This phase is poorly understood since it has been very difficult to model in mice and has been described occasionally in humans [56]. Studies on the cellular microenvironment of tumors in equilibrium revealed a higher proportion of $CD8^+$ T cells, NK cells, and γδTcells and a lower proportion of NKT cells, Tregs, and myelosuppressive dendritic cells as compared with tumors that escaped surveillance and undergoing overgrowth and progression [61]. These data indicate that the balance between immunosuppressive and antitumor effector functions is associated with maintaining the tumor in the dormancy state. T cells, IL12, and IFN-γ have been shown to be necessary in this phase; conversely, innate immunity is not; the latter appears as an obligate requirement for the elimination phase [62]. During this phase, the tumor mass is edited by the immune system and selection of highly or poorly immunogenic clones in such a genetically unstable cell population occurs, defining the fate of the tumor. If the immune pressure induces the selection of cell variants that are no longer recognized by the immune system, they acquire the ability to escape this recognition (*escape phase*) and, therefore, cancer develops. Otherwise, the equilibrium phase may potentially last for the entire lifetime, resulting in a definitive control of tumor growth. Several, complex and partly understood mechanisms are responsible for the escape, and encompass antigen loss variants/defects in the antigen presentation, resistance to immune effector mechanisms, and the development of an immunosuppressive tumor microenvironment [63]. Part of the escape mechanisms of NBL have been discussed above. Several other strategies developed by NBL cells to avoid immune-surveillance have been highlighted in the last two decades. They were shown to express high levels of gangliosides containing negatively charged epitopes that are poorly immunogenic or even immunosuppressive [64]. In addition, it has been documented that NBL can exploit protectin (CD59), a membrane protein that inhibits membrane attack complex (MAC) formation, to resist complement-mediated cytotoxicity (CMC) [65]. Moreover, the tumor can express and release inhibitory factors and proteins that induce apoptosis of T cells and NK cells (such as FasL, calprotectin, and HLA-G) [66–68].

The actual knowledge of the immune-editing process clearly reveals that, in order for the immune system to clear the tumor, immune tolerance has to be overcome. Immunotherapy finds its basis on these evidences, encompassing several different strategies aimed at breaking this tolerance and restoring the clearance of the tumor.

Interestingly, analyses performed on cancer patients treated with immunotherapies reveal that part or the entire immune-editing process reoccurs as an effect of the treatment, with patients entering the elimination phase, others showing evidence of a therapeutically induced equilibrium, and still others developing additional escape mechanisms [56]. The same mechanisms can even be present contemporarily in the same patient with different lesions displaying different responses [69].

13.3 Preclinical and Translational Approaches of Immunotherapy for Neuroblastoma

The main strategies explored to achieve the objective of the immune eradication of a clinically evident tumor include vaccination approaches to elicit specific immune responses to tumor antigens in the host; therapeutic administration of monoclonal antibodies to target and eliminate tumor cells; adoptive transfer of in vitro expanded, naturally arising or genetically engineered, tumor-specific lymphocytes.

13.3.1 Tumor Vaccination Strategies

Vaccination, a strategy aimed at inducing cytotoxic T lymphocytes (CTLs) able to recognize the desired antigens, has been, and remains, an effective strategy to protect animals and humans from infection for a long time [70, 71]. This approach has the advantage of being an "active" form of immunotherapy that acts by eliciting an immune response in the host, rather than by passively transferring it, therefore being, in principle, able to induce long-lasting memory and response. It can be effective especially for those tumors that are antigenic (i.e., they express TAAs), but not highly immunogenic (i.e., they fail to activate an effective immune response). In order to induce CTL responses, antigen presentation to the cytotoxic lymphocytes must occur, either through professional antigen-presenting cells (APCs) or by the tumor cell itself exerting an APC function. Several approaches of vaccination have been developed, and the strategy of choice depends on whether (1) the genetic sequence of the TAA is known, (2) the immunogenic epitopes recognized by the CTLs are known, or (3) tumor material is available and amenable to genetic modifications (Table 13.1).

Constructing an effective vaccine strategy for NBL, considering its highly immunosuppressive microenvironment and the multiple mechanisms of immune escape, is extremely daunting. Several preclinical studies have shown that DNA vaccines encoding NBL antigens offer a safe and effective therapy in murine models [72–74]. Huebener et al. developed a DNA vaccine targeting tyrosine hydroxylase, an enzyme highly expressed in NBL, delivered orally, using attenuated *Salmonella typhimurium* as a carrier [74]. The choice of this cellular carrier is aimed at helping stimulate the immune system through the presence of lipopolysaccharides on the bacterial

Table 13.1 Most relevant vaccination strategies for tumor immunotherapies

Vaccine strategy	Mechanism of action	Requirements	Advantages	Disadvantages
DNA vaccines	The sequence of a known TAA is injected inducing the expression of the encoded TAA and activating both CTL and humoral response	• Well characterized sequence of the TAA • Presence of APCs in the injected area	• Stable • Inexpensive • Simple to administer • No requirements for viral vectors	• Possible autoimmune disease • Weak responses
Dendritic cell (DC) vaccines	In vitro generation of DCs from the patient's precursors and loading with TAA peptides, tumor lysate/proteins, RNA, viral vectors or recombinant bacteria	• Identification of the immunogenic epitopes • Manufacturing facilities for generation of DCs	• Simple to administer • Inexpensive	• Possible autoimmune disease • Weak response • Possible time consuming manufacturing
Tumor vaccines	Ex vivo or in vivo genetic modifications of the tumor cells in order to render them more immunogenic, therefore improving one or multiple phases of the CTL activation and response	• Availability of tumor material • Tumor material amenable for genetic modifications • Manufacturing facility for gene modifications	Ex vivo • Early evaluation of transgene expression • Control of the number of transduced tumor cells injected In vivo • Fully representative of the whole tumor population • Elicitation of systemic responses that can eradicate metastatic tumors	Ex vivo • Possibly not fully representative of the in vivo tumor population In vivo • Low control of the number of transduced cells • Variability in the transduction of the different portion of large masses • Interpatient variability • Immunosuppressive microenvironment

membrane and CpG motifs within the bacterial genome, known to activate TLRs. This study demonstrated a clear antitumor effect of the approach, with reduction of the tumor growth and prevention of metastatic spread. Moreover, the induced immune responses were specific to NBL tissue and no infiltration of T cells was detected in normal tissues expressing tyrosine hydroxylase. Promising results were obtained using the same vector to deliver a minigene DNA vaccine encoding for survivin-derived peptides [75]. Using this approach in a syngeneic mouse model, the group of Fest et al. showed a reduction of both the tumor mass and the metastatic lesions and a significantly increased infiltration of CTLs in the tumors. Other target antigens explored have been the CTAs MAGE and NY-ESO1 and MYCN [76, 77]. Promising preclinical data were obtained using DCs pulsed with tumor lysate and modified to express IL4/GM-CSF or IL2 to boost the immune activation of CTLs [78, 79]. Finally, interesting preclinical results were obtained also with the use of tumor cell vaccination strategies, which are considered particularly appropriate for tumors such as NBL, considering that it can be relatively easily expanded in culture [80, 81]. In 2008, Croce et al. developed a vaccine based on NBL cells engineered to express IL21. When injected into immunocompetent mice, NBL-IL21 cells produced a significant reduction of tumor vascularity and improved the overall survival of tumor-bearing mice [82].

13.3.2 Monoclonal Antibodies

An important step in the development of immunotherapies has been the introduction of mAbs targeting TAAs. These biological agents act through the binding of the antigen and the induction of both an antibody-dependent cellular cytotoxicity (ADCC) and a complement-mediated cytotoxicity (CMC). Several antibodies designed to target tumor-specific antigens have been developed, and their efficacy has been variously tested in clinical trials. Examples of successful immunotherapies based on mAbs in solid cancers include the epidermal growth factor receptor antibody (cetuximab) for head and neck cancers and the human epidermal growth receptor 2 (HER2 or HER2/neu) antibody for breast cancer [83, 84]. Whereas the first mAbs were entirely derived from an animal host (mouse, rabbit, or chimeric) with the relative risk of immunization, leading to potentially fatal reactions and increased clearance from the serum when infused in humans, new generations mAbs have been humanized or are entirely human, reducing this risk [85].

In the context of NBL, antibodies targeting the cell-surface ganglioside GD2 have been developed and, based on the promising preclinical results, have been extensively explored in the clinical setting. As mentioned previously, GD2 is a disialoganglioside representing a good TAA target since it is largely and stably expressed on the cell membrane of human NBL cells, with little evidence of down-regulation or tumor escape in response to immunotherapies targeting this molecule [86]. Being an oncofetal antigen, GD2 is expressed during fetal development and in some normal tissues, mainly mature neurons, pain fibers and skin cells [87]. Three anti-GD2 IgG Ab have been extensively clinically tested: chimeric Ch14.18, murine 14G2a, and 3F824. All these mAbs have shown activity in preclinical studies, in particular when administered with IL2 and granulocyte-macrophage colony-stimulating factor (GM-CSF), but only chimeric Ch14.18 proved to be efficacious in a randomized clinical trial [88, 89]. A relevant understanding of the mechanisms of action of these mAbs has been provided by the clinical trials, showing a relevant role of NK- and granulocyte-mediated ADCC, and will be further discussed in the relative section [90].

For further improving the cytotoxicity of mAbs, they have been modified through the conjugation to cytokines, cytotoxic chemotherapeutic agents, radioisotopes, or toxins [91].

Immunocytokines are genetic fusion proteins derived from the combination of the humanized ch14.18 mAb with cytokines, aimed at targeting the tumor tissue and acting as immune-stimulants [92, 93]. Interestingly, in an immunocompetent murine model of metastatic NBL, the administration of the ch14.18-IL2 fusion protein showed a more efficient eradication of bone marrow and liver metastases than the administration of the equivalent mixture of the single components [94]. Moreover, the authors clearly showed that the eradication was mediated by NK cells since NK cell ablation abrogated entirely the antitumor effect, which remained, conversely, conserved when $CD8^+$ cells were deficient. Despite the interesting results observed in the preclinical models, the clinical translation revealed only modest therapeutic improvements, while significant increase of toxicities, including nerve pain, hypotension, and capillary leak syndrome was recorded, leading to the withdrawal of the approach [95].

The mostly studied and exploited TAA for NBL is undoubtedly the GD2 and, despite decades of research on this antigen, the remainder of the NBL cell-surface proteome (or *surfaceome*) remains unexplored. Other potential neuroblastoma cell-surface targets have been the O-acetylated GD2, GD3, ALK, L1 cell adhesion molecule (L1CAM), and B7-H3 [96–99].

The antigen B7-H3 is a member of the B7 family of immune regulators, such as CD80, CD86, PD-L1, and PD-L2 and, in addition to a subset of NBL tumors, is expressed on many normal tissues such as spleen, lymph nodes, thymus, and fetal liver, as well as other tumors [100]. The cognate ligand of B7-H3 has not been identified yet and is induced on activated T and NK cells, and blockade of this interaction results in reduced interferon-γ production and loss of cytotoxic activity of these cells. It represents a promising novel target for cancer immunotherapy [101].

In order to develop effective immune-based therapies for NBL, the identification of surface TAAs with limited expression on normal childhood tissues and, possibly, required for tumor sustenance is extremely important. Through an RNA sequence-based approach and a protein-level validation, associated with tumor functional studies, high-risk NBL tumors have been recently screened in order to respond to this unmet need [102]. Thanks to a multistep discovery and prioritization algorithm, the extracellular glycosylphosphatidylinositol (GPI) anchored signaling co-receptor glypican 2 (GPC2) was identified as a promising immunotherapeutic target, being highly expressed in NBL due to MYCN-driven mechanisms (such as transcriptional activation and/or somatic gain of the GPC2 locus). GPC2 was not detectable at relevant levels in normal childhood tissues (including normal neural crest-derived tissues) and required for tumor proliferation. Lastly, a GPC2 drug–conjugate antibody was developed; it showed a high affinity for the target and potent cytotoxic activity against tumor cells [100].

One of the main limitations of monoclonal antibodies relates to their inability to engage the most powerful agent of the immune system, namely T cells. In order to incorporate this essential component of the immune response, the bispecific T-cell engager (BiTE) technology has been developed. The mechanism of action of engagers relies on the formation of an immunological synapsis between T cells and tumor cells, resulting in an activation of T lymphocytes and the consequent induction of apoptosis of the tumor target [103]. BiTEs specific for CD3 and tumor antigens, such as CD19, HER2, or EGFR, successfully proved able to retarget T cells in several preclinical and clinical tumor models [104, 105]. In NBL, interesting preclinical results have been shown in vitro with the use of a BiTE directed against the neural cell adhesion molecule (NCAM, CD56), an antigen expressed on nearly 100% of NBLs [106]. This antigen is also expressed on NK cells and the group of Jensen et al. proved that, in the presence of NK cells, the NCAM-BiTE is able to induce T cells to proliferate and mount cytotoxic action against NCAM-positive NBL cells [107]. Although NK cells were almost completely depleted during T-cell activation, representing a possible pitfall of the strategy, they surprisingly observed a positive correlation between the number of NK cells present during T-cell activation and the strength of the cytotoxicity against NBL cells, suggesting the hypothesis of an "enhancement function" exerted by NK cells on T cells in this particular model [108]. GD-2-directed BiTE have also been developed and studied, showing a significantly improved tumor control and survival in the treated mice and a relevant infiltration of the tumor tissues with T cells and monocytes [109].

13.3.3 Adoptive Therapies

Although widely used to induce antitumor responses, cancer vaccines and monoclonal antibodies may be blocked in vivo by the multiple immune evasion strategies of the tumor. The generation and engineering of cells for adoptive immunotherapies offer several advantages over these strategies, including the following: (1) the characteristics of the cells, such as phenotype, activity, and specificity, can be evaluated and eventually tuned before infusion; (2) ex vivo expanded cells can be modified to express a marker, enabling their in vivo tracking; and (3) the cells can be engineered to improve their function or modify their antigen specificity. Adoptive therapies, therefore, encompass all the approaches that involve the adoptive transfer of manipulated immune cells targeting tumor cells in vivo. For NBL, the main strategies studied have been chimeric antigen receptor (CAR) T cells, NK cells, and NKT cells.

13.3.3.1 Adoptive T-Cell Therapies

Adoptive immunotherapy based on T cells has been under investigation for several years, arising from the use of non-gene-modified donor lymphocyte infusions (DLIs) for leukemia relapse after HSCT to optimize/implement the graft-versus-leukemia (GvL) effect [110]. This strategy has led to sustained remissions in patients with chronic myelogenous leukemia, while results in acute leukemia have been less successful [111]. Moreover, it has the significant risk of inducing graft-versus-host disease (GvHD). This risk could be removed by the use of autologous T cells but requires a means of breaking tolerance. The group of Rosenberg et al. provided a demonstration of the possibility of harnessing the cytotoxic ability of autologous T cells more than 20 years ago. In their clinical trial, they proved that tumor-infiltrating T cells adoptively infused after in vitro expansion in patients affected by metastatic melanoma had an antitumor effect, obtaining an objective response in 34% of the patients [112].

Through the antigen-specificity of mAb, the range of potential targets is extremely wide, including potentially any cell-surface molecule to which an antibody can be made, regardless of their nature (protein, glycoprotein, or glycolipid). As mentioned, an ideal target should be tumor specific, not expressed by normal cells, ubiquitously expressed on tumor cells and possibly required for tumor sustainment and expansion. Such ideal antigens are hard to find, but valuable alternatives include either antigens that are expressed at a different level on tumor cells compared with normal cells or that are expressed on a single-cell lineage whose function is replaceable. Considering the experience developed on the targeting of GD2 for NBL, this antigen represents an attractive target also for the development of more advanced adoptive T-cell approaches, such as the engineering of T cell with chimeric antigen receptor (CAR T cells).

The concept of combining the major histocompatibility complex (MHC)-independent antigen recognition of mAb and the effector function of T cells has been a complete revolution in the field of immunotherapy. Originally ideated by Eshhar et al. in 1989, it consists in the engineering of T cells to express a CAR resulting from the fusion of the heavy and light chain variable regions of a mAb to the cytotoxic zeta chain (ζ) of a T-cell receptor (TCR), named first-generation CAR (Fig. 13.3) [113]. In detail, the single-chain Ab fragments (scFv) are obtained from a variable heavy (VH) and a variable light (VL) chain isolated from an antibody. The signaling endo-domain is derived from the CD3ζ chain or the γ-chain of the

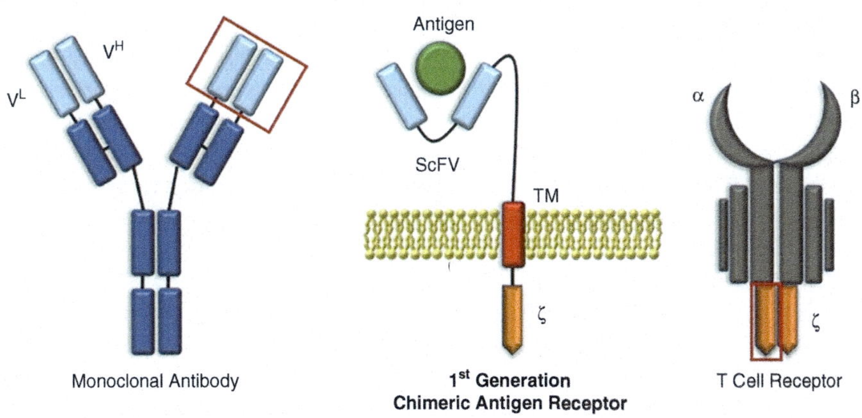

Fig. 13.3 First-generation CAR. The heavy and light chain variable regions of a monoclonal antibody are fused, through a spacer/hinge region and a transmembrane (TM) portion, with the ζ chain of a TCR to create a chimeric molecule that can be activated upon antigen recognition in an MCH-independent fashion

high-affinity IgE Fc receptor (FcεRI). The scFv determines the CAR antigen specificity and binds the target protein in an MHC-independent/unrestricted manner. Adjacent to the binding region, there is a hinge, sometimes derived from the CH2CH3 portion of immunoglobulin G1 (IgG1) that confers flexibility to the construct, in order to improve the binding. After engagement of the target, T cells are activated by the endo-domain signaling and induce the tumor cell lysis by activation of the cytotoxic machinery (granzyme-B and perforin) [111]. Using this strategy, it is now possible to target a wide range of tumor-associated targets and to potentially overcome the low immunogenicity of tumor related to the low levels of antigen and their poor presentation by MHC molecules at the tumor surface.

The advantages of CAR T cells over mAb are multiple and rely on the ability of CAR T cells to eliminate the tumor cells even at low levels of antigen expression, to self-amplify upon activation and to be better distributed in the tissues. Moreover, cytokine secretion upon T-cell activation by tumor antigen recruits additional components of the immune system, improving the antitumor response. Lastly, CAR T cells may enter the memory pool and provide long-lasting protection against tumor recurrence.

Engagement of the CAR by its ligand expressed by tumor cells results in tyrosine phosphorylation of immune-receptor activation motifs present in the cytoplasmic domain, initiating T-cell signaling and specific tumor cell lysis via the perforin/granzyme pathways. However, tumors rarely express costimulatory molecules. The presence of the signal 1 (ζ chain of the TCR) in the absence of signal 2 (costimulatory molecules signaling) enables CAR T cells to be activated and kill tumor cells, but not to proliferate and expand. This observation led to the development of second-generation CARs, incorporating signaling domains of the T-cell costimulatory molecules in frame with the CD3 ζ chain so that upon ligation, T cells both kill and proliferate [114]. Intracytoplasmic signaling domains of CD28, CD134 (OX40), CD137 (4-1BB), inducible costimulatory (ICOS), CD27, DAP10, or CD244 (2B4) in various combinations have been used [115, 116].

Unfortunately, it has been shown that, in the setting of solid tumors, second-generation CARs do not always expand properly after infusion into patients, and it is well accepted that antitumor efficacy requires adequate expansion and persistence in vivo [117]. Evidences of the primary role of T-cell exhaustion in limiting the antitumor efficacy of T cells in the setting of chronic antigen exposure are emerging [118, 119]. Recently, the central role of the CAR structure in predisposing chronic T-cell activation and exhaustion has been demonstrated, proving that CD28 costimulation augments, whereas 4-1BB costimulation reduces, exhaustion induced by persistent CAR signaling [120].

In the search for the optimal design for a CAR, even more potent constructs have been developed, containing two costimulatory domains (Fig. 13.4). These so-called third-generation CARs provide more potent proliferation in response to tumors than either first or second generations; moreover, higher T-cell resistance to several tumor evasion strategies was observed [121]. However, while the superiority of second-generation CAR over the first has been clearly proved, whether the incorporation of additional costimulatory domains in the third generation provides further benefits remains unknown [122].

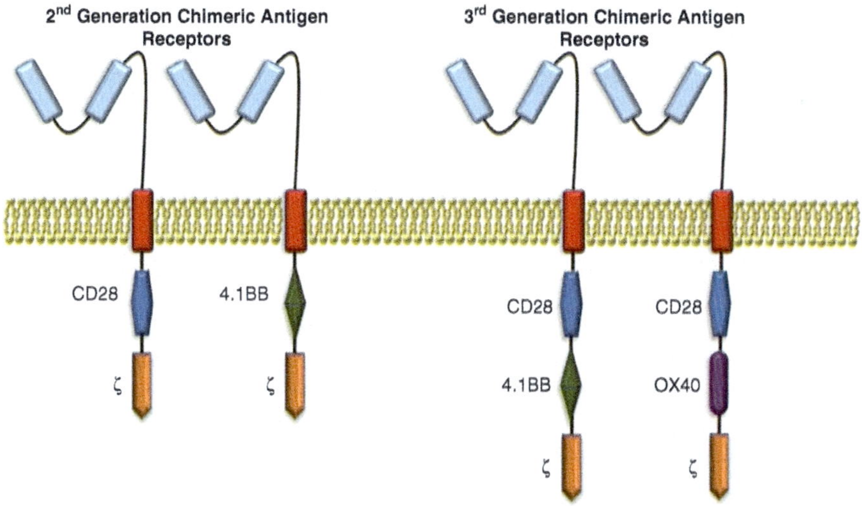

Fig. 13.4 Second- and third-generation CARs. Incorporation of the intracytoplasmic domains of costimulatory molecules (i.e., CD28, 4.1BB, OX40) generate second and third generations of CAR

The optimal design of a given CAR remains an area of active investigation and should be empirically evaluated case-by-case for the treatment of different malignancies [123].

In the setting of NBL, two main antigens have been targeted by CAR constructs: L1 cell adhesion molecule (L1CAM, mAb CE7) and GD2. L1CAM is a glycoprotein belonging to the immunoglobulin superfamily whose expression is relatively specific to NBL, although the molecule is also found on some cells of the central nervous system, sympathetic ganglia, and adrenal medulla, as well as on other types of cancer cells [124]. The L1CAM-CAR construct tested by Gonzalez et al. is a first-generation CAR that has been transduced in human T cells using naked DNA electrotransfer of the vector [125]. In the preclinical setting, this approach was shown to be effective, in vitro, in recognizing NBL cells and inducing their lysis, with release of Th1 cytokines, leading to the initiation of the clinical testing of the platform (see further for details) [122]. On the other side, the experience with GD2 CAR revealed a low persistence of first-generation CAR T cells and the need of further improving potency and persistence of these cells. Several strategies have been developed. Before moving to constructs of further generation, in fact, the use of Epstein–Barr virus (EBV)-specific CTLs instead of polyclonal activated T cells (ATCs) has been tested, to exploit the continuous antigenic stimulus of EBV-CTLs. This approach has been tested in the clinical setting, as explained further, showing an improved persistence of EBV-CTLs expressing the CAR construct [126]. Based on the well-known physiological mechanism of activation of T cells, requiring CD28 engagement followed by costimulation through other T-cell-signaling molecules, the same group developed a third-generation GD2 CAR incorporating the CD28 and OX40 costimulatory endodomains [127]. The introduction of the two costimulatory signals induced an increased and prolonged proliferation and cytokine release upon in vitro engagement of GD2⁺ NBL cells, and a potent cytotoxic activity against the tumor cells that is maintained after multiple encounters with NBL cells.

Despite the improvement obtained by the use of more potent constructs, however, it is clear that, in order to be effective in the treatment of solid tumors such as NBL, a CAR T-cell approach must take into account the relevant role of the tumor microenvironment and the relevant immunosuppressive properties displayed by the tumor. For this reason, Caruana et al. evaluated the interaction between CAR T cells and the tumor stroma through the analysis of the infiltrative ability of CAR T cells in the NBL context, revealing that ex vivo manipulation of these cells resulted into a reduced capacity to penetrate the tumor stroma [128]. In particular, cultured T cells were found to display an impaired degradation of the extracellular matrix (ECM) related to a culture-induced, downregulation of the enzyme heparanase (HSPE), responsible for the degradation of the main components of the ECM, the heparin sulfate proteoglycans. The authors also showed that forcing the expression of HPSE by the engineering of GD2 CAR T cells, facilitated tumor infiltration significantly enhances the antitumor activity [125].

13.3.3.2 Adoptive NK- and NKT-Cell Therapies

Based on the key roles played by NK and NKT cells in the antitumor immunity of NBL, these cells represent a promising platform for developing adoptive approaches. Moreover, NK cells display their antitumor effects without induction of GvHD, therefore representing an appealing strategy to develop *off-the-shelf* treatments. Several preclinical studies have shown the efficacy of NK cells for the treatment of NBL. The infusion of human NK cells, activated in vitro by selected cytokines, such as IL-2 or IL-15, improves the survival of mice in xenograft models [129, 130]. Some limitations of the approach, however, emerged also in the preclinical setting, including the low number of activated NK cells that reach the tumor sites as well as the low persistence of the cells, revealing the need for a further implementation of the strategy for its clinical application [131]. Strategies to induce a broader expansion and a stronger activation of NK cells ex vivo have been, therefore, developed, such as culturing and expanding with artificial APCs expressing IL-21 [132]. This approach provided promising results, determining the propagation of large numbers of NK cells that maintain potent antitumor activities. Because of this enhanced antitumor efficacy, mice bearing the NBL xenograft displayed a significantly improved survival. The anti-NBL activity of NK cells can be further enhanced by transducing the cells with a CAR construct targeting an antigen expressed by tumor cells. Interestingly, in an NBL xenograft model developed using an aggressive, drug-resistant NBL cell line, the infusion of NK cells transduced with a first-generation GD2-CAR mediated a significant antitumor response, proving the validity of the approach [133].

NKT cells can also be exploited for cancer treatment, considering their ability to induce NK-cell-mediated killing of NBL cells [134]. Several features make these cells an attractive platform for adoptive immunotherapies, such as their effective trafficking to tumor sites and their pleiotropic antitumor activity, mediated through direct killing of CD1d+ tumor cells, inhibition of TAMs, and transactivation of NK cells [135]. Therefore, human iNKT cells have been engineered with a third-generation GD2-CAR expressing 4.1BB and CD28 costimulatory domains and tested in a human xenograft model of metastatic NBL, showing a significant tumor control, translating into an increased survival of the mice [136]. Moreover, the group of Metelitsa identified a subset of NKT cells with a high proliferative potential, the CD62L$^+$ NKT cells. They clearly showed that the expansion and transduction of this subset of cells with a second-generation GD2-CAR provides significantly higher expansion of the cells and a superior persistence and therapeutic activity in vivo, as compared to the PBMCs-derived GD2-CAR$^+$ NKT cells [137].

13.4 Clinical Trials of Immunotherapy for Neuroblastoma

Taking into account the promising preclinical evidences previously discussed, several clinical trials have explored the different immunotherapy approaches in order to improve the grim prognosis of children affected by high-risk, relapsed/refractory NBL. The main challenge now lies in determining which patients are the most suitable to receive these immunotherapies and how we can use information about their tumors and microenvironments to inform us about the most effective treatment on a personalized basis.

13.4.1 Clinical Trials on NBL Vaccines

One of the first immunotherapy tested in patients has been based on different platforms of cancer vaccinations. Few clinical trials have been developed and/or are ongoing and are listed in Table 13.2. Despite the good safety profile and the feasibility of the approach, RNA-pulsed, DC-based vaccine showed scarce immune response, mainly humoral, and no objective response, revealing one of the main intrinsic limitations of these approaches, namely the strong immunosuppression of the patients at the time of administration impairs the possibility of inducing an effective antitumor immune response [143]. Similar results were obtained by the use of a similar strategy, namely tumor lysate pulsed DC [138].

More recently, in a phase I/II trial open at Memorial Sloan Kettering Cancer Center (Clinicaltrials.gov NCT00911560), relapsed patients have been treated in second or subsequent remission with a bivalent vaccine combining the antigens GD2 and GD3, covalently linked to the protein keyhole limpet hemocyanin (KHL) and associated to the immunologic adjuvant OPT-821 and to ß-glucan, a potent immune-stimulant. The results of the phase I trial showed a good safety profile of the treatment, exempt from major toxicities, and an encouraging antitumor immune effect, with 12/15 patients displaying antibody responses against GD2 and/or GD3 and 6/10 assessable patients with a disappearance of MRD; relapse-free survival at 24 months was reported to reach 80% ± 10% [142].

Table 13.2 Clinical trials using vaccine strategies for treatment of NBL

Vaccine	Comments	Reference #
Tumor RNA pulsed DC	11 patients with newly diagnosed stage 4 NBL. 2/3 pts. tested with tumor-specific humoral response; no objective responses	[129]
Tumor cell lysate pulsed DC	15 patients with pediatric solid tumors including neuroblastoma (3a), fibrosarcoma (1), PNET (2), renal cell cancer (1), osteosarcoma (1), inflammatory myofibroblastic sarcoma (1), hepatic sarcoma (1), desmoplastic round cell sarcoma (1), Ewing's sarcoma (2), clear cell sarcoma (1), Wilms' tumor (1) Outcome: 9 PD, 5 SD, 1 PR	[138]
Autologous neuroblastoma cells expressing IL-2	10 patients; 1 CR, 1 PR, 3 SD, 5 PD; 4/5 with clinical response had detectable antitumor T-cell response	[139]
Allogeneic neuroblastoma cells expressing IL-2	15 patients; 1 PR, 7 SD, 4 PD; no increase in direct cytotoxic effector function against immunizing cell line	[140]
Allogeneic neuroblastoma expressing IL-2 and lptn	21 patients; 2 CR, 1 PR; increased numbers of T and NK cells and eosinophils in peripheral circulation; induction of Th2 helper T cells	[141]
GD2/GD3-KHL combined with b-glucan	13 treated patients with NBL in ≥second CR/VGPR. Outcome: 12/13 patients remaining relapse-free at a median of 32 months; 1 relapse at 21 months; 6/10 disappearance of MRD. Still recruiting	[142]

Another vaccine strategy tested in clinical trials employed patient-derived, autologous, NBL tumor cells, engineered to express the T-cell stimulating cytokine IL-2 [139]. Tumor-specific immune response was elicited in 4/10 patients and 3 children showed tumor response (1 CR, 1 PR, 1 sustained SD). Also, this study did not show significant toxicity in any of the patients [142]. The feasibility of preparing individualized autologous vaccines for each patient is limited by the labor-intensive preparation of these products, and therefore, in order to develop an "*off-the-shelf*," universal, vaccine strategy, the same group tested, in a phase I trial, the same vaccine based on allogeneic, irradiated, NBL cell lines [140]. The results were, unfortunately, disappointing, with fewer antitumor immune responses than with the autologous strategy [139]. To improve the approach, the T-cell attractant lymphotactin has been added to the allogeneic vaccine with encouraging responses: not only tumor-specific, T-cell and humoral, immune responses were documented but also an increase in the circulating NK cells [141]. Moreover, 11/28 treated children showed objective responses, with 4 CR, 2 PR, and 5 SD, all of them heavily pretreated and with extensive disease [140].

Overall, the results obtained so far with vaccination strategies in pediatric NBL trials reveal that a subset of patients respond to this approach. Therefore, the question of identifying the variables predicting the occurrence of response in this subset of patients remains open, in order to predictively stratify the population and select the patients that have the chance to benefit from these approaches, on one side, and to develop new strategies that can be effective also in those patients that are actually considered non-responders, on the other side.

13.4.2 Clinical Trials on Monoclonal Antibodies

Targeted immunotherapy using a monoclonal antibody directed against GD2 represents an important advancement in the treatment of high-risk NBL and usually takes place after patients have received autologous stem-cell transplantation (auto-SCT).

As mentioned previously in the preclinical section, three version of the antibody have been developed. The first anti-GD2 mAb to be clinically tested was the murine IgG3 3F8, described in 1985 and first tested in a phase I trial in 1987, on 8 patients with refractory high-risk NBL [144]. The promising results of this first trial, namely two long-lasting CR, led to the further extension of the study to a phase II trial, with 16 more patients treated in relapse and obtaining one durable CR and one mixed response [145]. The subsequent shift to the use of the mAb 3F8 in patients with MRD after consolidation lead to more promising results, with 38% of the patients remaining free of progression for 40 to >130 months. Further improvement was obtained by combining the treatment with the administration of GM-CSF and isotretinoin, leading to 5-year PFS and OS of 62% and 81%, respectively, more than doubling the historical rates obtained with the standard of care [146, 147]. A major limitation of the approach emerged already with the first patients and is related to the development of human anti-mouse antibodies (HAMA), responsible for the elimination/inactivation of the antibody. Therefore, although, during the 1990s, a second murine anti-GD2 with promising antitumor efficacy had been evaluated in phase I and II trials, research on these first two mAbs ceased after the less immunogenic chimeric preparation ch14.18 became available [148, 149]. Two phase I trials reported highly encouraging results: the first showed 5/9 objective responses (2 CR, 2 PR, and 1 minor response) in relapsed/resistant high-risk NBL patients and no HAMA production; the second trial obtained 5/10 responses including 1 PR and 4 minor responses [150, 151]. The next phase of clinical development of ch14.18 occurred with the addition of GM-CSF (in the Pediatric Oncology Group—POG—trials) or GM-CSF, IL-2, and isotretinoin (in the Children's Oncology Group—COG—trial). Several phase I and II trials on multiple-relapsed patients first, and then after auto-SCT in frontline-treated patients, showed sustained responses [152–154]. In particular, the COG trial reported an estimated 3-year survival of approximately 78%, opening to the evaluation of the approach in a large, randomized, phase III trial. This study compared treatment with ch14.18, IL-2, GM-CSF plus isotretinoin with isotretinoin alone, at the end of the consolidation phase, and confirmed the efficacy of the approach in preventing NBL relapse among patients in first complete remission [88]. The study enrolled 226 patients and showed a 2-year EFS of 66% vs 46% for the immunotherapy arm vs the standard arm, respectively ($p = 0.01$); the 2-year overall survival was also significantly higher in the immunotherapy arm (86% vs 75%, $p = 0.02$). Based on these results, ch14.18 has become the standard of care in the COG centers. The recently closed phase III trial for high-risk NBL of the International Society of Paediatric Oncology European Neuroblastoma Group (SIOPEN) (EudraCT number 2006-001489-17; ClinicalTrial.gov NCT01704716) also includes the association of isotretinoin and the ch14.18 GD2-antibody in the post-consolidation maintenance phase of the treatment, randomizing patients to receive ch14.18, either alone or in combination with IL-2. The results of the trial have not yet been published.

GD2 mAbs have a more complex activity than the passive opsonization of NBL cells for ADCC and CMC. Based on the evidence that the clinical antitumor response to monoclonal antibodies has been associated with specific polymorphic-FcγR alleles, in the COG phase II trial, patients were genotyped for KIR, HLA, and FcγR to determine whether KIR receptor-ligand mismatch of specific FcγR alleles correlate with antitumor response. An association of an improved response and a KIR/KIR-ligand mismatch was documented, confirming the role of NK cells in this clinical response [155].

Noteworthy, several relevant treatment-related toxic effects were recorded in the clinical trials. The main toxicities included pain (reported to be of grade 3–4 in up to 52% of the patients in the randomized, phase III, clinical trial), hypotension, capillary leak syndrome, and hypersensitivity reactions [88]. Pain reactions tended to occur more frequently in the first cycle of treatment and has been related to the recognition of the GD2 antigen expressed by nociceptive fibers (determining a so-called "*on-target, off-tumor*" toxicity). Hypersensitivity reactions and capillary leak syndrome were more frequent during the courses involving the coadministration of IL-2, suggesting a cytokine-mediated pathogenesis. Other common side effects reported were fever, electrolytic alterations, liver dysfunction, diarrhea, iridoplegia (usually transient), urticaria, and hypoxia. Considering that IL-2 can induce adverse effects in patients, the European SIOPEN phase III trial included a randomization of the patients, in the maintenance phase with immunotherapy, in two arms: with or without coadministration of IL-2.

Considering the efficacy of GD2-mAb in binding to NBL cells, this strategy has been implemented to selectively target the metastatic sites that can be very hard to reach, such as the central nervous system (CNS). Therefore, following the demonstration of the feasibility of the approach in a phase I trial, the efficacy of 3F8 or the B7-H3 mAb radiolabeled with iodine-131 (^{131}I) and delivered intrathecally through an Ommaya device has been tested in patients with CNS metastases (ClinicalTrials.gov NCT00445965 and NCT00089245, respectively; the latter is actively recruiting) [156]. It has been reported that 17/21 treated patients remained free of CNS NBL and alive 7–74 months after CNS relapse, showing an increased survival and improved quality of life in these patients, considering that the treatment was well tolerated also by young patients [157].

Despite the improvement shown by these strategies, however, several pitfalls emerged. For instance, tumor cells can escape the toxic effects of mAb if the targeted antigen has a dim or heterogeneous expression or if the binding is suboptimal, thus failing to recruit the effector cells [158]. Moreover, mAbs are generally administered via intravenous (i.v.) infusion and their biodistribution can be altered by the presence of physical barriers; also, the relatively limited half-life reduces the exposition of the tumor to therapeutic levels of the compounds [159, 160].

13.4.3 Clinical Trials on Adoptive Therapies

The first phase I clinical trial using CARs for children with NBL investigated the feasibility, safety, and antitumor efficacy of a first-generation CAR targeting L1CAM in patients with relapsed/refractory disease [161]. Autologous $CD8^+$ CAR^+ T cells were generated by electroporating patient T cells and infused in refractory/relapsed high-risk NBL patients. Of the ten patients initially enrolled in the trial, only six could be treated: two patients became ineligible prior to cell infusion and in two additional children the cell product did not meet the release criteria. No grade IV or V toxicities were reported and only 1/6 antitumor response (PR) was detected, in the patient with MRD prior to infusion [160]. Importantly, short persistence of the CAR T cells in the blood was noted in all patients.

The results of a larger phase I clinical trial for patients with NBL and using a GD2-specific, first-generation CAR have been published preliminarily by Pule et al. in 2008 and subsequently updated in 2011 by Louis et al. [126, 162]. In order to improve the persistence of CAR T cells, in this study, the CAR was introduced by retroviral transduction not only into autologous ATCs but also into EBV-specific CTLs and both cell products were infused in 19 patients. Persistence, immunophenotypic changes, safety, and efficacy of the treatment were monitored. The treatment was well tolerated, with no dose-limiting toxicities (DLTs); mild pain at sites of disease and low-grade fever were only reported. Neither neurologic abnormalities nor peripheral neuropathy were experienced by any patient. Significant antitumor efficacy was detected in the 11 patients with evaluable disease at the time of enrollment (including 3 complete remissions—CR—1 partial response—PR—and 1 stable disease—SD) with a median OS of 931 days and a median follow-up of 329 days. Moreover, the analysis of the persistence of the CAR T cells revealed that the presence of both central memory cells and CD4 T-cell subsets in the product is critical for long-term CAR T-cell persistence and that the latter is significantly associated with improved tumor control [127]. Interestingly, since the infused ATCs and EBVs CAR T cells expressed genetically distinguishable CAR constructs, the authors showed that the initial persistence was greater in children given EBV-specific CTLs. This difference might be attributed to the physiologic costimulation received by EBVs T cells during engagement of the virus-specific endogenous TCR with APCs expressing viral antigens in seropositive recipients.

In view of these results, efforts have been made to increase the persistence of CAR T cells. Two main methods are under evaluation at the moment: the use of a lymphodepleting regimen prior to adoptive transfer and the utilization of second- and third-generation CARs.

The lymphodepletion proved able to create a better homeostatic environment for the transferred cells to expand [163]. In fact, it has become clear that the host's immune system needs to be properly conditioned in order to create an appropriate "lymphoid space" that is devoid of regulatory mechanisms. Thus, lymphodepletion enables the host to accommodate transferred T lymphocytes and gives these cells an advantage over other competing cellular populations [164].

As mentioned above, newer generation CARs have the ability to provide both activation and costimulation after binding, improving the antitumor activity of these cells and their survival. The use of second-generation CAR T cells directed against CD19 to target B-cell malignancies resulted in striking antitumor effects with high response rates and long-term persistence of the infused cells resulting in significantly improved EFS in heavily pretreated patients [165–168]. Several groups, including ours, are therefore testing the safety and efficacy of third-generation GD2 CAR T cells, variously associated with lymphodepleting regimens (Table 13.3). Recently, the results of a phase I trial on a third-generation GD2 CAR incorporating both the CD28 and the OX40 costimulatory endodomains, administered after a lymphodepleting regimen based on cyclophosphamide plus fludarabine, in patients with relapsed/refractory NBL have been published (ClinicalTrials.gov NCT01822652) [169]. No relevant toxicities were detected in any of the 11 treated patients and the use of the lymphodepleting chemotherapy was showed to induce a significant increase in the circulating levels of the homeostatic IL-15 and in the CAR T cells expansion by up to three logs. Antitumor responses, however, were modest at 6 weeks, and the association with a mAb targeting PD-1 in the last cohort of patients did not improve both persistence of the infused T cells and the antitumor response [168].

These results underline the need to further optimize this approach and to identify the best CAR construct design providing longer in vivo persistence and, ultimately, antitumor efficacy.

It must be noted, however, that more potent CAR T cells carry the risk of inducing more toxicity, in terms of cytokine release syndrome. Additional safety measures, such as the incorporation of a safety switch such as the inducible caspase 9 (iC9) in the construct, are therefore highly encouraged.

The iC9 suicide gene is an engineered human caspase 9, whose binding domain was modified with a drug-binding domain derived from human FK506-binding protein (FKBP). This chimeric caspase is quiescent inside cells until administration of a chemical dimerizing drug, AP1903 [170]. The dimerizer, an inert and nontoxic compound, induces the cross-linking and dimerization of the FKBP domains and the subsequent activation of the caspase cascade, which induces apoptosis of the cell within minutes to hours. The iC9 suicide gene is entirely human derived and therefore has a low immunogenic potential. It has been widely used in the clinic proving safe and effective, with a rapid clearance of iC9-expressing cells also *in vivo* [171, 172]. Our group has introduced the iC9 suicide gene in the CAR construct in order to increase the safety of these treatments by the means of a switch that can be rapidly activated in case of uncontrolled toxicity.

Table 13.3 Present clinical trials using CAR T cells against NBL

Approach	Status	NCT #	Phase	Sponsor	Locations	Year
GD2-CAR T cells	Recruiting	NCT02919046	I/II	Sinobioway Cell Therapy Co., Ltd.	• Nanjing Children's Hospital, China • Children's Hospital of Fudan University, Shanghai, China	2016–2020
Third generation iC9-GD2-CAR T cells	Recruiting	NCT03373097	I/II	Bambino Gesù Children's Hospital, IRCCS	• Bambino Gesù Children's Hospital, IRCCS, Rome, Italy	2017–2024
Second and third generation L1CAM-CAR T cells	Recruiting	NCT02311621	I	Seattle Children's Hospital	• Seattle Children's Hospital, Seattle, USA	2014–2017
Third generation iC9-GD2-CAR T cells	Active, not recruiting	NCT01822652	I	Baylor College of Medicine	• Houston Methodist Hospital, Houston, USA • Texas Children's Hospital, Houston, USA	2013–2015
Fourth generation GD2-CAR T cells	Recruiting	NCT02765243	II	Zhujiang Hospital	• Zhujiang Hospital of Southern Medical University, Guangzhou, China	2016–2019
GD2-CAR T cells	Recruiting	NCT02761915	I	Cancer Research UK	University College London (UCL), UK Great Ormond Street Hospital for Children, London, UK	2016–2023

13.4.4 Evaluation of Response According to the Immune-Related Response Criteria (irRC)

The mode of action of conventional cytotoxic agents implies a direct activity that leads to measurable, meaningful effects within a few weeks of initial administration. It is well established in the oncology field that the response achieved after the initial cycles of chemotherapy is predictive of the tumor response and ultimately of survival. Therefore, response criteria for solid tumors were developed by the WHO first and by the RECIST group later in 2000 [173, 174]. For NBL, the conventionally adopted International NBL Response Criteria (INRC) follow the same principle: these guidelines assume that an early increase in tumor growth and/or the appearance of new lesions indicate progressive disease (PD) and, therefore, drug failure [175].

The increasing clinical experience with immunotherapies, however, including vaccines, interleukins, mAbs, and checkpoint inhibitor–targeting drugs, reveals that the response observed with these agents might be different and display novel, unprecedented, patterns. The conventional response criteria might, therefore, be inadequate in the evaluation of the efficacy of these agents and in the prediction of long-term survival. Several studies have shown indeed that CR, PR, or SD can occur after an increase in tumor burden classified and judged as PD by conventional response criteria [176, 177].

In 2004 and 2005, a group of experts convened in a series of workshops to discuss their experiences with immunotherapeutic agents in cancer patients and draw some important conclusions, which can be summarized as follows: (a) the appearance of measurable antitumor activity may take longer for immune therapies than for cytotoxic therapies; (b) response to immune therapies may occur after conventional PD; (c) "allowance for clinically" insignificant PD is recommended, for example, in case of appearance of small new lesions in the presence of other responsive lesions; and (d) durable SD may represent antitumor activity [178].

Based on these observations, the immune-related response criteria (irRC) have been developed to provide more rigorous characterization of the atypical response patterns observed (specifically in the phase II development program for ipilimumab in melanoma) [176]. Four patterns of response to ipilimumab were observed and only two of these were captured by conventional response criteria: response in baseline lesions evident by week 12, with no new lesions, and stable disease followed by a slow, steady decline in tumor burden in some patients. The other two patterns were new and involved responses after an initial increase in total tumor burden and a reduction in total tumor burden during or after the appearance of new lesion(s). The initial increase in tumor burden may reflect either continued tumor growth until a sufficient immune response develops (*late-responding patients*) or transient immune-cell infiltrate with or without edema (*pseudo-progression*) [179]. For patients who seem to develop new lesions, they may represent T-cell infiltration into established, radiographically undetectable, tumor deposits present at baseline. As a result, inflammation in baseline lesions may be misinterpreted as PD.

Therefore, for the irRC, the antitumor response is based on total measurable tumor burden and both index and new measurable lesions are taken into account. At baseline, the total tumor burden is calculated on the index lesions and, at each subsequent tumor assessment, the new measurable lesions are incorporated into the total tumor burden. The change of the tumor burden relatively to the baseline measurements defines the response at each tumor assessment.

With these criteria, new lesions do not necessarily represent irPD if the total tumor burden does not increase by ≥25%. Moreover, if a patient is classified as having irPD at a tumor assessment, confirmation of irPD by a second scan at least 4 weeks apart is required, if the patient is clinically stable. In fact, this system allows for the identification of the late-responding patients, which have a trend toward response within 4 weeks after initial irPD, and of patients experiencing pseudo-progression. Data from the phase II study on ipilimumab in melanoma patients revealed that irRC can identify at least an additional 10% of patients with favorable survival among those characterized as WHO PD and for whom interruption of the ongoing immunotherapy and/or start of a new treatment would have represented a wrong therapeutic decision [178]. Similarly, a recent study on the evaluation of the treatment of patients with advanced melanoma with pembrolizumab revealed that atypical responses occurred in 7% of patients and that conventional RECIST might underestimate the benefit of pembrolizumab in approximately 15% of the patients, leading to premature cessation of treatment [180]. New clinical trials using immunotherapies are therefore strongly encouraged to include also the irRC in the evaluation of the response of the patients, in order to offer the best therapeutic approach to the patients.

References

1. Challis GB, Stam HJ. The spontaneous regression of cancer. A review of cases from 1900 to 1987. Acta Oncol. 1990;29:545–50.
2. Everson TC. Spontaneous regression of cancer. Ann N Y Acad Sci. 1964;114:721–35.
3. Papac RJ. Spontaneous regression of cancer: possible mechanisms. In Vivo. 1998;12:571–8.
4. Yamamoto K, et al. Marginal decrease in mortality and marked increase in incidence as a result of neuroblastoma screening at 6 months of age: cohort study in seven prefectures in Japan. J Clin Oncol. 2002;20:1209–14.
5. Sawada T, et al. Mass screening for neuroblastoma in Japan. Pediatr Hematol Oncol. 1991;8:93–109.
6. Erttmann R, et al. 10 years' neuroblastoma screening in Europe: preliminary results of a clinical and biological review from the Study Group for Evaluation of Neuroblastoma Screening in Europe (SENSE). Eur J Cancer. 1998;34:1391–7.
7. Woods WG, et al. A population-based study of the usefulness of screening for neuroblastoma. Lancet. 1996;348:1682–7.
8. Brodeur GM, Bagatell R. Mechanisms of neuroblastoma regression. Nat Rev Clin Oncol. 2014;11:704–13.
9. Muller CI, Trepel M, Kunzmann R, et al. Hematologic and molecular spontaneous remission following sepsis in acute monoblastic leukemia with translocation (9;11): a case report and review of the literature. Eur J Haematol. 2004;73:62–6.
10. Køstner AH, Johansen RF, Schmidt H, et al. Regression in cancer following fever and acute infection. Acta Oncol. 2013;52:455–7.

11. Wiemann B, Starnes CO. Coley's toxins, tumor necrosis factor and cancer research: a historical perspective. Pharmacol Ther. 1994;64:529–64.
12. Speeckaert R, van Geel N, Vermaelen KV, et al. Immune reactions in benign and malignant melanocytic lesions: lessons for immunotherapy. Pigment Cell Melanoma Res. 2011;24:334–44.
13. Redlinger RE, Mailliard RB, Lotze MT, et al. Synergistic interleukin-18 and low-dose interleukin-2 promote regression of established murine neuroblastoma in vivo. J Pediatr Surg. 2003;38:301–7.
14. Salcedo R, et al. Immunologic and therapeutic synergy of IL-27 and IL-2: enhancement of T cell sensitization, tumor-specific CTL reactivity and complete regression of disseminated neuroblastoma metastases in the liver and bone marrow. J Immunol. 2009;182:4328–38.
15. Salcedo R, et al. IL-27 mediates complete regression of orthotopic primary and metastatic murine neuroblastoma tumors: role for CD8+ T cells. J Immunol. 2004;173:7170–82.
16. Asgharzadeh S, et al. Clinical significance of tumor-associated inflammatory cells in metastatic neuroblastoma. J Clin Oncol. 2012;30:3525–32.
17. Larsson K, Kock A, Idborg H, et al. COX/mPGES-1/PGE2 pathway depicts an inflammatory-dependent high-risk neuroblastoma subset. Proc Natl Acad Sci U S A. 2015;112:8070–5.
18. Matthay KK, Maris JM, Schleiermacher G, et al. Neuroblastoma. Nat Rev Dis Primers. 2016;2:16708.
19. Metelitsa LS, Wu HW, Wang H, et al. Natural killer T cells infiltrate neuroblastomas expressing the chemokine CCL2. J Exp Med. 2004;199:1213–21.
20. Song L, Ara T, Wu H, et al. Oncogene MYCN regulates localization of NKT cells to the site of disease in neuroblastoma. J Clin Invest. 2007;117:2702–12.
21. Versteeg R, Kruse-Wolters KM, Plomp AC, et al. Suppression of class I human histocompatibility leukocyte antigen by c-myc is locus specific. J Exp Med. 1989;170:621–35.
22. Versteeg R, Noordermeer IA, Kruse-Wolters M, et al. C-myc down-regulates class I HLA expression in human melanomas. EMBO J. 1988;7:1023–9.
23. Raffaghello L, Prigione I, Bocca P, et al. Multiple defects of the antigenprocessing machinery components in human neuroblastoma: immunotherapeutic implications. Oncogene. 2005;24:4634–44.
24. Squire R, Fowler CL, Brooks SP, et al. The relationship of class I MHC antigen expression to stage IV-S disease and survival in neuroblastoma. J Pediatr Surg. 1990;25:381–6.
25. Forloni M, Albini S, Limongi MZ, et al. NF-κB, and not MYCN, regulates MHC class I and endoplasmic reticulum aminopeptidases in human neuroblastoma cells. Cancer Res. 2010;70:916–24.
26. Prigione I, Corrias MV, Airoldi I, et al. Immunogenicity of human neuroblastoma. Ann N Y Acad Sci. 2004;1028:69–80.
27. Seliger B, Cabrera T, Garrido F, et al. HLA class Iantigen abnormalities and immune escape by malignant T cells. Semin Cancer Biol. 2002;12:3–13.
28. Pistoia V, Morandi F, Bianchi G, et al. Immunosuppressive microenvironment in neuroblastoma. Front Oncol. 2013;3:1–8.
29. Venstrom JM, Zheng J, Noor N, et al. KIR and HLA genotypes are associated with disease progression and survival following autologous hematopoietic stem cell transplantation for high-risk neuroblastoma. Clin Cancer Res. 2009;15:7330–4.
30. Brandetti E, Veneziani I, Melaiu O, et al. MYCN is an immunosuppressive oncogene dampening the expression of ligands for NK-cell-activating receptors in human high-risk neuroblastoma. Oncoimmunology. 2017;6:e1316439.
31. Bottino C, Dondero A, Bellora F, et al. Natural killer cells and neuroblastoma: tumor recognition, escape mechanisms, and possible novel immunotherapeutic approaches. Front Immunol. 2014;5:56.
32. Cooper R, Khakoo Y, Matthay KK. Opsoclonus-myoclonus-ataxia syndrome in neuroblastoma: histopathologic features-a report from the Children's Cancer Group. Med Pediatr Oncol. 2001;36:623–9.

33. Altman AJ, Baehner RL. Favorable prognosis for survival in children with coincident opso-myoclonus and neuroblastoma. Cancer. 1976;37:846–52.
34. Rudnick E, Khakoo Y, Antunes NL, et al. Opsoclonus-myoclonus-ataxia syndrome in neuroblastoma: clinical outcome and antineuronal antibodies—a report from the Children's Cancer Group study. Med Pediatr Oncol. 2001;36:612–22.
35. Pranzatelli MR, Travelstead AL, Tate ED, et al. CSF B-cell expansion in opsoclonus-myoclonus syndrome: a biomarker of disease activity. Mov Disord. 2004;19:770–7.
36. Connolly AM, Pestronk A, Mehta S, et al. Serum autoantibodies in childhood opsoclonus-myoclonus syndrome: an analysis of antigenic targets in neural tissues. J Pediatr. 1997;130:878–84.
37. Blaes F, Fuhlhuber V, Korfei M, et al. Surface-binding autoantibodies to cerebellar neurons in opsoclonus syndrome. Ann Neurol. 2005;58:313–7.
38. Kirsten A, Beck S, Fühlhuber V, et al. New autoantibodies in pediatric opsoclonus myoclonus syndrome. Ann N Y Acad Sci. 2007;1110:256–60.
39. Candler PM, Dale RC, Griffin S, et al. Post-streptococcal opsoclonus-myoclonus syndrome associated with anti-neuroleukin antibodies. J Neurol Neurosurg Psychiatry. 2006;77:507–12.
40. Bataller L, Rosenfeld MR, Graus F, et al. Autoantigen diversity in the opsoclonus-myoclonus syndrome. Ann Neurol. 2003;53:347–53.
41. Korfei M, Fuhlhuber V, Schmidt-Woll T, et al. Functional characterisation of autoantibodies from patients with pediatric opsoclonus-myoclonus syndrome. J Neuroimmunol. 2005;170:150–7.
42. Morales La Madrid A, Rubin CM, Kohrman M, et al. Opsoclonus-myoclonus and anti-Hu positive limbic encephalitis in a patient with neuroblastoma. Pediatr Blood Cancer. 2012;58:472–4.
43. Fisher PG, Wechsler DS, Singer HS. Anti-Hu antibody in a neuroblastoma-associated paraneoplastic syndrome. Pediatr Neurol. 1994;10:309–12.
44. Meyer JJ, Bulteau C, Adamsbaum C, et al. Paraneoplastic encephalomyelitis in a child with neuroblastoma. Pediatr Radiol. 1995;25:S99–S101.
45. Mitchell WG, Blaes F. Cancer and autoimmunity: paraneoplastic neurological disorders associated with neuroblastic tumors. Semin Pediatr Neurol. 2017;24:180–8.
46. Facchetti P, Prigione I, Ghiotto F, et al. Functional and molecular characterization of tumor-infiltrating lymphocytes and clones thereof from major-histocompatibility-complex-negative human tumour: neuroblastoma. Cancer Immunol Immunother. 1996;42:170–8.
47. Gambini C, Conte M, Bernini G, et al. Neuroblastic tumors associated with opsoclonus-myoclonus syndrome: histological, immunohistochemical and molecular features of 15 Italian cases. Virchows Arch. 2003;442:555–62.
48. Kronenberg M. Toward an understanding of NKT cell biology: progress and paradoxes. Annu Rev Immunol. 2005;23:877–900.
49. Metelitsa LS, et al. Human NKT cells mediate antitumor cytotoxicity directly by recognizing target cell CD1d with bound ligand or indirectly by producing IL-2 to activate NK cells. J Immunol. 2001;167:3114–22.
50. Song L, Asgharzadeh S, Salo J, et al. Vα24-invariant NKT cells mediate antitumor activity via killing of tumor-associated macrophages. J Clin Invest. 2009;119:1524–36.
51. Maris JM. Recent advances in neuroblastoma. N Engl J Med. 2010;362:2202–11.
52. Cohn SL, Pearson AD, London WB, et al. The International Neuroblastoma Risk Group (INRG) classification system: an INRG Task Force report. J Clin Oncol. 2009;27:289–97.
53. Matthay KK, et al. Long-term results for children with high-risk neuroblastoma treated on a randomized trial of myeloablative therapy followed by 13-cis-retinoic acid: a children's oncology group study. J Clin Oncol. 2009;27:1007–13.
54. Barrett DM, Bagatell R. The beginning of the end of package deal therapy for patients with high-risk Neuroblastoma? J Clin Oncol. 2016;34:2437–9.
55. Mittal D, Gubin MM, Schreiber RD, et al. New insights into cancer immunoediting and its three component phase-elimination, equilibrium and escape. Curr Opin Immunol. 2014;27:16–25.

56. Rimoldi D, Romero P, Carrel S. The human melanoma antigen-encoding gene, MAGE-1, is expressed by other tumor cells of neuroectodermal origin such as glioblastomas and neuroblastomas. Int J Cancer. 1993;54:527–8.
57. Cheung IY, Barber D, Cheung NK. Detection of microscopic neuroblastoma in marrow by histology, immunocytology, and reverse transcription-PCR of multiple molecular markers. Clin Cancer Res. 1998;4:2801–5.
58. Schulz G, Cheresh DA, Varki NM, et al. Detection of ganglioside GD2 in tumor tissues and sera of neuroblastoma patients. Cancer Res. 1984;44:5914–20.
59. Gregorio A, Corrias MV, Castriconi R, et al. Small round blue cell tumours: diagnostic and prognostic usefulness of the expression of B7-H3 surface molecule. Histopathology. 2008;53:73–80.
60. Schreiber RD, Old LJ, Smyth MJ. Cancer immunoediting: integrating immunity's roles in cancer suppression and promotion. Science. 2011;331:1565–70.
61. Wu X, Peng M, Huang B, et al. Immune microenvironment profiles of tumor immune equilibrium and immune escape states of mouse sarcoma. Cancer Lett. 2013;340:124–33.
62. Koebel CM, Vermi W, Swann JB, et al. Adaptive immunity maintains occult cancer in an equilibrium state. Nature. 2007;450:903–7.
63. Mittal D, Gubin MM, Schreiber RD, et al. New insights into cancer immunoediting and its three component phases – elimination, equilibrium and escape. Curr Opin Immunol. 2014;27:16–25.
64. Shurin GV, et al. Neuroblastoma-derived gangliosides inhibit dendritic cell generation and function. Cancer Res. 2001;61:363–9.
65. Chen S, Caragine T, Cheung NK, et al. CD59 expressed on a tumor cell surface modulates decay-accelerating factor expression and enhances tumor growth in a rat model of human neuroblastoma. Cancer Res. 2000;60:3013–8.
66. Morandi F, et al. Bone marrow-infiltrating human neuroblastoma cells express high levels of calprotectin and HLA-G proteins. PLoS One. 2012;7:e29922.
67. Raffaghello L, et al. Downregulation and/or release of NKG2D ligands as immune evasion strategy of human neuroblastoma. Neoplasia. 2004;6:558–68.
68. Shurin GV, Gerein V, Lotze MT, et al. Apoptosis induced in T cells by human neuroblastoma cells: role of Fas ligand. Nat Immun. 1998;16:263–74.
69. Yuan J, Page DB, Ku GY, et al. Correlation of clinical and immunological data in a metastatic melanoma patient with heterogeneous tumor responses to ipilimumab theraoy. Cancer Immunol. 2010;10:1.
70. Gilboa E. The promise of cancer vaccines. Nat Rev Cancer. 2004;4:401–11.
71. Berzofsky JA, Terabe M, Oh S, et al. Progress on new vaccine strategies for the immunotherapy and prevention of cancer. J Clin Invest. 2004;113:1515–25.
72. Fest S, Huebener N, Weixler S, et al. Characterization of GD2 peptide mimotope DNA vaccines effective against spontaneous neuroblastoma metastases. Cancer Res. 2006;66:10567–75.
73. Lode HN, Pertl U, Xiang R, et al. Tyrosine hydroxylase-based DNA-vaccination is effective against murine neuroblastoma. Med Pediatr Oncol. 2000;35:641–6.
74. Huebener N, Lange B, Lemmel C, et al. Vaccination with minigenes encoding for novel 'self' antigens are effective in DNA-vaccination against neuroblastoma. Cancer Lett. 2003;197:211–7.
75. Fest S, Huebener N, Bleeke M, et al. Survivin minigene DNA vaccination is effective against neuroblastoma. Int J Cancer. 2009;125:104–14.
76. Bao L, Dunham K, Lucas K. MAGE-A1, MAGE-A3, and NY-ESO-1 can be upregulated on neuroblastoma cells to facilitate cytotoxic T lymphocyte-mediated tumor cell killing. Cancer Immunol Immunother. 2011;60:1299–307.
77. Sarkar AK, Nuchtern JG. Lysis of MYCN-amplified neuroblastoma cells by MYCN peptide-specific cytotoxic T lymphocytes. Cancer Res. 2000;60:1908–13.
78. Geiger JD, et al. Vaccination of pediatric solid tumor patients with tumor lysate-pulsed dendritic cells can expand specific T cells and mediate tumor regression. Cancer Res. 2001;61:8513–9.

79. Bowman L, et al. IL-2 adenovector-transduced autologous tumor cells induce antitumor immune responses in patients with neuroblastoma. Blood. 1998;92:1941–9.
80. Walker SR, Redlinger RE Jr, Barksdale EM Jr. Neuroblastoma-induced inhibition of dendritic cell IL-12 production via abrogation of CD40 expression. J Pediatr Surg. 2005;40:244–9.
81. Yan X, Johnson BD, Orentas RJ. Induction of a VLA-2 (CD49b)-expressing effector T cell population by a cell-based neuroblastoma vaccine expressing CD137L. J Immunol. 2008;181:4621–31.
82. Croce M, et al. Immunotherapy of neuroblastoma by an Interleukin-21-secreting cell vaccine involves survivin as antigen. Cancer Immunol Immunother. 2008;57:1625–34.
83. Specenier P, Vermorken JB. Cetuximab in the treatment of squamous cell carcinoma of the head and neck. Expert Rev Anticancer Ther. 2011;11:511–24.
84. Higgins MJ, Baselga J. Targeted therapies for breast cancer. J Clin Invest. 2011;121:3797–803.
85. Mirick GR, Bradt BM, Denardo SJ, et al. A review of human anti-globulin antibody (HAGA, HAMA, HACA, HAHA) responses to monoclonal antibodies. Not four letter words. Q J Nucl Med Mol Imaging. 2004;48:251–7.
86. Kramer K, Gerald WL, Kushner BH, et al. Disaloganglioside GD2 loss following monoclonal antibody therapy is rare in neuroblastoma. Med Pediatr Oncol. 2001;36:194–6.
87. Modak S, Cheung NK. Disialoganglioside directed immunotherapy of neuroblastoma. Cancer Investig. 2007;25:67–77.
88. Yu AL, Gilman AL, Ozkaynak MF, et al. Anti-GD2 antibody with GM-CSF, interleukin-2 and isotretinoin for neuroblastoma. N Engl J Med. 2010;363:1324–34.
89. Murray JL, et al. Phase I trial of murine monoclonal antibody 14G2a administered by prolonged intravenous infusion in patients with neuroectodermal tumors. J Clin Oncol. 1994;12:184–93.
90. Metelitsa LS, et al. Antidisialoganglioside/granulocyte macrophage-colony-stimulating factor fusion protein facilitates neutrophil antibody-dependent cellular cytotoxicity and depends on FcγRII (CD32) and Mac-1 (CD11b/CD18) for enhanced effector cell adhesion and azurophil granule exocytosis. Blood. 2002;99:4166–73.
91. Matthay KK, George RE, Yu AL. Promising therapeutic targets in neuroblastoma. Clin Cancer Res. 2012;18:2740–53.
92. Neal ZC, et al. Enhanced activity of hu14.18-IL2 immunocytokine against murine NXS2 neuroblastoma when combined with interleukin 2 therapy. Clin Cancer Res. 2004;10:4839–47.
93. Becker JC, Varki N, Gillies SD, et al. Long-lived and transferable tumor immunity in mice after targeted interleukin-2 therapy. J Clin Invest. 1996;98:2801–4.
94. Lode HN, Xiang R, Dreier T, et al. Natural killer cell-mediated eradication of neuroblastoma metastases to bone marrow by targeted interleukin-2 therapy. Blood. 1998;91:1706–15.
95. Shusterman S, et al. Antitumor activity of hu14.18-IL2 in patients with relapsed/refractory neuroblastoma: a Children's Oncology Group (COG) phase II study. J Clin Oncol. 2010;28:4969–75.
96. Wellstein A. ALK receptor activation, ligands and therapeutic targeting in glioblastoma and in other cancers. Front Oncol. 2012;2:192.
97. Carpenter EL, et al. Antibody targeting of anaplastic lymphoma kinase induces cytotoxicity of human neuroblastoma. Oncogene. 2012;31:4859–67.
98. Novak-Hofer I. The L1 cell adhesion molecule as a target for radioimmunotherapy. Cancer Biother Radiopharm. 2007;22:175–84.
99. Modak S, Kramer K, Gultekin SH, et al. Monoclonal antibody 8H9 targets a novel cell surface antigen expressed by a wide spectrum of human solid tumors. Cancer Res. 2001;61:4048–54.
100. Castriconi R, Dondero A, Augugliaro R, et al. Identification of 4Ig-B7-H3 as a neuroblastoma-associated molecule that exerts a protective role from an NK cell-mediated lysis. Proc Natl Acad Sci U S A. 2004;101:12640–5.
101. Lee Y-H, Martin-Orozco N, Zheng P, et al. Inhibition of the B7-H3 immune checkpoint limits tumor growth by enhancing cyto-toxic lymphocyte function. Cell Res. 2017;27:1034–45.
102. Bosse KR, Raman P, Zhu Z, et al. Identification of GPC2 as an oncoprotein and candidate immunotherapeutic target in high-risk neuroblastoma. Cancer Cell. 2017;32:295–309.

103. Offner S, Hofmeister R, Romaniuk A, et al. Induction of regular cytolytic T cell synapses by bispecific single-chain antibody constructs on MHC class I-negative tumor cells. Mol Immunol. 2006;43:763–71.
104. Topp MS, Kufer P, Gokbuget N, et al. Targeted therapy with the T-cell-engaging antibody blinatumomab of chemotherapy-refractory minimal residual disease in B-lineage acute lymphoblastic leukemia patients results in high response rate and prolonged leukemia-free survival. J Clin Oncol. 2011;29:2493–8.
105. Lutterbuese R, Raum T, Kischel R, et al. T cell-engaging BiTE antibodies specific for EGFR potently eliminate KRAS- and BRAF-mutated colorectal cancer cells. Proc Natl Acad Sci U S A. 2010;107:12605–10.
106. Bourne S, Patel K, Walsh F, et al. A monoclonal antibody (ERIC-1), raised against retinoblastoma, that recognizes the neural cell adhesion molecule (NCAM) expressed on brain and tumours arising from the neuroectoderm. J Neurooncol. 1991;10:111–9.
107. Jensen M, Ernestus K, Kemshead J, et al. The bi-specific CD3-NCAM antibody: a model to preactivate T cells prior to tumour cell lysis. Clin Exp Immunol. 2003;134:253–63.
108. Jensen M, Berthold F. Targeting the neural cell adhesion molecule in cancer. Cancer Lett. 2007;258:9–21.
109. Xu H, Cheng M, Guo H, et al. Retargeting T cells to GD2 pentasaccharide on human tumors using bispecific humanized antibody. Cancer Immunol Res. 2015;3:266–77.
110. Deol A, Lum L. Role of donor lymphocyte infusions in relapsed hematological malignancies after stem cell transplantation revisited. Cancer Treat Rev. 2010;36:528–38.
111. McLaughlin L, Cruz RC, Bollard CM. Adoptive T-cell therapies for refractory/relapsed leukemia and lymphoma: current strategies and recent advances. Ther Adv Hematol. 2015;6:295–307.
112. Rosenberg SA, Yannelli JR, Yang JC, et al. Treatment of patients with metastatic melanoma with autologous tumor-infiltrating lymphocytes and interleukin 2. J Natl Cancer Inst. 1994;86:1159–66.
113. Eshhar Z, Waks T, Gross G, et al. Specific activation and targeting of cytotoxic lymphocytes through chimeric single chains consisting of antibody-binding domains and the gamma or zeta subunits of the immunoglobulin and T-cell receptors. Proc Natl Acad Sci U S A. 1993;90:720–4.
114. Pule M, Finney H, Lawson A. Artificial T-cell receptors. Cytotherapy. 2003;5:211–26.
115. Maher J, Brentjens RJ, Gunset G, et al. Human T-lymphocyte cytotoxicity and proliferation directed by a single chimeric TCRzeta/CD28 receptor. Nat Biotechnol. 2002;20:70–5.
116. Imai C, Mihara K, Andreansky M, et al. Chimeric receptors with 4-1BB signaling capacity provoke potent cytotoxicity against acute lymphoblastic leukemia. Leukemia. 2004;18:676–84.
117. Robbins PF, Dudley ME, Wunderlich J, et al. Cutting edge: persistence of transferred lymphocyte clonotypes correlates with cancer regression in patients receiving cell transfer therapy. J Immunol. 2004;173:7125–30.
118. Woo SR, Turnis ME, Goldberg MV, et al. Immune inhibitory molecules LAG-3 and PD-1 synergistically regulate T-cell function to promote tumoral immune escape. Cancer Res. 2012;72:917–27.
119. Wherry EJ. T cell exhaustion. Nat Immunol. 2011;12:492–9.
120. Long AH, Haso WM, Shern JF, et al. 4-1BB costimulation ameliorates T cell exhaustion induced by tonic signaling of chimeric antigen receptors. Nat Med. 2015;21(6):581–93.
121. Loskog A, Giandomenico V, Rossig C, et al. Addition of the CD28 signaling domain to chimeric T-cell receptors enhances chimeric T-cell resistance to T regulatory cells. Leukemia. 2006;20:1819–28.
122. Savoldo B, Ramos CA, Liu E, et al. Brief report CD28 costimulation improves expansion and persistence of chimeric antigen receptor-modified T cells in lymphoma patients. J Clin Invest. 2011;121:1822–6.
123. Gill S, Maus MV, Porter DL. Chimeric antigen receptor T cell therapy: 25 years in the making. Blood Rev. 2015. pii: S0268-960X(15)00080-6.

124. Euer NI, Kaul S, Deissler H, et al. Identification of L1CAM, Jagged2 and Neuromedin U as ovarian cancer-associated antigens. Oncol Rep. 2005;13:375–87.
125. Gonzalez S, Naranjo A, Serrano LM, et al. Genetic engineering of cytolytic T lymphocytes for adoptive T-cell therapy of neuroblastoma. J Gene Med. 2004;6:704–11.
126. Pule MA, Savoldo B, Myers GD, et al. Virus-specific T cells engineered to coexpress tumor-specific receptors: persistence and antitumor activity in individuals with neuroblastoma. Nat Med. 2008;14:1264–70.
127. Pule MA, Straathof KC, Dotti G, et al. A chimeric T cell antigen receptor that augments cytokine release and supports clonal expansion of primary human T cells. Mol Ther. 2005;12:933–41.
128. Caruana I, Savoldo B, Hoyos V, et al. Heparanase promotes tumor infiltration and antitumor activity of CAR-redirected T lymphocytes. Nat Med. 2015;21:524–9.
129. Sivori S, Parolini S, Marcenaro E, et al. Involvement of natural cytotoxicity receptors in human natural killer cell-mediated lysis of neuroblastoma and glioblastoma cell lines. J Neuroimmunol. 2000;107:220–5.
130. Ferlazzo G, et al. Distinct roles of IL-12 and IL-15 in human natural killer cell activation by dendritic cells from secondary lymphoid organs. Proc Natl Acad Sci U S A. 2004;101:16606–11.
131. Castriconi R, Dondero A, Cilli M, et al. Human NK cell infusions prolong survival of metastatic human neuroblastoma-bearing NOD/scid mice. Cancer Immunol Immunother. 2007;56:1733–42.
132. Liu Y, Wu HW, Sheard MA, et al. Growth and activation of natural killer cells ex vivo from children with neuroblastoma for adoptive cell therapy. Clin Cancer Res. 2013;19:2132–43.
133. Seidel D, Shibina A, Siebert N, et al. Disialoganglioside-specific human natural killer cells are effective against drug-resistant neuroblastoma. Cancer Immunol Immunother. 2015;64:621–34.
134. Metelitsa LS, Naidenko OV, Kant A, et al. Human NKT cells mediate antitumor cytotoxicity directly by recognizing target cell CD1d with bound ligand or indirectly by producing IL-2 to activate NK cells. J Immunol. 2001;167:3114–22.
135. Metelitsa LS. Anti-tumor potential of type-I NKT cells against CD1d-positive and CD1d-negative tumors in humans. Clin Immunol. 2011;140:119–29.
136. Heczey A, Liu D, Tian G, et al. Invariant NKT cells with chimeric antigen receptor provide a novel platform for safe and effective cancer immunotherapy. Blood. 2014;124:2824–33.
137. Tian G, Courtney AN, Jen B, et al. CD62L+ NKT cells have prolonged persistence and antitumor activity in vivo. J Clin Invest. 2016;126:2341–55.
138. Geiger JD, Hutchinson RJ, Hohenkirk LF, et al. Vaccination of pediatric solid tumor patients with tumor lysate-pulsed dendritic cells can expand specific T cells and mediate tumor regression. Cancer Res. 2001;61:8513–9.
139. Bowman L, Grossmann M, Rill D, et al. IL-2 adenovector-transduced autologous tumor cells induce antitumor immune responses in patients with neuroblastoma. Blood. 1998;92:1941–9.
140. Bowman LC, Grossmann M, Rill D, et al. Interleukin-2 gene-modified allogeneic tumor cells for treatment of relapsed neuroblastoma. Hum Gene Ther. 1998;9:1303–11.
141. Rousseau RF, Haight AE, Hirschmann-Jax C, et al. Local and systemic effects of an allogeneic tumor cell vaccine combining transgenic human lymphotactin with interleukin-2 in patients with advanced or refractory neuroblastoma. Blood. 2003;101:1718–26.
142. Kushner BH, Cheung IY, Modak S, et al. Phase I trial of a bivalent gangliosides vaccine in combination with b-glucan for high-risk neuroblastoma in second or later remission. Clin Cancer Res. 2014;20:1375–82.
143. Caruso DA, Orme LM, Amor GM, et al. Results of a Phase I study utilizing monocyte-derived dendritic cells pulsed with tumor RNA in children with Stage 4 neuroblastoma. Cancer. 2005;103:1280–91.
144. Cheung NK, Lazarus H, Miraldi FD, et al. Ganglioside GD2 specific monoclonal antibody 3F8: a phase 1 study in patients with neuroblastoma and malignant melanoma. J Clin Oncol. 1987;5:1430–40.

145. Cheung NK, Kushner BH, Yeh SD, et al. 3F8 monoclonal antibody treatment of patients with stage 4 neuroblastoma: a phase II study. Int J Oncol. 1998;12:1299–306.
146. Cheung NK, Kushner BH, Cheung IY, et al. Anti-GD2 antibody treatment of minimal residual stage 4 neuroblastoma diagnosed at more than 1 year of age. J Clin Oncol. 1998;16:3053–60.
147. Cheung NV, Cheung IY, Kushner BH, et al. Murine anti-GD2 monoclonal antibody 3F8 combined with granulocyte-macrophage colony-stimulating factor and 13-cis-retinoic acid in high-risk patients with stage 4 neuroblastoma in first remission. J Clin Oncol. 2012;30:3264–70.
148. Handgretinger R, Baader P, Dopfer R. A phase 1 study of neuroblastoma with the anti-ganglioside GD2 antibody14.G2a. Cancer Immunol Immunother. 1992;35:199–204.
149. Frost JD, Hank JA, Reaman GH, et al. A phaseI/IB trial of murine monoclonal anti-GD2 antibody 14.G2a plus interleukin-2 in children with refractory neuroblastoma: a report of the Children's Cancer Group. Cancer. 1997;80:317–33.
150. Handgretinger R, Anderson K, et al. A phase I study of human/mouse chimeric antiganglioside GD2 antibody ch14.18 in patients with neuroblastoma. Eur J Cancer. 1995;31:261–7.
151. Yu AL, Uttenreuther-Fischer MM, Huang CS, et al. Phase 1 trial of a human-mouse chimeric anti-disialoganglioside monoclonal antibody ch14.18 in patients with refractory neuroblastoma and osteosarcoma. J Clin Oncol. 1998;16:2169–80.
152. Yu AL, Batova A, Alvarado C, et al. Usefulness of a chimeric anti-GD2 (ch14.18) and GM-CSF for refractory neuroblastoma: a POG phase II study. Proc ASCO. 1997;16:1846.
153. Ozkaynak MF, Sondel PM, Kraiolo MD, et al. Phase I study of chimeric human/murine anti-ganglioside GD2 monoclonal antibody with granulocyte-macrophage colony-stimulating factor in children with neuroblastoma immediately after hematopoietic stem-cell transplantation: a Children's Cancer Group study. J Clin Oncol. 2000;18:4077–85.
154. Gilman AL, Ozkaynak MF, Matthay KK, et al. Phase I study of ch14.18 with granulocyte-macrophage colony stimulating factor and interleukin-2 in children with neuroblastoma after autologous bone marrow transplantation or stem-cell rescue: a report from the Children's Oncology Group. J Clin Oncol. 2009;27:85–91.
155. Delgado DC, Hank JA, Kolesar J, et al. Genotypes of NK cell KIR receptors, their ligands, and Fcγ receptors in the response of neuroblastoma patients to Hu14.18-IL2 immunotherapy. Cancer Res. 2010;70:9554–61.
156. Kramer K, Humm JL, Souweidane MM, et al. Phase I study of targeted radio-immunotherapy for leptomeningeal cancers using intra-Ommaya 131-I-3F8. J Clin Oncol. 2007;25:5465–70.
157. Kramer K, Kushner BH, Modak S, et al. Compartmental intrathecal radioimmunotherapy: results for treatment for metastatic CNS neuroblastoma. J Neurooncol. 2010;97:409–18.
158. Christiansen J, Rajasekaran AK. Biological impediments to monoclonal antibody-based cancer immunotherapy. Mol Cancer Ther. 2004;3:1493–501.
159. Caruana I, Diaconu I, Dotti G. From monoclonal antobodies to chimeric antigen receptors for the treatment of human malignancies. Semin Oncol. 2014;41(5):661–6.
160. Klinger M, Benjamin J, Kischel R, et al. Harnessing T cells to fight cancer with BITE® antibody constructs – past developments and future directions. Immunol Rev. 2016;270(1):193–208.
161. Park JR, DiGiusto DL, Slovak M, et al. Adoptive transfer of chimeric antigen receptor re-directed cytolytic T lymphocyte clones in patients with neuroblastoma. Mol Ther. 2007;15:825–33.
162. Louis CU, Savoldo B, Dotti G, et al. Antitumor activity and long-term fate of chimeric antigen receptor-positive T cells in patients with neuroblastoma. Blood. 2011;118(23):6050–6.
163. Muranski P, Boni A, Wrzesinski C, et al. Increased intensity lymphodepletion and adoptive immunotherapy–how far can we go? Nat Clin Pract Oncol. 2006;3:668–81.
164. Klebanoff CA, Khong HT, Antony PA, et al. Sinks, suppressors and antigen presenters: how lymphodepletion enhances T cell-mediated tumor immunotherapy. Trends Immunol. 2005;26:111–7.
165. Kalos M, Levine BL, Porter DL. T cells with chimeric antigen receptors have potent antitumor effects and can establish memory in patients with advanced leukemia. Sci Transl Med. 2011;3(95):95ra73.

166. Davila ML, Riviere I, Wang X, et al. Efficacy and toxicity management of 19-28z CAR T cell therapy in B cell acute lymphoblastic leukemia. Sci Transl Med. 2014;6(224):224ra25.
167. Maude SL, Frey N, Shaw PA, et al. Chimeric antigen receptor T cells for sustained remissions in leukemia. N Engl J Med. 2014;371(16):1507–17.
168. Lee DW, Kochenderfer JN, Stetler-Stevenson M, et al. T cells expressing CD19 chimeric antigen receptors for acute lymphoblastic leukaemia in children and young adults: a phase 1 dose-escalation trial. Lancet. 2015;385(9967):517–28.
169. Heczey A, Lous CU, Savoldo B, et al. CAR T cells administered in combination with Lymphodepletion and PD-1 inhibition to patients with neuroblastoma. Mol Ther. 2017;25:2214–24.
170. Tey SK, Dotti G, Rooney CM, et al. Inducible caspase 9 suicide gene to improve the safety of allodepleted T cells after haploidentical stem cell transplantation. Biol Blood Marrow Transplant. 2007;13:913–24.
171. Di Stasi A, Tey S-K, Dotti G, et al. Inducible apoptosis as a safety switch for adoptive cell therapy. N Engl J Med. 2011;365:1673–83.
172. Zhou X, Di Stasi A, Tey SK, et al. Long-term outcome after haploidentical stem cell transplant and infusion of T cells expressing the inducible caspase 9 safety transgene. Blood. 2014;123(25):3895–905.
173. Miller AB, Hoogstraten B, Staquet M, et al. Reporting results of cancer treatment. Cancer. 1981;47:207–14.
174. Therasse P, Arbuck SG, Eisenhauer EA, et al. New guidelines to evaluate the response to treatment in solid tumors. J Natl Cancer Inst. 2000;92:205–16.
175. Castel V, García-Miguel P, Cañete A, et al. Prospective evaluation of the International Neuroblastoma Staging System (INSS) and the International Neuroblastoma Response Criteria (INRC) in a multicentre setting. Eur J Cancer. 1999;35(4):606–11.
176. van Buren N, Bonnet MC, Dréno B, et al. Tumoral and immunologic response after vaccination of melanoma patients with an ALVAC virus encoding MAGE antigens recognized by T cells. J Clin Oncol. 2005;23:9008–21.
177. Kruit WHJ, van Ojik HH, Brichard VG, et al. Phase 1/2 study of subcutaneous and intradermal immunization with a recombinant MAGE-3 protein in patients with detectable metastatic melanoma. Int J Cancer. 2005;117:596–604.
178. Wolchok JD, Hoos A, O'Day S, et al. Guidelines for the evaluation of immune therapy activity in solid tumors: immune-related response criteria. Clin Cancer Res. 2009;15:7412–20.
179. Hodi FS, Butler M, Oble DA, et al. Immunologic and clinical effects of antibody blockade of cytotoxic T lymphocyte-associated antigen 4 in previously vaccinated cancer patients. Proc Natl Acad Sci U S A. 2008;105:3005–10.
180. Hodi FS, Hwu WJ, Kefford R, et al. Evaluation of immune-related response criteria and RECIST v1.1 in patients with advanced melanoma treated with pembrolizumab. J Clin Oncol. 2016;34:1510–20.

Prognostic Factors and Risk Stratification

14

Meredith S. Irwin

14.1 Introduction

Prognostic factors have been used to guide neuroblastoma therapeutic approaches for more than three decades. The most commonly used and statistically well-validated prognostic clinical risk factors are age and stage, as well as components of histopathology. Additional prognostic biomarkers include *MYCN* status, ploidy or DNA tumour content, and segmental chromosome aberrations (SCA) [1, 2]. NGS-based studies have provided exciting early data examining prognostic roles for other genomic alterations. The majority of prognostic factors incorporated into current risk classification systems are patient and/or tumour characteristics at diagnosis. However, there are increasingly examples of measures of response to therapy that correlate with outcome, such as semi-quantitative MIBG score following induction chemotherapy or minimum residual disease (MRD) as detected by neuroblastoma tumour-specific transcripts in the peripheral blood or bone marrow at various time points. Ultimately, inclusion of response criteria into risk classifiers may follow the examples of other cancers such as MRD detection in ALL or PET-imaging avidity in patients with Hodgkin's Disease, both of which are used to refine prognosis and risk groups to further tailor therapy.

There are many clinical features and expression of genes, proteins and other biomarkers that have been reported to correlate with outcome. In the following sections, we will review the data supporting the most well-validated and robust prognostic factors and describe how they are used in international risk classification systems. It is important to recognize that the significance of any prognostic factor depends on the therapies received by patients. In other words, poor prognostic factors can be "treated away" by adopting more intensive therapies for patients defined

M. S. Irwin (✉)
Department of Paediatrics, Hospital for Sick Children, University of Toronto,
Toronto, ON, Canada
e-mail: meredith.irwin@sickkids.ca

S. Sarnacki, L. Pio (eds.), *Neuroblastoma*,
https://doi.org/10.1007/978-3-030-18396-7_14

as poor prognosis. The concept that treatment itself is a risk factor is important to consider when interpreting prognostic data over several decades, during which patients may have received different therapies.

14.2 Current Prognostic Factors in Neuroblastoma

In the following sections, we will review each of the well-validated clinical risk factors and biomarkers and present data for emerging biomarkers referencing the largest retrospective and prospective studies supporting the inclusion of these biomarkers as prognostic factors in risk classifiers. In each section, there will be discussion of the particular value of an individual prognostic factor in specific subset of patients (e.g. metastatic vs. non-metastatic) and how it may overlap with other risk factors. In the final part of this chapter we will describe the currently used international risk classifiers that incorporate subsets of these clinical and biological risk factors in order to predict prognosis, risk groups and guide choice of therapies.

14.2.1 Stage

Many studies have demonstrated that stage is a powerful independent prognostic marker. There have been multiple neuroblastoma staging systems, but since 1993, the International Neuroblastoma Staging System (INSS) had been used by most cooperative groups [3] (Table 14.1). Analyses of the INRG database of 8800 patients diagnosed between 1990–2002 demonstrated superior EFS for patients with non-metastatic (INSS 1, 2 and 3) as compared to metastatic neuroblastoma (INSS 4) (83% vs. 35%) [4]. The INSS is a post-surgical staging system that relies, in part, on degree of resection. Based on data from the SIOPEN, the INRG Staging System (INRGSS) was developed as a presurgical/pretreatment staging system in which loco-regional disease is categorized as resectable or unresectable based on the presence or absence of Image Defined Risk Factors (IDRFs), previously referred to as surgical risk factors (SRFs) [5] (see Chap. 7 and Table 14.2). L1 and L2 are loco-regional tumours with or without IDRFs, respectively [5–7]. The majority of L1 tumours are INSS 1 and 2, and most L2 tumours are INSS 3 [6]. INSS 4 (distant metastases) is equivalent to INRG M and there are only minor differences between 4S and MS including extending the age cut-off from 12 to 18 months. The INRG SS has been adopted by most groups and will be validated prospectively in clinical trials across North America and Europe.

14.2.2 Age

Age was one of the earliest neuroblastoma prognostic factors identified. Historically, patients <12 months have superior outcomes compared to those >12 months [4, 8–11]. Older patients, including rare adolescents and young adults, have a more

Table 14.1 International Neuroblastoma Staging System (INSS)

INSS stage[a]	
1	Localized tumor with complete gross excision, with or without microscopic residual disease; representative ipsilateral lymph nodes negative for tumor microscopically (nodes attached to and removed with the primary tumor may be positive)
2A	Localized tumor with incomplete gross resection; representative ipsilateral nonadherent lymph nodes negative for tumor microscopically
2B	Localized tumor with or without complete gross excision, with ipsilateral nonadherent lymph nodes positive for tumor; enlarged contralateral lymph nodes must be negative microscopically
3	Unresectable unilateral tumor infiltrating across the midline,[b] with or without regional lymph node involvement; or localized unilateral tumor with contralateral regional lymph node involvement; or midline tumor with bilateral extension by infiltration (unresectable) or by lymph node involvement[c]
4	Any primary tumor with dissemination to distant lymph nodes, bone, bone marrow, liver, skin, and/or other organs (except as defined for stage 4S)
4S	Localized primary tumor (as defined for stage 1, 2A or 2B) with dissemination limited to skin, liver, and/or bone marrow[d] (limited to infants <1 year of age)

[a]Multifocal primary tumors (e.g., bilateral adrenal primary tumors) should be staged according to the greatest extent of disease, as defined above, and followed by a subscript "M" (e.g. 3_M)
[b]The midline is defined as the vertebral column. Tumors originating on one side and crossing the midline must infiltrate to or beyond the opposite side of the vertebral column
[c]Proven malignant effusion within the thoracic cavity if it is bilateral or the abdominal cavity upstages the patient to INSS 3
[d]Marrow involvement in Stage 4S should be minimal, i.e., less than 10% of total nucleated cells identified as malignant on bone marrow biopsy or marrow aspirate. More extensive marrow involvement would be considered to be Stage 4

Table 14.2 International Neuroblastoma Risk Group Staging System (INRGSS)

Stage	Description
L1	Localized tumor not involving vital structures as defined by the list of image-defined risk factors and confined to one body compartment
L2	Locoregional tumor with presence of one or more image-defined risk factors (IDRFs) (see Chap. 7)
M	Distant metastatic disease (except stage MS)
MS	Metastatic disease in children younger than 18 months with metastases confined to skin, liver, and/or bone marrow

Note: Patients with multifocal primary tumors should be staged according to the greatest extent of disease as defined in the table

indolent course; however, studies have not identified any cut-offs (e.g. >5 or 10 years) that correlate with overall survival (OS) [12]. While the impact of age is independent of other risk factors, the subset of children >18 months with metastatic disease (stage 4/M) have the poorest outcome. Since age is a continuous variable analyses to determine optimal age, cut-offs have been performed using a COG cohort of >3600 patients. The most significant age cut-off was 460 days (15.1 months) [11]. Subsequently, the INRG determined that the age cut-off could be extended to 18 months, which increases the favourable group by approximately 11% [4, 11]. This cut-off is supported by additional studies, which demonstrate that for INSS 4 patients with *MYCN*-NA the 6-year EFS was 92% for <12 months, 74% for 12–18 months and 31% for >18 months [13]. The most difficult age range to determine risk group is the 12–18 months INSS 4 toddlers. Although the outcome for 12–18 months is superior to those >18 months, this group appears to be very heterogeneous. Retrospective studies suggest that one or more biomarkers, including SCAs, ploidy and/or histology, may help distinguish which toddlers with metastatic disease should receive more intensive high risk treatments [10, 13, 14]; however, prospective trials for these relatively rare patients have not confirmed which of these marker(s) can reliably distinguish Stage 4/M toddlers with high risk from those with intermediate-risk disease. Thus, current risk classifiers described below utilize different age cut-offs of 12 and 18 months to stratify patients, depending on the presence of additional prognostic factors such as stage.

14.2.3 MYCN Status

Amplification of the *MYCN* oncogene is the strongest independent negative prognostic factor for neuroblastoma. *MYCN*, localized on chromosome 2p24, is amplified in 16–25% of tumours and has been used in risk classification for more than two decades [15, 16]. *MYCNA* can be detected in double minutes (DMs), which are extra chromosomal chromatin bodies, or integrated into chromosomes to form homogeneously staining regions (HSRs); however, the effect of *MYCNA* on outcome is not influenced by the presence of DMs or HSRs [17]. *MYCN* status was initially detected using Southern blotting [15, 16], but more recently, the standard method used in most laboratories is fluorescence in situ hybridization (FISH) on tumour or metastatic bone marrow with infiltration of tumour cells (>30%). The international consensus for *MYCNA* is defined as >four-fold increase in the signal of the *MYCN* gene as compared to the signal detected for the control centromeric probe (for chromosome 2q) [18]. The international recommended guidelines are that *MYCN* copy number data should be reported as 4–10, >10 or >30 copies. The prognostic importance of *MYCN* copy gain and heterogeneity of amplification have been studied, but currently, there are not enough data to support separating out these small groups or using this information to inform risk classification schemas [19–21]. Newer techniques used to detect other copy number alterations (CNAs), including CGH (comparative genomic hybridization) or SNP (single nucleotide polymorphism) arrays may eventually replace FISH for detection of *MYCN* copy number.

MYCN, is one of three MYC genes (MYCN, c-myc, L-myc) and encodes a transcription factor that is involved in various cellular processes, including growth, differentiation, proliferation, apoptosis, metabolism and metastasis (reviewed in [22, 23]). MYCN has important roles in neural crest cells and sympathetic neurons during development and modulating its expression in neuroblastoma cells has effects on cell death, differentiation and chemosensitivity. Importantly, overproduction of MYCN transgene in neural crest precursors, alone or in conjunction with mutant forms of ALK, in mice and zebrafish results in the development of neuroblastoma [24–26]. The MYC family of transcription factors regulate thousands of genes and identifying specific targets of MYCN [27], mechanisms that regulate its ability to bind DNA and stability have been active areas of study in neuroblastoma. Although historically pharmacological targeting of MYCN had been challenging and considered "undruggable," newer strategies that focus on inhibiting MYC complexes, and specifically targeting the transcriptional co-factor BRD4, such as BET bromodomain inhibitors, have shown promising results in pre-clinical models [28]. Other drugs that target MYCN degradation via inhibition of Aurora Kinases also demonstrate MYCN selectivity in vitro and in animal models and have been tested in early phase clinical trials in children with relapsed neuroblastoma [29–31].

The majority of studies of MYC status in neuroblastoma have focused on MYCN; however, small retrospective studies suggest that high levels of MYC (c-MYC), as determined by immunohistochemistry (IHC), may also correlate with poor outcome, in particular in patients with tumours that have normal levels of MYCN [32, 33]. Further studies are needed to determine if c-MYC might have an independent prognostic role and thus could be integrated into future risk classifiers.

14.2.3.1 MYCN as Prognostic Factor

In the majority of large studies of patients with neuroblastoma, including the INRG [4], *MYCNA* is one of the most powerful independent risk factors that predicts poor outcome. In the original INRG cohort, the 5-year EFS for patients whose tumours harboured *MYCNA* was 29% as compared to 74% for those who had no amplification detected. This included patients of all ages and stages revealing the significance of *MYCNA* as an independent prognostic factor. Similarly, for patients diagnosed between 2007–2016 in Children's Oncology Group (COG), the 5-year EFS was 76.4% (*MYCN-NA*) compared to 48.1% (*MYCNA)* [19]. However, it is important to recognize that *MYCN* status also correlates with other clinical and biological features. Although, approximately 20% of all tumours harbour *MYCNA*, the incidence of *MYCNA* is higher in more advanced stage (INSS 3,4) disease (40%) as compared to 2–3% of loco-regional low stage (INSS 1,2) neuroblastoma [34]. In addition, *MYCNA* varies according to the primary tumour location and is more common in adrenal compared to thoracic tumours [35, 36]. *MYCNA* is also more commonly detected in tumours with unfavourable histological features such as high mitosis-karryorhexis index (MKI) [37–40], and other unfavourable genomic features such as diploidy [41–43] and presence of SCAs [14, 44]. Interestingly, while *MYCNA* correlates with a general pattern of SCA, alterations of specific loci, such as loss of heterozygosity (LOH) of 1p or 11q show distinctive patterns. 1p LOH is common in *MYCNA* tumours, while 11q LOH occurs almost exclusively in *MYCN*-NA tumours [45–49].

As discussed below in Sect. 14.4, the majority of high-risk (HR) neuroblastoma patients are >18 months with stage M/4. Within this cohort, the presence of *MYCNA* does not significantly affect overall outcome and thus is not used to further sub-stratify this common HR cohort. In contrast, based on numerous retrospective and prospective studies, the presence of *MYCNA* has a critical role in predicting outcome for the following subgroups of patients who have other more favourable characteristics: (1) infants (<12 months) and toddlers (12–18 months) with stage M/4, (2) patients with loco-regional INSS 2/3 (usually INRG L2).

Prior to the discovery of the importance of *MYCNA*, all stage 4/M patients were treated as HR. However, several European and North American studies demonstrated that infants <12 months with *MYCN-NA* tumours had an improved outcome compared to those with *MYCNA* [50–53]. These studies led to trials that demonstrated that classifying (and treating) infant patients with *MYCN-NA* tumours as intermediate risk (IR), with regimens that do not include stem cell transplant, maintain 5-year EFS rates of approximately 80% [51, 54].

Patients with loco-regional *MYCNA* have also been shown to have inferior outcomes than other patients with loco-regional disease regardless of age, stage or other factors. Most of these studies reported on outcomes based on INSS staging. The difference in 5-year EFS for INSS 1,2,3,4S patients based on *MYCN* status was 46 ± 4% vs. 87 ± 1% [4]. *MYCNA* also had prognostic significance for infants with loco-regional disease [55] and for the subsets of patients with resectable loco-regional disease (INSS 1,2) [34]. Currently, most patients with *MYCNA* are treated according to HR protocols, although for the rare INSS 1/INRG L1 patients with *MYCNA*, the approaches (and risk classification) are not consistent across all cooperative groups.

14.2.4 Histology

The International Neuroblastoma Pathology Classification (INPC) is based on a prognostic system that was initially developed by Shimada et al. [39] and uses morphological characteristics of the tumour cells (grade of differentiation) and stroma, mitosis-karyorrhexis index (MKI) and age to divide tumours into favourable (FH) or unfavourable histology (UH) categories. Large retrospective cooperative group studies have validated the prognostic significance of INPC FH/UH classification and have helped to identify specific subgroups of patients for whom histology may have particular relevance [39, 40, 56]. For example, in a COG study of INSS 1 and 2 patients, the majority of whom received surgery but no chemotherapy, FH correlated with an improved outcome as compared to those with UH (EFS 90 ± 3 vs. 72 ± 7%) [57]. UH is also prognostic for subsets of patients with INSS 3 *MYCN-NA* tumours. Although the 5-year EFS was 81% for the entire INSS 3 UH cohort in the INRG database, those patients >18 months had an inferior 5-year EFS (64% vs. 90%) [58]. These patients (>18 months) with unfavourable INPC and *MYCN-NA* are classified as HR in North America (COG), but intermediate risk according to SIOPEN and INRG classifiers. Since INPC uses age (which is an independent prognostic factor), other outcome analyses, including the INRG studies, have looked at separate components of histology such as grade of differentiation. The INRG risk classifier uses these components rather than the INPC, which is still used by the COG. In general, risk classifiers mostly utilize INPC or histology components mainly for loco-regional disease [4].

14.2.5 Ploidy

DNA ploidy (number of chromosome copies) has been shown to have prognostic importance, in particular in specific subgroups with otherwise favourable features. DNA content is most commonly analysed by flow cytometry, though it can also be determined using newer technologies that are being developed to detect copy number alterations in specific genes (e.g. CGH and SNP arrays). Diploid status (DNA index = 1) is often associated with other unfavourable features such as *MYCNA* and SCAs such as LOH or 1p or 11q. Hyperdiploid tumours (DNA index > 1) usually do not have structural abnormalities, but, instead, have gains or losses of whole chromosomes and are associated with more favourable outcomes [41, 42, 59]. Although in the INRG, ploidy was prognostic for the total neuroblastoma cohort (5-year EFS of 76% (hyperdiploid) vs. 55%, (diploid)), the independent significance for ploidy as a prognostic marker is highest in patients <18 months [4, 42, 59], and in particular has been shown to help distinguish those with differential outcomes among the 12–18 months toddlers with Stage 4/M *MYCN-NA* disease [10]. The status of ploidy has been recently used in trials for patients with IR neuroblastoma to determine therapy duration or number of chemotherapy cycles [18, 54, 60]. For most risk classification systems, including the INRG, ploidy is used only to distinguish risk group among <18 months patients with stage 4/M with *MYCN-NA* tumours [4]. Patients with DNA index >1 or =1 are classified as LR and IR, respectively.

14.2.6 Segmental Chromosome Aberrations

There are two general patterns for neuroblastoma genomes—(1) whole chromosome gains and losses or numerical chromosome alterations (NCAs) and (2) SCAs, which often include partial gains and losses of chromosome regions [44]. NCA and SCA patterns are associated with favourable and poor outcomes, respectively, and have been detected using both CGH and SNP arrays. Historically, most SCAs were analyzed individually by examining the gains or losses at specific chromosome loci (using PCR or FISH-based methods), and these loci were predicted to encode oncogenes and tumour suppressors, respectively. These included gain of 17 q, and 1p and 11q LOH. 17 q gain is detected in more than 50% of patients and is associated with other unfavourable characteristics [61, 62]. 1p36 LOH is detected in 23–30% of tumours and predicts poor outcome [45, 63]. 1p LOH correlates with other unfavourable features including *MYCNA*, unfavourable INPC and presence of metastases, and its use as a prognostic factor is strongest in infants and *MYCN-NA* patients [45, 64]. 11q LOH correlates with poor outcome, but in contrast to 17q gain and 1p LOH, 11q loss is more common in *MYCN-NA* tumours, supporting its use as an independent prognostic marker [45, 49, 65], which has been incorporated into the INRG risk classifier where it is specifically used in L2 and MS patients.

More recent studies, mainly from the SIOPEN and INRG, have analyzed the impact of SCAs and showed that presence of one or more SCAs is more significant than particular loci [66]. In addition to the specific loci mentioned above, other common SCAs in neuroblastoma include gains of 1q and 2p and losses of 3p, 4p and14q. The specific subgroups in which SCAs have been shown to have prognostic value include patients >12 months with unresectable loco-regional *MYCN-NA* tumours [67]and infants (<12 months) with unresectable loco-regional and metastatic *MYCN-NA* tumours [14].

While the only SCA included in the INRG risk classifier is 11qLOH (for L2 and MS patients), newer classifiers are incorporating the overall presence of ≥1 of the following SCAs (gains of 1q, 2p, 17q or losses of 1p, 3p, 4p, 11q, 14q.); however, prospective studies will be needed to validate whether all/ any SCAs predict outcome for homogeneously treated cohorts of patients. Currently, SCAs are detected in tumour tissue, but early studies suggest that cell-free DNA harvested from serum is another potential source for SCA detection [68, 69].

14.3 Emerging Prognostic Factors in Neuroblastoma

In addition to the well-validated risk factors used in current risk classifiers that are described above, there have been numerous reports of new biomarkers and other prognostic factors, many of which are being further studied to determine whether they improve our ability to distinguish different subgroups of LR, IR or HR neuroblastoma. In this section, we will present the subset of novel prognostic factors with the most data supporting possible integration into future risk classifiers.

14.3.1 Somatic Mutations

NGS technologies have elucidated the genomic landscape of newly diagnosed and, more recently, relapsed neuroblastoma. Although, in comparison to adult-onset tumours such as carcinomas, the number of mutations in neuroblastoma and other paediatric tumours is relatively low, some targetable genomic alterations have been identified [70].

Sequencing of DNA and RNA at diagnosis, has demonstrated that neuroblastoma harbour heterogeneous genomic alterations [71–73]. The most common copy number alteration at diagnosis is amplification of the *MYCN* oncogene (20%) (see Sect. 14.2.3) and the most frequent mutations are missense alterations of the receptor tyrosine kinase, anaplastic lymphoma kinase or *ALK* (8–10%). In addition to point mutations, amplifications of *ALK* are detected in 2–3% [74]. Alterations in *ATRX* are detected in up to 10% of patients, and are more common in older children and adults [71, 75, 76]. Other genes that have recurrent, but less frequent, mutations (<5%) include *PTPN11, MYCN,* and *p53*. At the time of relapse, there are additional changes that often include a higher number of mutations (tumour mutation burden) as well as clonal selection leading to increased allele frequency for certain alterations such as those involving ALK [77, 78]. The most common missense mutations at recurrence include genes that encode members of the RAS/MAPK pathway, including, but not limited to, *RAS* (*N-Ras*, *H-Ras*, *K-Ras*), *PTPN11*, *NF1* and activating *ALK* variants [79, 80]. Deletions and missense mutations of AT-rich interactive domain 1A and 1B (*ARID1a/1b*) were detected in11% of tumours, and in small cohorts there appears to be a correlation with poor outcome [73]. In addition to *ARID1A/1B*, mutations in other genes encoding chromatin remodelling proteins have also been identified in a small number of cases.

Thus far, no specific mutations have strong independent prognostic significance. ALK genomic alterations are identified in tumours from patients in all risk groups. In some studies, ALK variants are associated with adverse outcome, and high levels of ALK protein or amplification may correlate with inferior outcome, independent of mutation status [74, 81–83]. To date, ALK mutation status has not distinguished patient outcomes within risk categories and thus, ALK is unlikely to be used as an independent prognostic factor, but is a predictive factor for sensitivity to ALK tyrosine kinase inhibitors [74, 84, 85].

Most of the studies to date have focused on DNA sequencing, but early RNA and whole genome sequencing efforts have identified other potentially targetable alterations including fusions of TERT [86, 87], as discussed below.

14.3.1.1 Telomerase Pathway Alterations

Telomeres are repetitive nucleotide sequences on the ends of chromosomes and, in the majority of non-malignant cells, telomeres are not replicated sufficiently, leading to progressive chromosome shortening and ultimately senescence or cell death. Most cancer cells acquire telomere-lengthening mechanisms (TLMs). In neuroblastoma, mainly in HR tumours, TLMs that have been detected include high levels of expression of the catalytic subunit of the enzyme telomerase (TERT) due to *MYCNA* or *TERT* rearrangements [27, 86–88]. The subset of HR tumours without upregulated TERT often have activated alternative lengthening of telomeres (ALT), most commonly associated with *ATRX* mutations or deletions. The presence of TLM alterations, most notably TERT-fusions, correlates with poor outcome in two small studies of HR patients, suggesting a potential role as a prognostic biomarker to further distinguish outcome among HR patients to identify those with a particularly poor outcome and to determine whether TLMs might identify non-HR patients with otherwise favourable features who recur. Future retrospective and prospective studies are required to validate the role of different TLMs as prognostic biomarkers, independent of other well-studied risk factors. It will be important to use methods that distinguish different TLM alterations such as C-circle [89] to detect ALT phenotype, sequencing or IHC to detect ATRX alterations, RT-PCR or RNAseq to identify increased TERT expression and /or fusions. TLMs may also have roles as predictive biomarkers as studies in non-neuroblastoma cells demonstrate that the nucleoside analogue 6-thio-2′-deoxyguanosine [90] and ATR inhibitors [91] selectively target cells with high TERT or ALT activation, respectively.

14.3.2 Expression Signatures

Instead of focusing on specific genes as candidates for biomarkers, several studies have reported multigene expression profiles (GEPs) that can predict outcome. Many of the mRNA signatures include genes implicated in neuroblastoma tumorigenesis, neural development or immune responses and may reflect genes expressed in neuroblastoma or infiltrating immune cells. One goal of such studies is to further refine risk categories based on these GEPs. One of the largest studies identified a 59-gene signature that could predict survival independent of well-validated risk factors with an increased odds-ratio of 19.3 and 3.96 for PFS and OS, respectively [92]. Further studies have evaluated different gene classifiers, which range from 3 to more than 50 genes in unselected neuroblastoma patient cohorts that include patients from all risk groups [93–96]. There have been fewer reports identifying GEPs that can distinguish outcome within a particular risk group. Asgharzadeh et al. identified a 14-gene classifier that predicts poor outcome (EFS < 20%) in several HR *MYCN-NA* cohorts [97, 98]. Another study used publicly available datasets to identify a prognostic signature for the subset of patients with *MYCNA* neuroblastoma [99]. Furthermore, within LR and IR groups, Oberthuer et al. were able to improve the estimation of risk and optimize stratification by combining standard risk factors with GEPs [100]. Additional studies are also ongoing to determine whether microRNA profiles may also be prognostic [101–103]. Expression signatures will need to be validated in prospective clinical trials to determine whether they provide additional ability to discriminate risk groups.

14.3.3 Metastatic Burden and Response as Prognostic Factors

In addition to risk factors at diagnosis, there are studies that suggest that response to therapy predicts outcome and thus, might be incorporated into risk stratification systems and/or used to further tailor therapy. The main areas of focus to determine response have been imaging of metastatic sites and minimal residual disease (MRD) detection in peripheral blood(PB) and bone marrow(BM).

14.3.3.1 MIBG

Standard imaging of metastatic response requires I-^{123} or -^{131} MIBG (meta-iodobenzylguanidine) scans. Many different systems have been developed to semi-quantitatively score metastatic involvement by MIBG scan and retrospective studies have demonstrated that the relative score of metastatic involvement on MIBG scan at diagnosis and/or end of induction chemotherapy has prognostic value [104–107]. The two most common—Curie and SIOPEN—scores have been shown to have comparable ability to predict outcome. The largest and most recent studies have focused on determining whether a particular absolute score or relative score cut-off at different time points during treatment, most commonly at the end of induction, can be used to predict relapse and thus identify a cohort of patients with HR neuroblastoma with a particularly poor outcome. MIBG scans of 280 patients on COG A3973 Phase III trial were centrally reviewed. Patients with a curie score >2 at the end of induction had an inferior outcome when compared to those with a curie score of ≤2, and this effect was independent of other known prognostic factors such as *MYCN* status (3-year EFS: 15.4% ± 5.3% vs. 44.9% ± 3.9%) [104]. Although absolute curie scores at diagnosis were not prognostic, any MIBG avid disease post-autologous stem cell transplant (curie score > 0) predicted patients with a significantly worse outcome 3-year EFS: 28.9% ± 6.8% vs. 49.3% ± 4.9%). Similarly, data from 341 patients treated on SIOPEN/HR-NBL-1 study showed that SIOPEN cut-off scores >3 at diagnosis were predictive of inferior outcome (5-year EFS 47 ± 7% and 26 ± 3%) [108]. At the end of induction, the differences were 36 ± 4% versus 14 ± 4%. These findings suggest that metastatic response using semi-quantitative scores has strong predictive value in identifying patients who will go on to recur. Thus, there are clinical trial consortium groups considering the incorporation of semi-quantitative scores into risk stratification systems, and future trials may use this response to identify patients to treat with different therapies, including high dose MIBG.

14.3.3.2 MRD

Metastatic burden measured by the detection of tumour cells in the PB or BM has been shown to be prognostic at different points during treatment. The most common assay method for minimum residual disease (MRD) detection is reverse transcriptase polymerase chain reaction (RT-PCR) to measure the levels of two or more neuroblastoma cell-specific transcripts, which most commonly include PHOX2B and tyrosine hydroxylase (TH), at a sensitivity of approximately one tumour cell per ten million normal cells [109]. In the SIOPEN-HRNBL-1, high levels of TH and PHOX2BmRNA in PB of INSS 4 patients at diagnosis, but not end of induction, is prognostic with inferior 5-year EFS and OS of 0% as compared to EFS of 38% and OS of 25% in the patients with lower MRD [110]. MRD in BM and PB also predicted increased risk for recurrence specifically in the subset of infants (<12 months) and toddlers (12–18 months) [111]. For HR patients on the COG A3973 trial, the level of neuroblastoma mRNA detected in harvested PB stem cells after two cycles of chemotherapy correlated with outcome [112]. Additional studies have shown that levels of neuroblastoma mRNA transcripts in PB and/or BM at different time-points, including diagnosis, during induction, post consolidation and during treatment for relapse have been reported to be prognostic [113] (reviewed in [109]). The levels of combinations of TH, PHOX2B and other neuroblastoma-specific genes in PB and/or BM at different time-points needs to be validated in prospective trials of patients treated with modern era therapies in order to enable integration into risk classifiers.

14.4 Risk Classification

The improved understanding of neuroblastoma biology and biomarkers and their impact on prognosis, together with studies of large databases of patients with well annotated clinical features, has resulted in the development of risk stratification approaches that are used to predict outcomes and tailor therapies. Using many of the pretreatment clinical and biological risk factors discussed in Sect. 14.2, risk classification systems have been developed by most large clinical trials cooperative groups, including the Children's Oncology Group (COG) (Table 14.3) and the

Society of International Pediatric Oncology Neuroblastoma (SIOPEN) groups. In an effort to harmonize risk-based treatment approaches and the criteria used to stratify patients, the INRG developed a pretreatment classifier that has largely been adopted universally (Table 14.4) [4]. The analyses of 8800 patients diagnosed between 1990–2002 were used to identify seven prognostic risk factors (age, stage, MYCN status, ploidy, 11q LOH, and two histologic features) and these factors defined 16 groups of very low/low, intermediate and high risk based on their 5 year EFS rates. In this section, we review the features that define these risk groups in the INRG and COG and highlight the features that are different between the classifiers for specific subgroups (Fig. 14.1). Risk-based treatment approaches for these groups are outlined in detail in Chap. 12. Notably, the COG is currently revising their risk classifier (Table 14.3) to incorporate INRGSS, include additional biomarkers and modify certain groups based on newer outcome data for patients treated with modern era treatments, including immunotherapy. The current approach to risk classification of loco-regional and metastatic patients is shown in Fig. 14.1; however, treatment decisions also incorporate symptoms (usually for LR and stage 4S/MS patients). Although patients are divided into LR, IR and HR groups, the distinction

Table 14.3 COG Neuroblastoma Risk Stratification (version 1)

Risk group	Stage (INSS)[a]	Age	MYCN	Ploidy	INPC
Low risk	1	Any	Any	Any	Any
Low risk[b]	2a/2b	Any	Non-amp	Any	Any
High risk	2a/2b	Any	Amp	Any	Any
Intermediate risk	3	<547 days	Non-amp	Any	Any
Intermediate risk	3	≥547 days	Non-amp	Any	FH
High risk	3	Any	Amp	Any	Any
High risk	3	≥547 days	Non-amp	Any	UH
High risk	4	<365 days	Amp	Any	Any
Intermediate risk	4	<365 days	Non-amp	Any	Any
High risk	4	365–<547 days	Amp	Any	Any
High risk	4	365–<547 days	Any	DI = 1	Any
High risk	4	365–<547 days	Any	Any	UH
Intermediate risk	4	365–<547 days	Non-amp	DI > 1	FH
High risk	4	≥547 days	Any	Any	Any
Low risk[c]	4s	<365 days	Non-amp	DI > 1	FH
Intermediate risk	4s	<365 days	Non-amp	DI = 1	Any
Intermediate risk	4s	<365 days	Non-amp	Any	UH
High risk	4s	<365 days	Amp	Any	Any

Courtesy of Children's Oncology Group

Table 14.2: The Children's Oncology Group (COG) currently uses INSS stage, age, MYCN status (amp = amplification), DNA index (DI) or ploidy, and INPC histology (FH = favorable histology, UH = unfavorable histology) to determine patient's risk category as high, intermediate, or low

[a]COG currently modifying to Risk Classification system version 2.0 that will use INRG staging and will also incorporate Segmental Chromosome aberrations (SCAs)

[b]if <50% resection or patient is symptomatic then classified as Intermediate risk

[c]if presence of clinical symptoms patient is considered "Intermediate risk"

Table 14.4 International Neuroblastoma Risk Group (INRG) Consensus Pretreatment Classification schema

INRG stage	Age (months)	Histologic category	Differentiation grade	MYCN	11q LOH	Ploidy	Pretreatment risk group
L1/L2		GN maturing; GNB-intermixed					Very low
L1		Any except GN maturing, or GNB-intermixed		NA			Very low
L1		Any except GN maturing, or GNB-intermixed		AMP			High
L2	<18 months	Any except GN maturing, or GNB-intermixed		NA	NO		Low
L2	<18 months	Any except GN maturing, or GNB-intermixed		NA	YES		Intermediate
L2	≥18 months	GNB-nodular, neuroblastoma	Differentiating	NA	NO		Low
L2	≥18 months	GNB-nodular, neuroblastoma	Differentiating	NA	YES		Intermediate
L2	≥18 months	GNB-nodular, neuroblastoma	Poorly differentiated or undifferentiated	NA			Intermediate
L2	≥18 months	GNB-nodular, neuroblastoma		AMP			High
M	<18 months			NA		Hyperdiploid	Low
M	<12 months			NA		Diploid	Intermediate
M	12–<18 months			NA		Diploid	Intermediate
M	<18 months			AMP			High
M	≥18 months						High
MS	<18 months			NA	NO		Very low
MS	<18 months			NA	YES		High
MS	<18 months			AMP			High

Classification schema is based on analysis of 8800 patients in the INRG database (1990–2002). Risk groups are: very low risk (5-year EFS > 85%); low risk (5-year EFS > 75% to ≤85%); intermediate risk (5-year EFS ≥ 50% to ≤75%); high risk (5-year EFS < 50%). *GN* ganglioneuroma, *GNB* ganglioneuroblastoma, *Amp* amplified, *NA* not amplified; Staging of L1, L2, M, and MS described in Fig. 14.1b; *EFS* event-free survival

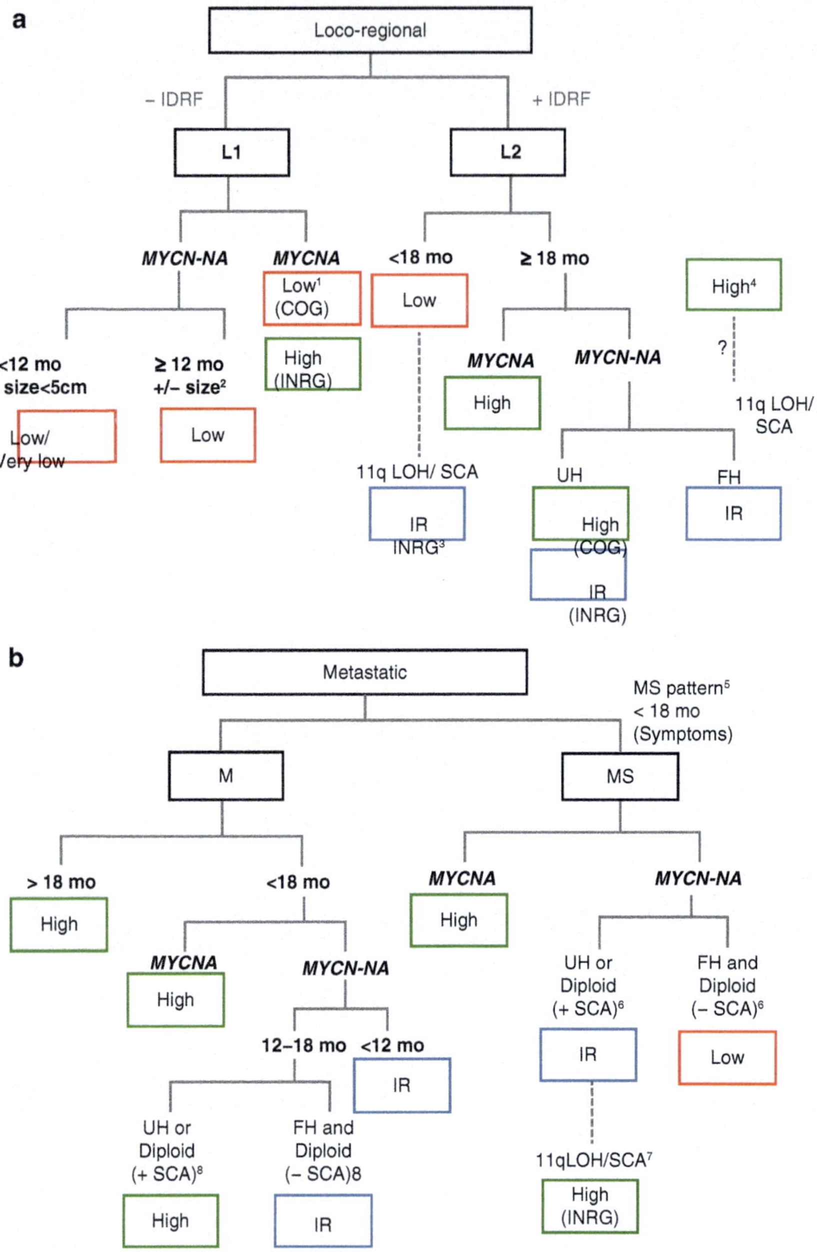

Fig. 14.1 (**a**) Risk assignments for loco-regional neuroblastoma. (**b**) Risk assignments for metastatic neuroblastoma

Shown in this schematic are the factors used to risk classify patients using the INRG staging system. Differences in risk classification for specific subsets between COG, SIOPEN and INRG are noted. Dashed line refers to incorporation of an additional factor to potentially alter risk assignment in one or more group. It should be noted that size of primary tumor may be used to assign risk group (and therapy) in some trials for L1 tumors. SCAs are increasingly incorporated into current classification systems between low and IR is becoming less significant and, instead, for the non-high risk group, most prognostic factors are used to tailor the type, and in certain cases, amount of therapy.

14.4.1 Low Risk (LR)

The majority of patients categorized as LR (and very low risk) are those with localized disease that is usually amenable to surgical resection due to the absence of IDRFs. These patients have survival rates of >95% [8, 57, 114–116]. Approximately 40% of patients are classified as LR and the majority are INSS 1, 2, 4S (usually INRG L1) without *MYCNA*. Most LR patients at diagnosis do not require chemotherapy, unless there are organ- or life-threatening symptoms. Many undergo partial or complete surgical resection and a subset can be safely observed without resection due to high likelihood of spontaneous regression [117]. Increasingly, prognostic biomarkers (e.g. SCAs) are used in COG and SIOPEN clinical trials to determine if asymptomatic young infants and toddlers with favourable biological features can be observed or receive less therapy [54, 60] and whether the small subset of patients with LR disease who recur can be identified with specific biomarkers.

14.4.2 Intermediate (IR)

Approximately 20% of patients meet current criteria for the IR group and their OS is approximately 90%. The majority of these patients are INSS 3 (mostly INRG L2) and infants with stage 4/M disease with favourable biology (mainly lack of *MYCNA*). In most cooperative group trials, IR patients receive between 2–8 cycles of chemotherapy and usually surgical resection. Based on small series in which biologically favourable localized IR patients were observed without chemotherapy [118, 119] increasingly, biological factors are being used to reduce therapy. Classification of IR patients is similar across cooperative groups with the exception of INSS 3 UH (without *MYCNA*) which are considered HR in COG but IR in SIOPEN trials [58]. The specific biomarkers used to distinguish HR and IR categories in Stage 4/M toddlers 12–18 months without *MYCNA* also vary among different trials. SCAs or newer biomarkers, including alterations of the telomerase pathway, may help predict outcome in these groups or predict the small subsets that will progress or recur following therapy.

14.4.3 High Risk (HR)

The 5 year EFS for the entire group of HR patients is approximately 50%, but improving [112, 120, 121]. More than 80% of these patients are Stage 4/M patients >18 months or Stage 4/M patients with *MYCNA* and the remainder are INSS 3(usually L2) with *MYCNA* (or UH in North America). Standard therapy for patients classified as HR includes chemotherapy, surgery, autologous stem cell transplant(s) and immunotherapy. The outcome for these patient subgroups within HR cohort varies and suggests that not all groups may require the same therapy or be eligible for more intensive treatments being evaluated on clinical trials. There are significant international efforts aimed at further discriminating cohorts of HR patients with the most inferior outcomes, often referred to as 'ultra-high risk' [122].

14.5 Conclusion

There has been significant progress in identifying prognostic factors to risk classify patients with neuroblastoma into LR, IR and HR groups. International collaborations and the INRG database have enabled the development of a universal risk classifier that will enable comparisons of results across clinical trials and allow for further refinement of risk groups. Current classifiers rely on biological and clinical prognostic risk factors at diagnosis. Revisions to risk-stratification systems will likely incorporate new biomarkers for specific subgroup, which will include novel genomic alterations and potentially imaging or MRD response to upfront therapies. Challenges moving forward include defining prognostic features for small rare subgroups, such as toddlers with *MYCN-NA*. The identification of prognostic factors within the HR cohort to distinguish patients with particularly poor outcomes may also facilitate intensification of therapy only for those subsets of HR patients. Finally, the discovery of novel genomic factors (somatic and germ line) that predict response to targeted therapies may require additional changes to the current paradigm by which patients are classified into LR, IR and HR groups to enable precision medicine strategies based on specific predictive biomarkers. These approaches may not only optimize our ability to determine prognosis, tumour response and guide therapy decisions but eventually may predict late effects and other sequelae of treatment regimens.

References

1. Irwin MS, Park JR. Neuroblastoma: pediatric paradigm for precision medicine. Pediatr Clin North Am. 2015;62:225–56.
2. Pinto NR, et al. Advances in risk classification and treatment strategies for neuroblastoma. J Clin Oncol. 2015;33:3008–17. https://doi.org/10.1200/JCO.2014.59.4648.
3. Brodeur GM, et al. Revisions of the international criteria for neuroblastoma diagnosis, staging, and response to treatment. J Clin Oncol. 1993;11:1466–77.
4. Cohn SL, et al. The International Neuroblastoma Risk Group (INRG) classification system: an INRG Task Force report. J Clin Oncol. 2009;27:289–97.
5. Cecchetto G, et al. Surgical risk factors in primary surgery for localized neuroblastoma: the LNESG1 study of the European International Society of Pediatric Oncology Neuroblastoma Group. J Clin Oncol. 2005;23:8483–9.
6. Monclair T, et al. The International Neuroblastoma Risk Group (INRG) staging system: an INRG Task Force report. J Clin Oncol. 2009;27:298–303.
7. Simon T, Hero B, Benz-Bohm G, von Schweinitz D, Berthold F. Review of image defined risk factors in localized neuroblastoma patients: results of the GPOH NB97 trial. Pediatr Blood Cancer. 2008;50:965–9. https://doi.org/10.1002/pbc.21343.

8. Simon T, Spitz R, Faldum A, Hero B, Berthold F. New definition of low-risk neuroblastoma using stage, age, and 1p and MYCN status. J Pediatr Hematol Oncol. 2004;26:791–6.
9. Schmidt ML, et al. Biologic factors determine prognosis in infants with stage IV neuroblastoma: a prospective Children's Cancer Group study. J Clin Oncol. 2000;18:1260–8.
10. George RE, et al. Hyperdiploidy plus nonamplified MYCN confers a favorable prognosis in children 12 to 18 months old with disseminated neuroblastoma: a Pediatric Oncology Group study. J Clin Oncol. 2005;23:6466–73.
11. London WB, et al. Evidence for an age cutoff greater than 365 days for neuroblastoma risk group stratification in the Children's Oncology Group. J Clin Oncol. 2005;23:6459–65.
12. Mosse YP, et al. Neuroblastoma in older children, adolescents and young adults: a report from the International Neuroblastoma Risk Group project. Pediatr Blood Cancer. 2014;61:627–35. https://doi.org/10.1002/pbc.24777.
13. Schmidt ML, et al. Favorable prognosis for patients 12 to 18 months of age with stage 4 nonamplified MYCN neuroblastoma: a Children's Cancer Group study. J Clin Oncol. 2005;23:6474–80.
14. Schleiermacher G, et al. Segmental chromosomal alterations lead to a higher risk of relapse in infants with MYCN-non-amplified localised unresectable/disseminated neuroblastoma (a SIOPEN collaborative study). Br J Cancer. 2011;105:1940–8. https://doi.org/10.1038/bjc.2011.472.
15. Brodeur GM, Seeger RC, Schwab M, Varmus HE, Bishop JM. Amplification of N-myc in untreated human neuroblastomas correlates with advanced disease stage. Science. 1984;224:1121–4.
16. Seeger RC, et al. Association of multiple copies of the N-myc oncogene with rapid progression of neuroblastomas. N Engl J Med. 1985;313:1111–6.
17. Moreau LA, et al. Does MYCN amplification manifested as homogeneously staining regions at diagnosis predict a worse outcome in children with neuroblastoma? A Children's Oncology Group study. Clin Cancer Res. 2006;12:5693–7.
18. Ambros PF, et al. International consensus for neuroblastoma molecular diagnostics: report from the international Neuroblastoma Risk Group (INRG) Biology Committee. Br J Cancer. 2009;100:1471–82.
19. Campbell K, et al. Association of MYCN copy number with clinical features, tumor biology, and outcomes in neuroblastoma: a report from the Children's Oncology Group. Cancer. 2017;123:4224–35. https://doi.org/10.1002/cncr.30873.
20. Berbegall AP, et al. Comparative genetic study of intratumoral heterogenous MYCN amplified neuroblastoma versus aggressive genetic profile neuroblastic tumors. Oncogene. 2016;35:1423–32. https://doi.org/10.1038/onc.2015.200.
21. Marrano P, Irwin MS, Thorner PS. Heterogeneity of MYCN amplification in neuroblastoma at diagnosis, treatment, relapse, and metastasis. Genes Chromosomes Cancer. 2017;56:28–41. https://doi.org/10.1002/gcc.22398.
22. Huang M, Weiss WA. Neuroblastoma and MYCN. Cold Spring Harb Perspect Med. 2013;3:a014415. https://doi.org/10.1101/cshperspect.a014415.
23. Ruiz-Perez MV, Henley AB, Arsenian-Henriksson M. The MYCN protein in health and disease. Genes (Basel). 2017;8 https://doi.org/10.3390/genes8040113.
24. Weiss WA, Aldape K, Mohapatra G, Feuerstein BG, Bishop JM. Targeted expression of MYCN causes neuroblastoma in transgenic mice. EMBO J. 1997;16:2985–95.
25. Zhu S, et al. Activated ALK collaborates with MYCN in neuroblastoma pathogenesis. Cancer Cell. 2012;21:362–73. https://doi.org/10.1016/j.ccr.2012.02.010.
26. Berry T, et al. The ALK(F1174L) mutation potentiates the oncogenic activity of MYCN in neuroblastoma. Cancer Cell. 2012;22:117–30. https://doi.org/10.1016/j.ccr.2012.06.001.
27. Valentijn LJ, et al. Functional MYCN signature predicts outcome of neuroblastoma irrespective of MYCN amplification. Proc Natl Acad Sci U S A. 2012;109:19190–5. https://doi.org/10.1073/pnas.1208215109.
28. Puissant A, et al. Targeting MYCN in neuroblastoma by BET bromodomain inhibition. Cancer Discov. 2013;3:308–23. https://doi.org/10.1158/2159-8290.CD-12-0418.

29. Gustafson WC, et al. Drugging MYCN through an allosteric transition in Aurora Kinase A. Cancer Cell. 2014;26:414–27. https://doi.org/10.1016/j.ccr.2014.07.015.
30. Brockmann M, et al. Small molecule inhibitors of Aurora-A induce proteasomal degradation of N-Myc in childhood neuroblastoma. Cancer Cell. 2013;24:75–89. https://doi.org/10.1016/j.ccr.2013.05.005.
31. DuBois SG, et al. Phase I study of the Aurora A kinase inhibitor alisertib in combination with irinotecan and temozolomide for patients with relapsed or refractory neuroblastoma: a NANT (new approaches to neuroblastoma therapy) trial. J Clin Oncol. 2016;34:1368–75. https://doi.org/10.1200/JCO.2015.65.4889.
32. Wang LL, et al. Neuroblastoma of undifferentiated subtype, prognostic significance of prominent nucleolar formation, and MYC/MYCN protein expression: a report from the Children's Oncology Group. Cancer. 2013;119:3718–26. https://doi.org/10.1002/cncr.28251.
33. Wang LL, et al. Augmented expression of MYC and/or MYCN protein defines highly aggressive MYC-driven neuroblastoma: a Children's Oncology Group study. Br J Cancer. 2015;113:57–63. https://doi.org/10.1038/bjc.2015.188.
34. Bagatell R, et al. Significance of MYCN amplification in international neuroblastoma staging system stage 1 and 2 neuroblastoma: a report from the International Neuroblastoma Risk Group database. J Clin Oncol. 2009;27:365–70.
35. Vo KT, et al. Clinical, biological and prognostic differences based on primary tumor site in neuroblastoma: a report from the International Neuroblastoma Risk Group (INRG) project. J Clin Oncol. 2014;32(28):3169–76.
36. Thompson D, et al. Identification of patient subgroups with markedly disparate rates of MYCN amplification in neuroblastoma: a report from the International Neuroblastoma Risk Group project. Cancer. 2016;122:935–45. https://doi.org/10.1002/cncr.29848.
37. Teshiba R, et al. Age-dependent prognostic effect by Mitosis-Karyorrhexis Index in neuroblastoma: a report from the Children's Oncology Group. Pediatr Dev Pathol. 2014;17:441–9. https://doi.org/10.2350/14-06-1505-OA.1.
38. George RE, et al. Relationship between histopathological features, MYCN amplification, and prognosis: a UKCCSG study. United Kingdom Children Cancer Study Group. Med Pediatr Oncol. 2001;36:169–76. https://doi.org/10.1002/1096-911X(20010101)36:1<169::AID-MPO1041>3.0.CO;2-U.
39. Shimada H, et al. The international neuroblastoma pathology classification (the Shimada system). Cancer. 1999;86:364–72.
40. Shimada H, et al. Identification of subsets of neuroblastomas by combined histopathologic and N-myc analysis. J Natl Cancer Inst. 1995;87:1470–6.
41. Bowman LC, et al. Genetic staging of unresectable or metastatic neuroblastoma in infants: a Pediatric Oncology Group study. J Natl Cancer Inst. 1997;89:373–80.
42. Look AT, et al. Clinical relevance of tumor cell ploidy and N-myc gene amplification in childhood neuroblastoma: a Pediatric Oncology Group study. J Clin Oncol. 1991;9:581–91.
43. Oppedal BR, Storm-Mathisen I, Lie SO, Brandtzaeg P. Prognostic factors in neuroblastoma. Clinical, histopathologic, and immunohistochemical features and DNA ploidy in relation to prognosis. Cancer. 1988;62:772–80.
44. Janoueix-Lerosey I, et al. Overall genomic pattern is a predictor of outcome in neuroblastoma. J Clin Oncol. 2009;27:1026–33.
45. Attiyeh EF, et al. Chromosome 1p and 11q deletions and outcome in neuroblastoma. N Engl J Med. 2005;353:2243–53.
46. Brodeur GM, et al. Molecular analysis and clinical significance of N-myc amplification and chromosome 1p monosomy in human neuroblastomas. Prog Clin Biol Res. 1988;271:3–15.
47. Maris JM, et al. Loss of heterozygosity at 1p36 independently predicts for disease progression but not decreased overall survival probability in neuroblastoma patients: a Children's Cancer Group study. J Clin Oncol. 2000;18:1888–99.
48. Mosse YP, et al. Neuroblastomas have distinct genomic DNA profiles that predict clinical phenotype and regional gene expression. Genes Chromosomes Cancer. 2007;46:936–49. https://doi.org/10.1002/gcc.20477.

49. Guo C, et al. Allelic deletion at 11q23 is common in MYCN single copy neuroblastomas. Oncogene. 1999;18:4948–57.
50. Tonini GP, et al. MYCN oncogene amplification in neuroblastoma is associated with worse prognosis, except in stage 4s: the Italian experience with 295 children. J Clin Oncol. 1997;15:85–93.
51. De Bernardi B, et al. Excellent outcome with reduced treatment for infants with disseminated neuroblastoma without MYCN gene amplification. J Clin Oncol. 2009;27:1034–40. https://doi.org/10.1200/JCO.2008.17.5877.
52. Minard V, et al. Adverse outcome of infants with metastatic neuroblastoma, MYCN amplification and/or bone lesions: results of the French society of pediatric oncology. Br J Cancer. 2000;83:973–9. https://doi.org/10.1054/bjoc.2000.1412.
53. Katzenstein HM, et al. Prognostic significance of age, MYCN oncogene amplification, tumor cell ploidy, and histology in 110 infants with stage D(S) neuroblastoma: the pediatric oncology group experience—a pediatric oncology group study. J Clin Oncol. 1998;16:2007–17.
54. Baker DL, et al. Outcome after reduced chemotherapy for intermediate-risk neuroblastoma. N Engl J Med. 2010;363:1313–23. https://doi.org/10.1056/NEJMoa1001527.
55. Rubie H, et al. N-Myc gene amplification is a major prognostic factor in localized neuroblastoma: results of the French NBL 90 study. Neuroblastoma Study Group of the Societe Francaise d'Oncologie Pediatrique. J Clin Oncol. 1997;15:1171–82. https://doi.org/10.1200/JCO.1997.15.3.1171.
56. Shimada H, et al. Histopathologic prognostic factors in neuroblastic tumors: definition of subtypes of ganglioneuroblastoma and an age-linked classification of neuroblastomas. J Natl Cancer Inst. 1984;73:405–16.
57. Strother DR, et al. Outcome after surgery alone or with restricted use of chemotherapy for patients with low-risk neuroblastoma: results of Children's Oncology Group study P9641. J Clin Oncol. 2012;30:1842–8. https://doi.org/10.1200/JCO.2011.37.9990.
58. Meany HJ, et al. Significance of clinical and biologic features in Stage 3 neuroblastoma: a report from the International Neuroblastoma Risk Group project. Pediatr Blood Cancer. 2014; https://doi.org/10.1002/pbc.25134.
59. Look AT, Hayes FA, Nitschke R, McWilliams NB, Green AA. Cellular DNA content as a predictor of response to chemotherapy in infants with unresectable neuroblastoma. N Engl J Med. 1984;311:231–5. https://doi.org/10.1056/NEJM198407263110405.
60. Park JR, et al. Children's Oncology Group's 2013 blueprint for research: neuroblastoma. Pediatr Blood Cancer. 2013;60:985–93. https://doi.org/10.1002/pbc.24433.
61. Bown N, et al. Gain of chromosome arm 17q and adverse outcome in patients with neuroblastoma. N Engl J Med. 1999;340:1954–61.
62. Meddeb M, et al. Additional copies of a 25 Mb chromosomal region originating from 17q23.1-17qter are present in 90% of high-grade neuroblastomas. Genes Chromosomes Cancer. 1996;17:156–65. https://doi.org/10.1002/(SICI)1098-2264(199611)17:3<156::AID-GCC3>3.0.CO;2-3.
63. Caron H, et al. Allelic loss of chromosome 1p as a predictor of unfavorable outcome in patients with neuroblastoma. N Engl J Med. 1996;334:225–30.
64. Riley RD, et al. A systematic review of molecular and biological tumor markers in neuroblastoma. Clin Cancer Res. 2004;10:4–12.
65. Spitz R, Hero B, Simon T, Berthold F. Loss in chromosome 11q identifies tumors with increased risk for metastatic relapses in localized and 4S neuroblastoma. Clin Cancer Res. 2006;12:3368–73. https://doi.org/10.1158/1078-0432.CCR-05-2495.
66. Schleiermacher G, et al. Segmental chromosomal alterations have prognostic impact in neuroblastoma: a report from the INRG project. Br J Cancer. 2012;107:1418–22. https://doi.org/10.1038/bjc.2012.375.
67. Defferrari R, et al. Influence of segmental chromosome abnormalities on survival in children over the age of 12 months with unresectable localised peripheral neuroblastic tumours without MYCN amplification. Br J Cancer. 2015;112:290–5. https://doi.org/10.1038/bjc.2014.557.

68. Chicard M, et al. Genomic copy number profiling using circulating free tumor DNA highlights heterogeneity in neuroblastoma. Clin Cancer Res. 2016;22:5564–73. https://doi.org/10.1158/1078-0432.CCR-16-0500.
69. Van Roy N, et al. Shallow whole genome sequencing on circulating cell-free DNA allows reliable noninvasive copy-number profiling in neuroblastoma patients. Clin Cancer Res. 2017;23:6305–14. https://doi.org/10.1158/1078-0432.CCR-17-0675.
70. Campbell BB, et al. Comprehensive analysis of hypermutation in human cancer. Cell. 2017;171:1042–1056 e1010. https://doi.org/10.1016/j.cell.2017.09.048.
71. Pugh TJ, et al. The genetic landscape of high-risk neuroblastoma. Nat Genet. 2013; https://doi.org/10.1038/ng.2529.
72. Molenaar JJ, et al. Sequencing of neuroblastoma identifies chromothripsis and defects in neuritogenesis genes. Nature. 2012;483:589–93. https://doi.org/10.1038/nature10910.
73. Sausen M, et al. Integrated genomic analyses identify ARID1A and ARID1B alterations in the childhood cancer neuroblastoma. Nat Genet. 2013;45:12–7. https://doi.org/10.1038/ng.2493.
74. Bresler SC, et al. ALK mutations confer differential oncogenic activation and sensitivity to ALK inhibition therapy in neuroblastoma. Cancer Cell. 2014;26:682–94. https://doi.org/10.1016/j.ccell.2014.09.019.
75. Suzuki M, et al. Treatment and outcome of adult-onset neuroblastoma. Int J Cancer. 2018; https://doi.org/10.1002/ijc.31399.
76. Cheung NK, et al. Association of age at diagnosis and genetic mutations in patients with neuroblastoma. JAMA. 2012;307:1062–71. https://doi.org/10.1001/jama.2012.228.
77. Bellini A, et al. Deep sequencing reveals occurrence of subclonal ALK mutations in neuroblastoma at diagnosis. Clin Cancer Res. 2015;21:4913–21. https://doi.org/10.1158/1078-0432.CCR-15-0423.
78. Schleiermacher G, et al. Emergence of new ALK mutations at relapse of neuroblastoma. J Clin Oncol. 2014; https://doi.org/10.1200/JCO.2013.54.0674.
79. Eleveld TF, et al. Relapsed neuroblastomas show frequent RAS-MAPK pathway mutations. Nat Genet. 2015;47:864–71. https://doi.org/10.1038/ng.3333.
80. Padovan-Merhar OM, et al. Enrichment of targetable mutations in the relapsed neuroblastoma genome. PLoS Genet. 2016;12:e1006501. https://doi.org/10.1371/journal.pgen.1006501.
81. Schulte JH, et al. High ALK receptor tyrosine kinase expression supersedes ALK mutation as a determining factor of an unfavorable phenotype in primary neuroblastoma. Clin Cancer Res. 2011;17:5082–92. https://doi.org/10.1158/1078-0432.CCR-10-2809.
82. De Brouwer S, et al. Meta-analysis of neuroblastomas reveals a skewed ALK mutation spectrum in tumors with MYCN amplification. Clin Cancer Res. 2010;16:4353–62. https://doi.org/10.1158/1078-0432.CCR-09-2660.
83. Duijkers FA, et al. High anaplastic lymphoma kinase immunohistochemical staining in neuroblastoma and ganglioneuroblastoma is an independent predictor of poor outcome. Am J Pathol. 2012;180:1223–31. https://doi.org/10.1016/j.ajpath.2011.12.003.
84. Bresler SC, et al. Differential inhibitor sensitivity of anaplastic lymphoma kinase variants found in neuroblastoma. Sci Transl Med. 2011;3:108ra114. https://doi.org/10.1126/scitranslmed.3002950.
85. Infarinato NR, et al. The ALK/ROS1 inhibitor PF-06463922 overcomes primary resistance to crizotinib in ALK-driven neuroblastoma. Cancer Discov. 2016;6:96–107. https://doi.org/10.1158/2159-8290.CD-15-1056.
86. Peifer M, et al. Telomerase activation by genomic rearrangements in high-risk neuroblastoma. Nature. 2015;526:700–4. https://doi.org/10.1038/nature14980.
87. Valentijn LJ, et al. TERT rearrangements are frequent in neuroblastoma and identify aggressive tumors. Nat Genet. 2015;47:1411–4. https://doi.org/10.1038/ng.3438.
88. Hertwig F, Peifer M, Fischer M. Telomere maintenance is pivotal for high-risk neuroblastoma. Cell Cycle. 2016;15:311–2. https://doi.org/10.1080/15384101.2015.1125243.
89. Henson JD, et al. The C-Circle Assay for alternative-lengthening-of-telomeres activity. Methods. 2017;114:74–84. https://doi.org/10.1016/j.ymeth.2016.08.016.

90. Mender I, Gryaznov S, Dikmen ZG, Wright WE, Shay JW. Induction of telomere dysfunction mediated by the telomerase substrate precursor 6-thio-2′-deoxyguanosine. Cancer Discov. 2015;5:82–95. https://doi.org/10.1158/2159-8290.CD-14-0609.
91. Flynn RL, et al. Alternative lengthening of telomeres renders cancer cells hypersensitive to ATR inhibitors. Science. 2015;347:273–7. https://doi.org/10.1126/science.1257216.
92. Vermeulen J, De Preter K, Laureys G, Speleman F, Vandesompele J. 59-Gene prognostic signature sub-stratifies high-risk neuroblastoma patients. Lancet Oncol. 2009;10:1030. https://doi.org/10.1016/S1470-2045(09)70325-0, S1470-2045(09)70325-0 [pii].
93. De Preter K, et al. Accurate outcome prediction in neuroblastoma across independent data sets using a multigene signature. Clin Cancer Res. 2010;16:1532–41.
94. Oberthuer A, et al. Customized oligonucleotide microarray gene expression-based classification of neuroblastoma patients outperforms current clinical risk stratification. J Clin Oncol. 2006;24:5070–8.
95. Oberthuer A, et al. Prognostic impact of gene expression-based classification for neuroblastoma. J Clin Oncol. 2010;28:3506–15. https://doi.org/10.1200/JCO.2009.27.3367, JCO.2009.27.3367 [pii].
96. Garcia I, et al. A three-gene expression signature model for risk stratification of patients with neuroblastoma. Clin Cancer Res. 2012–2023;18:2012. https://doi.org/10.1158/1078-0432.CCR-11-2483.
97. Asgharzadeh S, et al. Prognostic significance of gene expression profiles of metastatic neuroblastomas lacking MYCN gene amplification. J Natl Cancer Inst. 2006;98:1193–203. https://doi.org/10.1093/jnci/djj330., 98/17/1193 [pii].
98. Asgharzadeh S, et al. Clinical significance of tumor-associated inflammatory cells in metastatic neuroblastoma. J Clin Oncol. 2012;30:3525–32. https://doi.org/10.1200/JCO.2011.40.9169.
99. Hallett RM, Seong AB, Kaplan DR, Irwin MS. Transcript signatures that predict outcome and identify targetable pathways in MYCN-amplified neuroblastoma. Mol Oncol. 2016;10:1461–72. https://doi.org/10.1016/j.molonc.2016.07.012.
100. Oberthuer A, et al. Revised risk estimation and treatment stratification of low- and intermediate-risk neuroblastoma patients by integrating clinical and molecular prognostic markers. Clin Cancer Res. 2015;21:1904–15. https://doi.org/10.1158/1078-0432.CCR-14-0817.
101. Buckley PG, et al. Chromosomal and microRNA expression patterns reveal biologically distinct subgroups of 11q-neuroblastoma. Clin Cancer Res. 2010;16:2971–8. https://doi.org/10.1158/1078-0432.CCR-09-3215, 1078-0432.CCR-09-3215 [pii].
102. Chen Y, Stallings RL. Differential patterns of microRNA expression in neuroblastoma are correlated with prognosis, differentiation, and apoptosis. Cancer Res. 2007;67:976–83. https://doi.org/10.1158/0008-5472.CAN-06-3667.
103. De Preter K, et al. miRNA expression profiling enables risk stratification in archived and fresh neuroblastoma tumor samples. Clin Cancer Res. 2011;17:7684–92. https://doi.org/10.1158/1078-0432.CCR-11-0610.
104. Yanik GA, et al. Semiquantitative mIBG scoring as a prognostic indicator in patients with stage 4 neuroblastoma: a report from the Children's Oncology Group. J Nucl Med. 2013; https://doi.org/10.2967/jnumed.112.112334.
105. Matthay KK, et al. Correlation of early metastatic response by 123I-metaiodobenzylguanidine scintigraphy with overall response and event-free survival in stage IV neuroblastoma. J Clin Oncol. 2003;21:2486–91. https://doi.org/10.1200/JCO.2003.09.122.
106. Suc A, et al. Metastatic neuroblastoma in children older than one year: prognostic significance of the initial metaiodobenzylguanidine scan and proposal for a scoring system. Cancer. 1996;77:805–11.
107. Ady N, et al. A new 123I-MIBG whole body scan scoring method—application to the prediction of the response of metastases to induction chemotherapy in stage IV neuroblastoma. Eur J Cancer. 1995;31A:256–61.
108. Ladenstein R, et al. Validation of the mIBG skeletal SIOPEN scoring method in two independent high-risk neuroblastoma populations: the SIOPEN/HR-NBL1 and COG-A3973 trials. Eur J Nucl Med Mol Imaging. 2018;45:292–305. https://doi.org/10.1007/s00259-017-3829-7.

109. Brownhill SC, Burchill SA. PCR-based amplification of circulating RNAs as prognostic and predictive biomarkers – focus on neuroblastoma. Pract Lab Med. 2017;7:41–4. https://doi.org/10.1016/j.plabm.2016.04.003.
110. Viprey VF, et al. Neuroblastoma mRNAs predict outcome in children with stage 4 neuroblastoma: a European HR-NBL1/SIOPEN study. J Clin Oncol. 2014;32:1074–83. https://doi.org/10.1200/JCO.2013.53.3604.
111. Corrias MV, et al. A novel syngeneic murine model for thoracic neuroblastoma obtained by intramediastinal injection of tumor cells. Cancer Detect Prev. 2002;26:468–75.
112. Kreissman SG, et al. Purged versus non-purged peripheral blood stem-cell transplantation for high-risk neuroblastoma (COG A3973): a randomised phase 3 trial. Lancet Oncol. 2013;14:999–1008. https://doi.org/10.1016/S1470-2045(13)70309-7.
113. Marachelian A, et al. Expression of five neuroblastoma genes in bone marrow or blood of patients with relapsed/refractory neuroblastoma provides a new biomarker for disease and prognosis. Clin Cancer Res. 2017;23:5374–83. https://doi.org/10.1158/1078-0432.CCR-16-2647.
114. Alvarado CS, et al. Natural history and biology of stage A neuroblastoma: a Pediatric Oncology Group study. J Pediatr Hematol Oncol. 2000;22:197–205.
115. Perez CA, et al. Biologic variables in the outcome of stages I and II neuroblastoma treated with surgery as primary therapy: a Children's Cancer Group study. J Clin Oncol. 2000;18:18–26.
116. Simon T, Spitz R, Hero B, Berthold F, Faldum A. Risk estimation in localized unresectable single copy MYCN neuroblastoma by the status of chromosomes 1p and 11q. Cancer Lett. 2006;237:215–22. https://doi.org/10.1016/j.canlet.2005.06.001.
117. Nuchtern JG, et al. A prospective study of expectant observation as primary therapy for neuroblastoma in young infants: a Children's Oncology Group study. Ann Surg. 2012;256:573–80. https://doi.org/10.1097/SLA.0b013e31826cbbbd.
118. Hero B, et al. Localized infant neuroblastomas often show spontaneous regression: results of the prospective trials NB95-S and NB97. J Clin Oncol. 2008;26:1504–10. https://doi.org/10.1200/JCO.2007.12.3349.
119. Kushner BH, et al. Survival from locally invasive or widespread neuroblastoma without cytotoxic therapy. J Clin Oncol. 1996;14:373–81.
120. Ladenstein R, et al. Busulfan and melphalan versus carboplatin, etoposide, and melphalan as high-dose chemotherapy for high-risk neuroblastoma (HR-NBL1/SIOPEN): an international, randomised, multi-arm, open-label, phase 3 trial. Lancet Oncol. 2017;18:500–14. https://doi.org/10.1016/S1470-2045(17)30070-0.
121. Yu A, Gilman AL, Ozkaynak MF. A phase III randomized trial of the chimeric anti-GD2 antibody ch14.18 with GMCSF and IL2 as immunotherapy following dose intensive chemotherapy for high risk neuroblsatoma: Children's Oncology Group (COG) study ANBL0032. J Clin Oncol. 2009;27
122. Depuydt P, et al. Genomic amplifications and distal 6q loss: novel markers for poor survival in high-risk neuroblastoma patients. J Natl Cancer Inst. 2018; https://doi.org/10.1093/jnci/djy022.

Part IV

Surgery

15 Biopsy of Neuroblastoma

Dhanya Mullassery, Laurence Abernethy, Rajeev Shukla, and Paul D. Losty

Neuroblastoma is the most common extracranial solid tumour in childhood. This enigmatic tumour shows extremely divergent behaviour, ranging from spontaneous regression, through maturation into differentiated cell types, to extreme chemoresistance, resulting in high mortality. The prognosis and treatment stratification of patients with this tumour is currently based on the International Neuroblastoma Risk Group (INRG) Staging System, which categorizes cases into high, intermediate, low and very low risk groups. In this classification system, tumour histology (Shimada) and biology (MYCN, segmental and numerical chromosomal aberrations including 1p, 11q) play a vital role, in addition to the age and extent of disease. Therefore, the key role of adequate solid tumour biopsy in the diagnosis and prognostic decision-making of patients with neuroblastoma cannot be overemphasised.

The aim(s) of tumour biopsy are to firmly establish diagnosis and also to obtain adequate tissue for molecular testing and biologic risk stratification. There are generally three types of techniques deployed in the biopsy of neuroblastic tumours. Traditionally, European and North American paediatric cancer guidelines had advocated open surgical biopsy (OSB) in all suspected neuroblastic tumours. The approaches often utilised involved a mini-laparotomy, thoracotomy or open neck dissection, depending on the anatomical location of tumour. The proposed advantages of the open 'classical' surgical methods were to ensure wholly adequate sampling of different parts of the tumour lesion (to account for the known heterogeneity of this neoplasm) and to obtain adequate volume (minimum 1 cm^3) of tissue to

D. Mullassery
Great Ormond Street Hospital for Sick Children, London, UK

L. Abernethy · R. Shukla
Alder Hey Children's Hospital NHS Foundation Trust, Liverpool, UK

P. D. Losty (✉)
Alder Hey Children's Hospital NHS Foundation Trust, University of Liverpool, Liverpool, UK
e-mail: paul.losty@liverpool.ac.uk

S. Sarnacki, L. Pio (eds.), *Neuroblastoma*,
https://doi.org/10.1007/978-3-030-18396-7_15

suffice for the different histological and molecular biology techniques/tests required in addition to tissue tumour banking for vital multinational collaborative research. In patients harbouring metastatic tumours, the more superficial 'metastatic lesions' may be easily accessed as the source of tumour tissue for biopsy. Complications reported for open 'classical' surgical biopsy in neuroblastoma tumours include (1) intraoperative bleeding, (2) injury to adjacent anatomical organs, particularly bowel and post-operatively (3) adhesive intestinal obstruction, (4) need for blood transfusion(s) and (5) abdominal compartment syndrome. Post-operative hospital stay after open surgical biopsy is usually 48 h. The current defining role for open surgical biopsy is now relatively limited to (1) neuroblastic tumours in those patients with "no safe window" for image guided percutaneous access due to vital structures, i.e., gut or major blood vessels in the pathway of the biopsy trajectory site required or (2) in cases where there is lack of hospital staff adequately trained in interventional paediatric radiology wholly familiar with image-guided core biopsy techniques.

In recent years, image-guided core needle biopsy techniques have become well-established in specialist units worldwide, caring for children with solid tumour malignancies. Boston Children's Hospital, USA, in 1996, first published their centre's preliminary experience on the utility and feasibility of percutaneous needle biopsy for diagnosis of neuroblastoma. Several international centres, including Alder Hey Children's Hospital Liverpool, UK, have since published further defining reports confirming that core needle biopsy (CNB) has many advantages versus open surgical biopsy in terms of recording lower patient complication rates (%), particularly bleeding from tumour and the need for blood transfusion(s). There is now sufficient growing evidence to confirm image guided CNB also provides sufficient biological tissue material for all diagnostic purposes/testing in neuroblastoma. The risk of 'tumour seeding' following needle biopsy observed in some other solid malignancies has not been recorded in childhood neuroblastoma. A recent systematic review study has shown that almost 95% of all image-guided core needle biopsies for solid tumours provided adequate tissue sampling for the complete diagnosis of malignant childhood diseases. Importantly, post-operative hospital stay for CNB is much shorter compared to open 'classical' surgical biopsy, and usually no more than 6–12 h convalescence after the interventional radiology procedure. Although fine needle aspiration cytology (FNA) has been shown to be adequate for FISH analyses for neuroblastoma molecular genetic studies, these methods are generally not recommended by European and North American cancer protocols due to the limited amount of tissue material yielded for full histology required in neuroblastic tumours.

A third useful strategy deployed for neuroblastoma tumour biopsy is minimally invasive video-assisted core needle biopsy procedures, which have the advantage(s) of being able to access different regions of the gross tumour lesion, guided by laparoscopy or thoracoscopy.

All of the tumour biopsy methods for the diagnosis of neuroblastoma herein described requires the procedure to be performed safely under general anaesthesia. Regardless of the biopsy technique deployed, adequate preoperative patient preparation is essential, requiring informed signed consent from the patient's family with a full discussion of the risks/benefits of the procedure, including (1) optimisation of coagulation status and (2) availability of blood products as necessary. At the tumour board meeting, the multidisciplinary team members, including medical oncology, radiology, pathology and surgical oncologists should agree upon the optimal method of tumour biopsy on an individual patient basis, given the anatomical site of disease and other factors discussed.

15.1 Paediatric Radiology—Image-Guided Biopsy Neuroblastic Tumours

15.1.1 Indications for Image-Guided Percutaneous Biopsy

Image-guided percutaneous biopsy is a minimally invasive technique for obtaining tissue for diagnosis, which can be employed for suspected neuroblastoma, whether in a typical suprarenal location or at other sites, such as the thoracic, pelvic and paraspinal regions. Percutaneous biopsy may also be used for confirmation of suspected disease recurrence or metastatic disease, and to monitor residual disease following treatment.

Laboratory analysis of tissue obtained by biopsy is important not only for histological diagnosis but also risk stratification and determination of the biological characteristics of the tumour. This helps to inform therapeutic decision-making and the choice of the various modalities deployed in the treatment of newly diagnosed neuroblastoma, which include surgery, chemotherapy, radiotherapy, differentiation therapy, immunotherapy, and, in selected cases (notably infants with 4S disease), observation only. Most clinical trials now stratify neuroblastoma patients into low, intermediate or high-risk groups based on age of the patient, INSS stage, histology according to the INPC, MYCN status, and DNA ploidy. The biological heterogeneity of neuroblastoma tumours occurring in childhood has resulted in new therapeutic approaches directed at reducing intensity of treatment in tumours deemed to have favourable biology and an intensification of chemoradiotherapy in those lesions linked with an adverse prognosis. It is therefore paramount that biopsy techniques obtain sufficient tissue, representative of the whole of the tumour, to ensure that diagnosis and risk stratification of neuroblastoma are wholly accurate.

Fine needle aspiration for cytology is widely used as a minimally invasive diagnostic procedure for some types of tumours in adults, in whom carcinomas are most common, but are not generally recommended in paediatric oncology, as cytology is less suitable for distinguishing between the multiple types of small, round blue cell tumours encountered in children.

15.1.2 Imaging Modalities

Diagnosis and staging of neuroblastoma involves multi-modality imaging, often including ultrasound, radiography, CT, MRI and radionuclide imaging (I-MIBG,

Tc99 m methylene diphosphonate bone scan); all of these modalities may be valuable in planning the optimal site and approach for biopsy, and all available imaging should be carefully assessed before the procedure is performed.

Percutaneous biopsy is usually performed under direct ultrasound guidance, which allows continuous real-time visualisation of the position of the tip of the biopsy needle in relation to the tumour and adjacent organs. Colour Doppler facilitates identification of blood vessels and areas of high vascularity. However, in some situations, the field of view of ultrasound is limited, as ultrasound cannot penetrate bone and air-filled structures (such as lung and bowel). Young children are generally excellent ultrasound subjects because of relative lack of fat, but in older, overweight patients, an excess of fatty tissue may reduce the clarity of ultrasound images and, in the worst case, cause misregistration of needle position.

In difficult anatomical locations, and in very overweight patients, CT-guided biopsy or a combination of CT and ultrasound may be preferred. The field of view of CT is not limited by bone, lung, or air-filled bowel, and the position of the tip of the biopsy needle is clearly demonstrated, but CT involves exposure to ionising radiation and does not provide the same facility of real-time, continuous imaging as ultrasound.

MRI guided biopsy is possible, but requires special equipment, as no ferromagnetic objects or any devices that are not certified as MR compatible can be taken into an MRI scanner. In a strong magnetic field, such objects may become dangerous missiles, and absorption of radiofrequency energy may result in heating or electrical injury.

15.1.3 Patient Preparation

Percutaneous biopsy in children is usually performed under general anaesthesia, and is often combined with other procedures such as bone marrow aspirates and trephine biopsies, including central venous catheter insertion for vascular access. A multidisciplinary approach, involving close collaboration between radiologist, oncologist, surgeon, anaesthetist, pathologist and the nursing team is essential.

Awareness of the needs of the child and parents is of utmost importance, recognising that the diagnosis of a potentially life-threating tumour in the paediatric age group is extremely traumatic. The process of obtaining fully informed consent should not be rushed and may require more than one interview with the parents and other family members; it is important for the interventional radiologist to introduce themselves and to explain carefully their role.

The general medical condition of the child should be stabilised, with correction of anaemia and any coagulation disorder. Platelet count should ideally be in the normal range and INR (international normalised ratio) less than 1.5 before the procedure, and the necessary blood samples should have been taken to facilitate rapid blood transfusion in the event of serious haemorrhage.

15.1.4 Equipment

Semi-automated, spring-loaded biopsy devices make it possible to obtain diagnostic quality specimens, while minimising crush artefact and tissue fragmentation also reducing the risk of damage to surrounding tissues. A range of suitable high-precision biopsy devices are available—Fig. 15.1. Needle sizes in the range 15–18 G are generally most suitable, and variable needle throw length (typically 13–33 mm) enhances flexibility and precision; the best tissue samples are obtained with longer throw lengths, but shorter throw lengths are helpful for small lesions and difficult anatomical locations (for example, lesions in close proximity to bowel or large blood vessels).

Coaxial introduction through an introducer needle or sheath makes it possible to take multiple biopsies from different parts of the tumour, using a single point of entry, and to occlude the biopsy track with a haemostatic agent immediately in the event of serious haemorrhage or other high-risk situations.

15.1.5 Operative Technique (Figs. 15.2, 15.3, 15.4, 15.5, 15.6, 15.7, 15.8, and 15.9)

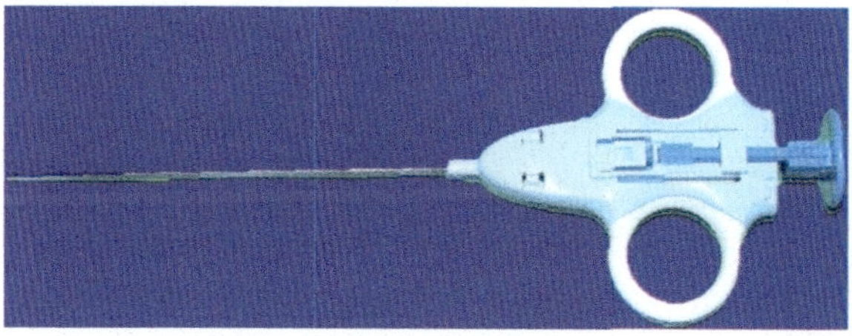

Fig. 15.1 Temno Evolution Co-axial Biopsy System (CareFusion, IL, USA)

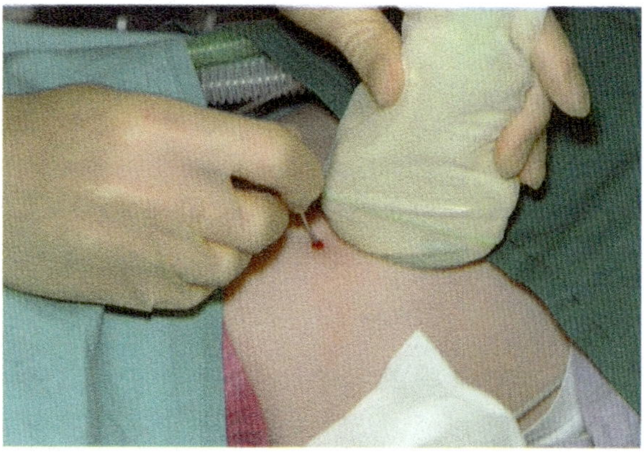

Fig. 15.2 Insertion of trocar and cannula under ultrasound guidance

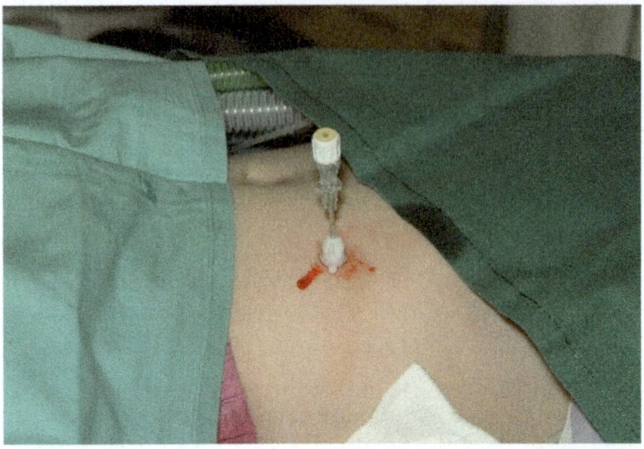

Fig. 15.3 Trocar and cannula in place

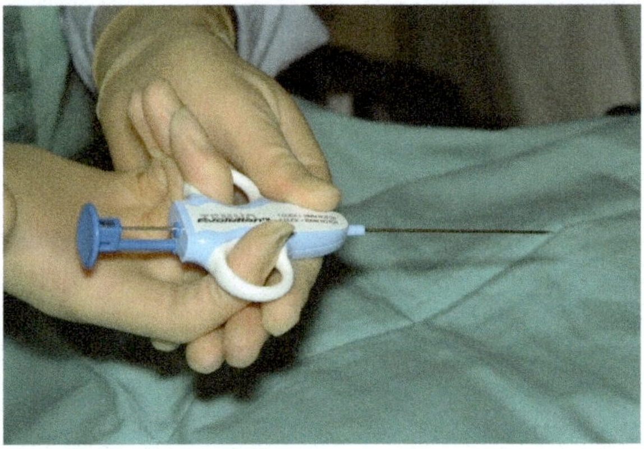

Fig. 15.4 Biopsy device prepared for use

Percutaneous biopsy procedures should be performed under strictly aseptic conditions, and in children, preferably, under general anaesthesia. The biopsy site is chosen with care using the available imaging and the site infiltrated with a long-acting local anaesthetic agent (such as levobupivacaine) to aid post-operative pain relief. A small skin incision is made with a scalpel blade, and the biopsy device is used to take multiple biopsies from different parts of the tumour from a single entry point, under direct ultrasound guidance. Fresh tissue samples are sent directly to histopathology or processed immediately by laboratory staff in the Interventional Radiology Suite. Haemostasis is then secured with gentle pressure. At the end of the procedure, ultrasound is used to check for signs of active bleeding or haematoma formation, and a sterile adhesive dressing applied to the needle biopsy wound site (no sutures should be required).

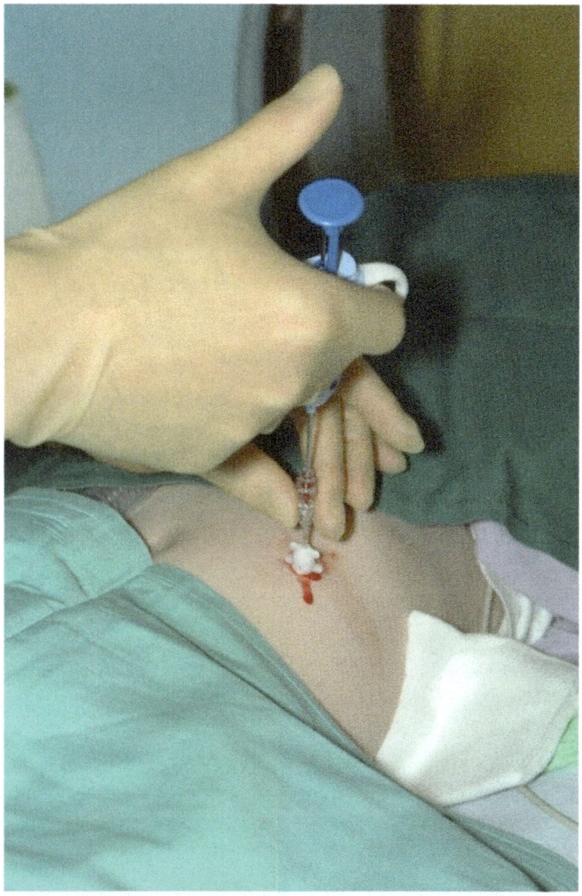

Fig. 15.5 Biopsy needle advanced through the cannula

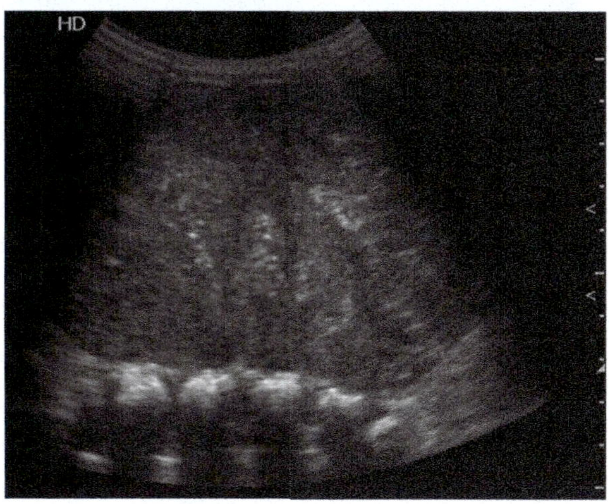

Fig. 15.6 Ultrasound image of paravertertabral neuroblastoma

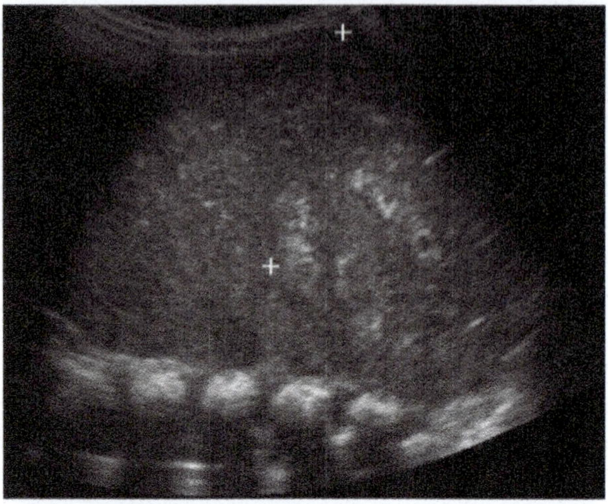

Fig. 15.7 Site chosen for percutaneous biopsy and depth measured

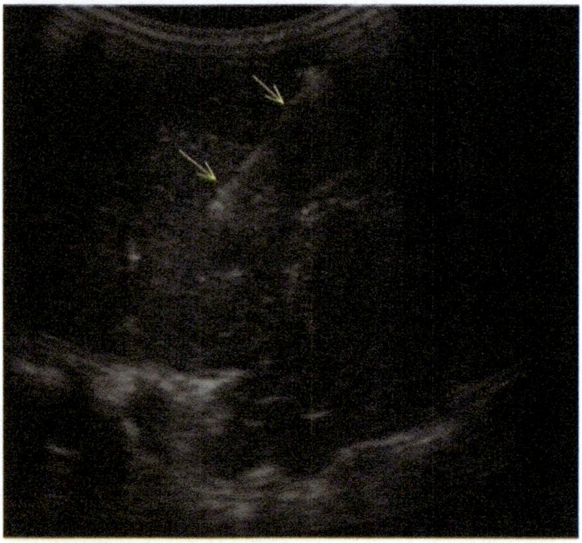

Fig. 15.8 Ultrasound image taken as the biopsy needle (arrows) is deployed

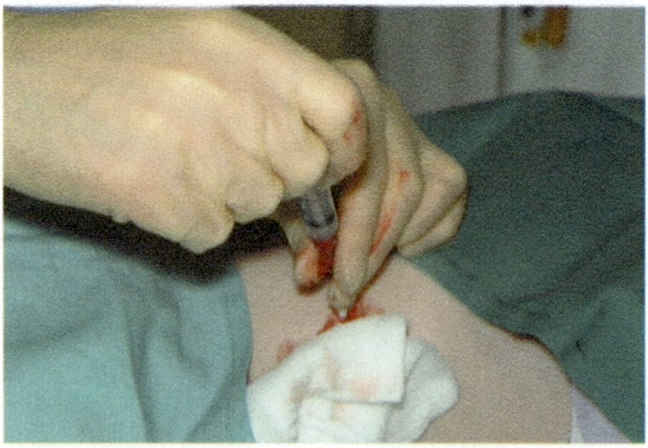

Fig. 15.9 Occlusion of biopsy track with haemostatic agent as the cannula is withdrawn

15.1.6 Monitoring and Aftercare

Following recovery from anaesthesia, bed rest and careful observation in the ward is recommended for a period of at least 6 h, to ensure adequate pain relief and regular monitoring of pulse and blood pressure to detect signs of internal bleeding.

15.1.7 Safety and Efficacy—Commentary

Open surgical biopsy was previously the preferred method to achieve an adequately sized tissue sample for complete histological and molecular characterisation of neuroblastoma. At Alder Hey Children's Hospital, Liverpool, after early success of initiating tumour needle biopsy, we developed the uniform practice of performing needle biopsy for all anatomically accessible neuroblastic paediatric solid tumours. All needle biopsies were of sufficient high quality for all the diagnostic procedures, including histopathology, immunohistochemistry, molecular pathology and cytogenetics, with biology crucially adequate for Shimada histological classification, including data on MYCN, 1p and 11q, 17 q, as well as tissue banking for future studies.

Heterogeneity is a characteristic hallmark of neuroblastoma, and it is well known that samples taken from different regions of a primary tumour are known to vary in terms of MYCN, 1p status, stromal, neuronal components and extent of differentiation. Percutaneous needle biopsy, with its capability to obtain cores from multiple sites within a tumour has many theoretical advantages over open biopsy in accurately determining disease risk. Several published series indicate that percutaneous image-guided needle biopsy yields adequate tissue sampling for the diagnosis, risk classification and staging of neuroblastoma and for tissue banking for future studies.

Patient safety is of paramount importance in comparing alternative biopsy methods. No biopsy method is completely without risk. Gupta et al. reported a duodenal injury and small bowel obstruction occurring in their series of 13 children having open biopsy. Six patients who had open biopsy also required blood transfusions within 5 days of biopsy. More recently, Hassan et al. published their early experience with open and needle biopsy and found a significantly higher number of major complications in patients having open biopsy.

The relatively slow uptake of minimally invasive image-guided percutaneous biopsy techniques for suspected neuroblastoma may have been due to concerns among paediatric surgeons and oncologists that needle biopsy has the potential to disseminate tumour in children, a very rare but documented complication in adult cancer(s). However, at time of writing, we are aware of no recorded instances of dissemination of neuroblastoma attributable to needle biopsy in recent years.

Percutaneous image-guided needle biopsy is therefore a safe and effective technique for diagnosis of neuroblastoma, and can reliably provide sufficient tissue for the full range of investigations, including histopathology, immunohistochemistry, molecular pathology and cytogenetics required for diagnosis and prognostic markers, as well as reserving vital tumour material for tissue banking/future collaborative studies.

15.2 Pathology—Specimen Handling/Analysis/Reporting

15.2.1 Specimen Handling

Tumour biopsy is undertaken to obtain the diagnosis of suspected neuroblastic tumours (NT) and gather full histological and molecular prognostic information relevant for treatment stratification. As the understanding of NT and its optimal management is still evolving, whenever possible, vital tissue material should also be saved for research purposes. Tumour biopsy material has to be carefully handled and processed in different ways for routine histopathology, cytogenetics and molecular pathology. With so much to do, it is crucial that the limited tumour tissue available from a biopsy is triaged adequately—Fig. 15.10.

Biopsies should be rapidly transferred to the pathology laboratory unfixed, and wrapped in saline soaked filter paper in a sterile container. In Liverpool, pathologists triage the tumour tissue sample (Fig. 15.10), making sure that there is sufficient material for histological diagnosis, touch preparations for fluorescence in situ hybridization (FISH) and snap frozen tissue for molecular biology. If transport time to the pathology laboratory is expected to be unduly delayed, adequate measures must be absolutely taken to maintain the integrity of tissue samples. An acceptable option here is that two separate biopsy tissue samples are submitted to the laboratory—(1) RPMI-1640 cell transport medium for a combination of DNA index (ploidy) and MYCN analysis and (2) 10% formalin for histopathologic analysis.

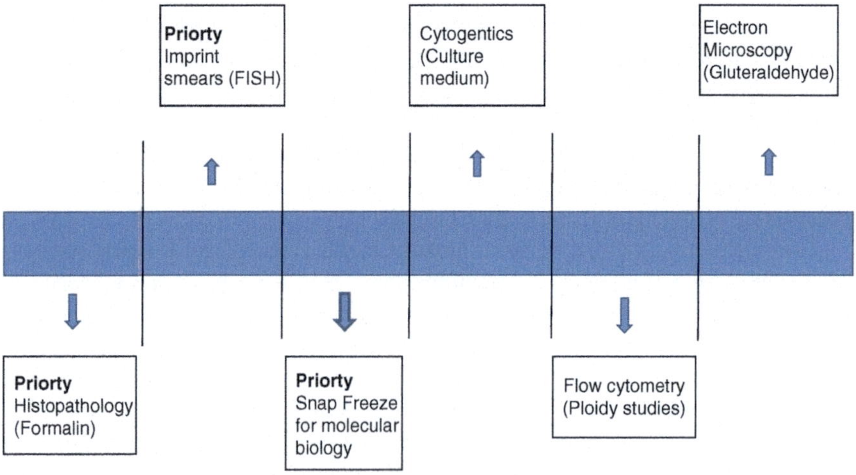

Fig. 15.10 Specimen triaging. Flow chart diagram illustrating neuroblastoma tissue biopsy specimen handling by pathology personnel

15.3 Morphology and Immunohistochemistry

Morphologically, neuroblastic tumours are heterogeneous lesions composed of varying combination of neuroblasts, maturing and mature ganglion cells, schwannian stroma and neuropil. The spectrum ranges from tumours exclusively composed of neuroblastic elements (neuroblastoma) to those with dominant schwannian stroma with no neuroblasts (ganglioneuroma)—Fig. 15.11a–d.

Diagnosis of neuroblastic tumours showing ganglionic differentiation and/or identifiable schwannian stroma is usually straight forward on morphology. On the other hand, diagnosis of undifferentiated neuroblastoma is often not possible on morphology alone. These lesions belong to the so called 'small round blue cell tumours' with wide differential diagnostic options, including rhabdomyosarcoma, peripheral primitive neuroectodermal tumour (PNET)/Ewing sarcoma(s), blastematous Wilms' tumour or blastic hematopoietic neoplasms. A panel of immunohistochemical markers, ultrastructural examination and/or molecular genetics studies is often required to rule in or rule out the diagnosis of NTs.

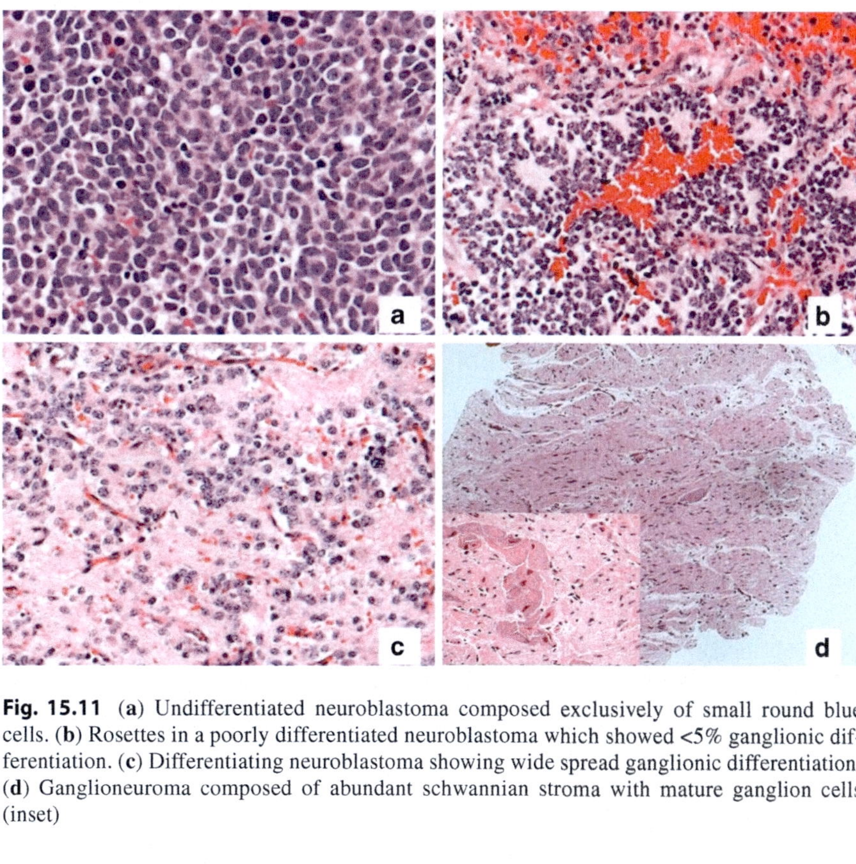

Fig. 15.11 (**a**) Undifferentiated neuroblastoma composed exclusively of small round blue cells. (**b**) Rosettes in a poorly differentiated neuroblastoma which showed <5% ganglionic differentiation. (**c**) Differentiating neuroblastoma showing wide spread ganglionic differentiation. (**d**) Ganglioneuroma composed of abundant schwannian stroma with mature ganglion cells (inset)

Table 15.1 Expression of markers in neuroblastoma and paediatric solid tumours

	Neuroblastoma	Rhabdomyosarcoma	Ewing's/PNET	DSRCT	Lymphoma
Desmin		++		++	
Myogenin		++			
Myo D1		++			
CD99			++	+	Occasional
NKX2.2			++		
Fli1			++	++	+
PHOX2	++				
NB84a	++		+	+	
CD45					+++
NSE	+		+		

15.3.1 Immunohistochemistry

Neuron specific enolase (NSE), chromogranin A, synaptophysin, Tyrosine hydroxylase, Protein gene product 9.5 (PGP9.5), GD2 (disialoganglioside), PHOX 2B and NB84 are positive in a variable proportion of neuroblastomas. As there may be aberrant positivity of certain markers in neuroblastoma and in other small round blue tumours, various neuronal markers and panels of antibodies should be used to obtain a firm diagnosis (Table 15.1). NB84, an antibody raised against an antigen from human neuroblastoma tissue is considered to be more sensitive but less specific than synaptophysin for neuroblastic differentiation. It can be positive in range of other SRCT's including Ewings/PNET and DSRCT. Phox2b has emerged as relatively specific marker in neuroblastoma. Similar to tyrosine hydroxylase (TH), it is a sympathoadrenal marker specific for neural crest tumours with neuronal/neuroendocrine differentiation.

15.3.2 Electron Microscopy (EM)

Neuroblastoma on EM ultrastructural examination shows round cells exhibiting neural differentiation featuring cell organelles, such as microtubules, neurofilaments, neurosecretory granules, glycogen and synaptic vesicles.

15.4 Classification and Grading of Neuroblastoma

Neuroblastic tumours are quite heterogeneous in terms of their biology, genetic, and morphologic characteristics. As per International Neuroblastoma Pathology Classification System (INPC), there are four major histological categories of Neuroblastic Tumours, i.e. Neuroblastoma, Ganglioneuroblastoma intermixed, Ganglioneuroma and Nodular Ganglioneuroblastoma. This is based on the relative composition(s) and distribution (nodular vs. diffuse) of neuroblastic and ganglioneuromatous components. There are further subcategories based on degree of ganglionic differentiation.

MKI is an important histological prognostic parameter. To determine MKI, sections of tumour should contain at least 5000 viable tumour cells from multiple microscopic fields. Technically, MKI is possible on needle core biopsies and often reported on biopsies. Because of tumour heterogeneity, it may not be truly representative—Fig. 15.12.

Histological subtypes are further linked to age and cellular proliferation index as defined by mitotic karyorrhexis index (MKI) to yield clinical prognostic groups as shown in the Table 15.2.

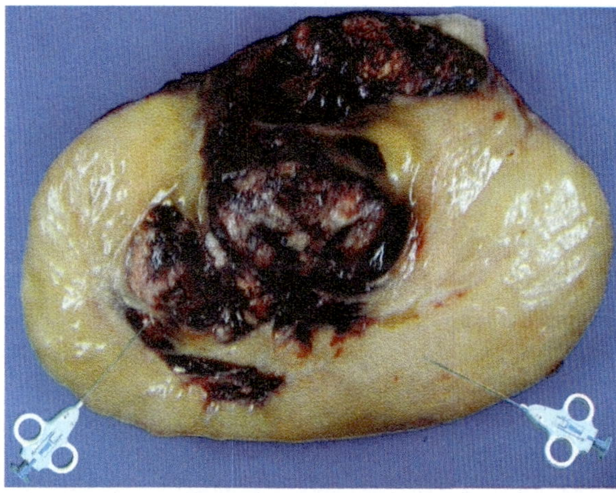

Fig. 15.12 Cut surface of nodular ganglioneuroblastoma with haemorrhagic nodule representing neuroblastoma component and rest of the tumour is benign ganglioneuromatous element. There is a theoretical possibility of sampling error. Schematic representation of biopsy system getting the diagnostic material (Lt. corner) and missing malignant component (Rt. corner)

Table 15.2 Histological neuroblastic tumour subtypes and prognosis

INPC histology	MKI	Age	Category
Ganglioneuroma mature/maturing	Any	Any	Favourable
Ganglioneuroblastoma intermixed	Any	Any	Favourable
Neuroblastoma undifferentiated	Any	Any	Unfavourable
Neuroblastoma poorly differentiated	>4%	Any	Unfavourable
	Any	>1.5	Unfavourable
	<4%	<1.5	Favourable
Neuroblastoma differentiating	Any	>5 years	Unfavourable
	<4%	<1.5	Favourable
	>4%	<1.5	Unfavourable
	<2%	1.5–5 years	Favourable
	>2%	1.5–5 years	Unfavourable
Ganglioneuroblastoma nodular			Favourable/unfavourable depending on morphology of neuroblastoma nodule

In clinical practice, tumour biopsy specimens greater than at least 1 cm^3, or biopsies with at least 5000 viable tumour cells are considered often adequate to provide INPC classification. Its value in treatment stratification has declined in recent years. The International Society of Paediatric Oncology Europe Neuroblastoma Group (SIOPEN) uses age, surgical risk factors defined by imaging and MYCN status for risk-group assignment. Histology is of value, but biologic features, such as MYCN status, chromosome 1p deletion, and abnormalities of chromosome 17q have a powerful impact on individual patient prognosis that far outweighs the histology in many instances. These genetic alterations can be assessed from tumour obtained through percutaneous biopsy methods.

15.5 Molecular Genetics

Various genetic abnormalities have been linked to the biologic behaviour of neuroblastic tumours. Neuroblastic tumours tend to show whole chromosome gains with few, if any, segmental chromosome aberrations and without gene amplification(s). Tumour cell hyperdiploidy (usually near-triploid DNA content), is also known to be associated with spontaneous maturation and possibly spontaneous regression.

Neuroblastomas with an unfavourable clinical behaviour frequently show segmental aberrations and/or high-level amplification of the MYCN locus. MYCN amplification has been shown to be strongly associated with rapid tumour progression and dismally poor prognosis in patients of all ages, regardless of stage of disease—Fig. 15.13.

Although MYCN status is central to the risk stratification systems, it is important to emphasise that the majority of metastatic neuroblastomas do not always show MYCN amplification. Other chromosomal aberrations have been assumed to predict unfavourable tumour behaviour, including deletion on chromosome regions 1p, 11q, 3p, 4p, 9p and 12p and unbalanced gain of the long arm of chromosome 17

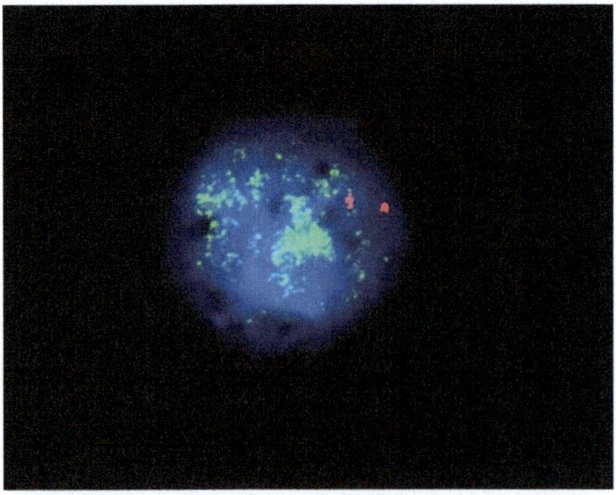

Fig. 15.13 FISH—Numerous green dots represent amplified MYCN. Two red dot show normal copy number for CEP 2 (centromeric region of chromosome 2) as control. (image courtesy Mr. Mark Atherton, Cheshire and Merseyside Genetics Service)

(17q21 to 17qter). Of these, 11q deletion has emerged as a powerful biomarker of outcome in cases without MYCN amplification, as it is inversely associated with MYCN amplification. The INRG database has confirmed this finding, and on the basis of these studies, 11q status has been included as an important prognostic criterion in the INRG classification system.

The International Neuroblastoma Risk Group Biology Committee (INRG) recommends the following parameters to assess three obligatory genetic markers required for the INRG Consensus Pretreatment Classification.

1. MYCN: I-FISH, PCR, aCGH, MLPA
2. 11q23: I-FISH, PCR; pan-/multigenomic techniques: aCGH (oligo, clone or SNP based); MLPA
3. Ploidy: Flow or static cytometry

An adequate amount of tumour material (i.e., 10^7 tumour cells) from at least two different regions of the tumour should be obtained. In collaboration with the Pathologist, the tumour cell content must be determined and recorded. The latter is an indispensable prerequisite to avoid false results and has to be carried out by the Pathologist. A tumour cell content of more than 60% is required for most molecular studies and more than 20% for ploidy measurement.

Differentiating/maturing tumours can have fewer tumour cells, and therefore, the interpretation of these data needs to be done with caution. It is recognised that, risk stratification of neuroblastoma is far from perfect and in future more genetics parameters will be included to classify these tumours more accurately. There is now a consensus recommendation by INRG to prospectively evaluate larger numbers of other markers (i.e. 1p, 2p, DDX1, NAG, ALK, 3p, 4p, 7q, 9p, 12p, 14q, 17q). For ongoing and future studies, the application or implementation of technologies that provide a more comprehensive picture of the tumour cell genome is essential. Therefore, the INRG Biology Subcommittee has also suggested using pan or multigenomic techniques, enabling an analysis of all relevant genomic loci.

Multiplex ligation-dependent probe amplification (MLPA) allows the simultaneous investigation of a large number of loci, covering all currently-known important aberrant regions found in neuroblastoma tumours in a single assay. The robust nature of the results and the relatively low cost of the MLPA kits make this technique very attractive for routine neuroblastoma analysis. Ultra-high density (UHD) SNP array techniques have high specificity and sensitivity and gives combined copy number and allele information, highly appropriate for the genomic diagnosis of neuroblastoma.

The INRG classification system will continue to evolve with the possible incorporation of molecular diagnostic data from neuroblastoma genome (DNA), transcriptome (RNA) and epigenome for personalised cancer treatment.

In closing, we would like to emphasize that vital co-operation amongst medical oncologists, paediatric oncology surgeons, interventional radiologists and pathologists is very essential in the expert multidisciplinary management of childhood neuroblastoma.

Suggested Readings

1. Hassan SF, Mathur S, Magliaro TJ, et al. Needle core vs open biopsy for diagnosis of intermediate- and high-risk neuroblastoma in children. J Pediatr Surg. 2012;47(6):1261–6.
2. Mullassery D, Sharma V, Salim A, Jawaid WB, Pizer BL, Abernethy LJ, Losty PD. Open versus needle biopsy in diagnosing neuroblastoma. J Pediatr Surg. 2014;49(10):1505–7.
3. Avanzini S, Faticato MG, Crocoli A, et al. Comparative retrospective study on the modalities of biopsying peripheral neuroblastic tumors: a report from the Italian Pediatric Surgical Oncology Group (GICOP). Pediatr Blood Cancer. 2017;64(5) https://doi.org/10.1002/pbc.26284.
4. Bittles MA, Hoffer FA. Interventional radiology and the care of the pediatric oncology patient. Surg Oncol. 2007;16(3):229–33.
5. Garrett KM, Fuller CE, Santana VM, Shochat SJ, Hoffer FA. Percutaneous biopsy of pediatric solid tumors. Cancer. 2005;104(3):644–52.
6. Hoffer FA, Chung T, Diller L, Kozakewich H, Fletcher JA, Shamberger RC. Percutaneous biopsy for prognostic testing of neuroblastoma. Radiology. 1996;200(1):213–6.
7. Robertson EG, Baxter G. Tumour seeding following percutaneous needle biopsy: the real story! Clin Radiol. 2011;66(11):1007–14.
8. Sebire NJ, Roebuck DJ. Pathological diagnosis of paediatric tumours from image-guided needle core biopsies: a systematic review. Pediatr Radiol. 2006;36(5):426–31.
9. Avanzini S, Faticato MG, Sementa AR, et al. Video-assisted needle core biopsy in children affected by neuroblastoma: a novel combined technique. Eur J Pediatr Surg. 2017;27(2):166–70.
10. Gupta A, et al. Analysis of needle versus open biopsy for the diagnosis of advanced stage pediatric neuroblastoma. Pediatr Blood Cancer. 2006;47:875–9.
11. Cohn SL, et al. The International Neuroblastoma Risk Group (INRG) classification system: an INRG Task Force report. J Clin Oncol. 2009;27:289–97.
12. Ambros PF, et al. International consensus for neuroblastoma molecular diagnostics: report from the International Neuroblastoma Risk Group (INRG) Biology Committee. Br J Cancer. 2009;9:1471–82.
13. Tornóczky T, Kálmán E, Kajtár PG, Nyári T, Pearson AD, Tweddle DA, Board J, Shimada H. Large cell neuroblastoma: a distinct phenotype of neuroblastoma with aggressive clinical behavior. Cancer. 2004;100(2):390–7.
14. Tornóczky T, Semjén D, Shimada H, Ambros IM. Pathology of peripheral neuroblastic tumors: significance of prominent nucleoli in undifferentiated/poorly differentiated neuroblastoma. Pathol Oncol Res. 2007;13(4):269–75.
15. Shimada H, Ambros IM, Dehner LP, Hata J, Joshi VV, Roald B. Terminology and morphologic criteria of neuroblastic tumors: recommendations by the International Neuroblastoma Pathology Committee. Cancer. 1999;86(2):349–63.
16. Miettinen M, Chatten J, et al. Monoclonal antibody NB84 in the differential diagnosis of neuroblastoma and other small round cell tumors. Am J Surg Pathol. 1998;22(3):327–32.
17. Bielle F, Fréneaux P, Jeanne-Pasquier C, Maran-Gonzalez A, Rousseau A, Lamant L, Paris R, Pierron G, Nicolas AV, Sastre-Garau X, Delattre O, Bourdeaut F, Peuchmaur M. PHOX2B immunolabeling: a novel tool for the diagnosis of undifferentiated neuroblastomas among childhood small round blue-cell tumors. Am J Surg Pathol. 2012;36(8):1141–9.
18. Warren M, Matsuno R, Tran H, Shimada H. Utility of Phox2b immunohistochemical stain in neural crest tumors and non-neural crest tumors in pediatric patients. Histopathology. 2018;72(4):685–96.
19. Kim NR, Ha SY, Cho HY. Utility of transmission electron microscopy in small round cell tumors. J Pathol Transl Med. 2015;49(2):93–101.
20. Cullinane CJ, Burchill SA, Squire JA, O'Leary JJ, Lewis IJ, Variend S, Burchill SA. Neuroblastoma. In: Molecular biology and pathology of paediatric cancer. Oxford: Oxford University Press; 2003.
21. Cecchetto G, Mosseri V, De Bernardi B, et al. Surgical risk factors in primary surgery for localized neuroblastoma: the LNESG1 study of the European International Society of Pediatric Oncology Neuroblastoma Group. J Clin Oncol. 2005;23:8483–9.

22. Ambros IM, Zellner A, Roald B, Amann G, Ladenstein R, Printz D, Gadner H, Ambros PF. Role of ploidy, chromosome 1p, and Schwann cells in the maturation of neuroblastoma. N Engl J Med. 1996;334:1505–11.
23. Perez CA, Matthay KK, Atkinson JB, Seeger RC, Shimada H, Haase GM, Stram DO, Gerbing RB, Lukens JN. Biologic variables in the outcome of stages I and II neuroblastoma treated with surgery as primary therapy: a children's cancer group study. J Clin Oncol. 2000;18:18–26.
24. Cohn SL, Pearson ADJ, London WB, Monclair T, Ambros PF, Brodeur GM, Faldum A, Hero B, Iehara T, Machin D, Mosseri V, Simon T, Garaventa A, Castel V, Matthay KK. The International Neuroblastoma Risk Group (INRG) classification system: an INRG task force report. J Clin Oncol. 2009;27(2):289–97.
25. Ambros PF, Ambros IM, Brodeur GM, Haber M, Khan J, Nakagawara A, Schleiermacher G, Speleman F, Spitz R, London WB, Cohn SL, Pearson ADJ, Maris JM. International consensus for neuroblastoma molecular diagnostics: report from the International Neuroblastoma Risk Group (INRG) Biology Committee. Br J Cancer. 2009;100(9):1471–82.
26. Attiyeh EF, London WB, Mosse YP, Wang Q, Winter C, Khazi D, McGrady PW, Seeger RC, Look AT, Shimada H, Brodeur GM, Cohn SL, Matthay KK, Maris JM. Chromosome 1p and 11q deletions and outcome in neuroblastoma. N Engl J Med. 2005;353:2243–53.
27. Villamon E, Piqueras M, Mackintosh C, Alonso J, de Alava E, Navarro S, Noguera R. Comparison of different techniques for the detection of genetic risk-identifying chromosomal gains and losses in neuroblastoma. Virchows Arch. 2008;453:47–55.
28. Ambros IM, Brunner C, Abbasi R, Frech C, Ambros PF. Ultra-high density SNParray in neuroblastoma molecular diagnostics. Front Oncol. 2014;4:202.

Surgical Techniques

16

James A. Saltsman III, Nicole J. Croteau, and Michael P. LaQuaglia

16.1 History and Current Indications for Surgery for Neuroblastoma

A role for surgery in neuroblastoma was first reported in the 1950s by key figures in the history of pediatric surgery. In 1953, Robert E. Gross noted in his seminal text, *The Surgery of Infancy and Childhood*, that for neuroblastoma "extensive and radical surgery has a definite place under certain circumstances and can lead to permanent cure" [1]. C. Everett Koop then explained the positive effect of tumor debulking on outcome in his 1955 article "Neuroblastoma in Childhood: Survival after Major Surgical Insult to the Tumor" published in the journal *Surgery* [2].

In the 1970s, there were major advances in pediatric imaging, surgical technique, anesthesia, blood banking, and critical care [3–6], all of which expanded the potential role for surgery in the treatment of neuroblastoma. Also during this time, a variety of different staging systems for the disease were developed in Europe, the United States, and Japan. With the establishment of pediatric oncology cooperative groups, multi-institutional data became available to guide international standardization of staging and surgical treatment of neuroblastoma. One such prospective study was published in 1988 by investigators from the Pediatric Oncology Group, (POG, a predecessor to the current Children's Oncology Group [COG]), which showed that certain localized neuroblastomas could be effectively treated with surgery alone, even with involvement of regional lymph nodes [7]. Around the same time, the International Neuroblastoma Staging System (INSS) was established, which grouped patients into stages (1, 2A, 2B, 3, 4, and 4S) based on the extent and location of tumor, as well as completeness of resection [8] (see Table 16.1).

J. A. Saltsman III · N. J. Croteau · M. P. LaQuaglia (✉)
Department of Surgery, Memorial Sloan Kettering Cancer Center, New York, NY, USA
e-mail: laquaglm@mskcc.org

S. Sarnacki, L. Pio (eds.), *Neuroblastoma*,
https://doi.org/10.1007/978-3-030-18396-7_16

Table 16.1 International Neuroblastoma Staging System (INSS) [8]

Stage	Definition
1	Localized tumor with complete gross excision, with or without microscopic residual disease; representative ipsilateral lymph nodes negative for tumor microscopically (nodes attached to and removed with the primary tumor may be positive)
2A	Localized tumor with incomplete gross excision; representative ipsilateral nonadherent lymph nodes negative for tumor microscopically
2B	Localized tumor with or without complete gross excision, with ipsilateral nonadherent lymph nodes positive for tumor. Enlarged contralateral lymph nodes must be negative microscopically
3	Unresectable unilateral tumor infiltrating across the midline, with or without regional lymph node involvement; or localized unilateral tumor with contralateral regional lymph node involvement; or midline tumor with bilateral extension by infiltration (unresectable) or by lymph node involvement
4	Any primary tumor with dissemination to distant lymph nodes, bone, bone marrow, liver, skin and/or other organs (except as defined for stage 4S)
4S	Localized primary tumor (as defined for stage 1, 2A or 2B), with dissemination limited to skin, liver, and/or bone marrow (limited to infants <1 year of age)

Table 16.2 International neuroblastoma risk group staging system [10]

Stage	Definition
L1	Localized tumor not involving vital structures as defined by the list of IDRFs and confined to one body compartment
L2	Locoregional tumor with the presence of one or more IDRFs
M	Distant metastatic disease (except stage MS)
MS	Metastatic disease in children younger than 18 months with metastases confined to skin, liver, and/or bone marrow

The International Neuroblastoma Risk Group (INRG) classification system was later developed to facilitate patient risk stratification prior to surgical intervention. In this system, nonmetastatic tumors are assessed using cross-sectional imaging for specific image-defined risk factors (IDRFs) that predict unresectability [9, 10] (see Tables 16.2 and 16.3). Both INSS and INRG staging systems have been combined with other factors, including patient age and tumor biology, to create the COG and INRG risk groupings. While these risk groupings are similar (and many patients fall into the same risk group in both systems), there are some important differences. As a result, readers should take note of the risk group stratification system used when evaluating the literature on surgical outcomes in various neuroblastoma risk groups [9].

Since early reports, the role of resection in neuroblastoma, in particular the extent of resection, has been controversial. With increased experience, the role of risk grouping has become paramount, and any analysis of surgery must stratify by risk group. Recent data suggest that low risk and intermediate risk neuroblastoma without IDRFs are treatable by resection alone [11]. Chemotherapy is usually required in intermediate risk tumors with image-defined risk factors. High-risk neuroblastoma remains an area of significant debate; however, recent reports from the

Table 16.3 Image-defined risk factors (IDRFs) in neuroblastoma [10]

Neck
Tumor encasing carotid and/or vertebral artery and/or internal jugular vein
Tumor extending to base of skull
Tumor compressing the trachea
Cervicothoracic junction
Tumor encasing brachial plexus roots
Tumor encasing subclavian vessels and/or vertebral and/or carotid artery
Tumor compressing the trachea
Thorax
Tumor encasing the aorta and/or major branches
Tumor compressing the trachea and/or principal bronchi
Lower mediastinal tumor, infiltrating the costovertebral junction between T9 and T12
Thoracoabdominal
Tumor encasing the aorta and/or vena cava
Abdomen/pelvis
Tumor infiltrating the porta hepatis and/or the hepatoduodenal ligament
Tumor encasing branches of the superior mesenteric artery at the mesenteric root
Tumor encasing the origin of the celiac axis and/or the superior mesenteric artery
Tumor invading one or both renal pedicles
Tumor encasing the aorta and/or vena cava
Tumor encasing the iliac vessels
Pelvic tumor crossing the sciatic notch
Any location
Intraspinal tumor extension when more than one third of the spinal canal in the axial plane is invaded and/or the perimedullary leptomeningeal spaces are not visible and/or the spinal cord signal is abnormal
Infiltration of adjacent organs/structures including pericardium, diaphragm, kidney, liver, duodenopancreatic block, and mesentery
Ipsilateral tumor extension within two body compartments (i.e., neck-chest, chest-abdomen, abdomen-pelvis)

COG and the International Society for Pediatric Oncology Europe—Neuroblastoma (SIOPEN) suggest that >90% resection of the primary tumor and regional lymphatics in high-risk cases improves local control [12, 13]. The findings of these studies support attempts at aggressive surgical resection in high risk patients, with the understanding that the reported benefits of this approach have, thus far, been limited to improved event-free survival (EFS) and reduced cumulative incidence of local progression (CILP) [13]. Detailed treatment protocols based on risk groupings are found in Chap. 12 of this text.

It should be understood that R0 resection is almost never feasible in neuroblastoma, and the goal of surgery in these patients is a macroscopic gross total resection of tumor (R1). Present data suggest that intermediate-risk neuroblastoma can be treated by an R2 resection that removes >50% of the primary mass, although greater resections are recommended, if safe and feasible [14].

Although the diagnosis of neuroblastoma can be established by bone marrow biopsy and the finding of urinary catecholamines, incisional biopsy is an integral diagnostic procedure that is required to establish risk group status, including histologic and molecular analysis of the tumor. With the exception of small, localized, and easily resectable tumors, the initial surgical procedure in all neuroblastoma patients should be incisional biopsy. If the patient's clinical status allows, the surgeon should obtain at least one cubic centimeter of viable tumor tissue in good condition for an adequate biopsy analysis. Additional information regarding biopsy technique and associated diagnostic procedures can be found in Chap. 16. Central line placement for delivery of chemotherapy, and staging bone marrow aspirations and biopsies can be conveniently performed at the same time as incisional biopsy.

16.2 Preoperative Preparation

It cannot be emphasized too strongly that these are very serious resections. They should be scheduled early in the day with a fresh operating room team and adequate preoperative preparation. Regardless of the staging system used, presurgical assessment of IDRFs should be completed using cross-sectional imaging for detailed operative planning (see Table 16.3 for a list of all IDRFs). Imaging should be available for reference in the operating room. Laboratory values, especially platelet and white blood cell counts, should be obtained preoperatively, and comorbidities like asthma or cardiac dysfunction should be addressed with appropriate specialty consultation. Consultation with other surgical subspecialties (e.g. vascular surgery or neurosurgery) should be initiated preoperatively in cases where the need for intraoperative collaboration is likely. Blood and blood products should be prepared and easily available. The pediatric intensive care unit (PICU) should be notified prior to the start of the resection, and a PICU bed should be available for the patient postoperatively.

16.3 Anesthesia Considerations

While specific anesthesia considerations vary based on the extent and anatomic location of the operation, resuscitative preparedness of the anesthesia team is critical to safe surgery. The anesthesiologist managing the patient during neuroblastoma resection should have experience with this kind of surgery. Single-lung ventilation may be required for thoracic and posterior mediastinal lesions. There is a risk of hypotension due to blood loss, as well as a risk of hypertensive crisis due to tumor catecholamine release. As such, adequate vascular access, and intraoperative arterial monitoring of blood pressure and gases is recommended. Blood products should be readily available in all cases. A nasogastric tube should be placed to facilitate identification of the esophagus.

16.4 Surgical Technique

As neuroblastoma can affect a variety of locations in the body, the specific surgical techniques for resection vary based on the anatomic site. Specific techniques for all common locations will be detailed below. In general, tumor dissection proceeds along the pseudocapsule of the mass. Sectioning of the tumor may be required to improve visualization or avoid injury to underlying vital structures, especially in cases of vascular encasement. This can be done without adverse consequences as long as the course of major vessels and nerves is determined.

16.4.1 Cervical Lesions

Most primary cervical lesions occur in infants younger than 1 year and have favorable biologic features. These patients occasionally present with various clinical findings consistent with Horner's syndrome and the parents should be informed that a permanent Horner's syndrome will be present postoperatively in almost all cases. To facilitate operative planning, it is important to assess the extent of a cervical lesion and determine whether the tumor invades the thoracic inlet prior to surgery. An MRI of this region with gadolinium will give excellent anatomic detail. Also, we have found that intraoperative neurophysiologic monitoring and stimulation is very helpful. The patient is placed in a dorsal recumbent position. The head of the table is somewhat elevated to reduce venous pressure and a silicone gel roll or towel is placed under the shoulders so that the head and neck are extended. The head is rotated toward the contralateral side to improve exposure. The entire neck and upper chest neck is sterilely prepped from the mastoid process to the nipples or lower. The general approach is through a transverse neck incision in Langer's lines and should extend from the posterior belly of the sternocleidomastoid to just beyond the anterior belly of the muscle for large lesions. Care should be taken to identify and preserve the great auricular nerve at the anterior edge of the sternocleidomastoid, as well as the spinal accessory nerve which may be in the field. Nerve stimulation should be used liberally during the dissection. Large lesions may require division of the sternocleidomastoid muscle for adequate exposure. This can be safely done just above the clavicle and greatly improves visualization. The mass is centered posteriorly in the paravertebral region and should be mobilized away from the carotid sheath structures first. The carotid artery or internal jugular vein may be encased, but can usually be separated away from the tumor by identifying an uninvolved area and working along the media of the vessels. The artery or vein is protected with a right-angle clamp or other instrument, and the encasing tongue of tumor is incised. Once the vessel wall is exposed, the tumor can be slowly peeled away using a clamp or Penfield dissector. Bleeding can be controlled with gentle finger pressure and small (6-0) monofilament sutures. Once the course of the vessels is known the vagus nerve should also be identified and the tumor then approached from the lateral by dissecting along the scalene muscle. The phrenic nerve should be identified and preserved. The trapezius is laterally retracted after the course of the spinal accessory nerve is known. In the case of grossly positive lymph nodes, a formal lymphadenectomy with a modified neck dissection technique should be performed (Fig. 16.1).

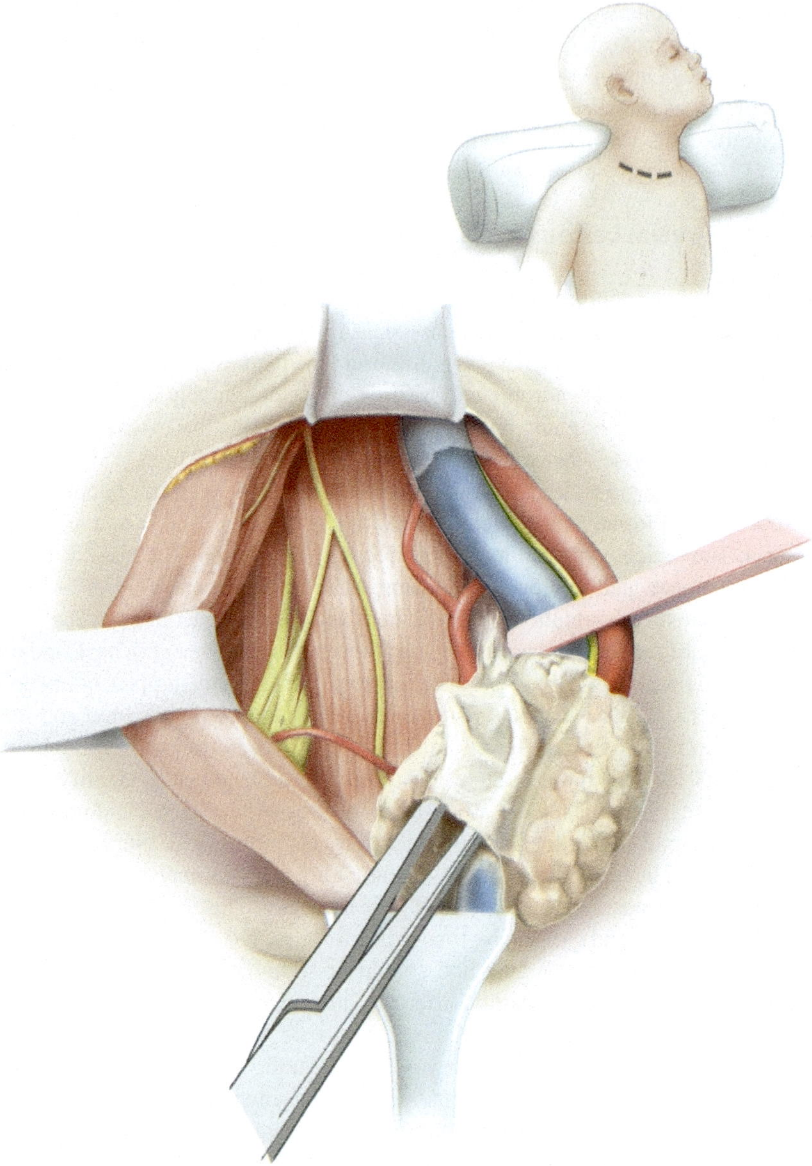

Fig. 16.1 The cervical incision is performed with the patient in the dorsal recumbent position with extension of the head and neck. The transverse neck incision is made above the clavicle, with division of the sternocleidomastoid muscle if needed. ©2018, Memorial Sloan Kettering Cancer Center

16.4.2 Cervicothoracic Lesions

Primary cervical lesions may extend into the chest through the thoracic inlet, which is a complex of nerves and vessels. Adequate exposure is integral to achieving gross total resection of these tumors. This can usually be achieved using some form of a cervical incision along with a total or partial median sternotomy in-continuity with an anterior thoracotomy (trap-door thoracotomy). The patient is placed in a dorsal recumbent position with the head of the table somewhat elevated and a small silicone gel roll or towel roll is placed under the shoulders so that the head and neck are extended. The arm, ipsilateral to the lesion, is abducted, and the contralateral arm tucked at the side. The head is rotated away from the lesion to expose the ipsilateral neck. The entire neck, chest and upper abdomen is prepped and draped. This should be extended as far laterally as possible (almost to the operating room table) to accommodate chest tube placement or extension of the incision. The neck incision can be transverse or along the anterior border of the sternocleidomastoid muscle and is extended into the sternal notch. The incision is then extended in the midline anterior to the sternum and then laterally across an ipsilateral anterior interspace. The incision is deepened and the anterior interspace and pleura entered. Since the innervation of the pectoralis major comes from above, it is advisable to select a lower interspace below the nipple (usually the fifth interspace) so that this muscle, when cut, is not denervated. This may also minimize the postoperative cosmetic impact. The pectoralis major muscle is divided near its insertion and the chest is entered. The internal mammary artery and veins are identified and divided and the retrosternal space bluntly dissected. Blunt dissection in the sternal notch allows complete isolation of the posterior wall of the sternum, which is now divided. The ipsilateral attachments of the strap muscles, and possibly the sternal head of the sternocleidomastoid may also be cut to improve exposure. The SCM should be repaired, but this is not necessary with the strap muscles (Fig. 16.2). A self-retaining retractor (often

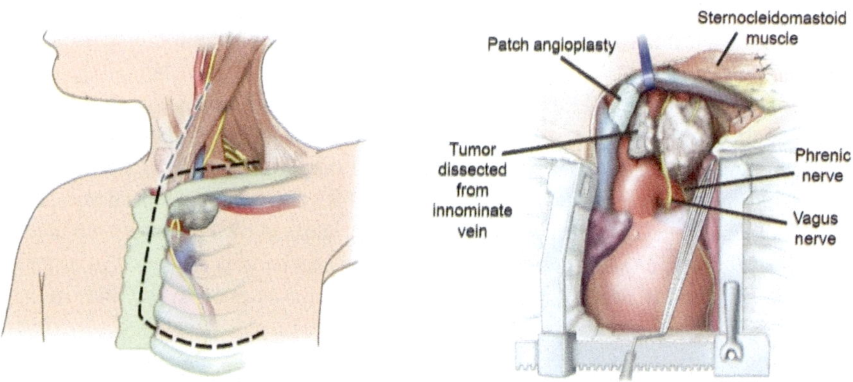

Fig. 16.2 (**a**) The trap-door incision requires the ipsilateral arm to be abducted 90° at the shoulder. (**b**) With full exposure of the cervicothoracic structures, gross total resection is possible in patients with primary cervical lesions that extend into the chest through the thoracic inlet and may involve vascular invasion. ©2018, Memorial Sloan Kettering Cancer Center

a Finochietto) is placed and nerves and vessels identified. This approach can be modified for lesions with a larger cervical component by extending the neck incision superior along the anterior border of the sternocleidomastoid. Nerve stimulation is often employed to monitor the vagus nerve and the brachial plexus. The tumor is often removed in pieces as encased vessels and nerves are dissected out. After complete resection of the tumor, one or two chest tubes are placed depending on the extent of the dissection and a cervical drain may also be used. The ribs are reapproximated and a standard closure is done.

Lesions that extend into both hemithoraces can be reliably exposed using a bilateral anterior thoracotomy (clamshell thoracotomy) at the fifth interspace. The patient is placed in the dorsal recumbent position with a roll behind the midportion of the chest. The arms are abducted to 90° at the shoulder and elbow and the patient is prepped from the chin to the umbilicus and transversely to the bilateral posterior axillary lines. An anterior curvilinear incision is made along the fifth interspace bilaterally from each anterior-axillary line, connecting at the midline. The pleural space is entered bilaterally and the mammary vessels are isolated, ligated, and divided. The retrosternal space is then bluntly dissected, and the sternum divided transversely with a sternal saw. A self-retaining retractor is placed, allowing for exposure of both pleural cavities, from the pulmonary hilum to the posterior aspect of the diaphragm. Dissection of the tumor proceeds, as in other cervicothoracic lesions, with careful attention to neurovascular structures. After dissection of the tumor is complete and hemostasis is assured, bilateral chest tubes are placed and the sternum is either approximated with wire or stabilized in the anterior-posterior dimension with a Steinmann pin. A standard closure is completed (Fig. 16.3).

16.4.3 Mediastinal Lesions

The posterior mediastinum is the second most common primary site for neuroblastomas. These lesions can generally be approached through a muscle-sparing posterolateral thoracotomy (Fig. 16.4). The patient is placed in a lateral decubitus position. The lower leg is flexed at the knee, and a pillow is placed between it and the extended upper leg. A rolled towel is placed under the axilla to support the shoulder and upper chest. The arm on the side of the thoracotomy is extended anteriorly and superiorly. The lower arm is extended forward and rested on an arm board perpendicular to the operating table. Skin incision starts midway between the medial border of the scapula and the vertebral spine. The incision is extended in a gentle curve below the inferior angle of the scapula and is continued to the mid-axillary line at the level of the submammary crease. Skin flaps are developed superiorly, inferiorly, and posteriorly over the trapezius muscle. The plane between the trapezius muscle and latissimus dorsi is opened, and the posterior border of the latissimus dorsi is freed from the chest wall teres major. The chest is then entered at the sixth interspace and a rib retractor is inserted. The latissimus dorsi and serratus anterior are retracted together anteriorly. This exposure provides excellent exposure

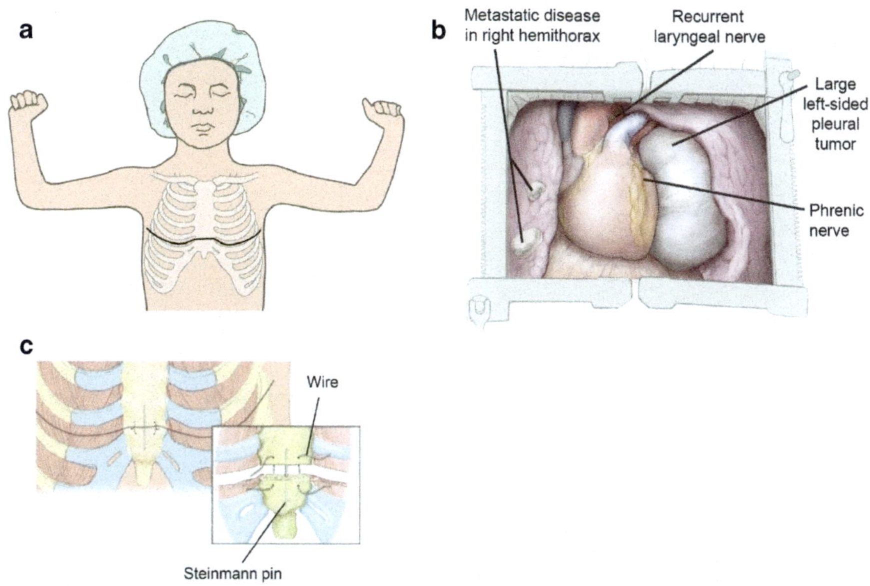

Fig. 16.3 (**a**) The clamshell incision is achieved with the patient's arms abducted 90° at the shoulder. (**b**) This illustration presents a patient with a large left-sided pleural tumor involving the pulmonary hilum with metastatic disease in the right hemithorax. (**c**) Closure of the sternum is achieved using a Steinmann pin and wires. ©2018, Memorial Sloan Kettering Cancer Center

to the posterior mediastinum to allow gross total resection of the majority of mediastinal neuroblastomas.

Infiltration through spinal foramina may require foraminotomy. The risk of proceeding with foraminectomy may outweigh the potential benefit of gross total resection, as patients with intermediate-risk disease and a small amount of residual disease still experience good outcomes. After complete resection of the tumor, the ribs are reapproximated, an appropriately-sized chest tube is left in place for drainage, and a standard closure is completed.

As with cervical lesions, injury to the stellate ganglion and resulting Horner's syndrome is a potential complication of resection of superior mediastinal tumors and should be discussed with the patient's parents/caregivers prior to surgery.

16.4.4 Upper Abdominal and Retroperitoneal Lesions

The majority of neuroblastomas originates from the adrenal gland or sympathetic ganglia and is found in the upper abdomen. There is frequent involvement of regional lymph nodes in the ipsilateral paraaortic or pericaval chains, as well as interaortocaval lymph nodes. The primary tumor and involved lymph nodes often create a confluent mass that encases but does not invade the great vessels of the abdomen. For these tumors, a thoracoabdominal approach is ideal (Fig. 16.5).

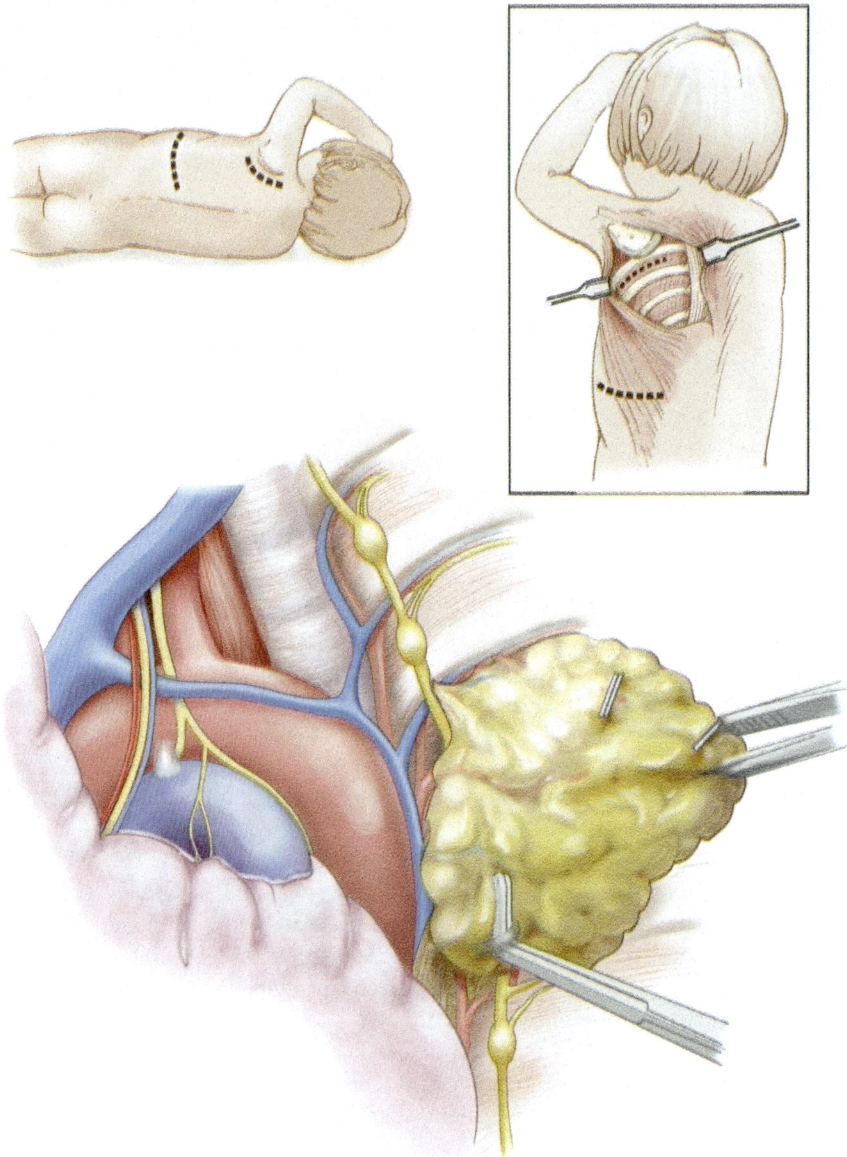

Fig. 16.4 Neuroblastoma lesions in the posterior mediastinum can be approached using a muscle-sparing posterolateral thoracotomy. ©2018, Memorial Sloan Kettering Cancer Center

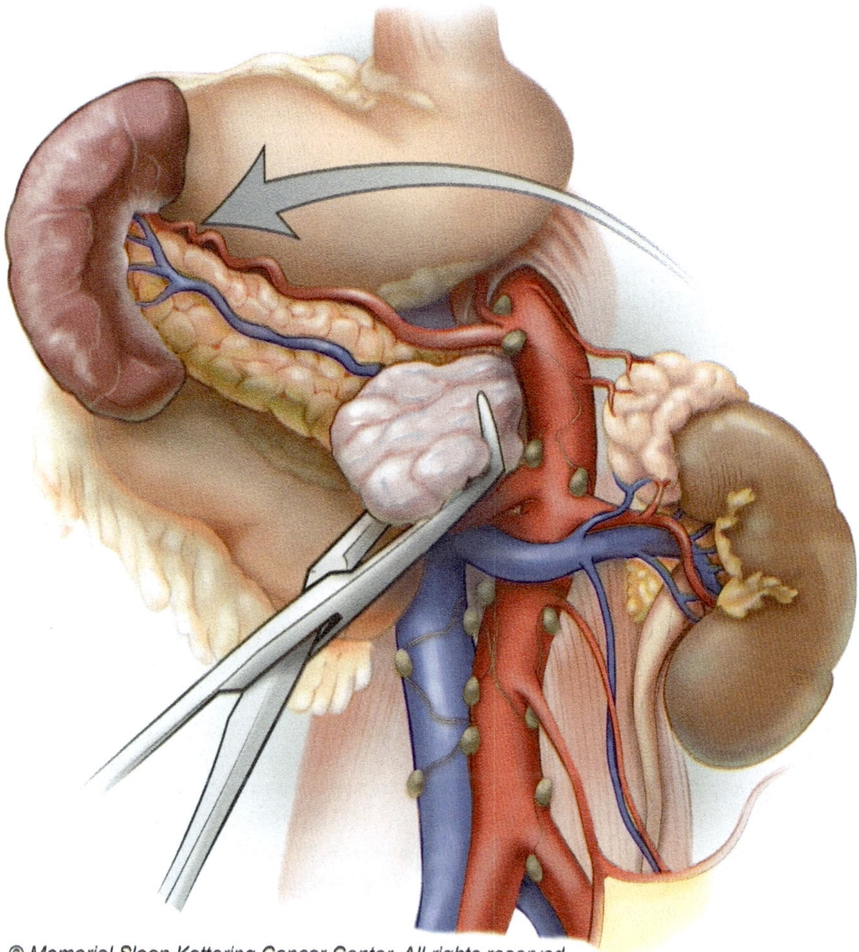

Fig. 16.5 For a majority of neuroblastomas, a thoracoabdominal approach facilitates exposure of the primary tumor, involved lymph nodes, and any encased major vessels of the abdomen. ©2018, Memorial Sloan Kettering Cancer Center

The patient is placed in a semilateral position with the affected side elevated. The ipsilateral arm is well-supported and extended superiorly and to the contralateral side. A roll is placed under the axilla to support the shoulder and upper chest. Additional support is placed in the lumbar region to produce mild hyperextension that enhances exposure. Padding is placed liberally to avoid nerve injury at all pressure points. A right-sided incision is used when the vena cava or right renal hilar vessels are infiltrated, while a left-sided incision is best for tumors involving the aorta, celiac axis, superior mesenteric artery, or left renal hilum. The thoracoabdominal incision allows for excellent exposure and control of encased visceral blood vessels.

The incision is initiated on the chest at the posterior axillary line along the eighth interspace on the left, and ninth interspace on the right. The incision is extended medially to the midline of the upper abdomen and then inferior as needed for adequate exposure. The intercostal space is entered and the diaphragm is divided radially. Care should be taken to avoid injury to the anterior and lateral divisions of the phrenic nerve. A Bookwalter self-retaining retractor is placed to facilitate wide exposure.

For a left-sided tumor, the dissection is initiated by dividing the peritoneum along the lateral peritoneal reflection. The splenorenal, and splenophrenic ligaments are also divided and the spleen along with the pancreas, stomach, descending colon, and the small bowel are reflected medially, exposing the entire retroperitoneum. For right-sided tumors, a Kocher maneuver is performed to mobilize the duodenum, and the ascending colon is then reflected medially. If tumor extends into the retrohepatic space, the liver can also be mobilized medially by dividing the right triangular ligament. Great care must be taken during this dissection, as vascular injury is possible when the aorta and visceral vessels are cleared.

Once the resection is complete, closure is begun with primary reapproximation of the diaphragm using nonabsorbable monofilament suture. The ribs are then reapproximated and an appropriately sized chest tube is left in place for drainage. The abdominal portion of the incision closure is completed in the standard fashion.

16.4.5 Pelvic Lesions

Similar to cervical lesions, primary pelvic tumors usually present with favorable biology and without distant metastases. However, these tumors can be challenging to resect due to encasement of iliac vessels and infiltration of the lumbosacral plexus. The patient is placed in a supine position and the abdomen is prepped from the costal margin to the pubis. A midline incision is made extending from the umbilicus to the pubic symphysis and deepened to enter the peritoneum. This approach provides good exposure of the pelvis and allows adequate control of the distal aorta and vena cava. Internal iliac vessels, if involved with tumor, may be ligated and resected without significant morbidity. Injury to pelvic nerve roots resulting in foot-drop is a common complication of pelvic tumor resection and should be discussed with parents prior to surgery.

16.5 Conclusion

While outcomes of many patients with neuroblastoma are strongly influenced by biological factors, extent of disease, and image-defined risk factors, surgery remains an integral part of managing patients with neuroblastoma. Appropriate surgical technique is essential for resection without damage to adjacent organs, nerves, and vasculature. In performing surgical procedures in such young patients, careful positioning and incision allow for adequate visualization of all internal anatomic structures and successful removal of the tumor. While an improved understanding of the molecular underpinnings of neuroblastoma and the refinement of patient risk stratification will undoubtedly contribute to better care of patients with neuroblastoma, surgery will continue to play an essential role in the management of the disease and determination.

References

1. Gross RE, Piotti E. The surgery of infancy and childhood: its principles and techniques. Philadelphia: Saunders; 1953, xxiv, 1000p
2. Koop CE, Kiesewetter WB, Horn RC. Neuroblastoma in childhood; survival after major surgical insult to the tumor. Surgery. 1955;38(1):272–8.
3. Harrison J, Myers M, Rowen M, Vermund H. Results of combination chemotherapy, surgery, and radiotherapy in children with neuroblastoma. Cancer. 1974;34(3):485–90.
4. Hollmann G, Lampert F. Carcinochemotherapy in pediatric surgery (author's transl). Langenbecks Arch Chir. 1975;339:95–8.
5. Stephen CR. Anesthesia for adrenal surgery. Urol Clin North Am. 1977;4:319–26.
6. Tsunooka H. Progress in diagnostic methods in pediatric surgery. Geka Chiryo. 1972;26(2):140–60.
7. Nitschke R, Smith EI, Shochat S, Altshuler G, Travers H, Shuster JJ, et al. Localized neuroblastoma treated by surgery: a Pediatric Oncology Group Study. J Clin Oncol. 1988;6(8):1271–9.
8. Brodeur GM, Pritchard J, Berthold F, Carlsen NL, Castel V, Castelberry RP, et al. Revisions of the international criteria for neuroblastoma diagnosis, staging, and response to treatment. J Clin Oncol. 1993;11(8):1466–77.
9. Cohn SL, Pearson AD, London WB, Monclair T, Ambros PF, Brodeur GM, et al. The International Neuroblastoma Risk Group (INRG) classification system: an INRG Task Force report. J Clin Oncol. 2009;27(2):289–97.
10. Monclair T, Brodeur GM, Ambros PF, Brisse HJ, Cecchetto G, Holmes K, et al. The International Neuroblastoma Risk Group (INRG) staging system: an INRG Task Force report. J Clin Oncol. 2009;27(2):298–303.
11. Monclair T, Mosseri V, Cecchetto G, De Bernardi B, Michon J, Holmes K. Influence of image-defined risk factors on the outcome of patients with localised neuroblastoma. A report from the LNESG1 study of the European International Society of Paediatric Oncology Neuroblastoma Group. Pediatr Blood Cancer. 2015;62(9):1536–42.
12. Holmes K, Sarnacki S, Poetschger U, Monclair T, Cecchetto G, Buffa P, et al., editors. Influence of surgical excision on survival of patients with high-risk neuroblastoma, report from study 1 of SIOP Europe (SIOPEN) [abstract PL012]. In: Advances in neuroblastoma research: ANR 2014 conference proceedings, Cologne, Germany. 2014.
13. von Allmen D, Davidoff AM, London WB, Van Ryn C, Haas-Kogan DA, Kreissman SG, et al. Impact of extent of resection on local control and survival in patients from the COG A3973 study with high-risk neuroblastoma. J Clin Oncol. 2017;35(2):208–16.
14. Kohler JA, Rubie H, Castel V, Beiske K, Holmes K, Gambini C, et al. Treatment of children over the age of one year with unresectable localised neuroblastoma without MYCN amplification: results of the SIOPEN study. Eur J Cancer. 2013;49(17):3671–9.

Surgical Strategies for High Risk Neuroblastoma

17

Sanjeev A. Vasudevan and Jed G. Nuchtern

17.1 History of Surgical Management of High Risk Neuroblastoma

The surgical management of high risk neuroblastoma has evolved from primary resection at diagnosis more than 3 decades ago, to a landmark paper written by Shamberger et al. showing that major surgical complications can be avoided with delayed surgery after neoadjuvant chemotherapy [1]. Interestingly, in the discussion when this paper was presented, it was proposed that the tumor is softer and necrotic prior to chemotherapy, making it possible to use an ultrasonic dissection technique to resect the tumor; however, post-chemotherapy, this was not possible due to the fibrotic nature of the tumor. Dr. Shamberger's response to this question was that

S. A. Vasudevan
Division of Pediatric Surgery, M. E. DeBakey Department of Surgery, Texas Children's Surgical Oncology Program, Baylor College of Medicine, Houston, TX, USA

Division of Surgical Research, M. E. DeBakey Department of Surgery, Baylor College of Medicine, Houston, TX, USA
e-mail: sanjeevv@bcm.edu

J. G. Nuchtern (✉)
Division of Surgical Research, M. E. DeBakey Department of Surgery, Baylor College of Medicine, Houston, TX, USA

Division of Pediatric Surgery, William J. Pokorny Professor of Pediatric Surgery, M. E. DeBakey Department of Surgery, Texas Children's Surgical Oncology Program, Baylor College of Medicine, Houston, TX, USA

Division of Global Surgery, William J. Pokorny Professor of Pediatric Surgery, M. E. DeBakey Department of Surgery, Texas Children's Surgical Oncology Program, Baylor College of Medicine, Houston, TX, USA
e-mail: nuchtern@bcm.edu

S. Sarnacki, L. Pio (eds.), *Neuroblastoma*,
https://doi.org/10.1007/978-3-030-18396-7_17

the fibrotic nature of the tumor is precisely what makes the surgery safer due to the decreased vascularity and achievable plains between the visceral arteries and the tumor. In this study they showed the blood loss was significantly less with this approach, thus setting the stage for the next three decades. In 1993, the famous British surgeon, Ed Kiely, published his series of 46 patients treated with aggressive resection of all visible retroperitoneal tumor by skeletonizing all of the visceral vessels [2]. He compared his cohort of patients with a group of 34 patients treated by other surgeons none of which underwent such extensive and complete resections. In this article, Mr. Kiely showed there was no difference in outcome amongst these patients and started to suggest that radical surgery may not change the outcome of high risk, metastatic patients. He concludes the paper by stating, "… the surgeon needs to be convinced that his/her efforts are worthwhile. The results reported here do not provide such reassurance."

After these first two studies published in the early 1990s, several follow-up studies were reported from very high volume programs including Children's Hospital of Philadelphia [3], Memorial Sloan Kettering Cancer Center [4], and a multi-institution study from Spain [5] with a combined total of 240 patients showing that extent of resection did not have an impact on overall survival in the INSS stage IV, >1 year of age group children that were recognized to be the highest risk group. In particular, in 1994, La Quaglia et al. reported a series of 70 high risk patients that did not show an independent effect of radical surgery on outcome [4]; however, a follow up paper in 2004 increased the numbers twofold to 141 patients and this analysis was the first to demonstrate a significant impact of extent of resection on survival [6]. This later study showed a local progression rate of 50% in the subtotal resection group, as opposed to 10% in the radical resection group ($p < 0.01$). Additionally, the overall survival was 50% in the radical resection group compared to 11% ($p < 0.01$). A complimentary CCG study soon followed by Adkins et al., showing surgical data on 539 high risk NB patients from the CCG-3891 trial [7]. This study showed a statistically significant increase in EFS in stage IV patients only, and this increase was modest (26% vs. 19%, $p = 0.0278$). Extent of resection did not have an impact on overall survival.

17.2 Current Surgical Approach to High Risk Neuroblastoma

Dr. La Quaglia's paper in 2004 led to a standard surgical approach to high risk neuroblastoma, in that most high volume centers across the US are routinely performing >95% resections with thorough skeletonization of the visceral blood vessels for thoracic, retroperitoneal, and pelvic neuroblastoma. The previous chapter focuses on specific surgical technique for the many primary locations for neuroblastoma. The following descriptions will be surgical approaches to the more common locations, thoracic, retroperitioneal, and pelvic, with an emphasis on surgical considerations for high risk disease.

17.2.1 Thoracic Lesions

In HR disease, often the thoracic component is either an extension of the retroperitoneal/abdominal lesion through the diaphragm hiatus along the aorta and bony spine or it can be a separate synchronous lesion in the paraspinous region. For the disease that extends from the retroperitoneum into the lower chest, we have been able to dissect the tumor away from the aorta and spine through the crus and hiatus. This technique should only be used for a minor amount of tumor in the lower chest that can be safely removed from the abdominal cavity, since this approach can have limited visibility of the thoracic aorta and esophagus. We have incised the diaphragm from this approach to improve the visibility and remove these tumors safely from the region. The other approach that offers very good exposure to this area is the left-sided thoracoabdominal approach described in the previous chapter. For synchronous, separate lesions in the paraspinous area, we usually approach these as we would localized thoracic disease with a video-assisted thoracoscopic approach (VATS). We have had great success in visualizing and extirpating these tumors with this approach. In addition, we have utilized this approach in a single setting with the bulk of the operation performed through a bilateral subcostal incision for the retroperitoneal tumor, followed by a VATS approach for the synchronous paraspinous, thoracic lesion. As previously mentioned, we pay special attention to the course of the thoracic duct particularly in the aortopulmonary window in a left apical paraspinous lesion. Additionally, in this area, the recurrent laryngeal, vagus, and phrenic nerves must be identified and preserved. Our general philosophy on tumor entering the neural foramina is to leave this portion alone and transect the tumor above the foramina either with bipolar cautery or harmonic scalpel to avoid thermal injury to the spinal cord. Additionally, in the lower thoracic spine, we assess the location of the artery of Adamkewicz in order to prevent injury and spinal ischemia (Fig. 17.1). For this lower thoracic paraspinous location, we often use spinal nerve monitoring to prevent any spinal cord ischemia or injury.

17.2.2 Retroperitoneal Lesions

Different approaches have been used for extensive retroperitoneal lymphatic spread from adrenal primaries. The thoracoabdominal approach is put forth as giving superior exposure from complete extirpation of the thoracoabdominal aorta, celiac trunk, SMA, and renal hilum. Others use a bilateral subcostal or transverse upper abdominal incision, giving access to the left and right retroperitoneum in tumors involving the central vasculature, as well as bilateral renal hilum or bilateral iliac vessels. The midline incision can be limiting in younger children since the transverse dimension is usually larger than the longitudinal dimension and the kidney on both sides often have to be completely mobilized and medialized in order to free up the more posterior renal artery from a tumor-encased hilum. We usually begin the procedure with

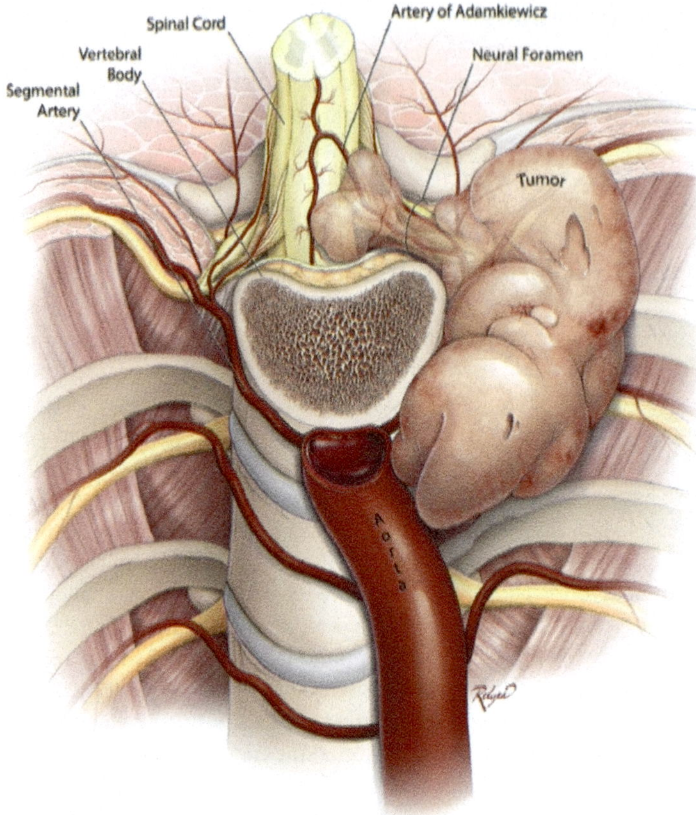

Fig. 17.1 Artery of Adamkewicz in relation to posterior mediastinal neuroblastoma. Image created by Katherine Relyea, MS, CMI and printed with permission from Baylor College of Medicine

left medial mobilization of the small/large bowel and spleen/pancreas. Sometimes, the pancreas is quite adherent to the central retroperitoneal portion of the tumor and is not as straightforward to mobilize. We gain access to the supraceliac aorta through the left crus and place a Rommel tourniquet for proximal control (Fig. 17.2). The general strategy is to debulk the tumor piecemeal. Given that the literature does not support en bloc removal of involved vasculature or organs, one should not attempt to remove the entire specimen in one piece. We begin with resection of the suprarenal/adrenal primary tumor bulk. This usually enables identification of the left crus and diaphragm in order to gain supraceliac control of the aorta, if it cannot be visualized earlier. Once the left crus and upper aorta are in view, one can then free up tumor working down the left side of the aorta toward the left renal hilum. This will enable initial identification of the celiac trunk just below the left crus and the SMA, a short distance distal to this. A thorough analysis of the preoperative CT/MRI should be performed with the radiologist to attain measurements of the distance from the celiac trunk to the SMA, the SMA to the renal arteries, the SMA to the

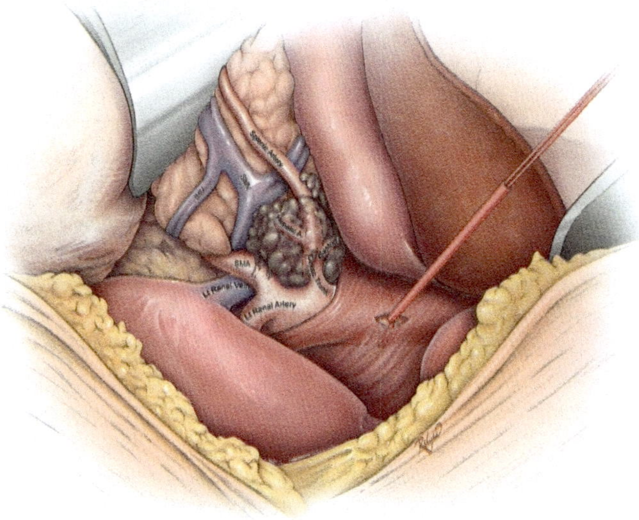

Fig. 17.2 Central retroperitoneal tumor relationships to major vessels. Image created by Katherine Relyea, MS, CMI and printed with permission from Baylor College of Medicine

IMA, and the SMA or IMA to the iliac bifurcation. Ultrasound and Doppler can be used intraoperatively to see "through" the encasing tumor to try and identify the location of these vessels. Once the origins of the celiac or SMA are identified from the aorta, a "bivalving" technique can be used by finding the plane between tumor and the adventitia of the vessel with a semi-blunt dissector, either a Gemini clamp or a gently-curved dissector. Once that plane is achieved and the vessel is kept underneath the clamp, cautery can be used on a higher setting for hemostasis to divide the tumor parenchyma above the clamp. In some cases, the periadventitial plane is obliterated and one may be compelled to pursue a sub-adventitial plane on these vessels or the aorta. We would caution this approach as this can weaken the vessel and increase the chance of vessel rupture or avulsion during surgery or in the postoperative period. We elect to leave small plaques of tumor in place, particularly on the celiac/SMA origin or distally. We are usually more aggressive with dissecting out the splenic artery and sometimes ligate the gastric artery; however, we often leave tumor on the hepatic artery to avoid any injury to this vessel as this amount of the tumor tends to be a very small percentage of the total tumor bulk. Special care should be taken when dissecting tumor in between the celiac trunk and SMA. This block of tumor usually abuts the uncinate process of the pancreas on the right, as well as the SMV; therefore, one should avoid taking pancreas tissue when dissecting this area of tumor. Also, proper identification of the portal vein/SMV from the right will prevent damage to this vessel during this portion of the dissection. Additionally, one has a tendency to pull on the small bowel viscera to expose this portion of tumor putting traction force on the SMA. As this vessel is skeletonized there is less and less additional surrounding tissue to absorb this force, eventually leading to an excessive amount of traction force directly on the SMA. This should be checked and monitored throughout this portion of the procedure to avoid avulsion of the vessel. The above portion of the dissection focusing on the central, retroperitoneal portion of the tumor is illustrated in Fig. 17.2 to show the relationships between the central tumor and the many major blood vessel branches.

A full Cattel-Braasch maneuver (right medial visceral rotation) is often required for these central tumors in order to fully expose the right renal hilum and the vena cava. A similar approach as detailed above should be followed for a right suprarenal tumor with central lymph node involvement. The vena cava is thin-walled as compared to the aorta, so special care must be taken to extirpate this vessel from encasing tumor. Particularly, the thin lumbar veins branching from the IVC tend to be very fragile and bleed significantly if avulsed. Many of these can be ligated. Some areas where there is no plane present for bivalving and dissection, a small rim of tumor can be left in place to prevent tearing the IVC. In our experience, the porta hepatis disease can be left alone if it constitutes a small percentage of the total tumor bulk due to the risk of damage to these vital structures. The disease in the "aortocaval" groove is dissected and removed in a similar piecemeal fashion. The underlying right renal artery and right side of the SMA must be identified and left unharmed when dissecting in this area. This area is also very lymphatic rich; therefore, we use suture ligation, hemoclips, or harmonic scalpel to seal these lymphatics to prevent chyle leakage. The right side of the aorta can be exposed from this area from the iliac bifurcation up to the IMA and then to the SMA. When dissecting posterior to the aorta either from the right or left, the lumbar arteries will be encountered, which can be ligated as needed. Often, if these vessels lie on the edge of the tumor or a small amount of encasing tumor, we bivalve tumor from around these vessels in an attempt to preserve them.

17.2.3 Pelvic Lesions

The primarily pelvic lesions can be approached through a lower midline incision or a Pfanennenstiel type incision, exposing the area about 1 cm above the pubic symphysis to give adequate exposure to the deep pelvis. This becomes more critical for the older patient as the pelvis is deeper. Lesions originating from the aortic bifurcation can encase both iliac artery and vein. The artery is often easily identified from the aorta and can be followed distally to the profunda/superficial femoral bifurcation. The vein is often more difficult to identify, being posterior to the artery and usually very fragile. This dissection must be performed very slowly and meticulously to avoid injury to this vessel. Preoperative ureteral stent placement is usually not required, and the ureter can be followed proximally to this area. The ureter should be circumferentially extirpated from the tumor with a bivalving technique as described above. The tumor is rarely adherent to the ureter and a plane can be identified. In our experience, small plaques of tumor can be left on the vessels at tightly adherent points to avoid injury. The iliac artery in younger children can spasm. We recommend having pulse oximetry on the leg most involved or both sides in order to continuously monitor distal perfusion and spasm. Topical papaverine or lidocaine can be used for spasm. Dissection of the tumor in the presacral space can be performed. One should be aware of the location of the hypogastric plexus in order to try and preserve these nerves, as well as, the sacral nerves for deeper pelvic tumors. We do not chase these tumors into the neural foramina as described above and are willing to leave small plaques of tumor in these areas to avoid nerve injury.

17.3 Extent of Resection for High Risk Neuroblastoma (Current Literature)

Since the 2004 paper by La Quaglia et al., several follow-up papers were published within the next 10 years, showing various single institution experiences with complete versus partial resection in high risk neuroblastoma. Among the most significant of these studies were a study of 124, greater than 1 year old stage 4 patients from St. Jude's Children's Research Hospital [8], a German study from their NB97 trial consisting of 278, greater than 18-month-old stage 4 patients [9], and finally a meta-analysis published by Mullassery et al. in 2014 [10]. None of these studies showed any increase in EFS or improvement in OS based on extent of resection in stage 4 patients. However, the meta-analysis did show a significant improvement in EFS and OS in stage 3 patients (non-metastatic) [10]. This finding was again shown in a follow-up study from the German, NB97 trial subanalysis, focusing on 179 patients with localized disease that were greater than 18 months old, of which 36 patients were HR and 23 IR [11]. Only the HR patients that underwent complete surgical resection had a dramatic improvement in EFS, local progression free survival and OS. However, again looking at all HR patients together in the COG A3973 study, there was only a longer EFS noted with >90% resection, but no effect on OS [12].

More recently, an international multicenter study was completed, analyzing 229 patients from seven centers in Europe and North America, all with high risk disease to test whether presence, change, or location of image defined risk factors (IDRF) influenced resectability of the primary tumor or EFS/OS. The results showed that there was a highly significant correlation with tumor size reduction and decrease in number of IDRF's with induction chemotherapy. This, however, did not translate to a correlation in frequency of ≥90% surgical resection of the primary tumor. In addition, the patients that did not receive ≥90% resection had significantly higher number of IDRF's at diagnosis and after neoadjuvant chemotherapy. The presurgery IDRFs that most significantly correlated with a <90% resection were those involving porta hepatis, aorta and branches, vena cava and branches, and both renal pedicles. The survival analysis revealed an event-free (EFS) and overall (OS) 5-year survival of 37.9% and 49%, respectively. There was no significant correlation between the absence or the presence of any IDRFs either at diagnosis or presurgery and EFS or OS. This was also true for the extent of resection and the absence or the presence of IDRFs associated with completeness of resection.

These studies together show that a surgical resection of some kind should be performed on metastatic NB, but the eventual overall outcome of these patients is highly dependent on biology and response to therapy rather than the extent of surgical resection. The principal of gross total resection leaving tumor in critical areas such as the porta hepatis or on the tightly adherent areas near the celiac trunk, SMA, or aorta appears to be a reasonable approach given the current data.

17.4 Timing of Surgery

In the current treatment protocols of the major international cooperative groups for high-risk NB, a minimal diagnostic biopsy procedure (open, minimally invasive, or image-guided needle core) is performed at initial presentation, and resection of the primary tumor is delayed until after three to five cycles of induction chemotherapy. (The exception to this approach would be the relatively rare INRGSS L1 tumor in a child with obvious metastatic disease.) This approach has evolved from several observations and represents a compromise based on the best evidence. The rationale for not attempting definitive resection of the primary tumor at the time of diagnosis comes from several studies demonstrating a higher rate of surgical complications when extirpation is performed at this time. Shamberger's 1991 paper [1] demonstrated a higher rate of complications with up-front versus delayed resections with no difference in overall survival between these groups. There are at least two potential explanations for this decrease in morbidity with delayed surgery. First, it is clear that the primary tumor almost always decreases in volume during induction chemotherapy, with the most significant decrease occurring after the first two cycles [13]. This decrease in volume alone likely explains some decrease in length of the surgery and intraoperative hemorrhage, independent of a reduction in IDRFs. A second explanation is the observed reduction in IDRFs during induction chemotherapy (see Sect. 17.3) and the correlation between the presence of IDRFs and the incidence of surgical complications [14, 15].

The optimal timing of definitive resection during induction chemotherapy is not certain. Given that the primary tumor volume does not change significantly after the third cycle of chemotherapy [13], it is unlikely that there are any changes in the IDRF's after this point in treatment. While it is possible that the tumor consistency changes in a positive way after this point, it is our anecdotal impression that extremely fibrotic tumors can be more difficult to safely dissect away from delicate blood vessels such as the renal artery. Furthermore, single institution studies from St. Jude suggest that resection earlier in induction may be associated with better prognosis, perhaps because there is less opportunity to develop resistant tumor clones when the largest mass of tumor cells is removed earlier in induction [8, 16]. In reality, the timing of surgical resection is often a compromise based on the logistics of stem cell harvesting, experimental therapy protocol arms, family convenience, and other factors.

17.5 Primary Tumor Response Criteria

It is important to have a rational system to assess primary tumor response to treatment. The International Neuroblastoma Response Criteria (INRC) represented the original system to assess tumor response. The primary tumor component of that response assessment was based on tumor volume. Thus, a very good partial response (VGPR) was a 90–99% reduction in tumor volume and a partial response was a >50% but less than 90% decrease in volume [17, 18]. More recently, we investigated whether change in tumor volume was preferable to change in the largest tumor diameter in measurement of primary tumor response to therapy. In a retrospective review of 229 high-risk NB patients from large centers in Europe and North America, two measures of tumor volume reduction, >50% and >65%, were compared to >30% reduction in largest tumor diameter (the RECIST guidelines) in response to induction chemotherapy in terms of the ability to predict extent of resection and event-free and overall survival [19]. In a multivariate analysis, no measure of primary tumor response was predictive of patient outcome or extent of resection. Based on these findings, the INRC was revised to use the >30% reduction in largest tumor diameter as the assessment of primary tumor response because it was easier to use than tumor volume measurements [20].

References

1. Shamberger RC, Allarde-Segundo A, Kozakewich HP, Grier HE. Surgical management of stage III and IV neuroblastoma: resection before or after chemotherapy. J Pediatr Surg. 1991;26:1113–7; discussion 1117–8.
2. Kiely EM. Radical surgery for abdominal neuroblastoma. Semin Surg Oncol. 1993;9:489–92.
3. Shorter NA, et al. The role of surgery in the management of stage IV neuroblastoma: a single institution study. Med Pediatr Oncol. 1995;24:287–91.
4. La Quaglia MP, et al. Stage 4 neuroblastoma diagnosed at more than 1 year of age: gross total resection and clinical outcome. J Pediatr Surg. 1994;29:1162–5; discussion 1165–6.
5. Castel V, et al. The role of surgery in stage IV neuroblastoma. J Pediatr Surg. 2002;37:1574–8.
6. La Quaglia MP, et al. The impact of gross total resection on local control and survival in high-risk neuroblastoma. J Pediatr Surg. 2004;39:412–7; discussion 412–7.
7. Adkins ES, et al. Efficacy of complete resection for high-risk neuroblastoma: a Children's Cancer Group study. J Pediatr Surg. 2004;39:931–6.
8. McGregor LM, et al. The impact of early resection of primary neuroblastoma on the survival of children older than 1 year of age with stage 4 disease: the St. Jude Children's Research Hospital Experience. Cancer. 2005;104:2837–46.
9. Simon T, Häberle B, Hero B, von Schweinitz D, Berthold F. Role of surgery in the treatment of patients with stage 4 neuroblastoma age 18 months or older at diagnosis. J Clin Oncol. 2013;31:752–8.
10. Mullassery D, Farrelly P, Losty PD. Does aggressive surgical resection improve survival in advanced stage 3 and 4 neuroblastoma? A systematic review and meta-analysis. Pediatr Hematol Oncol. 2014;31:703–16.
11. Fischer J, et al. Complete surgical resection improves outcome in INRG high-risk patients with localized neuroblastoma older than 18 months. BMC Cancer. 2017;17:520.
12. von Allmen D, et al. Impact of extent of resection on local control and survival in patients from the COG A3973 study with high-risk neuroblastoma. J Clin Oncol. 2017;35:208–16.

13. Medary I, et al. Kinetics of primary tumor regression with chemotherapy: implications for the timing of surgery. Ann Surg Oncol. 1996;3:521–5.
14. Cecchetto G, et al. Surgical risk factors in primary surgery for localized neuroblastoma: the LNESG1 study of the European International Society of Pediatric Oncology Neuroblastoma Group. J Clin Oncol. 2005;23:8483–9.
15. Monclair T, et al. Influence of image-defined risk factors on the outcome of patients with localised neuroblastoma. A report from the LNESG1 study of the European International Society of Paediatric Oncology Neuroblastoma Group. Pediatr Blood Cancer. 2015;62:1536–42.
16. Davidoff AM, et al. Radiographic assessment of resectability of locoregional disease in children with high-risk neuroblastoma during neoadjuvant chemotherapy. Pediatr Blood Cancer. 2005;44:158–62.
17. Brodeur GM, et al. International criteria for diagnosis, staging, and response to treatment in patients with neuroblastoma. J Clin Oncol. 1988;6:1874–81.
18. Brodeur GM, et al. Revisions of the international criteria for neuroblastoma diagnosis, staging, and response to treatment. J Clin Oncol. 1993;11:1466–77.
19. Eisenhauer EA, et al. New response evaluation criteria in solid tumours: revised RECIST guideline (version 1.1). Eur J Cancer. 2009;1990(45):228–47.
20. Bagatell R, et al. Assessment of primary site response in children with high-risk neuroblastoma: an international multicenter study. J Clin Oncol. 2016;34:740–6.

Surgical Strategies for Neuroblastoma with Spinal Canal Involvement

18

Luca Pio, Thomas Blanc, Christophe Glorion,
Stephanie Puget, Michel Zerah, and Sabine Sarnacki

18.1 Indications

Since 1984, neurological sign and symptoms at diagnosis of a child with Neuroblastoma with spinal canal involvement were started to be managed with urgent chemotherapy as described by Hayes et al. [1].

Corticoid therapy and chemotherapy in an urgency setting have proven to be effective in reducing neurologic sign and symptoms, in literature neurosurgical procedures as first treatment were more related to long term orthopaedic and neurologic sequelae, but these results are affected by a selection bias, in fact, in several studies, neurosurgical treatment was reserved for those patients with a more severe and rapid neurologic deteriorating condition at diagnosis [2].

In the last years, radiotherapy as first treatment was more and more abandoned in favour of chemotherapy and neurosurgery because of its effects on spinal growth, and development of post-irradiation thyroid problems in case of upper spine treatment [3–6].

L. Pio (✉) · T. Blanc · S. Sarnacki
Department of Pediatric Surgery, Necker - Enfants Malades Hospital, Assistance Publique Hopitaux de Paris, Paris, France

University of Paris, Paris, France
e-mail: luca.pio@aphp.fr

C. Glorion
Department of Orthopaedic Surgery, Hôpital Necker-Enfants Malades, University of Paris, Paris, France

Department of Pediatric Orthopedics, Hôpital Necker-Enfants Malades, Assistance Publique-Hôpitaux de Paris, Paris, France

S. Puget · M. Zerah
University of Paris, Paris, France

Department of Pediatric Neurosurgery, Hôpital Necker-Enfants Malades, Assistance Publique-Hôpitaux de Paris, Paris, France

S. Sarnacki, L. Pio (eds.), *Neuroblastoma*,
https://doi.org/10.1007/978-3-030-18396-7_18

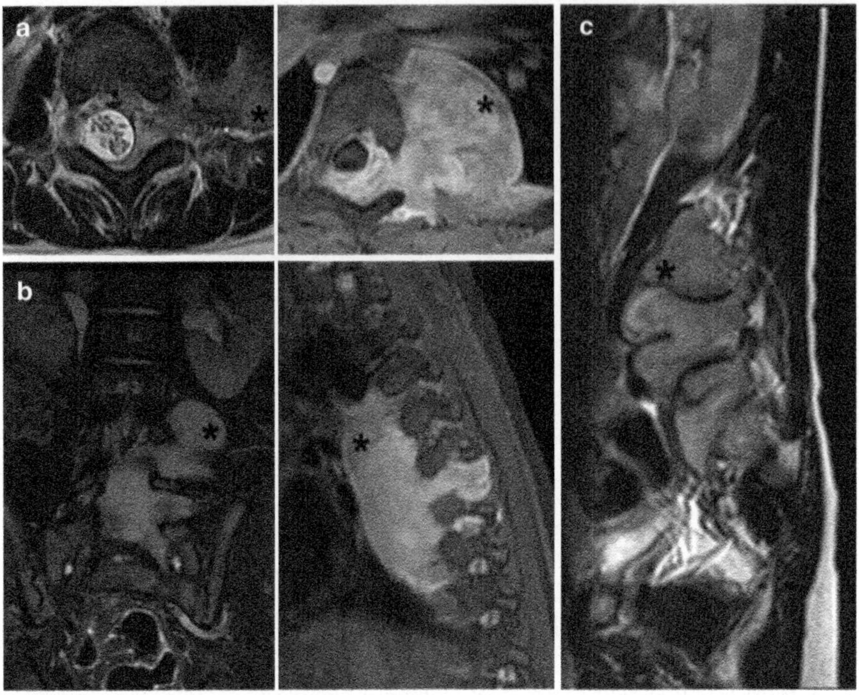

Fig. 18.1 Magnetic resonance imaging with spinal canal involvement. (**a**) Axial section; (**b**) coronal section. (**c**) sagittal section

Symptomatic patients represent 65% of children with Neuroblastoma with spinal canal involvement [7].

In case of asymptomatic patients, the surgical indication must take into account current protocols [8–10], and intraspinal tumour extension must be considered a surgical risk factor as stated by Brisse et al. in [11], in fact, an intraspinal tumour extension provided more than one-third of spinal canal in axial plane (Fig. 18.1), an absence of perimedullary leptomeningeal space visibility or an abnormal spinal cord signal intensity are considered as image-defined risk factors (IDRFs). In such cases, neoadjuvant chemotherapy is mandatory in order to try to reduce IDRFs.

Recently, a SIOPEN study described the modification of the IDRFs after chemotherapy, with a reduction of 100% in case of cervical spinal involvement, 16.7% for Dumbbel thoracic tumours and 46.7% for abdominopelvic spinal extension [12].

Even in the absence of large prospective studies, the actual recommendation of neurosurgery as first line treatment are the children with a rapid neurologic deterioration and differentiated tumours with a low rate of chemotherapy response or well differentiated neuroblastic tumours as ganglioneuroma.

General surgery is provided in case of thoracic, abdominal or pelvic extension.

An evaluation of pre-operative IDRFs is necessary also for the visceral surgeons in order to plan a correct surgical timing considering the chemotherapy efficacy and in order to set the proper surgical access.

18.2 Surgical Techniques

In the last years neurosurgery experienced a rapid evolution in terms of preoperative imaging, surgical devices and new techniques.

Magnetic resonance with new powerful 3Tesla system and new sequences provided a better preoperative surgical planification with more detailed anatomic and functional definitions and the possibility of reconstruction of several high definition three dimensional models.

The cavitron ultrasonic surgical aspirator (CUSA) radically changes the neurosurgeons attitudes in the last years with his effect of cavitation with tumour fragmentation providing at the same time suction and aspiration [13, 14].

CUSA was ameliorated in the last years optimizing ergonomics and then the instrument control and increased tissue selectivity and margin of control.

Neurosurgical techniques experienced a more conservative orientation, for many years laminectomy represented the neurosurgical gold standard technique with lamina complete removal with or without facet joint capsule preservation.

A long-terms spinal deformity sequelae rate was described by several studies with scoliosis, kyphosis, kyphoscoliosis, requiring in about 27% of cases a vertebral fusion surgical procedure [15–18]. Several independent risk factors for spinal deformity were identified as the age at surgery (<13 years old) with a high ligamentous laxity, the high proportion of cartilage and the horizontal facet orientation resulting in an alteration of skeletal development.

Preoperative scoliotic deformities, thoracolumbar involvement and extent of surgery (>4 discs) are others independent risk factors of spinal deformities following laminectomy [19, 20].

Laminotomy consists in the partial removal of the lamina, usually on one side. The support of the lamina is left in place with this technique, providing better results in terms of functional sequelae [21].

Recently Menger described a minimally invasive approach to perform pediatric laminectomy using 16 up to 22-mm instruments in order to have shorter hospital stays, smaller incision, less muscle disruption and reduced infection rates [22].

In recent years thoracic and abdominal paediatric surgery experienced a rapid development of minimally invasive procedures with an increasing number of thocacoscopic, laparoscopic and retroperitoneoscopic approaches [23–27].

A new era of minimally invasive surgery it is developing with the application of novel robotic systems also for the management of paediatric solid tumours [28].

Almost for the thoracic Neuroblastoma extension, thoracoscopy can give the advantage of a good exposition of the surgical site resulting in an absence of muscle dissection and subsequent better pain control and shorter hospital stay [29].

During thoracoscopy the surgeon must pay attention to avoid a deep dissection of the costo-vertebral space and limit the resection to the superficial neuroblatoma roots. An extended costo-vertebral dissection can result in a post-operative perispinal oedema with transitory or permanent neurological impairment.

The spinal canal neuroblastoma involvement must be treated by neurosurgeons before, in combination or after the general surgery procedures. To date in literature no data were provided regarding the timing and/or the association between neurosurgical and general surgical procedures.

18.3 Follow Up

Many follow-up studies reported 60–75% rates of long-term functional sequelae [20] with spinal deformities, neurological disorders (paraparesis, paralysis, sphincter disorders radicular permanent back pain).

In an era of multimodal strategy for paediatric solid tumours treatment an adequate follow-up must be provided with multiple specialized controls in addition to conventional oncologic follow up.

Orthopaedic follow up is fundamental to check the evolution of spinal development and for the early diagnosis and treatment of sequelae.

General surgeon must be involved to assess the eventually sphincter disfunction, faecal incontinence can be managed with peristeen [30, 31].

Urologic assessment will be necessary in case of neurologic bladder, and intermitted clean catheterisation with valuation of upper urologic system dilatation and bladder evaluation must be planned to preserve the renal function [32, 33].

Neurosurgical follow-up must evaluate the motor and sensitive neurological functions.

18.4 Conclusion

Surgical management of patient with intraspinal involvement of Neuroblastoma require a complex multimodal strategy with the involvement of different specialist [34].

Surgeons must take into the account that these patients represent not only a technical surgical challenge and preoperative and postoperative assessment must have an equivalence attention to reduce long term morbidities.

References

1. Hayes FA, Thompson EI, Hvizdala E, O'Connor D, Green AA. Chemotherapy as an alternative to laminectomy and radiation in the management of epidural tumor. J Pediatr. 1984;104(2):221–4.
2. Kraal K, Blom T, van Noesel M, Kremer L, Caron H, Tytgat G, van der Pal H. Treatment and outcome of neuroblastoma with intraspinal extension: a systematic review. Pediatr Blood Cancer. 2017;64(8) https://doi.org/10.1002/pbc.26451.
3. Sandberg DI, Bilsky MH, Kushner BH, Souweidane MM, Kramer K, Laquaglia MP, Panageas KS, Cheung NK. Treatment of spinal involvement in neuroblastoma patients. Pediatr Neurosurg. 2003;39(6):291–8.
4. Flandin I, Hartmann O, Michon J, Pinkerton R, Coze C, Stephan JL, Fourquet B, Valteau-Couanet D, Bergeron C, Philip T, Carrie C. Impact of TBI on late effects in children treated by

megatherapy for Stage IV neuroblastoma. A study of the French Society of Pediatric oncology. Int J Radiat Oncol Biol Phys. 2006;64(5):1424–31.

5. Armstrong GT, Stovall M, Robison LL. Long-term effects of radiation exposure among adult survivors of childhood cancer: results from the childhood cancer survivor study. Radiat Res. 2010;174(6):840–50.
6. Paulino AC, Mayr NA, Simon JH, Buatti JM. Locoregional control in infants with neuroblastoma: role of radiation therapy and late toxicity. Int J Radiat Oncol Biol Phys. 2002;52(4):1025–31.
7. Maris JM. Recent advances in neuroblastoma. N Engl J Med. 2010;362(23):2202–11.
8. Kohler JA, Rubie H, Castel V, Beiske K, Holmes K, Gambini C, Casale F, Munzer C, Erminio G, Parodi S, Navarro S, Marquez C, Peuchmaur M, Cullinane C, Brock P, Valteau-Couanet D, Garaventa A, Haupt R. Treatment of children over the age of one year with unresectable localised neuroblastoma without MYCN amplification: results of the SIOPEN study. Eur J Cancer. 2013;49(17):3671–9.
9. Pinto NR, Applebaum MA, Volchenboum SL, Matthay KK, London WB, Ambros PF, Nakagawara A, Berthold F, Schleiermacher G, Park JR, Valteau-Couanet D, Pearson AD, Cohn SL. Advances in risk classification and treatment strategies for neuroblastoma. J Clin Oncol. 2015;33(27):3008–17.
10. Smith V, Foster J. High-risk neuroblastoma treatment review. Children (Basel). 2018;5(9) https://doi.org/10.3390/children5090114.
11. Brisse HJ, McCarville MB, Granata C, Krug KB, Wootton-Gorges SL, Kanegawa K, Giammarile F, Schmidt M, Shulkin BL, Matthay KK, Lewington VJ, Sarnacki S, Hero B, Kaneko M, London WB, Pearson AD, Cohn SL, Monclair T. Guidelines for imaging and staging of neuroblastic tumors: consensus report from the International Neuroblastoma Risk Group Project. Radiology. 2011;261(1):243–57.
12. Avanzini S, Pio L, Erminio G, Granata C, Holmes K, Gambart M, Buffa P, Castel V, Valteau Couanet D, Garaventa A, Pistorio A, Cecchetto G, Martucciello G, Mattioli G, Sarnacki S. Image-defined risk factors in unresectable neuroblastoma: SIOPEN study on incidence, chemotherapy-induced variation, and impact on surgical outcomes. Pediatr Blood Cancer. 2017;64(11) https://doi.org/10.1002/pbc.26605.
13. Roth J, Korn A, Bitan-Talmor Y, Kaufman R, Ekstein M, Constantini S. Subcortical mapping using an electrified cavitron ultrasonic aspirator in pediatric supratentorial surgery. World Neurosurg. 2017;101:357–64.
14. Tang H, Zhang H, Xie Q, Gong Y, Zheng M, Wang D, Zhu H, Chen X, Zhou L. Application of CUSA excel ultrasonic aspiration system in resection of skull base meningiomas. Chin J Cancer Res. 2014;26(6):653–7.
15. De Bernardi B, Pianca C, Pistamiglio P, Veneselli E, Viscardi E, Pession A, Alvisi P, Carli M, Donfrancesco A, Casale F, Giuliano MG, di Montezemolo LC, Di Cataldo A, Lo Curto M, Bagnulo S, Schumacher RF, Tamburini A, Garaventa A, Clemente L, Bruzzi P. Neuroblastoma with symptomatic spinal cord compression at diagnosis: treatment and results with 76 cases. J Clin Oncol. 2001;19(1):183–90.
16. Kraal K, Blom T, Tytgat L, van Santen H, van Noesel M, Smets A, Bramer J, Caron H, Kremer L, van der Pal H. Neuroblastoma with intraspinal extension: health problems in long-term survivors. Pediatr Blood Cancer. 2016;63(6):990–6.
17. Simon T, Niemann CA, Hero B, Henze G, Suttorp M, Schilling FH, Berthold F. Short- and long-term outcome of patients with symptoms of spinal cord compression by neuroblastoma. Dev Med Child Neurol. 2012;54(4):347–52.
18. Angelini P, Plantaz D, De Bernardi B, Passagia JG, Rubie H, Pastore G. Late sequelae of symptomatic epidural compression in children with localized neuroblastoma. Pediatr Blood Cancer. 2011;57(3):473–80.
19. Yao KC, McGirt MJ, Chaichana KL, Constantini S, Jallo GI. Risk factors for progressive spinal deformity following resection of intramedullary spinal cord tumors in children: an analysis of 161 consecutive cases. J Neurosurg. 2007;107(6 Suppl):463–8.

20. Trahair T, Sorrentino S, Russell SJ, Sampaio H, Selek L, Plantaz D, Freycon C, Simon T, Kraal K, Beck-Popovic M, Haupt R, Ash S, De Bernardi B. Spinal canal involvement in neuroblastoma. J Pediatr. 2017;188:294–8.
21. Ozerov SS, Samarin AE, Andreev ES, Tereshchenko GV, Kachanov DY, Shamanskaya TV, Varfolomeeva SR. Neurosurgical aspects of the treatment of neuroblastoma patients. Zh Vopr Neirokhir Im N N Burdenko. 2016;80(3):50–7.
22. Menger R, Hefner MI, Savardekar AR, Nanda A, Sin A. Minimally invasive spine surgery in the pediatric and adolescent population: a case series. Surg Neurol Int. 2018;9:116.
23. Irtan S, Brisse HJ, Minard-Colin V, Schleiermacher G, Canale S, Sarnacki S. Minimally invasive surgery of neuroblastic tumors in children: indications depend on anatomical location and image-defined risk factors. Pediatr Blood Cancer. 2015;62(2):257–61.
24. Lacreuse I, Valla JS, de Lagausie P, Varlet F, Héloury Y, Temporal G, Bastier R, Becmeur F. Thoracoscopic resection of neurogenic tumors in children. J Pediatr Surg. 2007;42(10):1725–8.
25. Heloury Y, Muthucumaru M, Panabokke G, Cheng W, Kimber C, Leclair MD. Minimally invasive adrenalectomy in children. J Pediatr Surg. 2012;47(2):415–21.
26. Mattioli G, Avanzini S, Pini Prato A, Pio L, Granata C, Garaventa A, Conte M, Manzitti C, Montobbio G, Buffa P. Laparoscopic resection of adrenal neuroblastoma without image-defined risk factors: a prospective study on 21 consecutive pediatric patients. Pediatr Surg Int. 2014;30(4):387–94.
27. Fascetti-Leon F, Scotton G, Pio L, Beltrà R, Caione P, Esposito C, Mattioli G, Saxena AK, Sarnacki S, Gamba P. Minimally invasive resection of adrenal masses in infants and children: results of a European multi-center survey. Surg Endosc. 2017;31(11):4505–12.
28. Meehan JJ. Robotic surgery for pediatric tumors. Cancer J. 2013;19(2):183–8.
29. Fraga JC, Rothenberg S, Kiely E, Pierro A. Video-assisted thoracic surgery resection for pediatric mediastinal neurogenic tumors. J Pediatr Surg. 2012;47(7):1349–53.
30. Mosiello G, Marshall D, Rolle U, Crétolle C, Santacruz BG, Frischer J, Benninga MA. Consensus review of best practice of transanal irrigation in children. J Pediatr Gastroenterol Nutr. 2017;64(3):343–52.
31. Midrio P, Mosiello G, Ausili E, Gamba P, Marte A, Lombardi L, Iacobelli BD, Caponcelli E, Marrello S, Meroni M, Brisighelli G, Leva E, Rendeli C. Peristeen(®) transanal irrigation in paediatric patients with anorectal malformations and spinal cord lesions: a multicentre Italian study. Color Dis. 2016;18(1):86–93.
32. Li Y, Wen Y, He X, Li Y, Wu J, Feng J, Wang Q, Wen J. Application of clean intermittent catheterization for neurogenic bladder in infants less than 1 year old. NeuroRehabilitation. 2018;42(4):377–82.
33. Sturm RM, Cheng EY. The management of the pediatric neurogenic bladder. Curr Bladder Dysfunct Rep. 2016;11:225–33.
34. Pio L, Blanc T, de Saint Denis T, Irtan S, Valteau-Couanet D, Michon J, Brisse H, Galmiche-Rolland L, Joyeux L, Odent T, Harte C, Glorion C, Zerah M, Sarnacki S. Multidisciplinary surgical strategy for dumbbell neuroblastoma: a single-center experience of 32 cases. Pediatr Blood Cancer. 2019;2019:e27670.

Neuroblastoma: Minimally Invasive Surgery

19

Jörg Fuchs and Steven W. Warmann

19.1 General Considerations

19.1.1 Historical Development

Minimally invasive surgery (MIS) has been applied in children with cancer for over 20 years. Early multicenter trials or prospective studies reported that the vast majority of procedures were carried out in uncomplicated tumors or for biopsies. Initial experiences with MIS in neuroblastoma (NB) stem from that period [1–3]. With the development of surgical skills and technical equipment, more and more complex procedures were performed. Accordingly, the rate of tumor resections increased relevantly within the spectrum of MIS for oncological conditions. Despite the lack of randomized controlled trials regarding the role of MIS in NB, it is, meanwhile, widely accepted that under certain conditions, the minimally invasive approach is associated with comparable surgical and oncological results as the open approach. However, authors generally strongly emphasize a careful patient selection in order to achieve these results [4–8]. To date, the main emphasis regarding MIS in NB is on the definition of its exact role as compared to open procedures and on the formulation of guidelines in the protocols of national and international multicenter trials.

19.1.2 Imaging and Image-Defined Risk Factors (IDRF)

In addition to the regularities of imaging for NB (see Sect. 19.2), there are some peculiarities, which have to be taken into account for MIS in this tumor entity.

J. Fuchs (✉) · S. W. Warmann
Department of Pediatric Surgery and Pediatric Urology, University Children's Hospital Tübingen, Tübingen, Germany
e-mail: Joerg.Fuchs@med.uni-tuebingen.de; Steven.Warmann@med.uni-tuebingen.de

S. Sarnacki, L. Pio (eds.), *Neuroblastoma*,
https://doi.org/10.1007/978-3-030-18396-7_19

In localized NB, the presence of IDRF has an influence on survival rates and surgical complications [9]. IDRFs seem to have even more relevance for the minimally invasive approach than for open procedures. Numerous authors reported that the presence of IDRF does not preclude the possibility of gross total tumor resection in NB using the open approach [10–12]. On the other hand, recent reports postulated the absence of IDRF for a safe and effective minimally invasive resection of abdominal NB [13–16]. This fact is further underlined by the SIOPEN experience that there is no use in aspiring increased resection rates through prolonged chemotherapy, since, during chemotherapy, IDRF patterns remain unchanged in 50% of NB patients, while new IDRFs occur in approximately 20% [17]. Taken together, the presence of IDRF in L2-neuroblastoma does not represent a contraindication for a minimally invasive tumor resection. However, this subgroup represents a relevantly higher surgical challenge, also from a technical point of view; surgeons should therefore critically assess whether the minimally invasive approach is the correct choice for these tumors.

The techniques of diffusion-weighted imaging (DWI) and apparent diffusion coefficient (ADC) values seem to contain promising aspects with regard to tumor biopsy and resection. Recent reports described the ability of this imaging to distinguish ganglioneuroma from neuroblastoma/ganglioneuroblastoma and also to deliver quantitative data on tumor response to chemotherapy [18–20]. From the reported studies, a future development appears realistic, in which these additional imaging data contribute to directing not only surgical techniques but also the way of surgical approaches during tumor biopsy and resection. However, the exact impact of these recently introduced imaging techniques on the approach in NB surgery is yet to be assessed.

19.1.3 Surgical Principles

According to open procedures, possible applications for MIS in NB contain tumor biopsies, tumor resection, and oncological follow-up procedures/secondary procedures [21]. In this regard, the surgical principles of MIS in NB have to follow the guidelines for open procedures in respective cases. There is no justification for compromises in order to realize the minimally invasive technique.

Operative strategies must consider the patients' individual risk profiles. For example, tumor biopsy is reasonable as only a surgical step in some cases of newborn patients, although complete resection seems feasible with a moderate risk. In every case, indications for surgery and the corresponding approach should be established after an interdisciplinary decision-making process.

As in open surgery, surgeons must be prepared to face intraoperative hemorrhage. The minimally-invasive handling of bleeding during neuroblastoma surgery is possible to a certain extent. The principles of managing intraoperative bleeding minimally-invasively contain ad hoc closure of the vessel with an atraumatic forceps, intermittent increase of the endoscopic pressure within the abdomen or thorax, and usage of a suction/irrigation system for correctly identifying the site of vascular injury. Definite bleeding control should be realized using clips or monofilament sutures. Plaited sutures should be avoided, since they are more traumatic and may cause additional injury to the vessels.

Another aspect concerns lymph node sampling (LNS). Despite the fact that the exact role of LNS during NB surgery has not been definitely clarified, a report from the US National Cancer Data Base observed that LN harvesting is carried out significantly more often during open surgery than during MIS in children with NB [4]. Since this fact has been described in other pediatric tumor entities as well, MIS seems to prove difficult for LN sampling during tumor surgery in children [22]. However, it is noteworthy that in NB, the different rates of LNS did not result in significantly different survival rates.

Despite sporadic reports on port site metastases after minimally-invasive oncologic surgery in children, this complication does not seem to be a general issue [23, 24]. Nevertheless, maximal care has to be taken considering removal of any tumor specimen from the respective cavity after minimally-invasive procedures.

19.1.4 Outlook

Current proceedings of MIS in NB are still developing. Technical equipment as well as new technologies are being constantly evolved, leading to a wider spectrum of applications for the minimally-invasive approach.

Radioguided localization of NB during laparoscopy has recently been described. Following tumor labeling with ^{123}I-MIBG, this technique uses a specifically designed gamma-probe and has been found to be valuable during NB resection. The authors propose this approach for conditions in which the loss of tactile sense during laparoscopy becomes imminent [25].

Robot-assisted MIS has been described as a technique for several procedures in children; initial case presentations and case series also reported on the use of this technique in children with solid tumors. In several analyses, the authors observed that adrenalectomies were among the most frequent robot-assisted tumor resections in children. Neuroblastoma/ganglioneuroma accounted for a relevant number of cases in the analyzed studies; however, overall numbers are still extremely low [26, 27]. The authors concluded that currently the status of robot-assisted MIS for pediatric solid tumors is rather static and that, by now, there are no apparent index procedures. However, there is an ongoing development of this technique in oncolocial surgery in adults and it remains to be observed how the evolution will further proceed in the pediatric age group.

19.2 Abdominal Neuroblastoma

19.2.1 Indications/Contraindications for MIS

19.2.1.1 Biopsies

Biopsies of abdominal NB/ganglineuroma are regularly being carried out using MIS. Apart from general conditions precluding the minimally invasive technique as such, there do not seem to be major contraindications for the use of this technique for biopsies. Generally, a sufficient quantity and quality of tumor material can be obtained for histological and biological analyses from both midline as well as adrenal NB. There are no reports on significant disadvantages when compared to the open surgical approach [28, 29].

19.2.1.2 Tumor Resections

The most appropriate indication for minimally invasive abdominal NB resection is an adrenal tumor without the presence of IDRF (Fig. 19.1). Most studies reporting on equal surgical and oncological outcomes as compared to open surgery, propose this subgroup of tumors as eligible for MIS [16, 30]. Abdominal NB resected minimally-invasively are commonly smaller than tumors resected by open surgery. However, so far there has not been a certain tumor size, which was generally postulated as a limit for minimally invasive resection. It should be taken into consideration that handling of the tumor should not compromise the safety during operation, especially with regard to the management of large vessels. In selected cases, successful minimally invasive resection can be performed in paravertebral cases or in the presence of IDRF as well [15]. However,

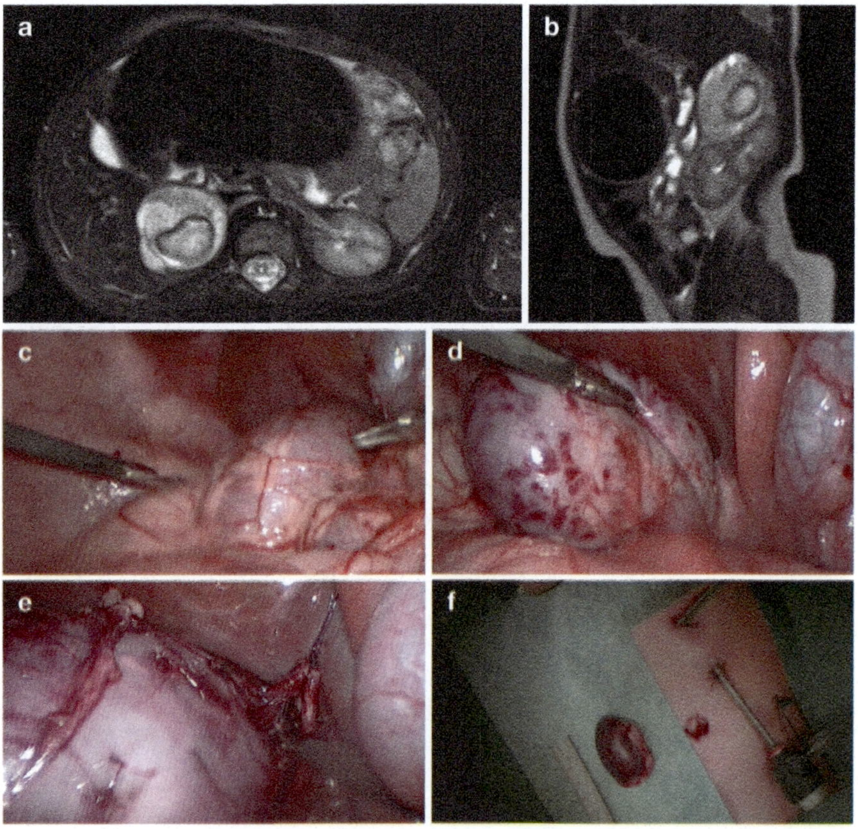

Fig. 19.1 Suprarenal right-sided neuroblastoma. (**a**, **b**) Preoperative MRI Scan. (**c**) Laparoscopic aspect of tumor before dissection. (**d**) Tumor dissection with mobilisation of the lower and lateral aspect. (**e**) Management of suprarenal vessels. (**f**) Trocar positions and tumor ante situ after complete resection

in these cases an exceptional expertise of the treating surgical team is essential in both fields: neroblastoma surgery and MIS. In general, contraindications for resection of NB using MIS comprise the presence of too complex IDRF with an expectable elevated risk for major surgical complications, lack of expertise of the operating surgeon, and the general contraindications for abdominal MIS in children and infants. In addition, MIS should be restrictively applied for tumor resection when an adrenocortical carcinoma (ACC) is suspected. Oncological outcome of ACC is poor, and even more so, when tumor spillage occurs during surgery. Therefore, a thorough preoperative assessment is essential for identifying this entity; the open resection has to be considered as surgical treatment of choice for ACC [6, 31, 32].

As in open surgery, decision making for minimally invasive resections of abdominal NB has to take the individual patient's conditions into account. General recommendations remain valid irrespective of the technical possibilities. Consequently, a patient stratified for observation should not undergo tumor resection just because there is a less invasive method of removing the tumor. On the other hand, in some instances, for example, in some cases of opsomyoclonus syndrome, MIS offers an elegant way of resecting tumors, which may be of little surgical challenge and would otherwise cause a large operative trauma when removed openly (Fig. 19.2). The definite decision when to apply MIS for resection of abdominal NB has to be made on an interdisciplinary platform, taking the above-mentioned aspects into consideration.

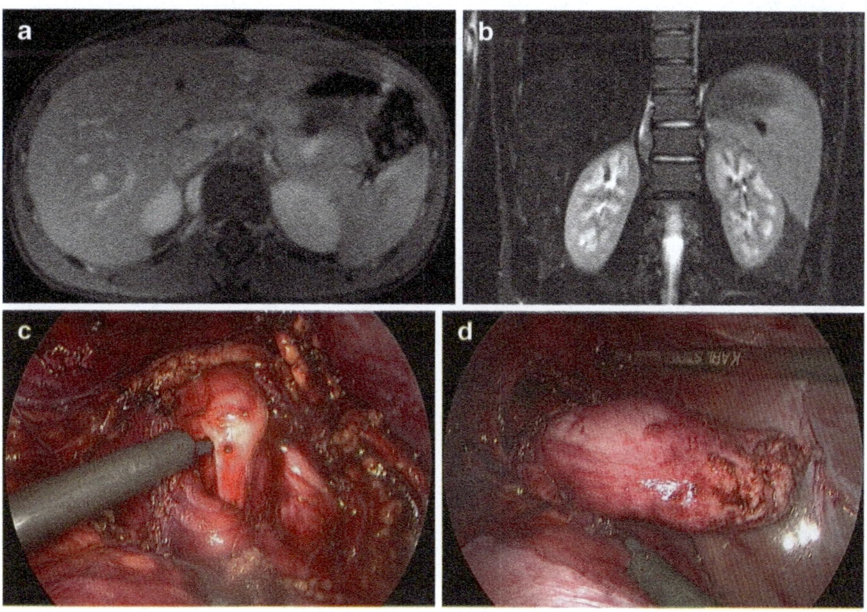

Fig. 19.2 Paravertebral right-sided abdominal neuroblastoma in a child with Opsomyoclonus Syndrome. (**a**, **b**) Preoperative MRI Scan. (**c**) Laparoscopic aspect of tumor and diaphragm during dissection. (**d**) Tumor mobilized before complete resection

19.2.2 Technical Aspects

Most authors prefer the laparoscopic approach for resecting adrenal NB minimally-invasively; however, the retroperitoneoscopic approach has also been described. Some analyses of the latter approach recommended a maximal tumor diameter of 4 cm as a limit for resection, whereas laparoscopic resections have also been reported for larger tumors. Provided there is sufficient expertise of the operating surgeon, both approaches seem to encounter no significant differences regarding surgical results and outcome. However, notably smaller patient numbers within the retroperitoneoscopic groups have to be taken into consideration in this regard [33–35].

Usually, three or four ports are used. Positioning of patients and placement of trocars are crucial for an optimal exposition of the operative field and should be thoroughly planned before surgery (Fig. 19.3). Retrieval of the tumors should be carried out using an abdominal bag. First choice for tumor removal from the abdominal cavity should be through one of the trocar orifices. Usually the subumbilical orifice is used, which can be enlarged and cosmetically reconstructed (Fig. 19.4). If this is not possible, an additional incision (most commonly Pfannenstiel incision) is necessary.

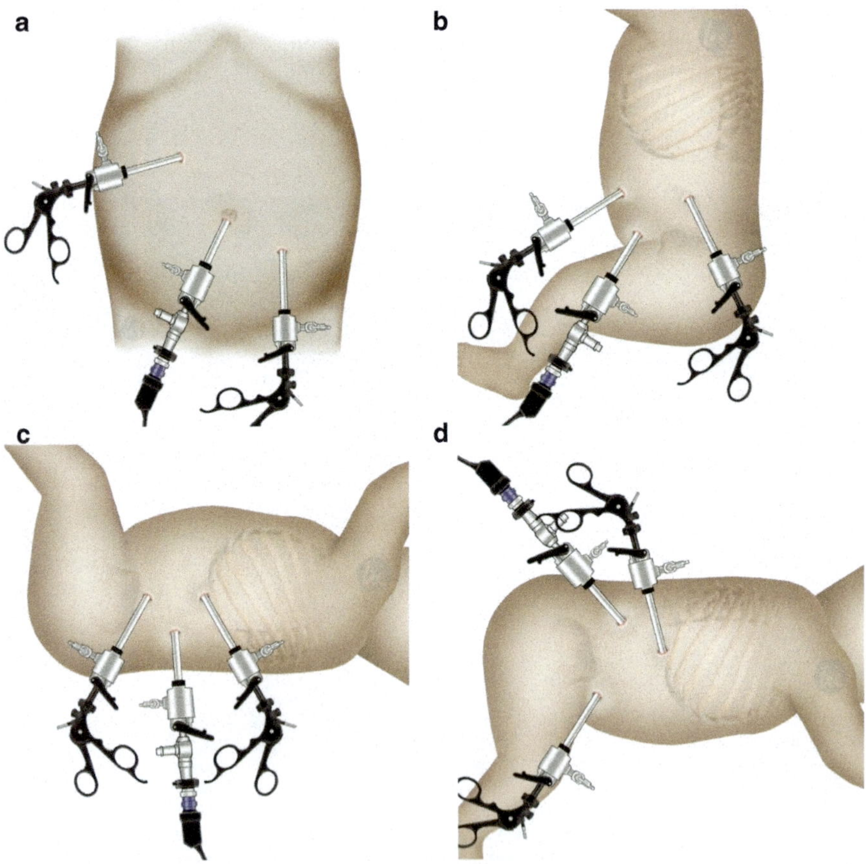

Fig. 19.3 Variation of patient positioning and trocar placement for surgery of a left-sided (**a-c**) or a right-sided (**d**) tumor: (**a**) Anterior laparoscopic, (**b**) Lateral laparoscopic, (**c**) Prone retroperitoneoscopic, (**d**) Lateral retroperitoneoscopic

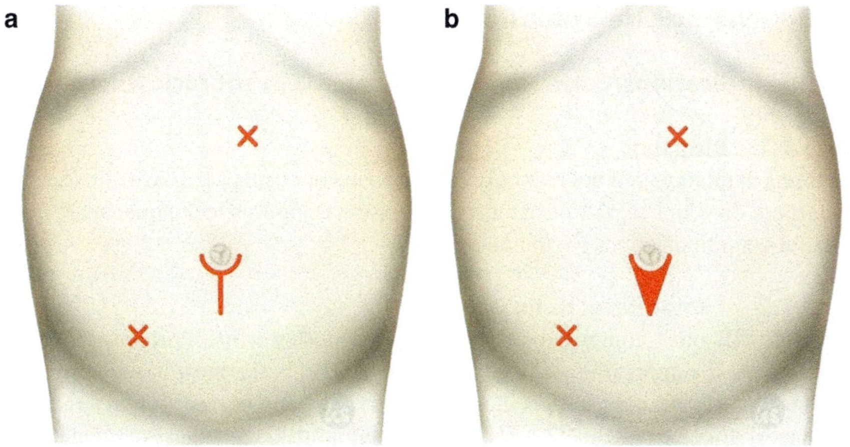

Fig. 19.4 Trocar placement and extension of the subumbilical access for surgery of a right-sided tumor. (**a**) Illustration of the subumbilical access for the camera port and two additional trocars. (**b**) Extension of the sub-umbilical access for retrieval of the tumor

Reports on resection of midline NB are rare [15, 35]. In this subgroup of NB patients, a higher rate of surgical complications, incomplete resections, and conversion to open surgery have been observed. Therefore, according to the considerations regarding IDRF and indications, MIS should be used reluctantly for resection of midline NB.

19.2.3 Complications

Typical complications of open NB surgery have also been reported for minimally-invasive procedures. Complication rates of minimally-invasive adrenal NB resections are comparable to those observed in open procedures [5, 30]. Precondition for achieving these results is a careful patient selection, together with experience and expertise of the surgical team.

19.2.4 Outcome

The oncological outcome of patients undergoing NB resection via MIS is comparable to those of open surgical procedures [5, 30, 35]. However, in this context, several aspects, possibly containing a relevant bias, have to be considered. NB undergoing MIS for resection are usually smaller than those removed by open surgery [28]. Furthermore, patients' cohorts are usually of unequal size with open surgery being by far more often performed; finally, NB patients undergoing minimally-invasive tumor resection are a highly selected subgroup, with favorable features concerning tumor characteristics and biology, as well as expertise of operating surgeons.

19.3 Thoracic Neuroblastoma

19.3.1 Indications/Contraindications for MIS in Thoracic NB

19.3.1.1 Biopsies

Biopsies in thoracic NB are regularly being carried out using MIS. As in abdominal NB, there does not seem to exist a restriction for using this technique, apart from general contraindications for thoracic MIS.

19.3.1.2 Tumor Resections

Thoracic NB most commonly occur within the posterior mediastinum [36]. For many of these tumors, the surgical resection represents the most important therapeutic step. Accordingly, MIS is increasingly used for tumor resection in a relevant number of affected patients [7, 15, 37]. As in abdominal NB, indications depend on localization and the conditions of IDRF. It seems noteworthy that localization within the lower mediastinum has to be regarded as IDRF, even in the absence of a vascular or bronchial affection [9].

In a relevant number of children suffering from Opsomyoclonus syndrome, a thoracic NB is the reason behind this neurologic condition (Fig. 19.5). Often, these tumors would not necessarily have to be removed for oncological reasons.

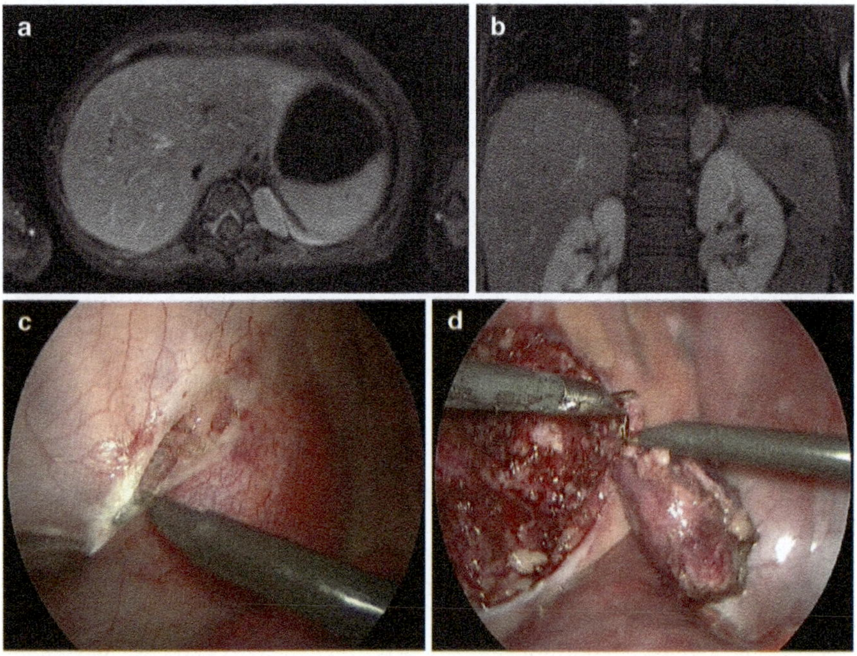

Fig. 19.5 Paravertebral left-sided thoracic neuroblastoma in a child with Opsomyoclonus Syndrome. (**a**, **b**) Preoperative MRI Scan. (**c**) Beginning of thoracoscopic tumor dissection with opening of the parietal pleura. (**d**) Tumor mobilized before complete resection

However, especially when conservative treatment measures did not bring an improvement, resection of these tumors might become necessary. In such cases, the minimally-invasive approach represents a good technique being associated with a comparably small operative trauma.

The proximity to the intervertebral nerve roots makes interdisciplinary operation planning necessary, including neurosurgical expertise in some cases. As in general, risk stratification of patients and biological characteristics of the tumors are especially important in these instances. Usually, it is not justified to risk major functional deficits during surgery; tumor resection should be limited by the level of the neuroforamina. In this regard, the surgical principles, as applied in open procedures, have to be also respected during MIS. Accordingly, lack of expertise with NB surgery or MIS represents an important contraindication for applying this technique in thoracic NB.

As in abdominal NB, the size of the tumors has to be critically assessed when considering minimally-invasive resection of a thoracic NB. On the one hand, handling of the tumors may lead to additional risks during surgery, especially with regard to the large vessels and mediastinal nerves; on the other hand, a sufficient opening of the thoracic wall has to be created for tumor removal. It is the responsibility of the operating surgeon to judge, up to what size the minimally-invasive resection of a thoracic NB is justified and reasonable.

19.3.2 Technical Aspects

The tumors most regularly occur in the posterior mediastinum. Therefore, children are positioned in a lateral decubitus or modified prone position. Three or four trocars are used for the procedures, their sizes varying between 3 and 10 mm, depending on the size of the patients. Trocars are placed forming a triangular shape, with the camera usually being positioned in the mid-axillary line. Especially during tumor resections, surgeons will benefit largely from contralateral single-lung ventilation. Collapse of the ipsilateral lung is achieved using a double-lumen endotracheal tube in older children as well as selective ipsilateral intubation or a bronchus blocker in smaller children. In infants, the intrathoracic pressure should be kept at moderate levels, since recent studies revealed relevant alterations of the cerebral conditions (namely, regional oxygen saturation, arterial $paCO_2$, and pH) during thoracoscopy with high intrathoracic CO_2 pressure [41].

Regularly, there is a covering pleural layer, which needs to be incised around the circumference of the lesions, usually using the monopolar hook. Further dissection can then be carried out releasing the tumor from its bed, especially taking care to manage intercostal, vertebral, and large mediastinal vessels (Fig. 19.6). Once fully mobilized, tumors can be retrieved in a plastic bag through an enlarged trocar site.

Special alertness is necessary in cases of tumors in the lower posterior mediastinum. These localizations possibly interfere with the course of the Adamkiewicz Artery. This vessel is usually located on the left side; however, it displays a wide

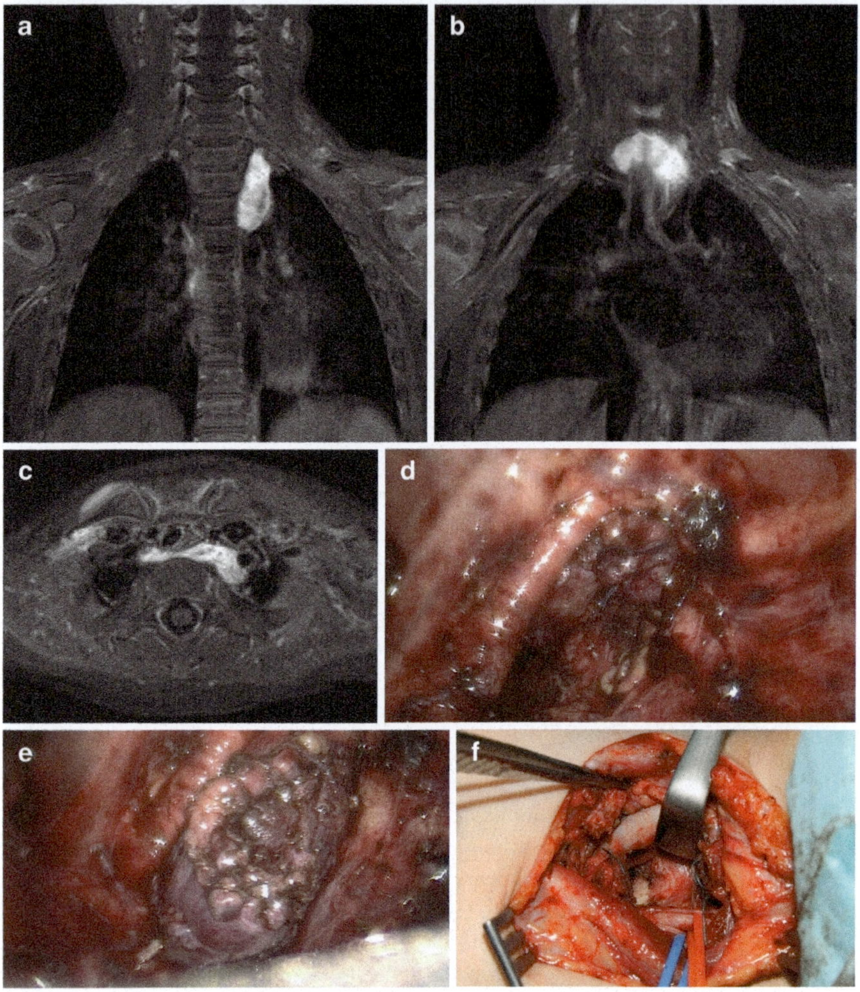

Fig. 19.6 Cervico-thoracic left-sided neuroblastoma in a child with Opsomyoclonus Syndrome. (**a-c**) Preoperative MRI Scan showing thoracic and cervical tumor compounds. (**d**) View during thoracoscopic tumor dissection; tumor released from the parietal Pleura. (**e**) End of thoracoscopic part; tumor transsected, tumor rest Marked with stitches. (**f**) Cervical tumor resectio: Tumot (Tu), Trachea (Tr), neuro-vascular bundle (NVB)

range of origin from T5-L2. Knowledge of its exact course and spatial relationship contributes to relevantly lower the risk for spinal injury during tumor resection. It can usually not be detected using standard cross-sectional imaging methods and therefore, an additional diagnostic workup (spinal angiography) should be considered in affected patients [38–41].

19.3.3 Complications

Reports on minimally-invasive resection of thoracic NB display complication rates and adverse events comparable to open procedures [7, 15, 42, 43]. Horner syndrome belongs to the most often-reported complications after this procedure. The Harlequin syndrome is a rare but notable complication after resection of neuroblastoma of the upper thorax, which is caused by a lesion to the sympathetic fibers and which is characterized by unilateral flushing and sweating of the face, neck, and upper chest. Horner and Harlequin Syndromes are sometimes seen in conjunction [44, 45].

However, the reason for the relatively low rate and severity of complications most likely is a careful patient selection together with a relevant expertise of operating surgeons.

19.3.4 Outcome

Comparative studies as well as retrospective analyses show that there is no difference in tumor recurrence, survival, or disease-free survival between open and minimally-invasive resections of thoracic NB [7, 15, 37, 43]. As in abdominal NB, a certain bias within the results can be postulated. Usually, surgeons performing MIS for thoracic NB are skilled in the minimally-invasive technique as well as in NB surgery. Furthermore, patients are usually selected with regard to age, tumor size, biology and histology, and other characteristics.

References

1. Holcomb GW 3rd, Tomita SS, Haase GM, Dillon PW, Newman KD, Applebaum H, et al. Minimally invasive surgery in children with cancer. Cancer. 1995;76:121–8.
2. Warmann S, Fuchs J, Jesch NK, Schrappe M, Ure BM. A prospective study of minimally invasive techniques in pediatric surgical oncology: preliminary report. Med Pediatr Oncol. 2003;40:155–7.
3. Yamamoto H, Yoshida M, Sera Y. Laparoscopic surgery for neuroblastoma identified by mass screening. J Pediatr Surg. 1996;31:385–8.
4. Ezekian B, Englum BR, Gulack BC, Rialon KL, Kim J, Talbot LJ, et al. Comparing oncologic outcomes after minimally invasive and open surgery for pediatric neuroblastoma and Wilms tumor. Pediatr Blood Cancer. 2018; https://doi.org/10.1002/pbc.26755.
5. Kelleher CM, Smithson L, Nguyen LL, Casadiego G, Nasr A, Irwin MS, et al. Clinical outcomes in children with adrenal neuroblastoma undergoing open versus laparoscopic adrenalectomy. J Pediatr Surg. 2013;48:1727–32.
6. Mir MC, Klink JC, Guillotreau J, Long JA, Miocinovic R, Kaouk JH, et al. Comparative outcomes of laparoscopic and open adrenalectomy for adrenocortical carcinoma: single, high-volume center experience. Ann Surg Oncol. 2013;20:1456–61.
7. Malek MM, Mollen KP, Kane TD, Shah SR, Irwin C. Thoracic neuroblastoma: a retrospective review of our institutional experience with comparison of the thoracoscopic and open approaches to resection. J Pediatr Surg. 2010;45:1622–6.
8. Boutros J, Bond M, Beaudry P, Blair GK, Skarsgard ED. Case selection in minimally invasive surgical treatment of neuroblastoma. Pediatr Surg Int. 2008;24:1177–80.

9. Monclair T, Mosseri V, Cecchetto G, De Bernardi B, Michon J, Holmes K. Influence of image-defined risk factors on the outcome of patients with localised neuroblastoma. A report from the LNESG1 study of the European International Society of Paediatric Oncology Neuroblastoma Group. Pediatr Blood Cancer. 2015;62:1536–42.
10. von Allmen D, Davidoff AM, London WB, Van Ryn C, Haas-Kogan DA, Kreissman SG, et al. Impact of extent of resection on local control and survival in patients from the COG A3973 study with high-risk neuroblastoma. J Clin Oncol. 2017;35:208–16.
11. Rich BS, McEvoy MP, LaQuaglia MP, Wolden SL. Local control, survival, and operative morbidity and mortality after re-resection, and intraoperative radiation therapy for recurrent or persistent primary high-risk neuroblastoma. J Pediatr Surg. 2011;46:97–102.
12. La Quaglia MP, Kushner BH, Su W, Heller G, Kramer K, Abramson S, et al. The impact of gross total resection on local control and survival in high-risk neuroblastoma. J Pediatr Surg. 2004;39:412–7.
13. Shirota C, Tainaka T, Uchida H, Hinoki A, Chiba K, Tanaka Y. Laparoscopic resection of neuroblastomas in low- to high-risk patients without image-defined risk factors is safe and feasible. BMC Pediatr. 2017;17:71.
14. Tanaka Y, Kawashima H, Mori M, Fujiogi M, Suzuki K, Amano H, et al. Contraindications and image-defined risk factors in laparoscopic resection of abdominal neuroblastoma. Pediatr Surg Int. 2016;32:845–50.
15. Irtan S, Brisse HJ, Minard-Colin V, Schleiermacher G, Canale S, Sarnacki S. Minimally invasive surgery of neuroblastic tumors in children: indications depend on anatomical location and image-defined risk factors. Pediatr Blood Cancer. 2015;62:257–61.
16. Mattioli G, Avanzini S, Pini Prato A, Pio L, Granata C, Garaventa A, Conte M, et al. Laparoscopic resection of adrenal neuroblastoma without image-defined risk factors: a prospective study on 21 consecutive pediatric patients. Pediatr Surg Int. 2014;30:387–94.
17. Avanzini S, Pio L, Erminio G, Granata C, Holmes K, Gambart M, et al. Image-defined risk factors in unresectable neuroblastoma: SIOPEN study on incidence, chemotherapy-induced variation, and impact on surgical outcomes. Pediatr Blood Cancer. 2017; https://doi.org/10.1002/pbc.26605.
18. Neubauer H, Li M, Müller VR, Pabst T, Beer M. Diagnostic value of diffusion-weighted MRI for tumor characterization, differentiation and monitoring in pediatric patients with neuroblastic tumors. Rofo. 2017;189:640–50.
19. Serin HI, Gorkem SB, Doganay S, Cıracı S, Unal E, Guzel M, et al. Diffusion weighted imaging in differentiating malignant and benign neuroblastic tumors. Jpn J Radiol. 2016;34(9):620–4.
20. Demir S, Altinkaya N, Kocer NE, Erbay A, Oguzkurt P. Variations in apparent diffusion coefficient values following chemotherapy in pediatric neuroblastoma. Diagn Interv Radiol. 2015;21:184–8.
21. Oberthür A, Berthold F, Hero B, Till H. Neuroblastoma. In: Fuchs, editor. Solide Tumoren im Kindesalter. Stuttgert: Schattauer; 2012. p. 77–110.
22. Warmann SW, Godzinski J, van Tinteren H, Heij H, Powis M, Sandstedt B, et al. Minimally invasive nephrectomy for Wilms tumors in children – data from SIOP 2001. J Pediatr Surg. 2014;49:1544–8.
23. Pentek F, Schulte JH, Schweiger B, Metzelder M, Schündeln MM. Development of port-site metastases following thoracoscopic resection of a neuroblastoma. Pediatr Blood Cancer. 2016;63:149–51.
24. Metzelder M, Ure B. Port-site metastasis after laparoscopic biopsy of a posttransplant Burkitt lymphoma in a child. Eur J Pediatr Surg. 2009;19:126–7.
25. Hishiki T, Saito T, Terui K, Mitsunaga T, Nakata M, Hayashi H, et al. Radioguided localization of neuroblastomas in laparoscopic surgery using (123)I- radiolabeled metaiodobenzylguanidine. Pediatr Blood Cancer. 2015;62:1297–9.
26. Uwaydah NI, Jones A, Elkaissi M, Yu Z, Palmer BW. Pediatric robot-assisted laparoscopic radical adrenalectomy and lymph-node dissection for neuroblastoma in a 15-month-old. J Robot Surg. 2014;8:289–93.

27. Cundy TP, Marcus HJ, Clark J, Hughes-Hallett A, Mayer EK, Najmaldin AS, et al. Robot-assisted minimally invasive surgery for pediatric solid tumors: a systematic review of feasibility and current status. Eur J Pediatr Surg. 2014;24:127–35.
28. Fuchs J. The role of minimally invasive surgery in pediatric solid tumors. Pediatr Surg Int. 2015;31:213–28.
29. Fuchs J, Schafbuch L, Ebinger M, Schäfer JF, Seitz G, Warmann SW. Minimally invasive surgery for pediatric tumors – current state of the art. Front Pediatr. 2014;2:48.
30. Fascetti-Leon F, Scotton G, Pio L, Beltrà R, Caione P, Esposito C, et al. Minimally invasive resection of adrenal masses in infants and children: results of a European multi-center survey. Surg Endosc. 2017;31:4505–12.
31. Hubertus J, Boxberger N, Redlich A, von Schweinitz D, Vorwerk P. Surgical aspects in the treatment of adrenocortical carcinomas in children: data of the GPOH-MET 97 trial. Klin Padiatr. 2012;224:143–7.
32. Miller BS, Ammori JB, Gauger PG, Broome JT, Hammer GD, Doherty GM. Laparoscopic resection is inappropriate in patients with known or suspected adrenocortical carcinoma. World J Surg. 2010;34:1380–5.
33. Theilen TM, Paran TS, Rutigliano D, Wexler L, Sonoda Y, LaQuaglia MP. Experience with retroperitoneoscopy in pediatric surgical oncology. Surg Endosc. 2011;25:2748–55.
34. Kouch K, Yoshida H, Matsunaga T, Ohtsuka Y, Okada T, Saito T, et al. Extirpation of mass-screened adrenal neuroblastomas by retroperitoneoscopy. Surg Endosc. 2003;17:1769–72.
35. Leclair MD, de Lagausie P, Becmeur F, Varlet F, Thomas C, Valla JS, et al. Laparoscopic resection of abdominal neuroblastoma. Ann Surg Oncol. 2008;15:117–24.
36. Warmann SW, Fuchs J. Mediastinal tumors. In: Fuchs, editor. Solide Tumoren im Kindesalter. Stuttgert: Schattauer; 2012. p. 69–76.
37. Lacreuse I, Valla JS, de Lagausie P, Varlet F, Héloury Y, Temporal G, et al. Thoracoscopic resection of neurogenic tumors in children. J Pediatr Surg. 2007;42:1725–8.
38. Neunhoeffer F, Warmann SW, Hofbeck M, Müller A, Fideler F, Seitz G, et al. Elevated intrathoracic CO2 pressure during thoracoscopic surgery decreases regional cerebral oxygen saturation in neonates and infants—a pilot study. Paediatr Anaesth. 2017;27:752–9.
39. Guziński M, Bryl M, Ziemińska K, Wolny K, Sąsiadek M, Garcarek JS. Detection of the Adamkiewicz artery in computed tomography of the thorax and abdomen. Adv Clin Exp Med. 2017;26:31–7.
40. Nordin AB, Fallon SC, Jea A, Kim ES. The use of spinal angiography in the management of posterior mediastinal tumors: case series and review of the literature. J Pediatr Surg. 2013;48:1871–7.
41. Boglino C, Martins AG, Ciprandi G, Sousinha M, Inserra A. Spinal cord vascular injuries following surgery of advanced thoracic neuroblastoma: an unusual catastrophic complication. Med Pediatr Oncol. 1999;32:349–52.
42. Fraga JC, Rothenberg S, Kiely E, Pierro A. Video-assisted thoracic surgery resection for pediatric mediastinal neurogenic tumors. J Pediatr Surg. 2012;47:1349–53.
43. Petty JK, Bensard DD, Partrick DA, Hendrickson RJ, Albano EA, Karrer FM. Resection of neurogenic tumors in children: is thoracoscopy superior to thoracotomy? J Am Coll Surg. 2006;203:699–703.
44. Irtan S, Auvrignon A. Harlequin syndrome after stellate ganglia neuroblastoma resection. J Pediatr. 2016;176:215.
45. Burlacu CL, Buggy DJ. Coexisting harlequin and Horner syndromes after high thoracic paravertebral anaesthesia. Br J Anaesth. 2005;95:822–4.

Robotic Surgery for Neuroblastoma 20

Luca Pio, Thomas Blanc, Girolamo Mattioli, Yves Heloury, and Sabine Sarnacki

In the last 20 years, minimally invasive surgery (MIS) has been introduced in the treatment of pediatric solid tumors [1–3]. The main indications are certainly neuroectodermic tumors, as this type of tumor could be fragmented without fearing peritoneal or thoracic spillage and/or port site engraftment [4]. This feature allows cutting the specimen in the bag before retrieval, avoiding an additional subpubic incision as it is mandatory in laparoscopic nephrectomy for Wilms tumor [5]. Most of the work describes the application of MIS for adrenal and paravertebral locations of NB [6–15]. Since the introduction of Image-Defined Risk Factors (IDRFs) [16], it has been widely accepted that MIS could be applied to NB without IDRFs and to tumors not exceeding a size larger than 5 cm in adrenal locations.

When considering the list of IDRFs [16], which could be related to the NB origin according to sympathetic anatomy [17], the most risky ones are certainly the encasement of superior mesenteric artery and coeliac axis. These tumors are usually high-risk NB, stage M and/or MYCN amplified, and these IDRFs remain usually the same despite induction chemotherapy [18, 19]. Open surgery remains a challenge for these perivascular locations and they are certainly an indubitable contraindication for any kind of MIS. NB of the stellate ganglia remains also a

L. Pio (✉) · T. Blanc · S. Sarnacki
Department Pediatric Surgery, Necker - Enfants Malades Hospital, Assistance Publique Hopitaux de Paris, Paris, France

University of Paris, Paris, France

G. Mattioli
Pediatric Surgery Department, Giannina Gaslini Research Institute, Genoa, Italy

Department of Neurosciences, Rehabilitation, Ophthalmology, Genetics, Maternal and Child Health (DINOGMI), University of Genoa, Genoa, Italy

Y. Heloury
Urology Department, Royal Children's Hospital, Parkville, VIC, Australia

Department of Pediatric Surgery and Urology, APHP Hôpital Necker-Enfants Malaldes, University of Paris, Paris, France

S. Sarnacki, L. Pio (eds.), *Neuroblastoma*,
https://doi.org/10.1007/978-3-030-18396-7_20

challenge in open surgery and is not suitable for MIS. Other vascular or nervous IDRFs may, however, be relative contraindications for MIS provided the vision and dissection could be improved by robotic assistance. This is the case of contact with renal vessels, aorta, or vena cava in the abdomen, contact with aorta and/or lower left paravertebral site in the thorax and presacral lesions in the pelvis.

Robotic-assisted resection of malignant tumors must follow the same oncologic principles than those applied to open and/or MIS surgery. In the case of neuroectodermic tumors, the completeness of resection is of utmost importance in low and intermediate tumors [20] and certainly plays an important role in high-risk tumors, although this is still widely debated [21].

In 2012, Meehan described the principles of the robotic approach in pediatric oncology [22]. He underlined the importance of patient positioning and trocars placement according to the tumor location in order to maximize the tumor exposure, while avoiding robotic arms collisions. It was also reported that, like in adult experience with robotic surgery [23, 24], the lack of tactile feedback was compensated by the 3D visualization offered by the robot (Figs. 20.1–20.4). Finally, robotics offer an

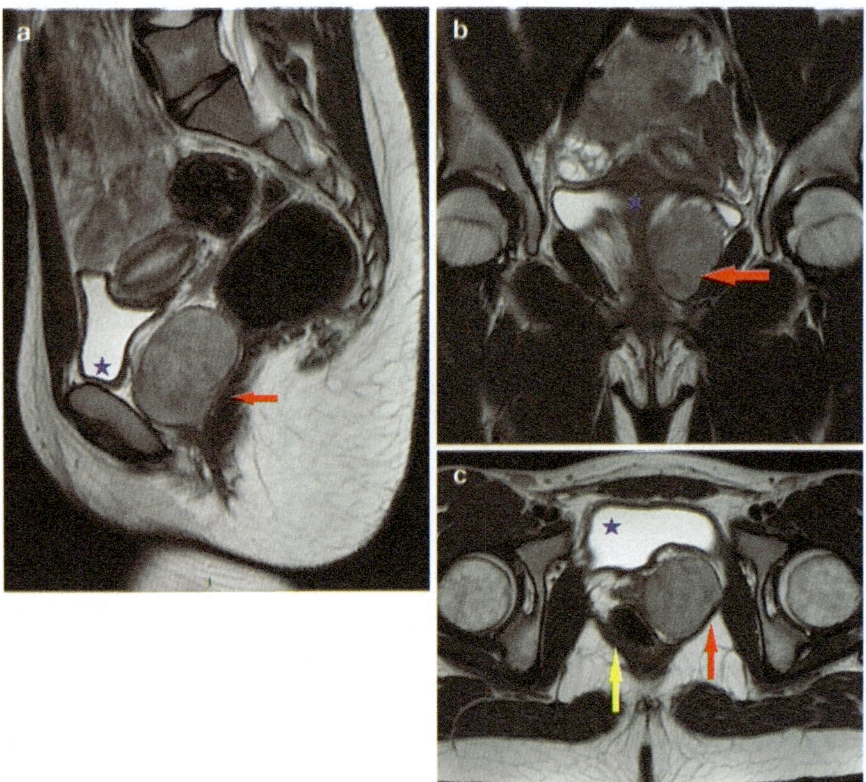

Fig. 20.1 Magnetic resonance findings of a pelvic paravaginal ganglioneuroma: (**a**) Coronal section, star: bladder, red narrow: neuroblastic tumor; (**b**) coronal section, star: uterus, red narrow: neuroblastic tumor; (**c**) axial section, star: bladder, red narrow: neuroblastic tumor, yellow narrow: rectum

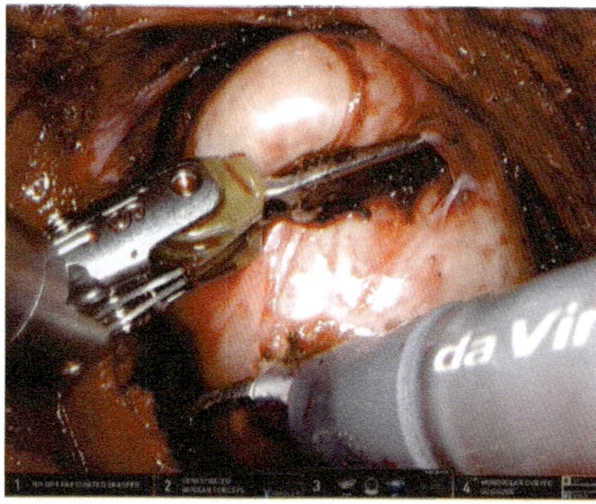

Fig. 20.2 3D image magnification of a pelvic ganglioneuroma

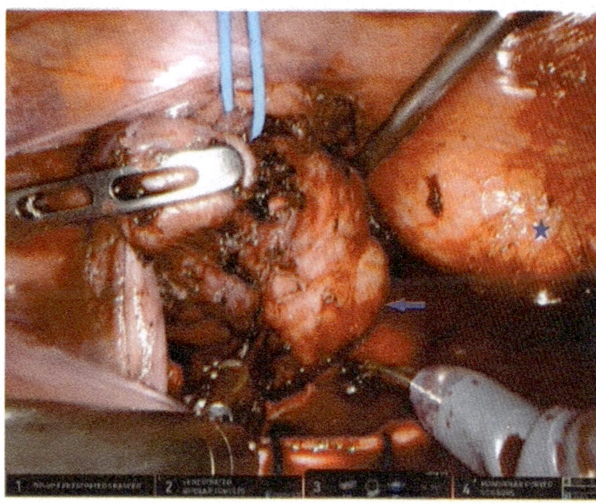

Fig. 20.3 Mobilization of the ganglioneuroma with a robotic grasper, dissection with a robotic monopolar scissor and hemostatic control with robotic bipolar forceps. Star: uterus; narrow: neuroblastic tumor

improvement on surgeon ergonomics (Fig. 20.5), which allows a more precise dissection and easy intracorporeal knotting, which may be required in case of vessel bleeding during tumor dissection.

Less than 30 cases of robotically-assisted NB resection have been currently reported in the literature. The first cases were reported by Meehan in 2008, with two thoracic neuroblastic tumors (one ganglioneuroma and one ganglioneuroblastoma) and three adrenal NB, one of which required conversion. No data were reported about tumor stage and IDRFs presence\absence [22]. Six years later, Uwaydah reported a successful resection of an adrenal NB without IDRFs by a robotic approach [25].

In 2017, Mattioli described his preliminary series of pediatric robotic-assisted procedures, including five neuroblastomas (one thoracic and four adrenal). One conversion to a laparoscopic procedure was reported for an adrenal NB with IDRFs [26].

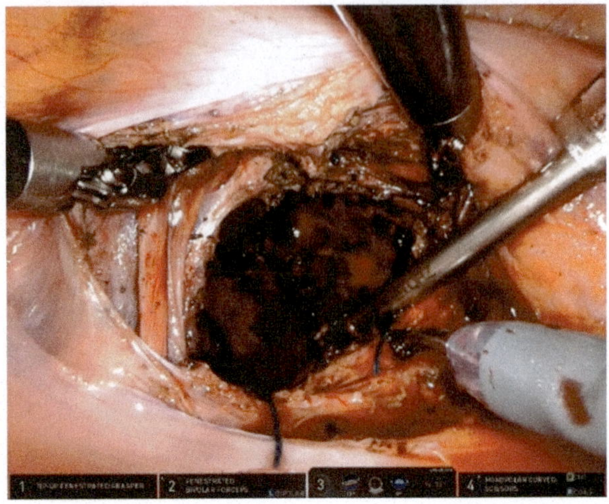

Fig. 20.4 Pelvic anatomy after ganglioneuroma removal

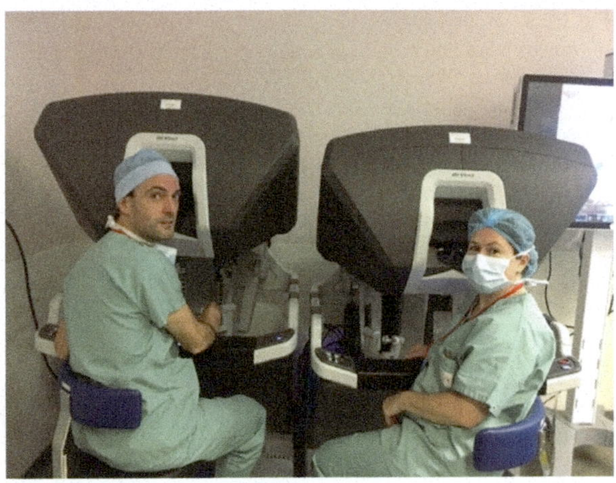

Fig. 20.5 Robotic double console setting

More recently, Meignan et al. [27] reported their experience in robotic-assisted resection of children's solid tumors. The series included 9 adrenal NB over 12 procedures with an R0 resection and no intraoperative complications. Our personal experience of 164 cases of robotic-assisted surgery over 23 months comprised six neuroectodermic tumors out of 41 solid tumors (personal communication). The add-value of robotics when compared to classical laparoscopic surgery was demonstrative in presacral and pelvic lesions, as well as in paravertebral NB extending in the intercostal spaces. Patients were discharged within 48 h.

One of the main limitations of robotic surgery is, first of all, the high cost of the equipment and maintenance and the need of specific training, with a learning curve that is, however, reduced when compared to classical MIS. Robotic-assisted surgery will certainly develop in the next years for pediatric cancers and may be of great interest in some locations of NB, where classical endoscopy has reached its limits.

20.1 Conclusions

To date, few data are available regarding indications and feasibility of the robotic approach for pediatric solid tumors. NB are good candidates, as tumors may be fragmented without jeopardizing the patient's outcome. Some advantages of robotic surgery compared to conventional MIS is 3D visualization, increased maneuverability allowing intracorporeal knotting, and adequate exposure may potentially extend the indication for NB surgery to tumors presenting with specific IDRFs, while ensuring security and carcinologic resection.

References

1. Holcomb GW 3rd, Tomita SS, Haase GM, et al. Minimally invasive surgery in children with cancer. Cancer. 1995;76:121–8.
2. Iwanaka T, Arai M, Kawashima H, et al. Endosurgical procedures for pediatric solid tumors. Pediatr Surg Int. 2004;20:39–42.
3. Saenz NC, Conlon KC, Aronson DC, LaQuaglia MP. The application of minimal access procedures in infants, children, and young adults with pediatric malignancies. J Laparoendosc Adv Surg Tech A. 1997;7:289–94.
4. Kelleher CM, Smithson L, Nguyen LL, Casadiego G, Nasr A, Irwin MS, Gerstle JT. Clinical outcomes in children with adrenal neuroblastoma undergoing open versus laparoscopic adrenalectomy. J Pediatr Surg. 2013;48(8):1727–32.
5. Bouty A, Burnand K, Nightingale M, Roberts A, Campbell M, O'Brien M, Heloury Y. What is the risk of local recurrence after laparoscopic transperitoneal radical nephrectomy in children with Wilms tumours? Analysis of a local series and review of the literature. J Pediatr Urol. 2018. Apr 12. pii: S1477–5131(18)30158-X.
6. Fraga JC, Rothenberg S, Kiely E, Pierro A. Video-assisted thoracic surgery resection for pediatric mediastinal neurogenic tumors. J Pediatr Surg. 2012;47(7):1349–53.
7. Peycelon M, Audry G, Irtan S. Minimally invasive surgery in childhood cancer: a challenging future. Eur J Pediatr Surg. 2014;24:443–9.
8. Cundy TP, Marcus HJ, Clark J, Hughes-Hallett A, Mayer EK, Najmaldin AS, Yang GZ, Darzi A. Robot-assisted minimally invasive surgery for pediatric solid tumors: a systematic review of feasibility and current status. Eur J Pediatr Surg. 2014;24:127–35.
9. De Lagausie P, Berrebi D, Michon J, et al. Laparoscopic adrenal surgery for neuroblastomas in children. J Urol. 2003;170:932–5.
10. Heloury Y, Muthucumaru M, Panabokke G, Cheng W, Kimber C, Leclair MD. Minimally invasive adrenalectomy in children. J Pediatr Surg. 2012;47(2):415–21.
11. Leclair MD, de Lagausie P, Becmeur F, et al. Laparoscopic resection of abdominal neuroblastoma. Ann Surg Oncol. 2008;15(1):117–24.
12. Theilen TM, Paran TS, Rutigliano D, Wexler L, Sonoda Y, LaQuaglia MP. Experience with retroperitoneoscopy in pediatric surgical oncology. Surg Endosc. 2011;25(8):2748–55.
13. Irtan S, Brisse HJ, Minard-Colin V, Schleiermacher G, Canale S, Sarnacki S. Minimally invasive surgery of neuroblastic tumors in children: indications depend on anatomical location and image-defined risk factors. Pediatr Blood Cancer. 2014;62(2):257–61. [Epub ahead of print].
14. Mattioli G, Avanzini S, Pini Prato A, Pio L, Granata C, Garaventa A, Conte M, Manzitti C, Montobbio G, Buffa P. Laparoscopic resection of adrenal neuroblastoma without image-defined risk factors: a prospective study on 21 consecutive pediatric patients. Pediatr Surg Int. 2014;30(4):387–94.
15. Kiely E. A technique for excision of abdominal and pelvic neuroblastomas. Ann R Coll Surg Engl. 2007;89(4):342–8.

16. Brisse HJ, McCarville MB, Granata C, Krug KB, Wootton-Gorges SL, Kanegawa K, Giammarile F, Schmidt M, Shulkin BL, Matthay KK, Lewington VJ, Sarnacki S, Hero B, Kaneko M, London WB, Pearson AD, Cohn SL, Monclair T, International Neuroblastoma Risk Group Project. Guidelines for imaging and staging of neuroblastic tumors: consensus report from the international Neuroblastoma Risk Group Project. Radiology. 2011;261(1):243–57.
17. Brisse HJ, Blanc T, Schleiermacher G, Mosseri V, Philippe-Chomette P, Janoueix-Lerosey I, Pierron G, Lapouble E, Peuchmaur M, Fréneaux P, Galmiche L, Algret N, Peycelon M, Michon J, Delattre O. Radiogenomics of neuroblastomas: relationships between imaging phenotypes, tumor genomic profile and survival. PLoS One. 2017;12(9):e0185190.
18. Irtan S, Brisse HJ, Minard-Colin V, Schleiermacher G, Galmiche-Rolland L, Le Cossec C, Elie C, Canale S, Michon J, Valteau-Couanet D, Sarnacki S. Image-defined risk factor assessment of neurogenic tumors after neoadjuvant chemotherapy is useful for predicting intra-operative risk factors and the completeness of resection. Pediatr Blood Cancer. 2015;62(9):1543–9.
19. Avanzini S, Pio L, Erminio G, Granata C, Holmes K, Gambart M, Buffa P, Castel V, Valteau Couanet D, Garaventa A, Pistorio A, Cecchetto G, Martucciello G, Mattioli G, Sarnacki S. Image-defined risk factors in unresectable neuroblastoma: SIOPEN study on incidence, chemotherapy-induced variation, and impact on surgical outcomes. Pediatr Blood Cancer. 2017;64(11) https://doi.org/10.1002/pbc.26605.
20. Murphy JM, La Quaglia MP. Advances in the surgical treatment of neuroblastoma: a review. Eur J Pediatr Surg. 2014;24(6):450–6.
21. von Allmen D, Davidoff AM, London WB, Van Ryn C, Haas-Kogan DA, Kreissman SG, Khanna G, Rosen N, Park JR, La Quaglia MP. Impact of extent of resection on local control and survival in patients from the COG A3973 study with high-risk neuroblastoma. J Clin Oncol. 2017;35(2):208–16.
22. Meehan JJ, Sandler A. Pediatric robotic surgery: a single-institutional review of the first 100 consecutive cases. Surg Endosc. 2008;22(1):177–82.
23. Martell J, Elmer T, Gopalsami N, Park YS. Visual measurement of suture strain for robotic surgery. Comput Math Methods Med. 2011;2011:879086.
24. Stitzenberg KB, Wong YN, Nielsen ME, Egleston BL, Uzzo RG. Trends in radical prostatectomy: centralization, robotics, and access to urologic cancer care. Cancer. 2012;118(1):54–62.
25. Uwaydah NI, Jones A, Elkaissi M, Yu Z, Palmer BW. Pediatric robot-assisted laparoscopic radical adrenalectomy and lymph-node dissection for neuroblastoma in a 15-month-old. J Robot Surg. 2014;8(3):289–93.
26. Mattioli G, Pini Prato A, Razore B, Leonelli L, Pio L, Avanzini S, Boscarelli A, Barabino P, Disma NM, Zanaboni C, Garzi A, Martigli SP, Buffi NM, Rosati U, Petralia P. Da Vinci robotic surgery in a pediatric hospital. J Laparoendosc Adv Surg Tech A. 2017;27(5):539–45.
27. Meignan P, Ballouhey Q, Lejeune J, Braik K, Longis B, Cook AR, Lardy H, Fourcade L, Binet A. Robotic-assisted laparoscopic surgery for pediatric tumors: a bicenter experience. J Robot Surg. 2018;12(3):501–8.

Complications of the Surgical Management of Children with Neuroblastoma

21

Andrew M. Davidoff

Survival for children with cancer has increased significantly over the past 50 years from an overall survival of 10% to nearly 90% currently. With this improvement in survival has come the recognition of therapy-related complications; significant long-term morbidity associated with therapy for childhood cancer has become increasingly appreciated as increasing numbers of children with cancer are becoming long-term survivors [1]. This, in turn, has led to an effort to minimize the morbidity, both acute and long term, from therapeutic interventions, including surgical procedures, while maintaining a high likelihood of cure. Surgery plays a critical role in the management of pediatric patients with cancer, particularly those with solid tumors. Yet it can contribute to the short term and chronic morbidity of therapy. Thus, an appreciation for the potential complications of surgery, both acute and long term, is critical when considering the risks and benefits of any procedure performed on a child with cancer.

Neuroblastoma is the most common extracranial solid tumor in children. Surgery plays a critical role in the treatment of these patients but surgery for neuroblastoma is also associated with a number of significant acute and long-term complications [2]. Complete resection of a localized neuroblastoma with favorable biology offers definitive therapy with generally excellent outcome, although the value of complete tumor removal may be overestimated because of the possibility that localized neuroblastomas may not require any therapy, including resection. The role of surgery is even less clear in the curative treatment of patients with high-risk, metastatic neuroblastoma [3], although a recent review of the COG experience suggests that ≥90% resection of the primary and regional disease is associated with significantly better event-free survival and a lower cumulative incidence of local progression [4]. However, overall survival in this study was not significantly impacted. Additionally, it has long been recognized that neuroblastoma resection, in part because of its frequently infiltrative growth pattern in young patients, can be associated with a high

A. M. Davidoff (✉)
Department of Surgery, St. Jude Children's Research Hospital, Memphis, TN, USA
e-mail: andrew.davidoff@stjude.org

S. Sarnacki, L. Pio (eds.), *Neuroblastoma*,
https://doi.org/10.1007/978-3-030-18396-7_21

complication rate [5–10]. Thus, it is crucial that surgeons consider the heterogeneous nature of neuroblastoma, and the molecular and biologic characteristics associated with good or bad prognoses, as well as the potential complications associated with neuroblastoma resection, when determining the role of surgery in any specific case [11]. An illustrative example is the very favorable overall outcome for infants with metastatic, single-copy *MYCN* disease, regardless of the extent of surgery, and the high risk of complications for infants undergoing major operations [12]. Clearly, the excellent prognosis for these patients should not be jeopardized by overly aggressive surgery that may lead to significant morbidity or even mortality.

Here we review the most common and significant surgical complications (Table 21.1) that occur with different operations for neuroblastoma. Generic

Table 21.1 Surgical complications

Surgical complications
Vascular complications
Hemorrhage
Need for vascular reconstruction
End-organ ischemia
Neurologic complications
Cord compression from intraspinal hematoma
Cord ischemia from interruption of artery of Adamkiewicz
Horner syndrome
Diaphragm paralysis
Sciatic nerve palsy
Urinary and/or fecal incontinence
Neurogenic bladder
Erectile dysfunction
Leg weakness
Solid organ complications
Enterotomy
Cystotomy
Renal loss
Atrophy
Renal artery spasm
Renal vein thrombosis
Nephrectomy
Ureteral injury
Compartment syndrome
Biliary complications
Bile leak
Bile duct stricture
Lymphatic complications
Chylothorax
Chylous ascites
Gastrointestinal complications
Diarrhea
Bowel obstruction
Intussusception
Adhesive
Musculoskeletal complications
Scoliosis

complications such as bleeding, infection, poor wound healing, and complications related to anesthesia will not be discussed in detail here.

21.1 Image-Defined Risk Factors

One way to anticipate the likelihood of complications following surgical resection of neuroblastoma is by assessing the presence or absence of image-defined surgical risk factors (IDRFs) on preoperative imaging. IDRFs are listed in Table 21.2 and generally reflect encasement of vital structures, primarily vessels and nerves, as determined by diagnostic imaging studies. Cecchetto et al. reported that the presence of one or more of these image-defined surgical risk

Table 21.2 Image-defined risk factors

Anatomic region	Description
Multiple body compartments	Ipsilateral tumor extension within two body compartments (i.e., neck and chest, chest and abdomen, or abdomen and pelvis)
Neck	Tumor encasing carotid artery, vertebral artery, and/or internal jugular vein
	Tumor extending to skull base
	Tumor compressing trachea
Cervicothoracic junction	Tumor encasing brachial plexus roots
	Tumor encasing subclavian vessels, vertebral artery, and/or carotid artery
	Tumor compressing trachea
Thorax	Tumor encasing aorta and/or major branches
	Tumor compressing trachea and/or principal bronchi
	Lower mediastinal tumor infiltrating costovertebral junction between T9 and T12 (may involve the artery of Adamkiewicz supplying the lower spinal cord)
Thoracoabdominal junction	Tumor encasing aorta and/or vena cava
Abdomen and pelvis	Tumor infiltrating porta hepatis and/or hepatoduodenal ligament
	Tumor encasing branches of superior mesenteric artery at mesenteric root
	Tumor encasing origin of celiac axis and/or origin of superior mesenteric artery
	Tumor invading one or both renal pedicles
	Tumor encasing aorta and/or vena cava
	Tumor encasing iliac vessels
	Pelvic tumor crossing sciatic notch
Intraspinal tumor extension	Intraspinal tumor extension (whatever the location) provided that more than one-third of spinal canal in axial plane is invaded, the perimedullary leptomeningeal spaces are not visible, or the spinal cord signal intensity is abnormal
Infiltration of adjacent organs and structures	Pericardium, diaphragm, kidney, liver, duodenopancreatic block, and mesentery

Adapted from: Monclair T, Brodeur GM, Ambros PF, et al. The International Neuroblastoma Risk Group (INRG) staging system: an INRG Task Force report. J Clin Oncol 2009; 27(2): 298–303 factors was associated with a greater risk of surgery-related complications and a lower complete resection rate, when attempting an initial resection of a localized neuroblastoma [13]. In 534 patients with localized, non-MYCN-amplified neuroblastomas studied, there was a 17% operative complication rate in patients with one or more IDRFs (L2), a rate significantly higher than the 5% incidence in patients without an IDRF (L1). In addition, surgery-related complications occurred more often in the neck compared with the thorax and abdomen (33.3% vs. 10.8% vs. 6.0%), given their proximity to the cranial nerves, critical vascular structures including the carotid and vertebral arteries and jugular veins, as well as the trachea [14, 15].

21.2 Vascular Injury

Neuroblastoma, particularly when it has unfavorable biologic features, commonly grows around major vessels (as well as encasing nerves and infiltrating surrounding organs and tissues). As a consequence of this propensity for vascular encasement, up to 10% of patients will suffer an injury to a major vascular structure during attempts at surgical tumor resection. This can result in significant blood loss, end-organ damage or loss due to ischemia, or the need for vascular reconstruction [16]. A critical step for avoiding injury to these vessels is their identification before they pass through the tumor, either in areas where the aorta and/or vena cava is uninvolved or at the takeoff of major branches from the aorta or vena cava. This should be done as early as possible in the conduct of an operation to minimize subsequent risk of vascular injury. The tumor is then usually removed piecemeal after freeing the circumference of the artery or vein. Removing a neuroblastoma in a piecemeal fashion does not violate any oncologic principals nor does leaving microscopic disease, or even a small amount of gross residual disease, in patients whose tumor has one or more image-defined risk factors. It is very difficult to identify the artery or vein by simply dissecting into the middle of the tumor in the hopes of finding the encased vessel before injuring it, and so this approach should be avoided. Additionally, the course of the vessels may be somewhat distorted and the vessels displaced by the tumor, making anticipation of their exact location difficult. Because vessel course may be distorted by large tumors, even readily apparent vessels are occasionally ligated and divided after mistaking them for vessels that can be sacrificed. Because of this, all sizable vessels should be tracked to their origin at the aorta or vena cava, and/or to the organ they supply/drain, in order to ensure their accurate identification. Finally, because of their thin wall and collapsibility, dissection along veins is often more difficult and dangerous than along thick-walled, muscular arteries. Even with meticulous dissection, however, significant blood loss and resultant transfusion requirement is common after resection of high-risk neuroblastoma with image-defined risk factors.

21.3 Neurologic Injury

Extension of neuroblastoma through neural foramina and into the spinal column is a fairly common occurrence, especially with paraspinal and thoracic primaries, and occurs in 7–15% of cases, although only about 20% are symptommatic [17]. In general, there is rarely an indication to remove the intraspinal tumor extension surgically, as the risks of resecting this residual disease, either from an anterior or posterior approach, appear to outweigh the benefits. Patients with favorable clinical characteristics and tumor biology have an excellent oncologic and neurologic prognosis despite leaving some gross residual disease in the neural foramina and spinal column. Patients with unfavorable clinical characteristics and tumor biology will receive intensive multimodality therapy, which is a critical component of successful treatment. However, children with intraspinal disease and acute, progressive neurologic deterioration may benefit from emergent laminotomy to remove expanding intraspinal tumor that is compressing the spinal cord [17]. Complications of aggressive surgery can include the development of an intraspinal hematoma and resultant cord compression, often due to injury to and failure to control (and sometimes recognize) injury to intercostal vessels (or small tumor vessels) that then retract into the spinal canal. Resection of intraspinal disease via a posterior approach (laminectomy or laminotomy) may result in scoliosis long term (discussed further below).

Direct injury to peripheral nerves can occur during the conduct of an operation for tumor resection, for the same reasons that vessels can be injured, as described above—being encased within tumor and not recognized during tumor mobilization and resection. Similarly, following the recommendations for avoiding vascular injury, identification of unencased nerve and then removing tumor from around the encased portion in a piecemeal fashion will help avoid this complication. And again, because leaving microscopic or even gross residual disease does not compromise oncologic principals or outcomes for neuroblastoma, purposeful resection of major nerves should be avoided. Direct injury to nerves may result in deficits including swallowing difficulties, diaphragm paralysis, sciatic nerve palsy, urinary and fecal incontinence, neurogenic bladder, erectile dysfunction, leg weakness, or nerve root injury, depending on the site of the primary tumor. A careful neurologic examination should be performed prior to surgery to document preexisting neurologic deficits.

Ischemia of the spinal cord can occur following resection of a paraspinal neuroblastoma, particularly inferiorly located posterior mediastinal tumors. This is due to injury to the artery of Adamkiewicz, an artery that arises off the aorta, typically at the level of the left 9–12th posterior intercostal artery, but whose origin can be variable, and which serves as the main blood supply to the spinal cord. Because of this, some authors have suggested the use of preoperative spinal angiography and intraoperative cord monitoring in certain circumstances, as they may help guide the conduct of tumor resection in avoiding injury to this critical artery [18].

21.4 Solid Organ Injury

Because of the propensity of unfavorable biology neuroblastoma to grow into surrounding tissues or organs, injury to the organ or its blood supply can occasionally occur as a consequence of neuroblastoma resection. However, for the most part, if recognized during the conduct of the operation, this is usually of little consequence. Enterotomies can usually be repaired with primary closure or resection of a short segment of bowel with primary reanastomosis. Because of this possibility some surgeons routinely use a preoperative bowel prep. Similarly, a gastrotomy, cystotomy, or rent in the liver can be closed primarily.

Compromise of the blood supply to these organs is also usually not problematic due to their generally redundant blood supply. However, the one significant exception is the kidney with its end artery blood supply. Because two of the most common locations for neuroblastoma are adrenal and retroperitoneal/periaortic (often in the region of the celiac axis), many neuroblastomas encase the renal vessels and/or invade the renal parenchyma. Every effort should be made to avoid nephrectomy when resecting a retroperitoneal neuroblastoma although resecting a small amount of renal parenchyma to remove the tumor may be indicated. Patients with favorable clinical characteristics and tumor biology generally have an excellent outcome regardless of the completeness of resection, while patients with unfavorable clinical characteristics and tumor biology need intensive multimodality therapy for which normal renal function is required in order to receive the full recommended doses. Nevertheless, for this latter group, some perform nephrectomy when it is required to achieve complete tumor resection, at reported rates of 5–10% [19, 20]. The benefit of this, when considering the impact on renal function and ability to tolerate high-dose chemotherapy, is uncertain, however.

Because neuroblastoma often grows into the renal hilum, encasing the renal vessels, kidney loss due to ischemia is not an uncommon occurrence, particularly in patients with high-risk disease. This complication occurs due to injury to the renal vasculature rather than to the kidney itself. This can be due to inadvertent ligation and division of the renal artery or vein, injury to either of these vessels that cannot be successfully repaired, or trauma to the artery from torque that results in spasm and renal ischemia. The latter may result in a "disappearing kidney," a term that refers to atrophy of a kidney likely due to vascular injury at the time of surgery. However, the consequence of this traumatic injury is generally not noted until later in a patient's clinical course, often months later, when follow-up imaging demonstrates a diminutive or completely absent kidney. The exact etiology for this complication is not well understood but is believed to involve spasm and/or intimal disruption of the renal artery due to excessive manipulation, particularly torque, on the vessel when trying to expose and resect lymphadenopathy from behind the renal vein. Thus, great care must be taken when removing tumor from around the renal vessels not to apply torque to the artery while retracting the tumor mass. Some advocate systemic renal-dose dopamine or intramural lidocaine in an attempt to prevent or break the spasm of the artery [21]. Thrombosis of the renal vein may also be associated with delayed loss of the kidney. As with occlusion of the renal artery, renal vein thrombosis may be associated with excessive manipulation of the vein during surgery or clamping or narrowing of the vein during attempts to repair a venotomy. Renal vein thrombosis is often heralded by hematuria several days after surgery. Ultrasound can confirm this as the etiology of delayed postoperative hematuria. Anticoagulation, thrombolysis, or thrombectomy may be attempted but is rarely associated with kidney salvage.

Occasionally neuroblastoma may invade the kidney, potentially leading to the misdiagnosis of Wilms tumor at presentation [22]. Distinguishing these tumor types is critical, as the surgical management for neuroblastoma and Wilms tumor differs significantly. The presence of constitutional symptoms, intratumoral calcification, or vascular encasement on preoperative imaging should heighten suspicion for neuroblastoma. In addition, laboratory evaluation, including urinary catecholamines, and radiographic studies, such as MIBG, should be completed prior to surgery when the etiology of an abdominal tumor is uncertain.

21.5 Biliary Injury

Among the most difficult neuroblastomas to resect are those located in the porta hepatis. In addition to potential injury to the vascular structures in the region, primarily the hepatic artery and portal vein, injury to the biliary tract can occur. This can happen due to direct bile duct injury and resultant bile leak or to ischemic injury to the biliary tree and delayed bile leak or bile duct stricture. Depending on the timing of injury recognition and the exact nature and extent of the injury, these complications can be managed by external drainage, stenting or dilatation, or with internal drainage with a hepaticojejunostomy.

21.6 Chylous Ascites/Chylothorax

Postoperative lymph leak is a well-recognized complication of neuroblastoma surgery that results from disruption of either mediastinal or retroperitoneal lymphatic channels during tumor resection [23]. Neuroblastoma often has an infiltrative growth pattern around major vessels where lymphatics are also residing, making them susceptible to injury or disruption when performing a perivascular dissection. Nonsurgical treatment of a postoperative chyle leak is effective for most patients. Management includes a low-fat diet or fasting to reduce lymph flow, the latter of which often requires the use of total parental nutrition. Drainage via tube thoracostomy or paracentesis may be required to alleviate compressive symptoms. Most patients respond to conservative management within 1–2 months although some will require operative intervention for failure of conservative management. Surgical options to abrogate a persistent chyle leak include primary direct surgical ligation, fibrin glue application, embolization, or creation of a peritoneovenous shunt. The exact duration that conservative therapy should be tried before surgical treatment is undertaken is controversial. Although most leaks will stop with conservative management, this may take a long time; thus, early ligation of the leakage site may be preferred in order to avoid metabolic complications, delay in restarting adjuvant therapy, and prolonged hospitalization [24].

21.7 Diarrhea

After resection of advanced abdominal neuroblastoma, children may have persistent diarrhea, perhaps resulting from disruption of the autonomic nerve supply to the gut during clearance of tumor from the major vessels of the retroperitoneum. In one series, 30% of patients had postoperative diarrhea [25]. Dissection around the superior mesenteric and celiac arteries was associated with a significantly higher incidence of diarrhea. Patients such as these may require long-term treatment with medication to slow intestinal peristalsis, and a few will have severe and unremitting diarrhea. The authors of that series hypothesized that (1) attenuation of inhibition of peristalsis resulting from disruption of the sympathetic nerve supply, (2) bile acid and fat malabsorption as a result of bacterial overgrowth in stagnant bowel loops caused by damage to the parasympathetic supply, and (3) disturbance in gut hormone activity caused by disruption of autonomic fibers all may contribute to the development of diarrhea.

21.8 Horner Syndrome

Horner syndrome, consisting of miosis (decreased pupil size), ptosis (drooping eyelid), and anhidrosis (decreased sweating on the ipsilateral side of the face) can be caused by disruption or trauma to the stellate ganglion which is located at the apex of the chest. This constellation of symptoms may be due to the presence of an apical thoracic tumor such as neuroblastoma, and may in fact be the presenting sign or symptom, or may occur as a consequence of resection of an apical neuroblastoma, with iatrogenic disruption during the course of tumor dissection. Because of this potential complication, which may be permanent, this possible outcome should be discussed with parents prior to surgery for an upper mediastinal neuroblastoma, after it has been determined that resection is critical for cure.

21.9 Bowel Obstruction

Although not unique to neuroblastoma resection, potential short- and long-term complications, common to all abdominal operations, is intestinal obstruction. Intussusception can occur in the immediate postoperative period. Postoperative intussusception is a rare complication after a variety of operations, but has an estimated incidence of 0.01–0.25% in children following laparotomy, particularly for resection of a retroperitoneal tumor such as neuroblastoma [26–28]. Early recognition in the postoperative period may be difficult because feeding intolerance may be attributed to postoperative ileus. Side effects of chemotherapy may also obscure the diagnosis [29]. However, delayed identification and management may result in significant morbidity and so a high index of suspicion should be maintained, particularly if oral intake had been tolerated initially after surgery. Ultrasound may be a useful study as the intussusception is most often ileoileal [30]. The etiology of postoperative intussusception is unclear. The theories to explain mechanisms include altered peristalsis, early postoperative adhesions, prolonged and excessive bowel manipulation, electrolyte disturbances in lengthy surgeries, anesthetic drugs, opioid analgesics, and neurogenic factors [31].

Long-term, bowel obstruction due to intestinal adhesions can occur after resection of a retroperitoneal neuroblastoma (and other tumors) [32]. Madenci et al. evaluated the occurrence of intestinal obstruction requiring surgery 5 or more years after cancer diagnosis in 12,316 5-year survivors in the Childhood Cancer Survivor Study. Late obstruction was reported by 165 survivors (median time from diagnosis, 13 years). The cumulative incidence of late obstruction at 35 years was 5.8% among survivors with abdominopelvic tumors. Treatment with abdominopelvic radiotherapy within 5 years of cancer diagnosis increased the rate of late obstruction. Importantly, the development of late obstruction increased subsequent mortality among survivors.

21.10 Scoliosis

Spinal curvature in children impacts not only musculoskeletal function and self-esteem, but it can also impact pulmonary function and exercise capacity long term. Scoliosis in children treated for neuroblastoma can result from the frequently paraspinal location of the primary tumor itself or from efforts at surgical extirpation [33]. In fact, scoliosis in a child without an obvious etiology should prompt an investigation for the possibility of a paraspinal tumor. In one institutional review, 58 children surviving a minimum of 5 years had overall 5-, 10-, and 15-year scoliosis-free rates of 87.6%, 79.0%, and 76.0%, respectively [34]. Twelve (21%) developed scoliosis at a median time of 51 months. The degree of scoliosis was mild (< or =20°) in 8 (67%). Four had scoliosis ranging from 30° to 66°. On multivariate analysis, both history of laminectomy and use of radiation therapy were found to be risk factors for development of scoliosis. Children who had a laminectomy were more likely to manifest scoliosis earlier (their median time to scoliosis was 23 months). Increasing RT dose was found to impact adversely on the development of scoliosis. In another study of children with symptomatic intraspinal neuroblastoma, seven of 24 assessable patients who had undergone laminectomy developed scoliosis, whereas spinal deformities were only detected in one of 49 assessable patients managed without laminectomy. Fewer orthopedic sequelae were observed in the children managed with chemotherapy than were seen in children managed with laminectomy [17]. Other studies have also shown that thoracotomy, particularly in younger patients, may be associated with the long-term development of scoliosis, including patients with thoracic neuroblastoma. In part because of this, minimally invasive approaches to neuroblastoma resection, including thoracoscopic and via laminotomy, are being increasingly used. Similarly, indications for and dose of radiation therapy are being reevaluated.

21.11 Compartment Syndrome

Compartment syndrome is a condition in which increased pressure within one of the body's compartments results in insufficient blood supply to tissue within that space. When considering neuroblastoma, this is most commonly within the abdomen and may affect perfusion of the kidneys and the lower extremities, in particular, or impair ventilation due to limited diaphragmatic excursion. Compartment syndrome occurs most frequently due to the large size of the primary abdominal tumor or to an extremely enlarged liver due to metastatic tumor burden in infants. However, it can occur in the postoperative setting due to tissue edema, particularly in the abdominal wall, due to significant fluid resuscitation during a long, complex neuroblastoma resection or to extensive intra-abdominal fluid buildup of blood, chyle, urine, or third-space losses. Evidence of poor tissue perfusion (acidosis, oliguria, lower extremity ischemia) or inadequate ventilation (hypercarbia) in the appropriate setting may raise the question of intra-abdominal compartment syndrome, which can be confirmed by measuring bladder pressure. An abdominal ultrasound may help distinguish abdominal wall edema from intra-abdominal fluid. Paracentesis or even opening the abdomen by reopening the abdominal incision may be required to relieve the consequences of abdominal compartment syndrome.

21.12 Summary

Surgery plays a critical role in the management of children with neuroblastoma. Yet, because of its propensity to invade surrounding structures and encase critical vessels and nerves, often in very young, small patients, it is associated with a number of potential complications, some of which are quite significant. The likelihood of having a complication with resection of a neuroblastoma relates to whether or not an image-defined risk factor is present. In addition, the prognosis for children with neuroblastoma can be anticipated based on the presence or absence of certain clinical and biologic risk factors. Thus, an appreciation for (1) the prognosis of the patient, (2) the image-defined risk factors, and (3) the potential complications of surgery, both acute and long term, is critical when considering the risks and benefits of any surgery performed on a child with neuroblastoma.

References

1. Bhakta N, Liu Q, Ness KK, Baassiri M, Eissa H, Yeo F, Chemaitilly W, Ehrhardt MJ, Bass J, Bishop MW, et al. The cumulative burden of surviving childhood cancer: an initial report from the St Jude Lifetime Cohort Study (SJLIFE). Lancet. 2017;390(10112):2569–82.
2. Kuroda T, Saeki M, Honna T, Kumagai M, Masaki H. Late complications after surgery in patients with neuroblastoma. J Pediatr Surg. 2006;41(12):2037–40.
3. Ziegler MM. Pediatric surgical oncology. Curr Opin Pediatr. 1990;2(3):579–84.
4. von Allmen D, Davidoff AM, London WB, Ryn CV, Haas-Kogan DA, Kreissman SG, Khanna G, Rosen N, Park JR, Quaglia MPL. Impact of extent of resection on local control and sur-

vival in patients from the COG A3973 study with high-risk neuroblastoma. J Clin Oncol. 2017;35(2):208–16.
5. Canete A, Jovani C, Lopez A, Costa E, Segarra V, Fernandez JM, Verdeguer A, Velazquez J, Castel V. Surgical treatment for neuroblastoma: complications during 15 years' experience. J Pediatr Surg. 1998;33(10):1526–30.
6. Azizkhan RG, Shaw A, Chandler JG. Surgical complications of neuroblastoma resection. Surgery. 1985;97(5):514–7.
7. Losty P, Quinn F, Breatnach F, O'Meara A, Fitzgerald RJ. Neuroblastoma—a surgical perspective. Eur J Surg Oncol. 1993;19(1):33–6.
8. Kiely EM. Radical surgery for abdominal neuroblastoma. Semin Surg Oncol. 1993;9(6):489–92.
9. Rich BS, McEvoy MP, Kelly NE, Oh E, Abramson SJ, Price AP, Cheung NK, La Quaglia MP. Resectability and operative morbidity after chemotherapy in neuroblastoma patients with encasement of major visceral arteries. J Pediatr Surg. 2011;46(1):103–7.
10. Cantos MF, Gerstle JT, Irwin MS, Pappo A, Farley S, Cheang T, Kim PC. Surgical challenges associated with intensive treatment protocols for high-risk neuroblastoma. J Pediatr Surg. 2006;41(5):960–5.
11. Davidoff AM. Neuroblastoma. Semin Pediatr Surg. 2012;21(1):2–14.
12. Schmidt ML, Lukens JN, Seeger RC, Brodeur GM, Shimada H, Gerbing RB, Stram DO, Perez C, Haase GM, Matthay KK. Biologic factors determine prognosis in infants with stage IV neuroblastoma: a prospective Children's Cancer Group study. J Clin Oncol. 2000;18(6):1260–8.
13. Cecchetto G, Mosseri V, De Bernardi B, Helardot P, Monclair T, Costa E, Horcher E, Neuenschwander S, Toma P, Rizzo A, et al. Surgical risk factors in primary surgery for localized neuroblastoma: the LNESG1 study of the European International Society of Pediatric Oncology Neuroblastoma Group. J Clin Oncol. 2005;23(33):8483–9.
14. Jackson JR, Tran HC, Stein JE, Shimada H, Patel AM, Marachelian A, Kim ES. The clinical management and outcomes of cervical neuroblastic tumors. J Surg Res. 2016;204(1):109–13.
15. Qureshi SS, Kembhavi S, Ramadwar M, Chinnaswamy G, Laskar S, Talole S, Desai S, Khanna N, Vora T, Kurkure P. Outcome and morbidity of surgical resection of primary cervical and cervicothoracic neuroblastoma in children: a comparative analysis. Pediatr Surg Int. 2014;30(3):267–73.
16. Paran TS, Corbally MT, Gross-Rom E, Rutigliano DN, Kayton ML, La Quaglia MP. Experience with aortic grafting during excision of large abdominal neuroblastomas in children. J Pediatr Surg. 2008;43(2):335–40.
17. Katzenstein HM, Kent PM, London WB, Cohn SL. Treatment and outcome of 83 children with intraspinal neuroblastoma: the Pediatric Oncology Group experience. J Clin Oncol. 2001;19(4):1047–55.
18. Nordin AB, Fallon SC, Jea A, Kim ES. The use of spinal angiography in the management of posterior mediastinal tumors: case series and review of the literature. J Pediatr Surg. 2013;48(9):1871–7.
19. Kiely EM. The surgical challenge of neuroblastoma. J Pediatr Surg. 1994;29(2):128–33.
20. Lim II, Goldman DA, Farber BA, Murphy JM, Abramson SJ, Basu E, Roberts S, LaQuaglia MP, Price AP. Image-defined risk factors for nephrectomy in patients undergoing neuroblastoma resection. J Pediatr Surg. 2016;51(6):975–80.
21. Fusaro F, Cecchetto G, Boglino C, Inserra A, Zanon GF, Giusti F, Dall'Igna P. Measures to prevent renal impairment after resection of retroperitoneal neuroblastoma. Pediatr Surg Int. 2002;18(5–6):388–91.
22. Dickson PV, Sims TL, Streck CJ, McCarville MB, Santana VM, McGregor LM, Furman WL, Davidoff AM. Avoiding misdiagnosing neuroblastoma as Wilms tumor. J Pediatr Surg. 2008;43(6):1159–63.
23. Qureshi SS, Rent EG, Bhagat M, Dsouza P, Kembhavi S, Vora T, Prasad M, Chinnaswamy G, Ramadwar M, Laskar S, et al. Chyle leak following surgery for abdominal neuroblastoma. J Pediatr Surg. 2016;51(9):1557–60.
24. Liu Y, Pan C, Tang JY, Chen J, Zhou M, Ye QD. What is the result: chylous leakage following extensive radical surgery of neuroblastoma. World J Pediatr. 2012;8(2):151–5.

25. Rees H, Markley MA, Kiely EM, Pierro A, Pritchard J. Diarrhea after resection of advanced abdominal neuroblastoma: a common management problem. Surgery. 1998;123(5):568–72.
26. Ein SH, Ferguson JM. Intussusception—the forgotten postoperative obstruction. Arch Dis Child. 1982;57(10):788–90.
27. Holcomb GW 3rd, Ross AJ 3rd, O'Neill JA Jr. Postoperative intussusception: increasing frequency or increasing awareness? South Med J. 1991;84(11):1334–9.
28. Pumberger W, Pomberger G, Wiesbauer P. Postoperative intussusception: an overlooked complication in pediatric surgical oncology. Med Pediatr Oncol. 2002;38(3):208–10.
29. Kaste SC, Wilimas J, Rao BN. Postoperative small-bowel intussusception in children with cancer. Pediatr Radiol. 1995;25(1):21–3.
30. VanHouwelingen LT, Seims AD, Ortega-Laureano L, Coleman JL, McCarville MB, Davidoff AM, Fernandez-Pineda I. Use of ultrasound in diagnosing postoperative small-bowel intussusception in pediatric surgical oncology patients: a single-center retrospective review. Pediatr Radiol. 2017;48(2):204–9.
31. Yang G, Wang X, Jiang W, Ma J, Zhao J, Liu W. Postoperative intussusceptions in children and infants: a systematic review. Pediatr Surg Int. 2013;29(12):1273–9.
32. Madenci AL, Fisher S, Diller LR, Goldsby RE, Leisenring WM, Oeffinger KC, Robison LL, Sklar CA, Stovall M, Weathers RE, et al. Intestinal obstruction in survivors of childhood cancer: a report from the childhood cancer survivor study. J Clin Oncol. 2015;33(26):2893–900.
33. Barrena S, Miguel M, de la Torre CA, Ramirez M, Diaz M, Martinez L, Perez-Grueso FS, Lassaletta L, Tovar JA. Late surgery for spinal deformities in children previously treated for neural tumors. Eur J Pediatr Surg. 2011;21(1):54–7.
34. Paulino AC, Fowler BZ. Risk factors for scoliosis in children with neuroblastoma. Int J Radiat Oncol Biol Phys. 2005;61(3):865–9.

Palliative Care

22

Alessandro Inserra and Alessandro Crocoli

22.1 Introduction

Over the last 50 years, the overall survival for children affected by cancer dramatically increased, with 5-year survival rate after diagnosis raised from 50% in late 1970s to 85% in 2010 [1, 2]. Interestingly, a more notable improvement has been observed for some tumors like acute lymphoblastic leukemia (5% in early 1950s to 90% in 2010) [3, 4], lymphomas (30% in 1960s to around 80% in 2010) [5, 6], and Wilms tumor (20–90%) [7, 8]. All those successes have been achieved since the concept of multidisciplinary treatment was introduced in the field of pediatric onco-hematology. For neuroblastoma, the 5-year survival rate increased over the same time, from 86% to 95% for children younger than 1 year and from 34% to 68% for children aged 1–14 years [9]. However, despite all those improvement in outcome and the fact that cancer is a rare condition in pediatric population, it is the second most common cause of death in children older than 12 months [10, 11]. In 2017, United States National Institute of Health-National Cancer Institute estimates that there will be 10,270 new diagnoses of cancer among children from 0 to 14 years of age, and 1190 patients are expected to die from the disease [10, 12]. In this respect, there are specific tumor groups that have disappointing survival rates, including metastatic solid tumors such as Ewing's sarcoma, rhabdomyosarcoma, osteosarcoma, and neuroblastoma. In other words, neuroblastoma accounts for about 15% of childhood cancer mortality, with higher percentage for high-risk patients.

Progression of disease determines impossibility to cure but not impossibility to have adequate and tailored treatment to control, when possible, the disease and to order to improve management of distressing symptoms, to guarantee earlier recognition of prognosis, and to reduce hospitalizations. The final goal is the promotion

A. Inserra (✉) · A. Crocoli
Operative Unit of General and Thoracic Surgery, Bambino Gesù Children's Hospital IRCCS, Rome, Italy
e-mail: alessandro.inserra@opbg.net

S. Sarnacki, L. Pio (eds.), *Neuroblastoma*,
https://doi.org/10.1007/978-3-030-18396-7_22

of both child and family living with inevitable life-shortening disease giving adequate and provision of "effective curative, life-prolonging and quality-of-life enhancing care" [13, 14]. In this respect, World Health Organization defines pediatric palliative care as care that "aims to improve the quality of life of patients facing life-threatening illnesses, and their families, through the prevention and relief of suffering by early identification and treatment of pain and other problems, whether physical, psychosocial, or spiritual" [15]. To be effective, it requires a broad multidisciplinary approach that includes the family and makes use of available community resources. Focusing on the therapeutical approaches available as palliative care, after diagnosis of recurrent/in progression neuroblastoma configuring terminal condition, physicians must face two major issues: control of symptoms which have direct influence on quality of life and necessity to provide adequate way and enable administration of different supportive care. In this respect, chemotherapy, surgery, and radiotherapy have different but essential functions in management of children affected by neuroblastoma in terminal phases of disease; in fact, patients relapsing after intensive therapy for advanced disease are very rarely cured by second-line treatment. Nonetheless, judicious use of chemotherapy and radiotherapy can be beneficial in terms of symptom control and prolongation of life, and supportive measures can often enhance the quality of life of terminally ill children.

22.2 Palliative Therapies

As previously reported, neuroblastomas are diverse in their clinical behavior. Certain factors influence the biologic behavior of these tumors and are helpful in predicting outcome; some are patient-related (e.g., age at the time of diagnosis), while the majority are tumor-related (disease stage, tumor histology, molecular and cytogenetic features). Most important factors influencing prognosis are age (>1 year), advanced stage (IV disease), and n-myc oncogene amplification [16, 17] with overall survival less 50%. Actually, half of the patients diagnosed with high-risk disease will necessitate of palliation for both progression of primary tumor and for metastatic relapse. For those children, control of disease is the cornerstone of palliative measures in order to maximize their quality of life with adequate symptoms management [18–20].

22.3 Chemotherapy

The use of oral etoposide, given daily for 3 weeks with a 7-day interval between courses, can sometimes produce disease stabilization even in heavily pretreated patients, although the response rate is disappointing [21]. As the capsules are very large and may be difficult to administer to children, the liquid intravenous preparation is preferred, although its unpleasant taste must be disguised. Rationale of this therapy is to obtain control of tumor growth with continuous/chronic, equally spaced, and low doses of etoposide as the administration according to such regimen, called metronomic, takes advantages of antiangiogenic effects and is not affected by toxicity induced according to maximum tolerated dose [22]. For these reasons, this regimen is well-tolerated and particularly suitable for children in a palliative setting, as the main advantage in treatment of metastatic neuroblastoma is the good response on pain induced by bone metastases. On the other hand, doses may need to be frequently adjusted in order to avoid myelotoxicity and subsequent high transfusion requirement [22, 23].

Five-day courses of intravenous irinotecan is another option for treatment of metastatic/advanced neuroblastoma as palliation: infusion does not require hyperhydration either before or after administration, gastrointestinal toxicity is low and well-tolerated, as well as the activity against tumor is effective also with dosages which do not impact bone marrow activity [24, 25]. Moreover camptothecins such as irinotecan and topotecan are known for their activity as radiation sensitizers [26, 27] in treatment of relapsed/refractory neuroblastoma with targeted radiopharmaceutical agents such as ^{131}I-MIBG [28]: this radionuclide is an effective and relatively nontoxic therapy when administrated at low dosage in selected patients with advanced disease in palliative settings. Sporadic reports [29, 30] showed encouraging results in control of pain induced by bone metastases, for both acceptable toxicity rate and significant reduction of opioid requirement during treatment of terminal patients, consequently improving their quality of life.

22.4 Radiotherapy

Approximately one half of prescribed radiotherapy is given for palliation of symptoms due to incurable cancer, also in pediatric patients. Distressing symptoms including pain, bleeding, and obstruction can often be relieved with minimal toxic effects [31]. Painful osseous metastasis is common in pediatric oncologic practice and symptomatic bone metastases obtain some pain relief with a low-dose, brief course of palliative radiotherapy. Other indications for use in pediatric setting for palliative purposes may include local control in brain tumors/metastases, spinal cord compression, dyspnea, and neurological issues [32].

Palliative radiotherapy—summary of indication [33]:

- Pain from bone or soft tissue metastases causing tissue or nerve root infiltration.
- Fungating or ulcerating tumor lesions.
- Impending or actual airway obstruction.
- Oncologic emergencies including spinal cord compression.
- Superior vena cava syndrome and superior mediastinal syndrome.
- Obstruction of stomach, gastrointestinal tract, bladder.
- Bleeding in the form of hemoptysis, gastric bleeding, or rectal/vaginal bleeding.
- Liver metastases causing pain or decreased infra-diaphragmatic excursion.
- Cranial nerve palsies or increased intracranial pressure from brain or leptomeningeal metastases.

Regarding neuroblastoma, several studies have been demonstrated over the last decades the role of radiotherapy for management of symptoms in palliative setting. Paulino [34] showed efficacy of external beam radiation therapy in treatment of metastases of liver, brain, bone, and soft tissue, with a median survival time of 10 weeks and complete/partial response to treatment in 79% of patients with bone lesions and 77% in soft tissue lesions. Author also claimed that fractioned external beam radiation therapy should be at least 2000 cGy whereas in children unable to undergo such treatment 400–800 cGy on painful single lesion should be delivered in palliation regimen [34]. Regarding bone metastases, some authors [35, 36] reported better outcome with response after single/multiple fractions of radiotherapy ranging between 80% and 90%. As a matter of fact, for neuroblastoma as for other children malignancies, data about different approaches (e.g., stereotactic models) as well as on efficacy of multiple dose fractioning schemes, optimal dose, timing (prophylactic or only in presence of symptoms), and setting (anesthesia, mild sedation, etc.) in palliative regimens are scant [2, 36] and still need further studies to be validated.

Another important issue of radiation therapy is the toxicity: Mak et al. [2] reported encouraging results in terms of symptoms/disease control with low and well-tolerated toxicity rate (grades 1–2 in 21% of treatments), thus consenting to maintain high and upstanding quality of life, necessary prerequisite for palliative care. For these reasons radiotherapy should be considered not only as primary therapy but also for palliative purposes in patients affected by progressive neuroblastoma [2, 34, 37].

22.5 Surgery

Role of surgery in management of patients affected by neuroblastoma is well-known, even if its profile changes according to the different clinical situations. In this respect, primary resection is the cornerstone of treatment for localized disease while surgical strategies and approaches should be carefully balanced with the risk of potentially life-threatening complications related with sacrifice of major vessel and/or vital organs for high-risk patients. As a consequence, children with advanced/refractory neuroblastoma had always history of previous multiple surgical procedures which determines higher risk of bowel obstruction [38]; moreover, progression of abdominal disease as well as radiation enteritis may also be other causes of this condition which may require careful surgical evaluation especially in palliation setting [20]. In fact, in case of severe worsening of performance status (dehydration/dyselectrolytemia for continuous vomiting, respiratory failure for abdominal distension, etc.), intestinal diversion should be considered as a palliative procedure with the purpose to improve quality of life, both relieving from symptoms and avoiding rapid life-threatening complications (e.g., perforation). On the other hand, ostomies represent also useful solution in case of nutritional issues; gastrostomy/jejunostomy should be planned in patients who are incapable of adequate oral intake (esophageal mucositis/stenosis, progression in chest/neck disease, etc.), thus avoiding necessity of nasogastric/jejunal tube as further discomfort (pain, secretion, irritation, etc.) [39–42].

Nutritional support may be delivered as parenteral nutrition, also in patients referred to home/hospice settings of care. In this respect, adequate central venous access is a necessary prerequisite especially for these patients. Devices to be eventually positioned in children undergoing palliative care should be carefully evaluated and chosen taking into account different factors: age of patient, history of previous vascular access, performance status, coagulation disorders, and experience of both family and caregivers in management of central venous lines [43].

Highly pretreated children may also experience, in their terminal phase of the disease, urinary complications such as obstructions [44]. Pelvic primitive/recurrent tumors and periureteral fibrosis induced by radiation therapy/chemotherapy are the main causes and the prognosis of such condition in rapidly poor for the development of acute renal failure. Strategies for management of urinary obstruction should be tailored on the single patient, according to the performance status and the quality of life, and may include open urinary diversion, retrograde ureteral stenting, and nephrostomy placement (percutaneous or surgical) [20].

Another important issue of patients with terminal neuroblastoma is management of pain, which could be caused by skeletal involvement or by compression/infiltration from the tumor [45]. Refractory pain is the most common symptom in end-stage disease and despite the development of more specific and aggressive pharmacological solutions (including a more liberal use of opioids over the last decades) with non-negligible influence on quality of life [46, 47]. In fact, one-third of patients undergone to prolonged medical therapy for pain control develop drug-resistant symptoms, thus necessitating of a different and often more invasive management. Surgical procedures to control pain include implant of systems for epidural/intrathecal drug infusion [48–50] as well as peripheral nerve block/neurolysis. Percutaneous CT-guided neurolysis should be recommended in fact in case of abdominal intractable pain for recurrent central neuroblastoma with invasion of celiac plexus [20]. More invasive procedures, such as cordotomy and myelotomy, have been progressively replaced over the last years by neuromodulation, which is the equivalent of surgical ablation performed by interruption of nerves. High-frequency electrical stimulation of target nerves determines interference in function, thus resulting in interruption of the nervous pathway transmitting nociceptive signals. Other advantages of neuromodulation are the possibility to customize the treatment on the single patient, adjusting stimulation intensity and frequency. On the other hand, implant of neuromodulation device is a surgical procedure which can be contraindicated/not tolerated in patients with poor performance status and terminal disease [20, 50].

22.6 Role of Clinical Trials

Individualized cancer therapies may include, especially for pediatric cancer patients, participation to clinical trials; those therapies may offer sometimes advantages in terms of quality of life especially in advanced disease. As per adult patients, clinical trials may allow to access to promising innovative settings of care also to children who failed first-/second-line treatments and have poor choice of other ones. Last but not least, enrolling a patient into a trial is also a contribute to the improvement in outcome of future patients as the highly regulated setting of such studies is the cornerstone of research of new therapies.

Focusing on pediatric patients, the most important issue for investigators is the selection of treatments to propose as a trial, since the number of patients is smaller compared to adult numbers. As a matter of fact, the likelihood of success of a project is the principal factor influencing its role in treatment of pediatric malignancies, since not every agent and/or combination with proven efficacy in adult patients can be tested in children. As noted by Bond and Pritchard [51], new agents to be included in clinical trial have usually been previously tested and found to be useful in adult cancer patients or may also be chosen for testing after response in preclinical models as a specific activity against pediatric tumors or based on a novel mechanism of action or favorable drug-resistance profile. Drug availability or predicted future drug availability is an important factor in the selection of agents for pediatric trials. Because pediatric cancers are uncommon, agents that are also effective in adult cancer types are more likely to continue to be produced.

Phase 1 and phase 2 clinical trials are experimental trials and are not expected to result in a cure, while phase 3 trials evaluate a new drug or drug combination in comparison with the current standard treatment, usually within randomized evaluation: they include a control arm, which represents the current best treatment, and an experimental arm, which has additional treatments or has been tested in a phase 2 setting.

Regarding palliative therapy for recurrent/advanced neuroblastoma, previously mentioned use of irinotecan and topotecan in a 5-day course [24, 52] has been shown to be effective in highly pretreated patients. However, no clinical trial for palliative therapies in neuroblastoma is currently under investigation.

On the other hand, there are several studies both under ITCC and under NIH governance investigating different therapies for recurrent/relapsed, progressive and refractory disease as neuroblastoma is a tumor with high rate of recurrence after first-line chemotherapy [53].

References

1. Smith MA, Seibel NL, Altekruse SF, Ries LA, Melbert DL, O'Leary M, et al. Outcomes for children and adolescents with cancer: challenges for the twenty-first century. J Clin Oncol. 2010;28(15):2625–34.
2. Mak KS, Lee SW, Balboni TA, Marcus KJ. Clinical outcomes and toxicity following palliative radiotherapy for childhood cancers. Pediatr Blood Cancer. 2017;65(1) https://doi.org/10.1002/pbc.26764.
3. Farber S. Chemotherapeutic studies of tumors, including leukemia, in children. Am J Dis Child. 1950;79(5):961–2.
4. Noone AM, Cronin KA, Altekruse SF, Howlader N, Lewis DR, Petkov VI, et al. Cancer incidence and survival trends by subtype using data from the surveillance epidemiology and end results program, 1992–2013. Cancer Epidemiol Biomark Prev. 2017;26(4):632–41.
5. Hooper WC, Holman RC, Strine TW, Chorba TL. Hodgkin disease mortality in the United States: 1979–1988. Cancer. 1992;70(5):1166–71.

6. Karalexi MA, Georgakis MK, Dessypris N, Ryzhov A, Zborovskaya A, Dimitrova N, et al. Mortality and survival patterns of childhood lymphomas: geographic and age-specific patterns in Southern-Eastern European and SEER/US registration data. Hematol Oncol. 2017;35(4):608–18.
7. Farber S. Chemotherapy in the treatment of leukemia and Wilms' tumor. JAMA. 1966;198(8):826–36.
8. Pritchard-Jones K, Moroz V, Vujanic G, Powis M, Walker J, Messahel B, et al. Treatment and outcome of Wilms' patients: an analysis of all cases registered in the UKW3 trial. Ann Oncol. 2012;23(9):2457–63.
9. Smith MA, Altekruse SF, Adamson PC, Reaman GH, Seibel NL. Declining childhood and adolescent cancer mortality. Cancer. 2014;120(16):2497–506.
10. Ward E, DeSantis C, Robbins A, Kohler B, Jemal A. Childhood and adolescent cancer statistics, 2014. CA Cancer J Clin. 2014;64(2):83–103.
11. Kowalczyk JR, Samardakiewicz M, Pritchard-Jones K, Ladenstein R, Essiaf S, Fitzgerald E, et al. European survey on standards of care in paediatric oncology centres. Eur J Cancer. 2016;61:11–9.
12. Siegel RL, Miller KD, Jemal A. Cancer statistics, 2017. CA Cancer J Clin. 2017;67(1):7–30.
13. Humphrey L, Kang TI. Palliative care in pediatric patients with hematologic malignancies. Hematology Am Soc Hematol Educ Program. 2015;2015:490–5.
14. Feudtner C, Friebert S, Jewell J, Friebert S, Carter B, Feudtner C, Hood M, Imaizumi S, Komatz K, SECTION ON HOSPICE AND PALLIATIVE MEDICINE AND COMMITTEE ON HOSPITAL CARE. Pediatric palliative care and hospice care commitments, guidelines, and recommendations. Pediatrics. 2013;132(5):966–72. https://doi.org/10.1542/peds.2013-2731.
15. American Academy of Pediatrics. Committee on Bioethics and Committee on Hospital Care. Palliative care for children. Pediatrics. 2000;106(2 Pt 1):351–7.
16. Ahmed AA, Zhang L, Reddivalla N, Hetherington M. Neuroblastoma in children: update on clinicopathologic and genetic prognostic factors. Pediatr Hematol Oncol. 2017;34(3):165–85.
17. Evans AE, Albo V, D'Angio GJ, Finklestein JZ, Leiken S, Santulli T, et al. Factors influencing survival of children with nonmetastatic neuroblastoma. Cancer. 1976;38(2):661–6.
18. Weaver MS, Heinze KE, Bell CJ, Wiener L, Garee AM, Kelly KP, et al. Establishing psychosocial palliative care standards for children and adolescents with cancer and their families: an integrative review. Palliat Med. 2016;30(3):212–23.
19. Himelstein BP, Hilden JM, Boldt AM, Weissman D. Pediatric palliative care. N Engl J Med. 2004;350(17):1752–62.
20. Inserra A, Narciso A, Paolantonio G, Messina R, Crocoli A. Palliative care and pediatric surgical oncology. Semin Pediatr Surg. 2016;25(5):323–32.
21. Kushner BH, Kramer K, Cheung NK. Oral etoposide for refractory and relapsed neuroblastoma. J Clin Oncol. 1999;17(10):3221–5.
22. Pasquier E, Kieran MW, Sterba J, Shaked Y, Baruchel S, Oberlin O, et al. Moving forward with metronomic chemotherapy: meeting report of the 2nd International Workshop on Metronomic and Anti-Angiogenic Chemotherapy in Paediatric Oncology. Transl Oncol. 2011;4(4):203–11.
23. Parikh NS, Howard SC, Chantada G, Israels T, Khattab M, Alcasabas P, et al. SIOP-PODC adapted risk stratification and treatment guidelines: recommendations for neuroblastoma in low- and middle-income settings. Pediatr Blood Cancer. 2015;62(8):1305–16.
24. Kushner BH, Kramer K, Modak S, Cheung NK. Five-day courses of irinotecan as palliative therapy for patients with neuroblastoma. Cancer. 2005;103(4):858–62.
25. Osone S, Hosoi H, Tsuchiya K, Misawa A, Iehara T, Sugimoto T. Low-dose protracted irinotecan as a palliative chemotherapy for advanced neuroblastoma. J Pediatr Hematol Oncol. 2008;30(11):853–6.
26. Gaze MN, Chang YC, Flux GD, Mairs RJ, Saran FH, Meller ST. Feasibility of dosimetry-based high-dose 131I-meta-iodobenzylguanidine with topotecan as a radiosensitizer in children with metastatic neuroblastoma. Cancer Biother Radiopharm. 2005;20(2):195–9.
27. Park JR, Scott JR, Stewart CF, London WB, Naranjo A, Santana VM, et al. Pilot induction regimen incorporating pharmacokinetically guided topotecan for treatment of newly

diagnosed high-risk neuroblastoma: a Children's Oncology Group study. J Clin Oncol. 2011;29(33):4351–7.
28. DuBois SG, Allen S, Bent M, Hilton JF, Hollinger F, Hawkins R, et al. Phase I/II study of (131) I-MIBG with vincristine and 5 days of irinotecan for advanced neuroblastoma. Br J Cancer. 2015;112(4):644–9.
29. Kang TI, Brophy P, Hickeson M, Heyman S, Evans AE, Charron M, et al. Targeted radiotherapy with submyeloablative doses of 131I-MIBG is effective for disease palliation in highly refractory neuroblastoma. J Pediatr Hematol Oncol. 2003;25(10):769–73.
30. Weyl Ben-Arush M, Ben Barak A, Bar-Deroma R, Ash S, Goldstein G, Golan H, Houri H, Waldman D, Nevo N, Bar Shalom R, Berniger A, Nevelsky A, Toren A, Yaniv I, Kuten A. Targeted therapy with low doses of 131I-MIBG is effective for disease palliation in highly refractory neuroblastoma. Israel Med Assoc J. 2013;15(1):31–4.
31. Rahn DA 3rd, Mundt AJ, Murphy JD, Schiff D, Adams J, Murphy KT. Clinical outcomes of palliative radiation therapy for children. Pract Radiat Oncol. 2015;5(3):183–7.
32. Varma S, Friedman DL, Stavas MJ. The role of radiation therapy in palliative care of children with advanced cancer: clinical outcomes and patterns of care. Pediatr Blood Cancer. 2017;64(5) https://doi.org/10.1002/pbc.26359.
33. Vern-gross T. Pediatric palliative radiation oncology. In: Lutz S, Chow E, Hoskin P, editors. Radiation oncology in palliative cancer care. Chichester, UK: John Wiley & Sons, Ltd; 2017. p. 220–37.
34. Paulino AC. Palliative radiotherapy in children with neuroblastoma. Pediatr Hematol Oncol. 2003;20(2):111–7.
35. Deutsch M, Tersak JM. Radiotherapy for symptomatic metastases to bone in children. Am J Clin Oncol. 2017;27(2):128–31.
36. Caussa L, Hijal T, Michon J, Helfre S. Role of palliative radiotherapy in the management of metastatic pediatric neuroblastoma: a retrospective single-institution study. Int J Radiat Oncol Biol Phys. 2011;79(1):214–9.
37. Bhasker S, Bajpai V, Turaka A. Palliative radiotherapy in paediatric malignancies. Singap Med J. 2008;49(12):998–1001.
38. Aguayo P, Ho B, Fraser JD, Gamis A, St Peter SD, Snyder CL. Bowel obstruction after treatment of intra-abdominal tumors. Eur J Pediatr Surg. 2010;20(4):234–6.
39. Parbhoo DM, Tiedemann K, Catto-Smith AG. Clinical outcome after percutaneous endoscopic gastrostomy in children with malignancies. Pediatr Blood Cancer. 2011;56(7):1146–8.
40. Buderus S, Sonderkötter H, Fleischhack G, Lentze MJ. Diagnostic and therapeutic endoscopy in children and adolescents with cancer. Pediatr Hematol Oncol. 2012;29(5):450–60.
41. Sacks N, Hwang WT, Lange BJ, Tan KS, Sandler ES, Rogers PC, et al. Proactive enteral tube feeding in pediatric patients undergoing chemotherapy. Pediatr Blood Cancer. 2014;61(2):281–5.
42. Huhmann MB, August DA. Nutrition support in surgical oncology. Nutr Clin Pract. 2009;24(4):520–6.
43. Crocoli A, Tornesello A, Pittiruti M, Barone A, Muggeo P, Inserra A, et al. Central venous access devices in pediatric malignancies: a position paper of Italian Association of Pediatric Hematology and Oncology. J Vasc Access. 2015;16(2):130–6.
44. Lambert SM. Transitional care in pediatric urology. Semin Pediatr Surg. 2015;24(2):73–8.
45. van den Beuken-van Everdingen MH, de Rijke JM, Kessels AG, Schouten HC, van Kleef M, Patijn J. Prevalence of pain in patients with cancer: a systematic review of the past 40 years. Ann Oncol. 2007;18(9):1437–49.
46. Wolfe J, Grier HE, Klar N, Levin SB, Ellenbogen JM, Salem-Schatz S, et al. Symptoms and suffering at the end of life in children with cancer. N Engl J Med. 2000;342(5):326–33.
47. Theunissen JM, Hoogerbrugge PM, van Achterberg T, Prins JB, Vernooij-Dassen MJ, van den Ende CH. Symptoms in the palliative phase of children with cancer. Pediatr Blood Cancer. 2007;49(2):160–5.
48. Tobias JD. Applications of intrathecal catheters in children. Paediatr Anaesth. 2000;10(4):367–75.

49. Rauck RL, Cherry D, Boyer MF, Kosek P, Dunn J, Alo K. Long-term intrathecal opioid therapy with a patient-activated, implanted delivery system for the treatment of refractory cancer pain. J Pain. 2003;4(8):441–7.
50. Deer TR, Levy R, Prager J, Buchser E, Burton A, Caraway D, et al. Polyanalgesic consensus conference—2012: recommendations to reduce morbidity and mortality in intrathecal drug delivery in the treatment of chronic pain. Neuromodulation. 2012;15(5):467–82; discussion 82.
51. Bond MC, Pritchard S. Understanding clinical trials in childhood cancer. Paediatr Child Health. 2006;11:148–50.
52. Santana VM, Furman WL, Billups CA, Hoffer F, Davidoff AM, Houghton PJ, et al. Improved response in high-risk neuroblastoma with protracted topotecan administration using a pharmacokinetically guided dosing approach. J Clin Oncol. 2005;23(18):4039–47.
53. Amoroso L, Haupt R, Garaventa A, Ponzoni M. Investigational drugs in phase II clinical trials for the treatment of neuroblastoma. Expert Opin Investig Drugs. 2017;26:1281–93.

The manufacturer's authorised representative in the EU is Springer Nature Customer Service Centre GmbH, Europaplatz 3, 69115 Heidelberg, Germany. If you have any concerns regarding our products, please contact ProductSafety@springernature.com

Printed and bound by CPI Group (UK) Ltd, Croydon, CR0 4YY
30/07/2026
02181718-0001